Study Guide

for

Kinn's **The Medical Assistant**

An Applied Learning Approach

TENTH EDITION

Alexandra Patricia Young, BBA, RMA, CMA

Adjunct Instructor
Everest College, Arlington Midcities Campus
Arlington, Texas
Professional Writer
Grand Prairie, Texas

Amy DeVore BA, CMA

Instructor
Butler County Community College
Butler, Pennsylvania

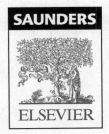

SAUNDERS

ELSEVIER

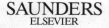

SAUNDERS
ELSEVIER

11830 Westline Industrial Drive
St. Louis, Missouri 63146

STUDY GUIDE FOR KINN'S THE MEDICAL ASSISTANT:
AN APPLIED LEARNING APPROACH

ISBN-13: 978-1-4160-3835-1
ISBN-10: 1-4160-3835-3

Notice

Knowledge and best practice in this field are constantly changing. As new research and experience broaden our knowledge, changes in practice, treatment and drug therapy may become necessary or appropriate. Readers are advised to check the most current information provided (i) on procedures featured or (ii) by the manufacturer of each product to be administered, to verify the recommended dose or formula, the method and duration of administration, and contraindications. It is the responsibility of the practitioner, relying on their own experience and knowledge of the patient, to make diagnoses, to determine dosages and the best treatment for each individual patient, and to take all appropriate safety precautions. To the fullest extent of the law, neither the Publisher nor the Authors assume any liability for any injury and/or damage to persons or property arising out or related to any use of the material contained in this book.

The Publisher

ISBN-13: 978-1-4160-3835-1
ISBN-10: 1-4160-3835-3

Executive Editor: Susan Cole
Developmental Editor: Celeste Clingan
Publishing Services Manager: Patricia Tannian
Senior Project Manager: Sarah Wunderly
Design Direction: Julia Dummitt

Printed in United States
Last digit is the print number: 9 8 7 6 5 4 3 2

Working together to grow
libraries in developing countries

www.elsevier.com | www.bookaid.org | www.sabre.org

ELSEVIER | BOOK AID International | Sabre Foundation

To The Student

This study guide was created to assist you in achieving the objectives of each chapter in *Kinn's: The Medical Assistant: An Applied Learning Approach* and in establishing a solid base of knowledge in medical assisting. Completing the exercises in each chapter in this guide will help to reinforce the material studied in the textbook and learned in class.

Study Hints for All Students
Ask Questions!
There are no stupid questions. If you do not know something or are not sure about it, you need to find out. Other people may be wondering the same thing but may be too shy to ask. The answer could mean life or death to your patient. That is certainly more important than feeling embarrassed about asking a question.

Chapter Objectives
At the beginning of each chapter in the textbook are learning objectives that you should have mastered when you finish studying that chapter. Write these objectives in your notebook, leaving a blank space after each. Fill in the answers as you find them while reading the chapter. Review to make sure your answers are correct and complete. Use these answers when you study for tests. This should also be done for separate course objectives that your instructor has listed in your class syllabus.

Vocabulary
At the beginning of each chapter in the textbook are vocabulary terms that you will encounter as you read the chapter. These vocabulary terms are in bold the first time they appear in the chapter.

Summary of Learning Objectives
Use the Summary of Learning Objectives at the end of each chapter in the textbook to help with review for exams.

Reading Hints
When reading each chapter in the textbook, look at the subject headings to learn what each section is about. Read first for the general meaning. Then reread parts you did not understand. It may help to read those parts aloud. Carefully read the information given in each table and study each figure and its legend.

Concepts
While studying, put difficult concepts into your own words to determine whether you understand them. Check this understanding with another student or the instructor. Write these concepts in your notebook.

Class Notes

When taking lecture notes in class, leave a large margin on the left side of each notebook page and write only on right-hand pages, leaving all left-hand pages blank. Look over your lecture notes soon after each class, while your memory is fresh. Fill in missing words; complete sentences and ideas; and underline key phrases, definitions, and concepts. At the top of each page, write the topic of that page. In the left margin, write the key word for that part of your notes. On the opposite left-hand page, write a summary or outline that combines material from both the textbook and the lecture. These can be your study notes for review.

Study Groups

Form a study group with some other students so you can help one another. Practice speaking and reading aloud. Ask questions about material you are not sure about. Work together to find answers.

References for Improving Study Skills

Good study skills are essential for achieving your goals in medical assisting. Time management, efficient use of study time, and a consistent approach to studying are all beneficial. There are various methods for reading a textbook and for taking class notes. Some methods that have proven helpful can be found in *Saunders Health Professional's Planner*.

Additional Study Hints for English as a Second Language (ESL) Students Vocabulary

If you find a nontechnical word you do not know (e.g., drowsy), try to guess its meaning from the sentence (e.g., With electrolyte imbalance, the patient may feel fatigued and drowsy). If you are not sure of the meaning or if it seems particularly important, look it up in the dictionary.

Vocabulary Notebook

Keep a small alphabetized notebook or address book in your pocket or purse. Write down new nontechnical words you read or hear along with their meanings and pronunciations. Write each word under its initial letter so you can find it easily, as in a dictionary. For words you do not know or for words that have a different meaning in medical assisting, write down how they are used and how they sound. Look up their meanings in a dictionary or ask your instructor or first-language buddy. Then write the different meanings or usages that you have found in your book, including the medical assisting meaning. Continue to add new words as you discover them.

First-Language Buddy

ESL students should find a first-language buddy—another student who is a native speaker of English and who is willing to answer questions about word meanings, pronunciations, and culture. Maybe, in turn, your buddy would like to learn about your language and culture. This could be useful for his or her medical assisting experience as well.

Contents

INTRODUCTION

UNIT ONE: INTRODUCTION TO MEDICAL ASSISTING

UNIT TWO: ADMINISTRATIVE MEDICAL ASSISTING

UNIT THREE: HEALTH INFORMATION IN THE MEDICAL OFFICE

UNIT FOUR: BILLING AND CODING PROCEDURES

Procedure Checklists

CHAPTER 1

Becoming a Successful Student

Vocabulary Review

Match the following terms and definitions.

1. _____ The constant practice of considering all aspects of a situation when deciding what to believe or what to do

2. _____ Those actions that identify the medical assistant as a member of a healthcare profession, including dependability, respectful patient care, initiative, positive attitude, and teamwork

3. _____ How an individual looks at information and sees it as real

4. _____ The way that an individual perceives and processes information to learn new material

5. _____ How an individual internalizes new information and makes it his or her own

6. _____ The process of considering new information and internalizing it to create new ways of examining information

7. _____ Sensitivity to the individual needs and reactions of patients

A. Learning style

B. Reflection

C. Professional behaviors

D. Processing

E. Empathy

F. Perceiving

G. Critical thinking

Skills and Concepts

True and False: Indicate which statements are true (T) and which statements are false (F).

8. _____ The best way to deal with conflict situations is through open, honest, assertive communication.

9. _____ The first step in conflict resolution is examination of pros and cons.

10. _____ Conflicts should be resolved immediately.

11. _____ Sometimes you will not be able to solve problems or a conflict may not be important enough for you to act to change the situation.

12. _____ It is best if you attempt to solve the conflict in a private place at a prescheduled time.

13. _____ You need to understand the problem and gather as much information about the situation as possible before you decide to act.

14. _____ As a future member of the healthcare team, you will frequently face problems and conflict.

Time Management

Answer the following questions.

15. List five time management skills.

a. _____

b. _____

c. _____

d. _____

e. _____

Which of these do you think will require the most effort on your road to becoming a medical assistant? How can you better prepare yourself for the challenges ahead?

_____

_____

16. Describe five strategies for breaking the cycle of procrastination.

a. _____

b. _____

c. _____

d. _____

e. _____

What barriers cause you to procrastinate? How can you prepare yourself to avoid procrastination?

_____

_____

Study Skills

Examine your own note-taking ability. Review the note-taking strategies in Chapter 1, and record the ideas that you plan to incorporate into your academic goals for this term.

_____

_____

_____

Case Studies

Read the case studies and answer the questions.

1. Dr. Weaver is running late seeing patients this afternoon. Sara Kline has been waiting in the examination room for Dr. Weaver for 30 minutes. She peeks her head out of the examination room doorway and demands to know what is taking so long. How should you, the medical assistant, approach this patient? How do you calm her down and explain the physician's situation without compromising other patients' confidentiality? What are some things you can do for the patient to make the wait not seem so long?

_____

_____

_____

_____

_____

_____

2. Victoria Graham, a 68-year-old woman with diabetic retinopathy, arrives today for diabetes disease management education. How might the medical assistant approach Ms. Graham's learning style? What are some possible barriers, and how can the medical assistant help Ms. Graham overcome them?

_____

_____

_____

_____

_____

_____

Workplace Applications

1. You are the office manager for a busy family practice office. Over the past week you have noticed that one of your employees has been 15 minutes late every day. Should you approach this employee? If so, how would you manage the situation? What are the main points you would want to stress to this employee? Are there any consequences? What follow-up, if any, should be done?

_____

_____

_____

2. Physicians' offices are extremely busy with many daily demands. How should one prepare for proper time management? Why is it necessary to prioritize tasks? What are some ideas the medical assistant can use to get the most out of the day and stay organized?

_____

_____

_____

3. Connie is the manager of a busy family practice office. The insurance clerk has complained that the receptionist takes too many smoking breaks and accepts too many personal calls while at work. What type of information should Connie obtain before approaching the situation? How should this situation be handled? Where? Who should be present?

_____

_____

_____

4. After being on vacation for a week, Laura returns to the office to find her desk piled high with tasks that require attention. Laura decides to get organized and make a list of the items that need attention. Prioritize the tasks from "most important and urgent" to "needs to be done later today" and "may be done later this week." Explain your answers.

   a. Make staff schedule for next week

   b. Pull patient charts for the laboratory results the office received this morning for the physician's review

   c. Call and order immunization vaccines (the staff has informed you that they are on the last vial)

   d. Call and confirm the patient appointments for tomorrow

   e. Order general stock supplies (e.g., bandages, gauze, needles, and sharps containers)

   f. Review the insurance reimbursements the practice received for last month, and address any claims that have not been paid

   g. File charts

   h. Edit the physician's schedule for a meeting scheduled next month

_____

_____

_____

Chapter 1 Quiz

Name: _____

1. List three examples of professional behaviors.

   _____

   _____

   _____

2. Describe three ways to use effective time management.

   _____

   _____

   _____

3. Define *procrastination*, and describe how it is a barrier for time management.

   _____

   _____

   _____

4. _____ is the process of sorting out conflicting information, weighing the knowledge you possess about that information.

   _____

5. What are some test-taking strategies you can recommend to other students?

   _____

   _____

   _____

6. Describe a "cycle map" and how it may be put into practice in your own life.

   _____

   _____

   _____

7. Compare and contrast the method of perceiving and processing.

   _____

   _____

   _____

CHAPTER 4

Professional Behavior in the Workplace

Vocabulary Review

Fill in the blanks with the correct vocabulary terms from this chapter.

1. Dr. Babinski struggles with _____, often putting off doing tasks that should be completed.

2. Anna has worked as a medical assistant for almost 30 years, and her professionalism and compassion are above _____.

3. Susan Bessler is a CMA who has supervised externships for almost 10 years; she expects students to display _____ when performing their duties at her clinic.

4. _____ is one of the most important attributes that medical assistants should display as they go about their duties.

5. James has learned that he must use _____ when dealing with the patients in the clinic, being careful not to reveal any confidential information to an unauthorized third party.

6. Roberta _____ the notes from the last staff meeting to all employees.

7. A few of the _____ that the professional medical assistant should employ include loyalty, initiative, and courtesy.

8. Because Julia has been dishonest about her reasons for missing work, her _____ has been called into question.

9. Kristen has a pleasant _____ when working with patients.

10. Medical assistants receive pay that is usually _____ with their experience and training.

11. Jessica holds drawings for small gifts at her staff meetings, which helps to raise employee _____.

12. Gene evokes a professional _____ when talking with patients that encourages them to place their trust in him.

13. Medical assistants must take _____ when they are performing both externship and job duties.

14. _____ is a cause for immediate dismissal from employment.

15. The phrase office politics has a negative _____.

Skills and Concepts

Part I: Short Answer Questions

Briefly answer the following questions.

16. List the eight characteristics of the professional medical assistant.

a. _____

b. _____

c. _____

d. _____

e. _____

f. _____

g. _____

h. _____

17. List five obstructions to professionalism.

a. _____

b. _____

c. _____

d. _____

e. _____

18. Define teamwork in your own words.

_____

_____

_____

_____

_____

Part II: Practicing Professional Behavior

Answer the following questions.

19. Karen has developed a friendship with Angela, who has a wonderful personality but does not always do her share in the family practice clinic where they work together. Dr. Rabinowitz shares with Karen that Angela is going to be terminated on Friday, and has asked Karen to take over some of Angela's duties until a replacement is found. How can Karen demonstrate loyalty to her employer in this situation? To her friend, Angela?

_____

_____

_____

_____

_____

20. Martin Smith is a patient who always disrupts the clinic. He constantly complains about everything from the moment he enters until the moment he leaves. Karen is at the desk when he arrives to check out and pay his bill. When she tells him that he has a previous balance from a claim that his insurance did not pay, he argues that Karen filed the claim incorrectly. Karen is not in charge of filing insurance claims and did not handle any part of the claim in question. How can she be courteous to this patient?

_____

_____

_____

_____

_____

21. Karen works in the office laboratory. She is often asked questions about insurance and billing that she must refer to other personnel. How should Karen efficiently request information or assistance for the patient from other office personnel?

_____

_____

_____

_____

22. Karen and her fiancé ended their relationship last week. How can she deal with personal stressors while she is in the workplace?

_____

_____

_____

_____

23. A patient needs to be scheduled for an outpatient endoscopic examination. When Karen gives the instruction sheet to the patient, she suspects from his reaction that the patient is unable to read. How can Karen professionally handle this situation without causing embarrassment to the patient?

_____

_____

_____

_____

_____

24. Which of the characteristics of professionalism is your greatest strength? Explain why.

_____

_____

_____

_____

_____

25. Which of the five obstructions to professionalism will be most difficult for you to overcome? Explain why.

_____

_____

_____

_____

_____

Case Study

Read the case study and answer the questions that follow.

Aaron is a new medical assistant in Dr. Roye's family practice. He was an exceptional student and he consistently performed well on his externship, receiving commendations from the externship office manager as well as a written recommendation from the physician. One month after he started his job, Bethany asked him to make a bank deposit for her, usually a duty that she performed daily. Bethany told him that she was leaving the bank deposit in Aaron's bottom left drawer at his desk. When Aaron looked for the deposit at the end of the day, it was not anywhere in his desk—he looked in every drawer, and even took the drawers out to make certain that it had not fallen behind them. All of the employees looked for the deposit, which was not found. No one was able to reach Bethany on the phone. The next morning when Aaron opened his left bottom desk drawer, the deposit bag was there, but it was empty. Bethany had already reported to the physician that the deposit had not been made. The physician calls Aaron to his office to discuss the situation.

What do you think happened?

_____

_____

_____

How can you deal with employees who are determined to cause problems for others in the clinic?

_____

_____

_____

How can situations such as this be proven effectively when one is unsure about exactly what happened?

_____

_____

_____

Workplace Application

Professionalism is a word used often with regard to medical personnel. What does professionalism mean? Write a report on the meaning of professionalism, and highlight a person whom you believe is the epitome of professionalism in the medical field. This person could be an instructor, a physician, or some other healthcare worker that you have come to know. Be specific about the ways that professionalism is apparent in his or her actions and speech.

Internet Activities

1. Find four articles on medical professionalism. What seems to be the primary issues when attempting to maintain professionalism in medical facilities?

2. What are some ways that medical professionalism is taught in medical schools? Do these methods apply to medical assistants?

Chapter 4 Quiz

Name: _____

1. Which of the following words is misspelled?

   a. Characteristic

   b. Compitence

   c. Commensurate

2. Office politics are always negative.

   a. True

   b. False

3. To intentionally put off something that should be done is called:

   a. initiative

   b. procrastination

   c. professionalism

   d. discretion

4. Insubordination can be grounds for termination.

   a. True

   b. False

5. A _____, by definition, is talk or widely disseminated opinion with no discernible source or a statement that is not known to be true.

6. The process of working well with others to achieve mutual goals is called

   _____.

7. In subordination might be justified if you are asked to perform an illegal act.

   a. True

   b. False

8. Which of the following words is misspelled?

   a. Demeanor

   b. Discretion

   c. Disemminated

   d. Detrimental

CHAPTER 5

Interpersonal Skills and Human Behavior

Vocabulary Review

Fill in the blanks with the correct vocabulary terms from this chapter.

1. Jill commented that the new office policies are confusing and _____.

2. Giving a patient an injection against his or her will could be considered _____.

3. Shane's remark was insulting and _____.

4. Whitney _____ denied leaving the narcotics cabinet unlocked.

5. With the increasing number of lawsuits, medical personnel can conclude that our society is quite _____.

6. Angry employees who are being terminated might turn _____ in a short time span.

7. The notion that large individuals are lazy is an example of a(n) _____.

8. Sayed uses positive _____ while he is training a new employee.

9. Rahima demonstrates _____ when she attempts to get her way in every situation.

10. Paula has learned that she uses _____ _____ when she feels threatened by her supervisor.

11. Karen felt intense _____ when her grandmother died.

12. _____ helps Angela to make certain that she understands exactly what a patient meant.

13. Roberto was eventually terminated for using _____ with several of the patients in the clinic.

14. Bobbie attended a seminar last week and learned about _____, which included the study of the spatial separation that individuals naturally maintain.

15. Sue Ann definitely felt out of her _____ _____ when she was asked to be a guest speaker at a regional AAMA meeting.

16. Mrs. Robinson is able to _____ her words quite distinctly.

17. Dr. Kirkham warned that no employee should speak to the _____ about any of his celebrity patients.

18. Rodman has a(n) _____ _____ at work because he speaks so little English.

19. It is important to consider the patient's _____ of the staff, clinic, and physician.

20. Dr. Rockwell took Julia off of phone duty because the high _____ of her voice was disconcerting to many patients.

Skills and Concepts

Part I: Open-Ended and Closed-Ended Questions

Label the following questions or statements as either open-ended or closed-ended.

21. _____ Are you taking blood pressure medication?

22. _____ Are you allergic to aspirin?

23. _____ Would you tell me about your past surgeries?

24. _____ Do you have asthma?

25. _____ What types of attempts have you made to stop smoking?

26. _____ Explain what you feel when your migraines begin.

27. _____ Do you have hospitalization insurance?

28. _____ Do you want a morning or afternoon appointment?

29. _____ How are you feeling today?

30. _____ What type of trouble do you have when swallowing pills?

Part II: Defense Mechanisms

Match the following defense mechanisms with the appropriate statements.

31. _____ "Everyone forgets to clock in from lunch once in a while. Why am I being singled out and written up?"

32. _____ "I refuse to believe that I'm HIV positive. I've only had sex with two people in the past 5 years."

33. _____ "I would do a better job at work, but I can't do everything in 1 day like I'm expected to."

34. _____ "I know that the office manager is angry with me because I've been late, and I should talk to her, but I just can't deal with that stress right now."

a. verbal aggression

b. projection

c. sarcasm

d. compensation

e. physical avoidance

f. regression

g. apathy

h. rationalization

i. displacement

j. repression

k. denial

35. _____ "Why are you attacking me about not filling out the narcotics log? You certainly aren't the perfect medical assistant!"

36. _____ "I know my blood sugar is high, and I have tried to avoid sugar, but at least I'm doing my exercises twice a week."

37. _____ "Dr. Roberts only yells at me because he's stressed about his patient load."

38. _____ "It doesn't matter what I do to please my family. They hate me anyway, and there's nothing I can do about it."

39. _____ "I have enough on my mind and don't need my co-workers complaining that I'm not doing my share of the work!"

40. _____ "I can't bear to go to Memorial Park for our office picnic because that's where my ex-husband told me he wanted a divorce."

41. _____ "Sure she looks good, if you like people from the 60s!"

Part III: Barriers to Communication

Determine which of the five barriers to communication applies in each example given.

42. Cylinda has lived in the south all of her life, and when Bruce came to work at the office, his brusque attitude made her feel defensive. She was so offended by his manner of speaking that she began to avoid him in the hallways and during breaks. He constantly spoke of how much more he'd been paid in New York and stressed the efficiency of the clinic where he formerly worked. Cylinda considers him a typical Northerner, and her dislike of him is based largely on the fact that he is different from her and most of the people she knows.

_____

43. Aretha dreads the days that Rahima Bathkar comes to the office. She is a pleasant patient, but Aretha cannot understand her well and feels as if she is not providing Rahima with the care that she deserves. She is always worried that she is missing some information that the physician needs to know to properly diagnose and treat the patient. Aretha takes extra time with her, but because there is no one to interpret for Rahima when she cannot find the right word in her broken English, Aretha is concerned.

_____

44. Allan and Rebecca Poe are an elderly couple; they visit the clinic twice a month for Rebecca's diabetes. Rebecca is blind in one eye and cannot read easily. Allan has vision problems as well, so the staff must read any documents that they are required to sign to them to assure that they understand the information contained in the documents.

_____

45. Tommy Lightman approached the office manager because he was concerned about the manner in which Sarah spoke to him in the office. He expressed that Sarah was quite short with him last Tuesday and seemed very distracted as she talked with him in the examination room before the physician came in to treat him. He also said that the physician seemed to spend less time with him that day than usual. Tommy was concerned that he was not wanted in the clinic and wanted to have his records sent to another physician. The office manager checked the appointment book and realized that Tommy was in the office last Tuesday at 11 o'clock, which was the exact time that another patient was being transported to the hospital because of heart failure.

_____

46. Teresa has a difficult time dealing with Orlando Guiterrez. He comes for appointments twice a month and is trying desperately to lose weight. He currently weighs 435 lb. He is a pleasant person, but Teresa has been raised to believe that those who are overweight are lazy individuals. She tries to avoid caring for him when he visits the clinic.

_____

Part IV: Dealing with Barriers to Communication

Reread the scenarios in the previous section, and explain how each situation could be professionally handled by the medical assistant using good communications skills.

47. How can Cylinda develop a positive working relationship with Bruce?

_____

_____

_____

_____

48. What can Aretha do to improve communication with Rahima?

_____

_____

_____

_____

49. How can the medical assistant make Rebecca Poe feel more comfortable with her disability in the physician's office?

_____

_____

_____

_____

50. What can Sarah and the office manager do to change Tommy's perception about the incident that happened during his last office visit?

_____

_____

_____

_____

51. What does Teresa need to do personally in order to deal with those patients that she doesn't care for who visit the clinic?

_____

_____

_____

_____

Part V: Communication During Difficult Times

Read the following descriptions, and suggest effective ways to communicate with the patient. Identify whether the patient is probably experiencing anger, shock, grief, or a combination of these emotions.

52. Joanna Taylor has just been brought to the physician's office after learning that her 16-year-old son was killed in a car accident. She is not responding to questions.

_____

_____

_____

53. Lafonda Williams has come to the physician's office because of injuries she sustained when her estranged husband assaulted her.

_____

_____

_____

54. Jackson Holland is seeing the physician today for antidepressants because of work-related stress as well as difficulty dealing with the death of his elderly mother.

_____

_____

_____

55. James Ackard comes to the physician's office for treatment for a work-related injury.

_____

_____

_____

Part VI: Death and Dying

List the stages of grief in proper order.

56. _____

57. _____

58. _____

59. _____

60. _____

Part VII: Maslow's Hierarchy of Needs

Draw and label the Hierarchy of Needs as shown in Figure 5-9 in the text.

Part VIII: The Process of Communication

Draw and label the transactional communication model as shown in Figure 5-4 in the text.

Case Study

Read the case study and answer the questions that follow.

Janet has tried for months to reach Mr. Robinson, a cancer patient who comes to the clinic every 3 weeks. He does not have any family in the local area and feels that no one is interested in him or the problems he faces. He is estranged from both of his daughters, whom he has told to stay out of his life. They have not seen or spoken to him in over 10 years. Each visit, Mr. Robinson complains about how worthless his family is and how they have all deserted him in his time of need. However, Janet knows from reviewing the chart that Mr. Robinson was insistent that his daughters stay out of his life.

How involved should Janet get in this patient's life?

_____

_____

_____

How can she deal with Mr. Robinson's attitude during his office visits?

_____

_____

_____

Does Janet or the physician have the right to contact the daughters and discuss Mr. Robinson's condition with them?

_____

_____

_____

Workplace Application

Solicit 10 volunteers to come to the classroom and role-play patients and co-workers. Develop several personalities by writing a synopsis of the chief complaints and general personality traits. Allow each student to experience each "patient" or "co-worker" and react to them using professional interpersonal behavior and good human relations skills. Discuss the activity in class, and talk about what this role-play activity can teach medical assisting students.

Internet Activities

Use the Internet to answer the following questions.

1. How many different career fields do human relations and interpersonal skills affect?

_____

_____

_____

2. Define *organizational behavior*.

_____

_____

_____

3. How are human relations and interpersonal skills practiced in classrooms?

_____

_____

_____

Write a classroom policy that stresses positive interpersonal skills and human relations. Share this policy with the class.

Chapter 5 Quiz

Name: _____

1. Which of the following words means a sharp or ironic response intended to hurt someone?

   a. Litigious

   b. Paraphrasing

   c. Sarcasm

   d. Vehemently

2. _____ means easily aroused, tending to erupt in violence.

3. The description of the study of the phenomena of death and of psychologic methods of coping with death is called *thanatology*.

   a. True

   b. False

4. According to Maslow, basic physiologic needs must be met before higher level needs can be addressed.

   a. True

   b. False

5. _____ ended questions are likely to provide more information to the medical assistant.

6. _____ means to speak evil of or curse.

7. An older child who starts sucking his or her thumb during a stressful period might be demonstrating regressive behavior.

   a. True

   b. False

8. Which of the following defense mechanisms results in the inability to remember a painful event?

   a. Denial

   b. Repression

   c. Regression

   d. Apathy

9. Human beings generally need about _____ hours of sleep each night.

10. The final stage of grief is _____.

CHAPTER 6

Medicine and Ethics

Vocabulary Review

Fill in the blanks with the correct vocabulary terms from this chapter.

1. Melissa believes that one of her roles as a medical assistant is to be a patient _____, supporting both the patient and his or her family members during illnesses.

2. Ben has conflicting views about _____ and is unsure as to whether he would want the option to die with dignity if he had an incurable, debilitating disease.

3. Jill understands that the _____ of her actions while she is at work could affect whether a patient complies with the physician's instructions.

4. _____ allows the medical assistant to consider his or her personal feelings about various ethical issues before being faced with those decisions while working with actual patients.

5. _____ or handicapped patients need special understanding and patience from those who are employed in medical facilities.

6. Bianca is an infertile patient who is participating in _____ _____ to research a new drug that may help her to conceive a child.

7. The members of the Council on Ethical and Judicial Affairs issue _____ about medical situations, similar to the way that the Supreme Court Justices consider matters that are brought before the court.

8. _____ is a devotion to the truth.

9. Kristy considers being friendly toward the patients in the clinic as her _____ and a vital part of her job performance.

10. When a person has breached an ethical standard, _____ may be necessary to atone for the action.

Skills and Concepts

Part I: Making Ethical Decisions

List the five steps of ethical decision making.

11. _____

12. _____

13. _____

14. _____

15. _____

For the following scenarios, determine the type of ethical problem presented, the agent(s), the course of action, and the outcome. Although these situations may present more than one ethical problem, choose only one possibility for each exercise.

Two sisters have gathered at a medical facility to discuss with the attending physician the course of action that they should take regarding their dying father. Mr. Roberts, the patient, is no longer responsive. Cassandra wishes to continue all possible medical treatment to keep her father alive. Janet insists that her father would not wish to have his life prolonged by artificial means. Mr. Roberts did not leave either sister with a power of attorney and has no written record of his wishes regarding this issue.

16. Type of ethical problem

_____

17. Agent(s)

_____

18. Course of action (suggest one)

_____

19. Outcome (suggest one)

_____

20. How can the medical assistant refrain from inflicting his or her own opinions on patients?

_____

_____

Dr. Patrick is the chief of staff at a regional medical center. His specialty is oncology, and the hospital is considering the construction of a cancer center as part of a multimillion-dollar project. One of Dr. Patrick's partners, Dr. Adams, is vehemently opposed to the project because of the cost to the local taxpayers who support the hospital. Dr. Adams has threatened to leave the practice unless Dr. Patrick votes against the project. Dr. Patrick wants the center to be built but also realizes that if Dr. Adams leaves, the practice will suffer a drastic loss of income.

21. Type of ethical problem

_____

22. Agent(s)

_____

23. Course of action (suggest one)

_____

24. Outcome (suggest one)

_____

25. How would you handle an ethical decision that has an equal number of pros and cons?

_____

_____

_____

Part II: Types of Ethical Problems

Identify the type of ethical problem that each diagram represents.

26.

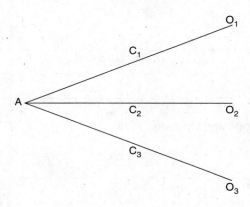

27.

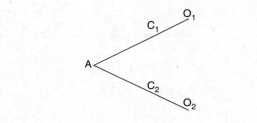

28.

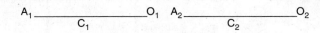

29.

A———C——||——O

Part III: Opinions on Medicoethical Issues

Write your personal opinion regarding the following medicoethical issues. After writing your opinion, consider differing opinions by writing a brief opposing argument.

30. Abortion

_____
_____
_____

31. Abortion: Opposing Opinion

_____
_____
_____

32. Stem Cell Research

_____
_____
_____

33. Stem Cell Research: Opposing Opinion

_____
_____
_____

34. Human Cloning

_____
_____
_____

35. Human Cloning: Opposing Opinion

_____
_____
_____

36. Genetic Counseling

_____

_____

_____

37. Genetic Counseling: Opposing Opinion

_____

_____

_____

38. Physician-Assisted Suicide

_____

_____

_____

39. Physician-Assisted Suicide: Opposing Opinion

_____

_____

_____

Part IV: Ethics and the Medical Assistant

40. Describe the behavior of an ethical medical assistant in your own words.

_____

_____

_____

Part V: Rights and Duties

Identify the following as a right, a duty, or neither.

41. Healthcare services for all Americans

    right   duty   neither

42. Owning a gun when licensed

    right   duty   neither

43. Providing care to an elderly parent

    right   duty   neither

44. Nondiscrimination

    right   duty   neither

45. Life

    right   duty   neither

46. Are there times when a right or duty in the preceding list is invalid or could be argued to be so? Explain your answer.

    _____

    _____

    _____

Part VI: Confidentiality

47. List several physical places within the physician's office where confidentiality could potentially be breached.

    _____

    _____

    _____

48. What are the usual consequences of breach of patient confidentiality?

    _____

    _____

    _____

49. Explain why confidentiality is critical in the medical environment.

    _____

    _____

    _____

Case Studies

Read the case studies and answer the questions that follow.

Robert is an HIV-positive patient. His employer invites the local blood bank to come to the workplace every 6 months and conduct a blood drive. Robert has declined donating in the past because of his HIV status but often feels pressured by co-workers to give blood. None of them is aware that he is HIV positive. How do blood banks handle this situation today? Does Robert have alternatives that will resolve the situation? Explain your answer.

    _____

    _____

    _____

Cameron works for Dr. Christian and works hard to obtain the trust of the patients. Mrs. Rainer confides to Cameron that she has been smoking against Dr. Christian's advice and asks Cameron not to tell the physician that she is smoking. How should Cameron handle this situation? What should she tell the patient?

_____

_____

_____

Workplace Application

Stepping into the medical environment, where confidentiality is so important, may be a difficult adjustment for some new medical assistants. In any medical facility you must think before speaking. At times, discussion of patients and their conditions will not be appropriate. How can you change your way of thinking and be constantly aware of the constraints that patient confidentiality places on discussion of patient information?

Internet Activities

1. Peruse the HIPAA website and download the quick fact sheets. Study this information to gain a basic knowledge of HIPAA guidelines before studying the law in more detail in Chapter 16.

2. Discuss ethics in the classroom. How do medical assisting students perform ethically while completing their education? Research this issue on the Internet, and talk about it in class.

3. Read the preamble and the nine principles of medical ethics on the American Medical Association website. Discuss each one. What changes would you make to these principles? Are they applicable to the situations faced in the medical world today?

Chapter 6 Quiz

Name: _____

1. The ethical duty that involves doing good or producing good is called _____.

2. The ethical duty that involves a devotion to the truth is called _____.

3. CEJA is a part of the:

   a. AAMA

   b. AMA

   c. AMT

4. The access to genetic information prompts many concerns and presents ethical, legal, and moral questions.

   a. True

   b. False

5. The law requires that abuse be reported to the proper authorities, and if a physician fails to do so, he or she has also breached ethical standards.

   a. True

   b. False

6. Guidelines surrounding confidentiality are some of the less important requirements of working in the physician's office.

   a. True

   b. False

7. Something that is done, collected, or occurs after death is referred to as being

   _____

8. The earliest written code of ethics was called the _____

9. Who decides what is ethical?

   _____

10. Information that is a part of the public record is said to be in the public _____.

CHAPTER 7

Medicine and Law

Vocabulary Review

Fill in the blanks with the correct vocabulary terms from this chapter.

1. Dr. Parker insists that a medical assistant be present during all of his patient examinations in order to avoid any _____ of wrongdoing or abuse.

2. Many physician offices require patients to sign a(n) _____ agreement that means disagreements may be settled by a qualified third party.

3. If a person contributes to a patient's poor condition, he or she may be charged with _____.

4. Dr. Samantha Beddingfield was called to court to discuss her knowledge of malpractice cases as a(n) _____.

5. When a patient offers his or her arm to have blood drawn, he or she has _____ consent.

6. A doctor of _____ studies the law.

7. Dr. Cartwright failed to follow the care of a hospital patient to whom he was assigned and may be guilty of _____ and/or _____.

8. Civil cases must be proved by a(n) _____ of the _____.

9. Criminal cases must be proved by _____ _____.

10. Roger Askew is bringing a case against a physician in the death of his wife during surgery, making him the _____ in the case.

11. Something put into one's own words is _____.

12. A court must have _____ over a case before it can hear the arguments and make a judgment.

13. If Alisha writes down comments that are untrue and inflammatory about another person, she might be accused of _____.

14. City court is often called _____ court.

15. City regulations are often called city _____.

16. If either side in a lawsuit is unhappy with the results, in most cases the decision can be _____.

17. Vince suffered a loss of use of his arm after surgery, loss of wages by being rendered unable to work, and loss of his ability to earn a living. These losses are called _____ in court.

18. The constitutional guarantee that legal proceedings will be fair is called _____.

19. Judge Roberts has 12 cases on the _____ for the day.

20. The person who stands accused of a crime in court is called the _____.

21. The person who stands accused in a civil trial is called the _____.

22. Alyssa may be held _____ for damaging her boyfriend's car.

23. An intentional attempt to injure another person is called _____.

24. The unlawful use of force or violence against another person is called _____.

25. A(n) _____ is a major crime, such as rape or murder.

26. Consent that is detailed and usually in writing is called _____ consent.

27. Judge Conlin uses previous cases as models to determine his decisions on current cases. The previous cases are called _____.

28. Barbara Harris was served a(n) _____, which required her to appear in court.

29. The document requiring that records be produced in court is called a(n) _____ _____.

30. The final decision of the judge or jury is called the _____.

Skills and Concepts

Part I: Classifications of Law

Fill in the blanks with the correct answers.

31. The three basic categories of criminal law discussed in this chapter include:

    a. _____

    b. _____

    c. _____

32. The three basic categories of civil law discussed in this chapter include:

    a. _____

    b. _____

    c. _____

33. A law that is minor in nature and usually a breach of municipal regulations is called a(n) _____.

34. Civil law involves cases that are brought to court by _____.

35. Criminal law involves a crime against the _____ or _____.

36. Medical professional liability falls under what category of civil law? _____

Part II: Anatomy of a Medical Professional Liability Lawsuit

Complete the following lists or statements.

37. List the four elements of a valid, legal contract.

   a. _____

   b. _____

   c. _____

   d. _____

38. List the three steps involved in the creation of the physician-patient relationship.

   a. _____

   b. _____

   c. _____

39. What must a letter of withdrawal of care state?

   a. _____

   b. _____

   c. _____

40. How should a letter of withdrawal be mailed? _____

41. Does the letter of withdrawal have to explain to patients the reason that the physician chose to withdraw from care of the patient? Explain your answer.

   _____

   _____

   _____

42. Explain what is meant by having jurisdiction over a case.

   _____

   _____

   _____

43. What is the ultimate appellate court in the United States?

   _____

44. Explain the difference between a deposition and an interrogatory.

   _____

   _____

   _____

45. List three of the five ways to determine if a subpoena is valid.

    a. _____

    b. _____

    c. _____

46. Briefly explain how a person called to testify in court should dress.

    _____

    _____

    _____

47. What is a defendant in a civil trial often called? _____

Part III: Medical Professional Liability and Negligence

Find the words in the list in the following puzzle.

```
Y  S  R  Z  S  T  F  P  E  M  Z  S  T  D  B  P  X  K  F  Q  W  U  T  F
M  R  K  O  F  U  N  H  C  H  A  F  C  B  M  N  G  J  K  M  M  T  E  U
Y  R  O  T  U  B  I  R  T  N  O  C  T  F  E  W  X  L  A  B  J  D  Y  O
M  R  U  T  T  P  A  A  Q  M  S  N  B  I  L  E  V  U  Y  K  I  W  Y  S
S  D  E  L  A  N  O  I  S  S  E  F  O  R  P  G  S  G  J  L  U  G  S  R
B  E  C  N  A  S  A  E  F  L  A  M  O  I  Y  V  P  G  H  K  W  P  E  G
V  N  N  K  Y  B  N  J  M  A  B  X  H  H  T  R  E  P  X  E  I  Z  W  S
T  I  A  Q  F  Y  E  E  U  U  E  A  T  I  U  A  I  M  B  S  Q  H  O  U
B  C  S  A  P  H  G  N  P  W  H  A  K  D  D  O  G  S  E  P  H  F  R  B
T  I  A  I  H  I  L  E  O  M  Z  H  E  I  M  V  B  E  J  M  N  B  K  M
S  D  E  R  E  L  I  C  T  I  O  N  A  C  Z  M  F  G  L  J  E  F  F  Z
C  E  F  F  O  F  G  N  G  Q  T  C  N  V  F  Q  K  A  T  L  D  G  S  S
K  M  S  R  U  R  E  A  S  O  N  A  B  L  E  X  E  M  P  L  A  R  Y  S
B  W  I  C  I  D  N  S  W  Z  G  Q  G  D  V  E  D  A  T  L  I  R  N  N
K  X  M  V  E  Z  C  A  C  S  U  V  N  I  I  V  H  D  T  O  M  R  R  T
R  D  F  C  L  O  E  E  A  P  O  N  D  K  T  X  I  J  W  K  L  M  K  I
Q  K  E  K  H  U  D  F  W  D  W  G  S  K  I  I  Y  R  U  D  E  W  U  S
L  D  R  P  X  Z  F  N  P  A  Z  R  B  V  N  F  L  P  Y  P  X  V  M  I
L  Y  Y  S  O  J  S  O  P  L  D  G  Q  U  U  V  G  P  E  F  R  U  J  P
A  V  P  J  X  X  J  N  C  L  W  U  I  S  P  S  N  N  I  P  A  V  F  T
D  B  W  T  R  U  V  R  V  C  Z  Q  D  X  O  W  U  F  E  Q  S  T  W  Z
```

Act	Duty	Nonfeasance
Allegation	Exemplary	Professional
Compensatory	Expert	Prudent
Contributory	Litigation	Punitive
Damages	Malfeasance	Reasonable
Decedent	Misfeasance	
Dereliction	Negligence	

Part IV: Short Answer Questions

Fill in the blanks with the correct answers.

48. The formal action of a legislative body is called a(n) _____.

49. The performance of an act that is wholly wrongful and unlawful is _____.

50. The agency that regulates safety in the workplace is _____.

51. A law enacted by the legislative branch of a government is called a(n) _____.

52. The failure to perform an act that should have been performed is _____.

53. A solemn declaration made by a witness under oath in response to interrogation by a lawyer is called _____.

54. The pretense of curing disease is called _____.

55. The improper performance of a legal act is _____.

56. Something that is easily understood or recognized by the mind is called a(n) _____.

57. An authoritative decree or direction usually set forth by a municipal regulation is called a(n) _____.

58. The law that promotes accuracy in medical laboratories is _____.

Part V: Inside the Courtroom

Circle T or F to indicate whether the statement is true or false.

59. T   F   Lying under oath constitutes perjury.

60. T   F   Arriving late to the courtroom is acceptable if the witness has a good excuse.

61. T   F   Attorneys usually discover new information when questioning their clients in the courtroom.

62. T   F   A sustained objection means that the judge disagrees with the objection and will allow the question to stand.

63. T   F   It is not necessary to use "ma'am" or "sir" in the courtroom when addressing the judge.

64. T   F   If a question is confusing to a witness, he or she should ask the attorney to restate or repeat the question.

65. T   F   Discovery is pretrial disclosure of pertinent facts or documents pertaining to a case.

66. T   F   Arbitration is a cost-saving alternative to trial.

Part VI: The Four D's of Negligence and Damages

67. A patient was given the wrong medication. No adverse effects occurred. Which of the four D's is missing? Why does this affect the possibility of a lawsuit?

_____

_____

_____

68. A car accident occurs at an intersection outside of a physician's office during normal business hours. Do the physician and staff have a duty to provide direct care for the injured persons? Why or why not?

    _____

    _____

    _____

69. A patient is treated for low back pain caused by a fall at the local mall. The patient sues the physician because the pain is unresolved. Which of the four D's would be the most difficult for the patient's attorney to prove? Why?

    _____

    _____

    _____

70. A medical assistant mislabeled a vial of blood that was sent to an outside laboratory. Because of this mistake, a child was given the wrong diagnosis and later died. The child's family sued the medical assistant, the physician, and the hospital that owned the practice. The child's family was awarded four million dollars. What type of damages is this?

    _____

    _____

    _____

71. A female patient was awarded punitive damages after a physician sexually molested her during her annual pelvic examination. What are punitive damages designed to do? Do you feel that the amount of punitive damages should be limited to a specific monetary amount?

    _____

    _____

    _____

Case Study

Read the case study and answer the questions that follow.

A 10-year-old girl was brought to a physician's office with a complaint of a headache after cheerleader practice in mid-August. The clinic was a freestanding minor emergency center and not the child's regular physician's office. The girl and the adult who had brought the child to the clinic—the girl's aunt—both denied that she had been in any type of accident and stated that her only complaint was the headache and being tired and hot. The adult mentioned that she also seemed a bit disoriented during the drive to the clinic. She didn't recall having been at cheerleader practice less than an hour earlier. The child told the physician that she had been a cheerleader for 6 years and that she really liked her coach.

The outside temperatures had reached 101° that day. The physician examined the patient and suggested that she be taken home to rest and rehydrate. No prescriptions were written, and the girl left the clinic.

Two hours later the girl could not be roused from sleeping and was immediately taken to the emergency room at the closest hospital by her aunt. The girl's mother met them at the hospital just in time to be told that the girl had slipped into a coma. The physician suspected that she had experienced heat stroke. The aunt was shocked and mentioned that she had taken the girl to a clinic earlier, questioning why this diagnosis was not considered at that time. The mother of the child immediately called the clinic and berated the physician for putting her child into a coma.

What went wrong in this case? Who is responsible for the child's condition? Is this a "good" malpractice case?

_____

_____

_____

_____

_____

_____

_____

_____

_____

Workplace Application

Research the laws that apply to medical clinics in your state. If possible, interview an office manager about the laws that apply to local clinics and ask what challenges exist in trying to comply with them. Share what you learn with the class.

Internet Activities

1. Use the Internet to find the place in your area where a small claims case would be filed. Obtain the paperwork necessary to file a claim. Create a fictional case, and complete the paperwork as if you plan to file it in court.

2. Research mediators in your local area using the Internet. Find the name and contact information for at least three. With your instructor's permission, contact a mediator and ask him or her to speak to the class.

3. Research medical malpractice attorneys in your local area using the Internet. Find the name and contact information for at least three. With your instructor's permission, contact one of the attorneys and invite him or her to speak to the class on how the medical assistant can help to avoid medical malpractice claims.

Chapter 7 Quiz

Name: _____

1. A patient rolls up his sleeve for a blood draw. Which type of consent does this illustrate?

   a. Informed

   b. Implied

   c. Expressed

2. Name an agency that deals with administrative law _____.

3. In a medical professional liability litigation, the physician is the:

   a. plaintiff

   b. bailiff

   c. defendant

   d. respondent

4. Consideration is an exchange of something of value, such as the physician's time.

   a. True

   b. False

5. Schedule II drugs include narcotics and Ritalin.

   a. True

   b. False

6. Informed consent includes knowledge of alternate treatments and risks.

   a. True

   b. False

7. A _____ of limitations is a period after which a lawsuit cannot be filed.

8. A person who is younger than 18 or 21 and can give legal consent for medical procedures and conduct other business dealings is called a(n)

   _____.

9. The agency that regulates controlled substances is:

   a. FDA

   b. OSHA

   c. HIPAA

   d. DEA

10. Medical licensure can be obtained through

    a. examination

    b. reciprocity

    c. endorsement

    d. all of the above

CHAPTER **8**

Computer Concepts

Vocabulary Review

Fill in the blanks with the correct vocabulary terms from this chapter.

1. Jacob uses a(n) _____ _____ to write data onto a blank compact disk and stores the CD as a backup for the clinic's blank forms.

2. To assist him with patient diagnosis, Dr. Matthews uses software that is equipped with a type of _____ _____.

3. The smallest unit of information inside the computer is called a(n) _____.

4. Olivia installed new _____ _____ on the office computers that will allow patients to check in without the assistance of a receptionist.

5. Ethan has asked that all of the computer users in the clinic clear the computer _____ periodically so that websites stored there will be erased and the system will run faster.

6. Isabella is proficient at using _____ because she has studied this object-oriented programming language.

7. The office manager asked Samantha to print a(n) _____ _____ of the minutes of the meeting for each person attending.

8. Daniel likes to change the _____ in the different sections of the clinic's patient newsletter to make it more readable and attractive.

9. A picture that represents a program or an object on the computer is called a(n) _____.

10. Information entered into and used by the computer is called _____.

11. Tyler is responsible for the operation of the clinic's _____, which manages shared network resources.

12. Information that is processed by the computer and transmitted to a monitor or printer is called _____.

13. Christian was able to easily connect a(n) _____ to his home computer, which allows information to be transmitted over telephone lines and allows him to connect to the Internet.

14. Any type of storage of files used to prevent their loss in the event of hard disk failure is called _____.

15. Victoria created a(n) _____ to place on Dr. Anthony's website that advertises the makeup they offer to patients who have had plastic surgery.

16. A(n) _____ is a removable device with a magnetic surface that is capable of storing documents; also called a *diskette*.

17. A disk _____ loads programs or data stored on a disk into the computer.

18. Natalie sends several _____ messages daily to patients and business associates.

19. The _____ tracks all patient information, including addresses, phone numbers, and details about insurance coverage.

20. Megan purchased a(n) _____ _____ to backup the patient database and archive computer files.

Skills and Concepts

Part I: Matching Exercises

Match the following terms with their definitions.

21. _____ Approximately one billion bytes   a. terabyte

22. _____ Approximately one trillion bytes   b. bit

23. _____ Eight bits   c. megabyte

24. _____ Binary digits   d. byte

25. _____ Approximately 1024 bytes   e. kilobyte

26. _____ Approximately one million bytes   f. gigabyte

Part II: Input, Output, and Storage Devices

Label each of the following as an input, output, or storage device.

27. Mouse	Input	Output	Storage
28. Keyboard	Input	Output	Storage
29. Printer	Input	Output	Storage
30. Scanner	Input	Output	Storage
31. Speakers	Input	Output	Storage
32. CD-ROM	Input	Output	Storage
33. Zip drive	Input	Output	Storage
34. Touch screen	Input	Output	Storage
35. Floppy disk	Input	Output	Storage
36. Flash drive	Input	Output	Storage

Part III: Parts of the Computer

Provide the name of the computer part described in the sentences below.

37. Central unit of the computer that contains the logic circuitry and carries out the instructions of the computer's programs

_____

38. Main circuit board of the computer

_____

39. Devices that are inserted into a computer that give it added capabilities

_____

40. Device used to display computer-generated information

_____

41. Magnetic disk inside the computer that can hold several hundred gigabytes of information and is used to store the application software that runs on the computer

_____

42. Device used to take information from one CD-ROM and write it to another CD-ROM

_____

43. Device over which data can be transmitted via telephone lines or other media, such as coaxial cable

_____

44. Allows music or MIDI files to be heard from the computer

_____

45. Software that is installed on a computer to allow a hardware device to function

_____

Part IV: The Computer as a Co-worker

List seven ways that computers assist workers in medical offices.

46. _____
47. _____
48. _____
49. _____
50. _____
51. _____
52. _____

Part V: Basic Computer Functions

Describe how the following functions are performed on the computer.

53. Open a document

_____

_____

54. Save a document

_____

_____

55. Rename a document

_____

_____

56. Cut and paste text

_____

_____

57. Copy text

_____

_____

58. Exit a program

_____

_____

59. Turn the computer on

_____

_____

60. Turn the computer off

_____

_____

Part VI: Short Answer Questions

Provide the answers to the questions in the blanks below.

61. The three elements that differentiate microprocessors are:

   a. _____

   b. _____

   c. _____

62. Explain peripheral devices, and give one example of a peripheral device.

   _____

   _____

63. What is the function of a browser?

   _____

   _____

64. Define computer networking.

   _____

   _____

65. Why is computer security so important in today's medical office?

   _____

   _____

Part VII: File Formats and Printer Types

Match the following terms with their definitions.

66. _____ Inexpensive printer that provides a moderate-quality hard copy

67. _____ File format that supports color and is often used for scanned images

68. _____ Bitmapped graphics that are compiled by a graphics image set in rows or columns of dots

69. _____ Printer output similar to that of a photocopier; capable of complex graphics

70. _____ Characters in this file format are represented by their ASCII codes

71. _____ File type that is commonly used for photographs

a. .doc

b. .gif

c. Laser

d. .jpeg

e. .bmp

f. Dot matrix

g. .txt

h. Ink jet

i. .rtf

j. Multifunctional

72. _____ File type that combines ASCII codes with special commands that distinguish variations

73. _____ File usually created by a word processor for various documents, including letters and forms

74. _____ Printer that uses a heating element that is energized during the printing process

75. _____ Type of printer that serves as a scanner, fax, and copier

Case Study

Read the case study and answer the questions that follow.

Brooke Comis works for Dr. Tomms as a clinical medical assistant. She is a former office computer specialist who worked in the computer field for 12 years before she entered medical assisting school. She changed career fields because of the work prospects in technology and acted on her dream to enter the medical field. Unfortunately, she is the only person in the office who is knowledgeable about computers, the Internet, and networking. Whenever a computer is not functioning correctly or a problem occurs with the network, Dr. Tomms summons Brooke and expects her to fix it. When the physician decided to buy new computers, he expected Brooke to assemble all of them and set up a new network. Brooke gets more and more irate each time she is asked to perform these duties, because she is not compensated other than her normal hourly pay. She knows that if Dr. Tomms paid someone to do this work, it would cost him more than her monthly salary. Brooke is not certain how to approach this situation with the physician. What should she do first? How should she approach the physician? Should she refuse to perform computer work? What could happen if she refuses?

Workplace Application

Assume that you have been selected to order a new computer system for the physician. Clinic personnel include three physicians, six administrative personnel, and four clinical assistants, plus you, the office manager. Describe the minimum equipment needed. Consider printers, Internet access, scanners, and wireless needs. Investigate computers using the Internet, and prepare a folder with photos and/or specifications that detail the equipment you have selected.

Internet Activities

Use the Internet to locate a company that sells computers in your geographic area. Explore the site. Find a computer that you might consider purchasing, then answer the following questions.

1. How much RAM and ROM does the system have?

_____

_____

2. What is the clock speed?

_____

_____

3. What is the baud rate of the modem?

_____

_____

4. What software, if any, comes with the system?

_____

_____

5. What is the total cost before taxes are applied?

_____

_____

Chapter 8 Quiz

Name: _____

1. Clock speed is measured in _____.

2. A DSL modem can operate while the phone is in use.

   a. True

   b. False

3. What is a major advantage of a laser printer?

   _____

   _____

4. Name two pieces of hardware.

   a. _____

   b. _____

5. LAN stands for _____

   _____.

6. What are applications, in relation to computers?

   _____

   _____

7. A megabyte contains _____ of data.

8. A printer is an output device.

   a. True

   b. False

9. A zip drive is a _____ device.

10. A gigabyte contains _____ of data.

CHAPTER 9

Telephone Techniques

Vocabulary Review

Fill in the blanks with the correct vocabulary terms from this chapter.

1. Taylor Medical USA sells durable medical equipment and supplies to the public, so the company is considered to be a(n) _____.

2. Julie is careful of her _____, because she wants her voice to be clear and effective when she is speaking on the telephone.

3. Cassie's voice has a nice _____, which is a change in pitch or loudness when speaking.

4. Dr. LeGrand wishes to _____ her relationships with patients of different cultures so that she can understand their needs.

5. The office manager cautions the medical assistants to avoid _____, because most patients do not understand complicated medical terms.

6. The highness or lowness of sound is called its _____.

7. Laura _____ will be at work on time and will stay until the last patient leaves.

8. When speaking on the phone or in public, Dr. Conn knows that he should avoid _____ speech to keep the listeners interested and enthusiastic about what he has to say.

9. The medical assistants at Wray Medical and Surgical Clinic are proficient at _____.

10. Being placed on hold for an extended period of time becomes quite _____.

11. The utterance of articulate, clear sounds is _____.

12. It is pleasant to hear a person speak with _____.

13. Dr. Beard ordered the laboratory tests _____ so that the results would be reported to him immediately.

14. Mackenzie has learned to be _____ when she speaks with patients on the phone, so that she maintains a good relationship with them.

15. Dr. Lightfoot prefers that the receptionist _____ all of his calls so that he can concentrate on the patients in the office during their examinations.

Skills and Concepts

Part I: Answering Incoming Calls and Taking Phone Messages

Read the following incoming calls. In the space below, write three questions that the medical assistant could ask the caller based on the information he or she has given. Then, use the telephone message forms to take an accurate message for each caller. The calls in quotations are taken from voicemail. After determining the questions that could be addressed with the caller, indicate what actions need to be taken to properly follow through. Although you are not required to list questions that are clinical in nature, you may include clinical questions if you would like.

Staff Members at Dr. Julie Beard's Office

Physician	Dr. Julie Beard
Office Manager	Julia Carpenter
Clinical Medical Assistant	Trina Martinez
Clinical Medical Assistant	Dean Howell
Scheduling Assistant	Stephanie Dickson
Receptionist	Ginny Holloway
Insurance Biller and Medical Records	Gloria Richardson

16. "Hello, this is Peter Young. I saw Dr. Beard on Monday about a rash on my forearms. This thing isn't getting any better, and the cream she prescribed for me isn't helping the itching, and it's very uncomfortable. Is there anything else we can do to help it? My number is 972-555-9873." The message was received at 8:30 AM on Thursday, February 3.

Who should receive this message?

_____

Questions to ask the patient when returning this call:

a. _____

b. _____

c. _____

What action should be taken after speaking to the patient?

_____

_____

_____

17. Gerald Morris called Dr. Beard's office to ask whether his insurance has paid for his last office visit. He is an established patient and has worked as a city police officer for more than 10 years. After asking to place Mr. Morris on hold, you pull up his account on the computer. No insurance payment has been credited to his account, and there is a note indicating that his insurance was not in effect at the time of his office visit. Mr. Morris' phone number is 972-555-8824. He requests a call back as he is concerned about this information. This message was taken at 3:45 PM on September 4.

Who should receive this message?

_____

Questions to ask the patient when returning this call:

a. _____

b. _____

c. _____

What action should be taken after speaking to the patient?

_____

_____

_____

18. "Hello, this is Savannah Yarborough. I visited with your receptionist earlier today, and she indicated that one of the medical assistants has resigned and you will have a position available in
a few weeks. I am very interested in interviewing and presenting myself as a candidate for the
job. I am a certified medical assistant with 6 years' experience. Please give me a call at your
convenience at 817-555-9902. I look forward to speaking with you and perhaps scheduling an
interview." This message was taken at 1:30 PM on May 1.

Who should receive this message?

_____

Questions to ask when returning this call:

a. _____

b. _____

c. _____

What action should be taken after speaking to Ms. Yarborough?

_____

_____

_____

19. Mr. Juan Ross called today at 10:15 AM to get his prescription for Ambien refilled. His pharmacy
is Wolfe Drug, and the drugstore phone number is 214-555-4523. He is allergic to penicillin. Mr.
Ross' phone number is 214-555-2377. Mr. Ross' message was received on July 23.

Who should receive this message?

_____

Questions to ask the patient when returning his call:

a. _____

b. _____

c. _____

What action should be taken after speaking to the patient?

_____

_____

_____

20. Mr. Benjamin Adams called to speak to the office manager to express his dissatisfaction with the times that he was offered for an appointment. His job is strict about attendance, and he cannot leave work until 4:00 PM. He has requested appointment times after 4:00 PM, but the scheduling assistant tells him that he cannot have an appointment any later than 4:00 PM. Mr. Adams is concerned that he will not be able to be at the clinic at that exact time, and he is frustrated that the clinic is not more responsive to his needs. He called at 2:15 PM on March 14. His phone number at work is 972-555-6343, and his cell phone number is 214-555-8080.

Who should receive this message?

_____

Questions to ask the patient when returning the call:

a. _____

b. _____

c. _____

What action should be taken after speaking to the patient?

_____

_____

_____

21. "This is Ms. Garrett from Blue Cross/Blue Shield, and it's 10:00 AM on June 5. I am calling to discuss employee benefits for the coming year with the office manager. BCBS provides insurance coverage for your clinic employees. Would you please have the office manager return my call when she has a few moments to talk? My number is 800-555-0024, extension 415. Thank you!"

Who should receive this message?

_____

Questions to ask when returning the call:

a. _____

b. _____

c. _____

What action should be taken after speaking to Ms. Garrett?

_____

_____

_____

22. "This is Sarah at Cline Meador Lab with a stat lab report. It's 9:35 AM on November 16. The patient's name is Laura Williamson, and her WBC count is 18,000. Please notify Dr. Beard immediately. The lab phone number is 800-555-3333, and my extension is 255. If he has any questions, please have him give me a call. Thanks."

Who should receive this message?

_____

Questions to ask or information to verify when returning the call:

a. _____

b. _____

c. _____

What action should be taken after speaking to Sarah?

_____

_____

_____

23. Judy Jordan has migraine headaches and occasionally takes hydrocodone to relieve the pain. Dr. Beard leaves the office for the weekend at noon on Friday, and office policy dictates that he is not to be paged except in cases of emergency. Patients with routine or lesser health issues are to be instructed to either make an appointment to come in and see the physician or go to the emergency room. Judy calls at 4:45 PM on Friday afternoon, March 9, after Dr. Beard has left the office. She requests that the staff authorize a refill for her pain medicine and insists on speaking to the office manager, who is currently in a meeting. Her phone number is 214-555-9822.

Who should receive this message?

_____

Questions to ask or information to verify when returning the call:

a. _____

b. _____

c. _____

What action should be taken in this situation?

_____

_____

_____

24. Gary Burritt is moving out of state, so he calls the office because he needs a copy of his medical records. Dr. Beard prefers to send medical records directly to the receiving physician. Mr. Burritt's phone number is 512-555-6679. Today's date is December 20, and this message was received at 11:45 AM.

Who should receive this message?

_____

Questions to ask or information to verify when returning the call:

a. _____

b. _____

c. _____

What action should be taken in this situation?

_____

_____

_____

25. Allan Jenkins is calling from the cleaning service to let the office manager know what supplies he needs. He leaves a message stating that they are out of window cleaner, paper towels, liquid cleanser, and floor cleaner. He says that she does not have to call him back, but they will be cleaning again on Friday evening and will need the supplies at that time. This message was received on Wednesday, April 7 at 8:10 AM. The caller leaves his phone number, 903-555-2378, in case the office manager has questions.

Who should receive this message?

_____

What action should be taken in this situation?

_____

_____

_____

26. "Hello. My name is Christina Cawtel, and I was referred to your office by Dr. Preston for an evaluation of an ovarian cyst. Today is Wednesday, October 4, and it is 8 AM. I would like to make an appointment for early next week if possible. My phone number is 817-555-9325. Oh, and by the way, I need to know if you are a provider for Aetna, because my company just changed to their managed care plan. I probably need to have a mammogram, too, and want to see if you will order it before I come in for the appointment. Thanks."

Who should receive this message?

_____

Questions to ask or information to verify when returning the call:

a. _____

b. _____

c. _____

What action should be taken in this situation?

_____

_____

_____

27. "My name is Janeen Shaw and I am Dr. Beard's patient. It is just before 2:00 PM, and I am trying to reach you as soon as you open your office after lunch. I am having a hard time breathing, and I have stomach pains. I am hurting all over my upper body, on my chest, my arms, my neck . . . just everywhere. I'm sweating, and I'm very nauseated. I'm 45, and I'm almost never ill. I wanted to find out if I can come in for an appointment today. Please call me back as soon as possible. My phone number is 601-555-3423. Thank you . . . please call as soon as you can. I really feel awful."

Who should receive this message?

_____

Questions to ask or information to verify when returning the call:

a. _____

b. _____

c. _____

What action should be taken in this situation?

_____

_____

_____

Part II: Handling Difficult Calls

Briefly explain how the following callers and types of calls should be handled.

28. Angry callers

_____

_____

_____

29. Sales calls

_____

_____

_____

30. Emergency calls

_____

_____

_____

31. Unauthorized inquiry calls

_____

_____

_____

32. Callers with complaints

_____

_____

_____

Part III: Using a Telephone Directory

Using your local telephone directory, locate the following telephone numbers for your city or community.

33. Nonemergency number for the police department

_____

34. General information number for the nearest airport

_____

35. Local tax office

_____

36. American Red Cross office

_____

37. Acute care hospital

_____

38. Mental health and mental retardation center

_____

39. Meals on Wheels

_____

40. American Cancer Society

_____

Part IV: Answering the Telephone

Use the local telephone directory to find telephone numbers for the following medical specialty offices in your area. Call these offices to determine how they answer the telephone. Explain the purpose of your call to the staff member who answers the phone, and record the phone greeting they use in the space provided below.

41. Ophthalmologist

_____

42. Oncologist

_____

43. General practitioner

_____

44. Chiropractor

_____

45. Cosmetic surgeon

_____

46. Dermatologist

_____

Part V: Short Answer Questions

Fill in the blank with the correct answer.

47. Selecting which calls will be forwarded to the physician immediately is a process called

_____.

48. A study by Harvard University claims that the physician's _____ of voice has a direct link to medical professional liability claims.

49. The medical assistant should not eat, drink, or _____ while answering the office telephone.

50. The mouthpiece of the telephone handset should be held _____ inch(es) from the lips.

51. The medical assistant must maintain patient _____ at all times, even when on the telephone.

52. Telephone calls should be answered by the _____ ring.

53. Unsatisfactory progress reports from patients should be directed to the _____.

54. _____ calls help the physician to communicate with family members in different parts of the country.

55. Medical offices should have a set of clearly written _____ that can be read to the caller who requests the information.

Part VI: Time Zones

Determine the correct times.

56. When it is 3:00 PM in Dallas, Texas, it is _____ in Los Angeles, California.

57. When it is 2:00 PM in Washington state, it is _____ in New York City.

58. When it is 5:00 PM in Las Cruces, New Mexico, it is _____ in Flint, Michigan.

59. When it is 4:00 PM in Augusta, Maine, it is _____ in Columbia, South Carolina.

60. When it is 11:00 AM in Biloxi, Mississippi, it is _____ in Chicago, Illinois.

Part VII: Telephone Technique

Give answers for the following statements.

61. List five questions that might be asked of a patient who calls with an emergency situation:

    a. _____

    b. _____

    c. _____

    d. _____

    e. _____

62. The phrase that often calms an angry patient is _____ _____

    _____ _____.

63. Explain the procedure for transferring a phone call.

    _____

    _____

    _____

64. What should the medical assistant do if a caller refuses to identify himself or herself?

    _____

    _____

    _____

65. List the seven components of a proper telephone message.

a. _____

b. _____

c. _____

d. _____

e. _____

f. _____

g. _____

Case Study

Denise has been the receptionist for a moderately large clinic for the past 3 months. She replaced Dorothy, who retired. Denise has been overwhelmed with the calls to the clinic, and the office manager has spoken to her twice about missing calls. Denise insists that she is constantly on the phone answering and transferring calls. She is beginning to lose faith in herself, but as she considers why she is failing at her job, she realizes that two new physicians have joined the practice since Dorothy left, and numerous calls come to the clinic for those two physicians. Denise wants to suggest to the office manager that perhaps the time has come for a second receptionist, but she is unsure how to broach the subject. How can Denise begin her conversation with the office manager? What should she not do or say?

_____

_____

_____

Workplace Application

Contact a clinic office manager and determine if he or she would allow you to shadow the office receptionist for a day. Take note of the types of calls that come into the clinic and how they are handled. Discuss the results of the visit with the class.

Internet Activities

1. Investigate telephone techniques and skills on the Internet and bring three tips to class. Share these with your classmates.

2. After researching information on the Internet, write a report that explains why the telephone is so important in making a good first impression.

3. Research the way that telephones actually work. Prepare a brief report for the class.

4. Research the way that Internet connections are made through phone systems. Prepare a brief report for the class.

Chapter 9 Quiz

Name: _____

1. The quality of being clear is

   _____ .

2. When it is 2:00 PM in Atlanta, it is
   _____ in Los Angeles.

3. The medical assistant must make certain that
   he or she is speaking to the right person on
   the phone when relating medical information
   to a patient.

   a. True

   b. False

4. Telephone systems that are answered by a
   recorded voice with a series of options are
   called _____ .

5. Lunch-hour and after-hours calls are
   frequently handled by a(n)

   _____ .

6. Provide three examples of emergency calls:

   a. _____

   b. _____

   c. _____

7. A change in voice pitch is called a(n)

   _____ .

8. Speech of an unvaried pitch is

   _____ .

9. Being tactful means to avoid offensive
   comments in speech.

   a. True

   b. False

10. List two ways to deal with an angry caller:

    a. _____

    b. _____

CHAPTER **10**

Scheduling Appointments

Vocabulary Review

Fill in the blank with the correct vocabulary term from this chapter.

1. Angela arranged for a short time _____ between Dr. Patrick's speaking engage-
ment and his first afternoon appointment so that he would have time for lunch.

2. Gayle gained _____ in computers by taking Saturday classes on the newest
software.

3. A(n) _____ noise came from the autoclave when it was turned on this morning, so
Pamela called service personnel to repair the machine.

4. Olivia realized that she needed to take a(n) _____ medical terminology course
before she could register for anatomy and physiology.

5. All of the medical assistants in the facility know that a(n) _____ _____
must be noted in the medical record, as well as the appointment book.

6. Before using an appointment book, establish the _____ by marking all times that
the physician is unavailable, so that patients will not be scheduled during those times.

7. A patient from a neighboring clinic caused a(n) _____ in the hallway as he left,
because he disagreed with a billing statement.

8. _____ _____ are those who have been seen as patients in the clinic
more than once.

9. The _____ among the staff at Dr. Wykowski's office has become strained since the
office manager was terminated.

10. Cooperation and willingness to help other staff members is a(n) _____ part of the
success of a practice.

Skills and Concepts

Part I: Appointment Reminder Cards

Practice completing appointment reminder cards on the forms provided.

11. Gayle Jackson has an appointment for August 23, 20XX, at 3 PM with Dr. Lupez.

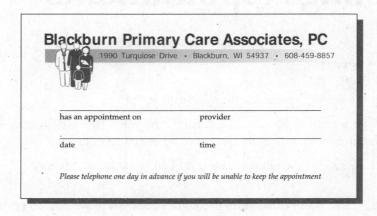

12. Debra Odom has an appointment for May 1, 20XX, at 9 AM with Dr. Hughes.

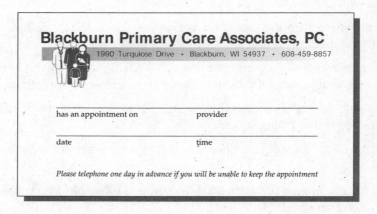

13. Katrina Shaw has an appointment for June 13, 20XX, at 11:45 AM with Dr. Hughes.

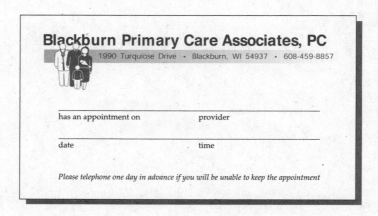

14. Joni Perry has an appointment for September 12, 20XX, at 2:40 PM with Dr. Lawler.

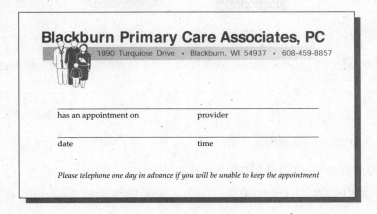

Blackburn Primary Care Associates, PC
1990 Turquiose Drive • Blackburn, WI 54937 • 608-459-8857

has an appointment on _____   provider _____

date _____   time _____

Please telephone one day in advance if you will be unable to keep the appointment

15. Savannah York has an appointment for December 15, 20XX, at 4:30 PM with Dr. Lupez.

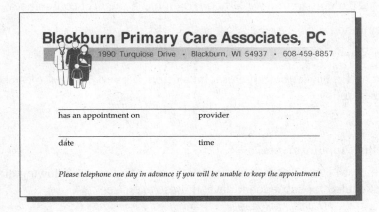

Blackburn Primary Care Associates, PC
1990 Turquiose Drive • Blackburn, WI 54937 • 608-459-8857

has an appointment on _____   provider _____

date _____   time _____

Please telephone one day in advance if you will be unable to keep the appointment

Part II: Guides for Scheduling

16. What three items must be considered when scheduling appointments?

   a. _____

   b. _____

   c. _____

17. Why is patient need an important consideration when planning services that the clinic will offer?

_____

_____

18. How can the medical assistant handle a physician who habitually spends more than the allotted time with patients?

_____

_____

19. List one advantage and one disadvantage to using an appointment book for scheduling.

    Advantage _____

    Disadvantage _____

20. List one advantage and one disadvantage to using a computer for scheduling.

    Advantage _____

    Disadvantage _____

Part III: Advance Preparation and Establishing a Matrix

Prepare Appointment Page #1 (Work Product 10-1) according to the following directions.

21. The date is Monday, October 13, 20XX.

22. Drs. Lawler and Hughes have hospital rounds from 8 to 9 AM.

23. Dr. Lupez sees patients from 8 AM to noon, then has a medical conference.

24. Lunch is from noon until 2 PM.

25. Dr. Lawler has a 4 PM meeting at the hospital.

26. Dr. Hughes and Dr. Lawler both prefer a break from 3:15 to 3:30 PM to catch up on telephone calls and other duties.

Part IV: Scheduling Appointments

Prepare Appointment Page #2 (Work Product 10-2) according to the following directions. Appointments can be scheduled for subsequent days in these exercises.

27. The date is Tuesday, October 14, 20XX.

28. Lunch is from noon until 2 PM.

29. Dr. Lawler will be out Tuesday afternoon.

30. Dr. Hughes is out of town speaking at a conference.

31. Tracey and Keith Jones would like an appointment with Dr. Lawler right before lunch. Both are new patient physical examinations, and they would like to come to the office at the same time so that they can also discuss family planning.

32. John Edgar, Lydia Perry, and June Trayner are established patients who need follow-up appointments with Dr. Lupez.

33. Wayne Harris needs a new patient appointment with Dr. Lawler as early as possible.

34. Lucy Fraser needs an appointment with Dr. Lawler or Dr. Hughes and has to make the appointment after 3:30 PM, because she picks up her children from school.

35. Asa Nordholm, Carrie Jones, and Seicho Ando need follow-up appointments with Dr. Lawler.

36. Talia Perez called and is having trouble with her new blood pressure medication. The soonest she can get off work and come to the clinic is 2:15 PM.

37. Paula Nolen needs an allergy shot in the morning.

38. Amy Wainwright needs a well-woman examination and can come to the clinic any time before 3 PM.

39. Pam Billingsley wants to come to the clinic in the later afternoon for a return check about her migraine headaches.

40. Adam Angsley needs an appointment with Dr. Lawler in the afternoon.

Prepare Appointment Page #3 (Work Product 10-3) according to the following directions. Appointments can be scheduled for subsequent days in these exercises.

41. The date is Wednesday, October 15, 20XX.

42. All of the physicians are in the office today.

43. Lunch is from noon until 2 PM.

44. Dr. Lawler has three rechecks today, with Ella Jones, Fred Linstra, and Mary Higgins.

45. Winston Hill is an established patient coming in for an annual physical with Dr. Lawler. His neighbor can drive him to the clinic for a 2 PM appointment.

46. Elnar Rosen, an established patient, needs a physical with Dr. Hughes at around 10:15 AM.

47. A staff meeting is scheduled for 9 AM.

48. A representative from Allied Medical Supply is demonstrating a self-scheduling computer program at 4:30 PM for all staff members.

49. Bob Jones needs a morning appointment with Dr. Lupez.

50. Talia Perez is extremely nauseated and needs to return to the clinic today.

51. Robin Tower is a new patient who wishes to see Dr. Lawler or Dr. Hughes.

52. Audrey Rhodes is a new patient who wishes to see Dr. Lawler.

53. Victor Garner is a follow-up patient whom Dr. Lupez saw last week in the hospital. He is new to the clinic.

54. Charlie Robinson missed his appointment today at 11 AM with Dr. Hughes.

55. Peter Blake calls to see if he can be seen by one of the physicians at 11:15 AM.

Prepare Appointment Page #4 (Work Product 10-4) according to the following directions. Appointments can be scheduled for subsequent days in these exercises.

56. The date is Thursday, October 16, 20XX.

57. Dr. Hughes is not in the office because his daughter is having a baby.

58. Lunch is from noon until 2 PM.

59. All patients must be seen in the morning because the clinic is closed on Thursday afternoons.

60. Cassie LeGrand is coming to the clinic as a new patient to see Dr. Lupez.

61. Cassandra LeBrock is coming to the clinic as an established patient to see Dr. Lupez.

62. Raymond Smith wants to make an appointment at 1:45 PM with Dr. Lawler.

63. Benjamin Charles requests an appointment with Dr. Lupez at 3:45 PM.

Prepare Appointment Page #5 (Work Product 10-5) according to the following directions.

64. The date is Friday, October 17, 20XX.

65. Dr. Lupez is the only provider in the office today.

66. Lunch is from noon until 2 PM.

67. Cassie LeGrand returns today for laboratory work and to consult with Dr. Lupez for surgery.

68. Bruce Wells is scheduled for a follow-up appointment at 10:15 AM.

69. Ronald Trayhan calls to make an appointment with Dr. Lupez for 2:30 PM.

70. Dr. Hughes calls to ask Dr. Lupez to see one of his young patients, Barbara Scott, at 3 PM for a high fever.

71. Stanley Allred calls for an appointment to see Dr. Lupez at 3 PM.

Part V: Types of Scheduling

Briefly describe each type of scheduling, and list one advantage and one disadvantage of each.

72. Scheduled appointments

_____

_____

73. Open office hours

_____

_____

74. Flexible office hours

_____

_____

75. Wave scheduling

_____

_____

76. Modified wave scheduling

_____

_____

77. Double booking

_____

_____

78. Grouping procedures

_____

_____

79. Advance booking

_____

_____

Part VI: Special Circumstances

80. How can the medical assistant deal with patients who are consistently late for appointments?

_____

_____

81. How does the medical assistant handle a patient who arrives at the clinic to see the physician but does not have an appointment?

_____

_____

Part VII: Verifying Appointments

82. Write a brief script that could be used to verify patient appointments and that does not violate patient privacy.

_____

_____

_____

_____

Part VIII: Scheduling Inpatient and Outpatient Admissions and Procedures

Complete the referral forms in Work Products 10-6 to 10-9 for the following patients. Create fictional demographic information.

83. Cassie LeGrand is to report to Mercy Hospital for excision of a nasal polyp on Tuesday, October 24, 20XX. Dr. Lupez is her attending physician. Surgery is scheduled for Tuesday at 2 PM. She will need blood work that morning. The procedure is considered outpatient, and Cassie will go home later that day if she does well. ICD code: 471.0 (Work Product 10-6).

84. Bob Jones arrives at Presbyterian Hospital to have an MRI on his right knee on Friday, November 2, 20XX. He needs an early morning appointment. ICD code: 715.8 (Work Product 10-7).

85. Lucille Saxton is to be admitted to the hospital for surgery because of a bowel obstruction. Her surgery date is June 14, 20XX, and she must be admitted a day in advance for laboratory work and a chest x-ray examination. ICD code: 560.9 (Work Product 10-8).

86. Pam Burton needs to be admitted for several tests because of her recurrent irritable bowel syndrome. She will be in the hospital for at least 3 days and should check in on July 23, 20XX in the afternoon, so that she will have taken nothing by mouth (NPO) before the blood tests are performed and x-ray films are taken the following morning. ICD Code: 564.1 (Work Product 10-9).

Case Study

Janie Haynie consistently arrives at the clinic between 15 and 45 minutes late. She always has a "good" excuse, but she could make her appointments on time if she had better time management skills. The office manager has mentioned to Paula, the receptionist, that Janie is to be scheduled at 4:45 PM and if she is late, she will not be seen by the physician. Paula books Janie's next three appointments at that time, and Janie actually arrives early. However, on the fourth appointment, Janie arrives at 5:50 PM, and Paula knows that it is her responsibility to tell Janie that she cannot see the physician. How does Paula handle this task? Is there more than one option?

_____

_____

_____

Workplace Application

Choose five clinics and call the receptionist at each. Tell them that you are studying scheduling in medical assisting school and are interested in the scheduling method that they use. Tally the results that each classmate obtains, then graph or chart the results for the class on one document. Discuss the frequency of the various methods of scheduling.

Internet Activities

1. Research scheduling software on the Internet, and select a software package that would be functional for a physician's office. Gather information about the features and benefits, and present the information to the class.

2. Research information about the different types of scheduling and how effective they are in physician offices. Determine the type of scheduling that is most ideal for a family practice clinic. Present the ideas to the class.

3. Research self-scheduling software, and determine the advantages and disadvantages of allowing patients to schedule appointments on the Internet. Present the information to the class, or write an informative report about the findings.

Chapter 10 Quiz

Name: _____

1. A person who fails to keep an appointment is sometimes referred to as a(n) _____.

2. A returning patient is called a(n) _____ patient.

3. A situation requiring haste or caution is said to reguire a(n) _____.

4. One of the advantages of computerized scheduling is that more than one person can schedule patients at a time.
   a. True
   b. False

5. A facility that accepts only walk-in appointments is using the type of scheduling called _____ _____.

6. Scheduling two patients to arrive at the same time is _____.

7. Chronically late patients should be scheduled at the _____ of the day.

8. Failed appointments should be noted in the _____ record.

9. Patients should be notified and an offer made to reschedule if the physician is running more than _____ minutes late.

10. _____ representatives bring information about various drugs to clinics and often leave samples for the physician to dispense to patients.

11. The medical assistant should offer the patient different _____ when scheduling him or her for appointments, such as "morning" or "afternoon."

WORK PRODUCT 10-1

Name: _____

Advance Preparation and Establishing a Matrix

Complete Appointment Page #1 using the information in Part III.

			DAY / DATE							
			8 00 10 20 30 40 50							
			9 00 10 20 30 40 50							
			10 00 10 20 30 40 50							
			11 00 10 20 30 40 50							
			12 00 10 20 30 40 50							
			1 00 10 20 30 40 50							
			2 00 10 20 30 40 50							
			3 00 10 20 30 40 50							
			4 00 10 20 30 40 50							
			5 00 10 20 30 40 50							

Bibbero Systems Form 56-7310

WORK PRODUCT 10-2

Name: _____

Scheduling Appointments

Complete Appointment Page #2 using the information in Part IV, Questions 27-40.

			DAY							
			DATE							
			8	00 10 20 30 40 50						
			9	00 10 20 30 40 50						
			10	00 10 20 30 40 50						
			11	00 10 20 30 40 50						
			12	00 10 20 30 40 50						
			1	00 10 20 30 40 50						
			2	00 10 20 30 40 50						
			3	00 10 20 30 40 50						
			4	00 10 20 30 40 50						
			5	00 10 20 30 40 50						

Bibbero Systems Form 56-7310

WORK PRODUCT 10-3

Name: _____

Scheduling Appointments

Complete Appointment Page #3 using the information in Part IV, Questions 41-55.

			DAY							
			DATE							
			8 00 10 20 30 40 50							
			9 00 10 20 30 40 50							
			10 00 10 20 30 40 50							
			11 00 10 20 30 40 50							
			12 00 10 20 30 40 50							
			1 00 10 20 30 40 50							
			2 00 10 20 30 40 50							
			3 00 10 20 30 40 50							
			4 00 10 20 30 40 50							
			5 00 10 20 30 40 50							

Bibbero Systems Form 56-7310

WORK PRODUCT 10-4

Name: _____

Scheduling Appointments

Complete Appointment Page #4 using the information in Part IV, Questions 56-63.

			DAY DATE							
			8 00 10 20 30 40 50							
			9 00 10 20 30 40 50							
			10 00 10 20 30 40 50							
			11 00 10 20 30 40 50							
			12 00 10 20 30 40 50							
			1 00 10 20 30 40 50							
			2 00 10 20 30 40 50							
			3 00 10 20 30 40 50							
			4 00 10 20 30 40 50							
			5 00 10 20 30 40 50							

Bibbero Systems Form 56-7310

WORK PRODUCT 10-5

Name: _____

Scheduling Appointments

Complete Appointment Page #5 using the information in Part IV, Questions 64-71.

			DAY								
			DATE								
			8	00							
				10							
				20							
				30							
				40							
				50							
			9	00							
				10							
				20							
				30							
				40							
				50							
			10	00							
				10							
				20							
				30							
				40							
				50							
			11	00							
				10							
				20							
				30							
				40							
				50							
			12	00							
				10							
				20							
				30							
				40							
				50							
			1	00							
				10							
				20							
				30							
				40							
				50							
			2	00							
				10							
				20							
				30							
				40							
				50							
			3	00							
				10							
				20							
				30							
				40							
				50							
			4	00							
				10							
				20							
				30							
				40							
				50							
			5	00							
				10							
				20							
				30							
				40							
				50							

Bibbero Systems Form 56-7310

WORK PRODUCT 10-6

Name: _____

Scheduling Inpatient and Outpatient Admissions and Procedures

Complete the referral form using the information in Part VIII, Question 83.

BLACKBURN PRIMARY CARE ASSOCIATES, P.C.
1990 Turquoise Drive • Blackburn, WI 54937
Phone 608-459-8857 • Fax 608-459-8860
Referral Form Effective Jan. 1, 20XX

Patient Name _____ **Phone #** _____
SS # _____ **DOB** _____
Diagnosis (ICD-9 Required) _____
Insurance Type _____
Referring Physician _____ **Phone** _____
Office Contact _____ **Fax** _____

REFERRAL FOR:
❑ Consult Only
❑ Evaluation and Treatment
❑ Inpatient Surgery
❑ Inpatient Admission
❑ Outpatient Surgery
❑ Outpatient Lab
❑ Outpatient X-ray
❑ Procedure Only
❑ Chiropractic
❑ Physical Therapy
❑ Back in Action Rehabilitation Program
❑ Psychophysiologic Evaluation
❑ Biofeedback
❑ Other _____

Comments
_____
_____
_____
_____
_____
_____
_____

REFERRAL TIMEFRAME:
❑ First Available Appt (within 5 business days)
❑ Stat (within 24 hr)

PROVIDER:
❑ Ron Lupez, M.D.
❑ Donald Lawler, M.D.
❑ Robert Hughes, D.O.
❑ Neil Stern, D.C.
❑ Joel Lively, P.T.

PLEASE INCLUDE THE FOLLOWING:
❑ Copy of Insurance Card
❑ Demographic Information
❑ Treatment Notes
❑ Diagnostic Reports

HOSPITAL/FACILITY
❑ Mercy Hospital
❑ Presbyterian Hospital
❑ Outpatient Surgical Complex
❑ Health and Wellness Center

Scheduled By _____

Appt Date/Time _____ Physician _____

WORK PRODUCT 10-7

Name: _____

Scheduling Inpatient and Outpatient Admissions and Procedures

Complete the referral form using the information in Part VIII, Question 84.

BLACKBURN PRIMARY CARE ASSOCIATES, P.C.
1990 Turquoise Drive • Blackburn, WI 54937
Phone 608-459-8857 • Fax 608-459-8860
Referral Form Effective Jan. 1, 20XX

Patient Name _____ **Phone #** _____
SS # _____ **DOB** _____
Diagnosis (ICD-9 Required) _____
Insurance Type _____
Referring Physician _____ **Phone** _____
Office Contact _____ **Fax** _____

REFERRAL FOR:
❑ Consult Only
❑ Evaluation and Treatment
❑ Inpatient Surgery
❑ Inpatient Admission
❑ Outpatient Surgery
❑ Outpatient Lab
❑ Outpatient X-ray
❑ Procedure Only
❑ Chiropractic
❑ Physical Therapy
❑ Back in Action Rehabilitation Program
❑ Psychophysiologic Evaluation
❑ Biofeedback
❑ Other _____

Comments
_____
_____
_____
_____
_____
_____
_____

REFERRAL TIMEFRAME:
❑ First Available Appt (within 5 business days)
❑ Stat (within 24 hr)

PROVIDER:
❑ Ron Lupez, M.D.
❑ Donald Lawler, M.D.
❑ Robert Hughes, D.O.
❑ Neil Stern, D.C.
❑ Joel Lively, P.T.

PLEASE INCLUDE THE FOLLOWING:
❑ Copy of Insurance Card
❑ Demographic Information
❑ Treatment Notes
❑ Diagnostic Reports

HOSPITAL/FACILITY
❑ Mercy Hospital
❑ Presbyterian Hospital
❑ Outpatient Surgical Complex
❑ Health and Wellness Center

Scheduled By _____

Appt Date/Time _____ Physician _____

WORK PRODUCT 10-8

Name: _____

Scheduling Inpatient and Outpatient Admissions and Procedures

Complete the referral form using the information in Part VIII, Question 85.

BLACKBURN PRIMARY CARE ASSOCIATES, P.C.
1990 Turquoise Drive • Blackburn, WI 54937
Phone 608-459-8857 • Fax 608-459-8860
Referral Form Effective Jan. 1, 20XX

Patient Name _____ Phone # _____
SS # _____ DOB_____
Diagnosis (ICD-9 Required) _____
Insurance Type _____
Referring Physician _____ Phone _____
Office Contact _____ Fax _____

REFERRAL FOR:
❑ Consult Only
❑ Evaluation and Treatment
❑ Inpatient Surgery
❑ Inpatient Admission
❑ Outpatient Surgery
❑ Outpatient Lab
❑ Outpatient X-ray
❑ Procedure Only
❑ Chiropractic
❑ Physical Therapy
❑ Back in Action Rehabilitation Program
❑ Psychophysiologic Evaluation
❑ Biofeedback
❑ Other _____

Comments
_____
_____
_____
_____
_____
_____

REFERRAL TIMEFRAME:
❑ First Available Appt (within 5 business days)
❑ Stat (within 24 hr)

PROVIDER:
❑ Ron Lupez, M.D.
❑ Donald Lawler, M.D.
❑ Robert Hughes, D.O.
❑ Neil Stern, D.C.
❑ Joel Lively, P.T.

PLEASE INCLUDE THE FOLLOWING:
❑ Copy of Insurance Card
❑ Demographic Information
❑ Treatment Notes
❑ Diagnostic Reports

HOSPITAL/FACILITY
❑ Mercy Hospital
❑ Presbyterian Hospital
❑ Outpatient Surgical Complex
❑ Health and Wellness Center

Scheduled By _____

Appt Date/Time _____ Physician _____

WORK PRODUCT 10-9

Name: _____

Scheduling Inpatient and Outpatient Admissions and Procedures

Complete the referral form using the information in Part VIII, Question 86.

BLACKBURN PRIMARY CARE ASSOCIATES, P.C.
1990 Turquoise Drive • Blackburn, WI 54937
Phone 608-459-8857 • Fax 608-459-8860
Referral Form Effective Jan. 1, 20XX

Patient Name _____ **Phone #** _____
SS # _____ **DOB** _____
Diagnosis (ICD-9 Required) _____
Insurance Type _____
Referring Physician _____ **Phone** _____
Office Contact _____ **Fax** _____

REFERRAL FOR:
❑ Consult Only
❑ Evaluation and Treatment
❑ Inpatient Surgery
❑ Inpatient Admission
❑ Outpatient Surgery
❑ Outpatient Lab
❑ Outpatient X-ray
❑ Procedure Only
❑ Chiropractic
❑ Physical Therapy
❑ Back in Action Rehabilitation Program
❑ Psychophysiologic Evaluation
❑ Biofeedback
❑ Other _____

Comments
_____
_____
_____
_____
_____
_____

REFERRAL TIMEFRAME:
❑ First Available Appt (within 5 business days)
❑ Stat (within 24 hr)

PROVIDER:
❑ Ron Lupez, M.D.
❑ Donald Lawler, M.D.
❑ Robert Hughes, D.O.
❑ Neil Stern, D.C.
❑ Joel Lively, P.T.

PLEASE INCLUDE THE FOLLOWING:
❑ Copy of Insurance Card
❑ Demographic Information
❑ Treatment Notes
❑ Diagnostic Reports

HOSPITAL/FACILITY
❑ Mercy Hospital
❑ Presbyterian Hospital
❑ Outpatient Surgical Complex
❑ Health and Wellness Center

Scheduled By _____

Appt Date/Time _____ Physician _____

Patient Reception and Processing

Vocabulary Review

Fill in the blanks with the correct vocabulary terms from this chapter.

1. Thomas noticed that the staff had _____ their supplies of gauze pads, so he ordered a case using the medical supplier's online system.

2. Jerri _____ the 1″ syringes so that Thomas would know to order more of them for the clinic.

3. Dr. Raleigh installed a(n) _____ system so that he could speak to the medical assistants both in the front and in the back offices from the examination rooms.

4. Medical assistants must be aware of the _____ that patients have of the office staff and take steps to ensure that it is a positive one.

5. Susan filed the laboratory reports in _____ order.

6. _____ information includes the patient's address, insurance information, and email address.

7. Any _____ offered to a patient should be within the physician's orders, so make certain that a beverage with sugar is not offered to a diabetic.

8. Angela uses _____ devices to help her remember the duties to complete before leaving the office.

9. Employees prefer to work in an office with a(n) _____ environment.

10. Dr. Lawson has a(n) _____ desire to serve his patients and promote wellness.

Skills and Concepts

Part I: The Office Mission Statement

11. Create a mission statement for a fictional family practice.

_____

_____

_____

_____

Part II: The Reception Area

12. Why is the first impression of the physician's office so important to patients?

_____

_____

_____

_____

13. List five items that might be found in the patient reception area.

a. _____

b. _____

c. _____

d. _____

e. _____

14. If a computer is provided in the reception area, what cautionary measure should be taken to ensure patient privacy?

_____

_____

_____

_____

15. Describe the ideal receptionist for a physician's office.

_____

_____

_____

_____

Part III: Registration Procedures

16. List six items of demographic information found on a patient information sheet.

a. _____

b. _____

c. _____

d. _____

e. _____

f. _____

Part IV: Consideration for Patient's Time

17. Why might a crowded waiting room be a sign of inefficiency instead of physician popularity?

    _____

    _____

    _____

18. Delays greater than _____ minutes should be explained to patients, and they should be allowed to reschedule if they desire to do so.

19. There should be no more than _____ to _____ patients in the reception area at any given time.

20. What feelings do patients often experience when waiting in the physician's office?

    _____

    _____

    _____

Part V: Patient Confidentiality

21. How can the medical assistant help avoid a breach of patient confidentiality by the placement of charts in wall holders?

    _____

    _____

    _____

    _____

22. How can the medical assistant help avoid a breach of patient confidentiality while using sign-in sheets?

    _____

    _____

    _____

    _____

Part VI: Patient Checkout

Write out a verbal response to the following patients in the checkout process.

23. Suzanne Anton is ready to leave the clinic, and she owes a copay of $25 plus a past due balance of $10 that her insurance did not pay. She questions the $10 balance.

    _____

    _____

    _____

24. Randy Stephens is leaving the clinic but is angry about his visit with the physician, who insists that he lose 40 pounds. He reluctantly pays his copay and needs to schedule a follow-up appointment for 1 month, during which time the physician wants him to have lost 5 pounds by following a strict diet.

_____

_____

_____

25. Mrs. Alfred Williams has come to the clinic for a checkup. She is being treated by the physician for colon cancer and is usually cheerful, despite her prognosis. Today she seems distressed and hesitates before paying her bill of $65.

_____

_____

_____

Part VII: The End of the Day

26. Paige is preparing for the next work day. What are some tasks that will help her prepare for tomorrow's patients?

_____

_____

_____

27. List several routine tasks for closing an office.

_____

_____

_____

28. How can the medical assistant gain confidence in asking for payments and co-payments?

_____

_____

_____

Part VIII: Evaluating Reception Areas

Visit several reception areas in physician's offices, hospitals, and/or clinics. Take note of the appearance and amenities in these facilities. Rate each reception area on a scale of 1 to 10. Total the figures to determine the "best" reception area.

AREA	Locations				
Cleanliness					
Color scheme					
Seating					
Lighting					
Comfort					
Amenities					
Noise level					
Total					

Case Study

Jill is the receptionist for Drs. Boles and Bailey, who are psychiatrists. Each week Sara Ables comes to her appointments but brings her two small children, Joey and Julie, ages 8 and 6 years, respectively. When Sara goes back for her appointment, the children are almost uncontrollable in the reception area. Although there are never more than two patients waiting, the kids are a serious disruption in the clinic. When Jill mentioned the problem to Dr. Boles, he said that Sara really needed the sessions and that Jill should try to work with Sara on this issue. What can Jill do to remedy the situation?

_____

_____

_____

Workplace Application

Design a registration form for a fictional clinic that includes all information necessary for a new patient. Be creative with logos and fonts. Make the form attractive and easy to understand.

Internet Activities

1. Search for innovations in patient reception on the Internet, including computers that allow patients to perform self–check-in for appointments. Present information to the class on one of the systems.

2. Find examples of office mission statements online. Compare them, and write a brief report about the contents of the various statements.

3. Research the Americans with Disabilities Act. Determine what accommodations must be made in reception areas to comply with this law. Present the information to the class.

Chapter 11 Quiz

Name: _____

1. List two activities that the medical assistant should complete before patients begin to arrive.

   a. _____

   b. _____

2. By spelling patient names _____, the medical assistant will find difficult ones easier to pronounce.

3. After the medical records for the day are pulled, the records should be arranged alphabetically.

   a. True

   b. False

4. What are some reasons that the medical assistant should not offer coffee or water to patients while they are waiting?

   _____

   _____

   _____

5. Registration forms allow the medical assistant to collect a patient's _____ information.

6. List two items that should be found in an adequate reception area.

   a. _____

   b. _____ .

7. List two activities that the medical assistant should complete before leaving the office for the day.

   a. _____

   b. _____

8. Using the patient's name often helps to develop patient _____.

9. Patients should not have to wait to see the physician for more than _____ minutes without an explanation.

10. _____ patients take up more of the physician's time than is justified.

CHAPTER 12

Office Environment and Daily Operations

Vocabulary Review

Fill in the blanks with the correct vocabulary terms from this chapter.

1. Julia noticed some _____ in the inventory when comparing last month's totals with the current month's totals.

2. Rhonda prefers that all _____ _____ be initialed by the person who checks in the package.

3. Dr. Hughes is _____ when dealing with conflicts within the office by talking with staff members and looking for ways to compromise.

4. Sarah enjoys developing a(n) _____ for office expenditures each fiscal year.

5. Items on _____ frustrate the office manager because of the follow-up required to make certain the item eventually arrives at the clinic.

6. When Douglas neglected to pay the supply bill by the due date, he _____ late charges and increased the total due by 2%.

7. The office manager was able to _____ a confrontation with the patient who complained about the bill by addressing his concerns in a cordial way.

8. By _____ websites that she uses frequently, Ann is able to find medical suppliers and research the best prices quickly.

Skills and Concepts

Part I: Opening the Office

Provide short answers to the following questions.

9. List six duties that should be completed before patient arrival.

   a. _____

   b. _____

   c. _____

   d. _____

e. _____

f. _____

10. What parts of the medical record should be checked to see if additional forms need to be added before a patient arrives for an office visit?

_____

_____

_____

11. Explain the precautions that should be taken with prescription pads.

_____

_____

_____

12. Why is patient traffic flow an important consideration in the office environment?

_____

_____

_____

Part II: The Office Environment

13. List 10 expenses that the physician's office incurs on a month-to-month basis.

a. _____

b. _____

c. _____

d. _____

e. _____

f. _____

g. _____

h. _____

i. _____

j. _____

14. List six tasks that the medical assistant can do between patients or during slower periods.

a. _____

b. _____

c. _____

d. _____

e. _____

f. _____

15. Explain the purpose of white noise.

_____

_____

_____

16. List three things related to the office environment that the medical assistant can do to help the physician save money.

a. _____

b. _____

c. _____

17. Explain why the number of individuals with keys and alarm codes should be limited in the medical office.

_____

_____

_____

Part III: Medical Waste and Regular Waste

Note whether each of the following items should be classified as medical or regular waste.

18. Gauze used to stop bleeding after venipuncture

_____

19. Tissues used in the reception room to clean eyeglasses

_____

20. Blood tubes containing blood that has already been tested

_____

21. Used syringes

_____

22. Paper towels used to clean a mirror in a patient restroom

_____

Part IV: Equipment Inventory

Complete an inventory of either administrative or clinical equipment at the school using the form in Work Product 12-1. Give the form to the instructor when finished.

Part V: Supply Inventory

Complete an inventory of either administrative or clinical supplies at the school using the form in Work Product 12-2. Give the form to the instructor when finished.

Part VI: Purchase Orders

Complete two purchase orders using an office supply catalog, newspaper ad, or the Internet. Complete one purchase order for supplies (things that are used up on a routine basis); complete the other for equipment (things that are reusable and usually of value).

Name _____

Date _____

PURCHASE ORDER   No. 1554

Bill to:

Blackburn Primary Care Associates. PC
1990 Turquoise Drive
Blackburn, WI 54937

Ship to:

Blackburn Primary Care Associates, PC
1990 Turquoise Drive
Blackburn, WI 54937

Vendor: _____
_____
_____

Terms: _____

ORDER #	DESCRIPTION	QTY.	COLOR	SIZE	UNIT PRICE	TOTAL PRICE
					SUBTOTAL	
					TAX	
					SHIPPING	
					TOTAL	

Name _____

Date _____

PURCHASE ORDER   No. **1554**

Bill to: **Ship to:**

Blackburn Primary Care Associates. PC   Blackburn Primary Care Associates, PC
1990 Turquoise Drive   1990 Turquoise Drive
Blackburn, WI 54937   Blackburn, WI 54937

Vendor: _____

_____

_____

Terms: _____

ORDER #	DESCRIPTION	QTY.	COLOR	SIZE	UNIT PRICE	TOTAL PRICE
					SUBTOTAL	
					TAX	
					SHIPPING	
					TOTAL	

Part VII: Maintenance Logs

Use the form in Work Product 12-3 to compile a log of the administrative equipment in your class-room. Follow the example given on the first line. Give the form to the instructor when you are finished.

Case Study

Read the case study and answer the questions that follow.

Dianna had worked at the Family Clinic for 6 years in the front office. When a new medical assistant, Kiran, was hired to work the phones and schedule appointments, Dianna noticed that she was not following the office policy and caused several problems with the schedule. Some patients were very late in seeing the physician; this was unusual for the office, so complaints were made. Dianna volunteered to work with Kiran to help her to schedule according to policy. She noticed that Kiran accessed the Internet and her email frequently, but that did not seem to detract from setting appointments. Kiran promised to perform according to office policy, but after 3 weeks, the problems continued. What should happen in this situation?

_____
_____
_____

Why is the scheduler such an important position in the facility?

_____
_____
_____
_____
_____

Workplace Application

Set up an interview with an office manager, and discuss the cost of running a medical practice from month to month. Discuss the biggest expenses that the physician pays each month. Report what you discover to the class.

Internet Activities

1. Find three medical suppliers on the Internet, and compare their prices for each of the following items. Use local suppliers if information is available online about their products.

Item	Suppliers	Price #1	Price #2	Price #3
1 case of 4×4 gauze pads				
1 gallon of isopropyl alcohol				
1 case of table paper				

2. Research medical office layout designs on the Internet, and design an office. Include a color scheme and floor plan. Present the design to the class using a computer presentation, poster, or handouts.

3. Research three local medical facilities on the Internet, looking for information such as company reports, financial information, company profiles, news, and current affairs. Write a report on one of the facilities to share with the class.

4. Research information on fire extinguishers, including their operation and the types for different uses. Prepare a report on the findings.

Chapter 12 Quiz

Name: _____

1. What happens to the two copies of the appointment schedule that are made each day?

   _____

   _____

   _____

2. Why must special care be taken with prescription pads?

   _____

   _____

   _____

3. What side of the hallway should be used when walking from place to place?

   _____

   _____

   _____

4. All office tasks should be detailed in either of which of the following?

   a. _____

   b. _____

5. Name two expenses to be included in office budgeting.

   a. _____

   b. _____

6. Is the product with the best price always the least expensive? Why or why not?

   _____

   _____

   _____

7. What is outsourcing?

   _____

   _____

   _____

8. The document that is inside a box shipment is called a _____.

9. What is the difference between an invoice and a statement?

   _____

   _____

   _____

10. Is email considered to be written communication?

   _____

   _____

   _____

WORK PRODUCT 12-1

Name: _____

Equipment Inventory

Complete the form below according to the instructions in Part IV.

Blackburn Primary Care
Associates, PC
1990 Turquoise Drive
Blackburn, WI 54937

Phone: 608-459-8857
Fax: 608-459-8860
E-mail:
blackburnom@blackburnpca.com
www.blackburnpca.com

BLACKBURN PRIMARY CARE ASSOCIATES, P.C.

Equipment Inventory List

Purpose:

Date:

Description	Check/P.O. #	Purchased From	Date Purchased	Serial Number	Warranty	Value
					Total	

WORK PRODUCT 12-2

Name: _____

Supply Inventory

Complete the form below page according to the instructions in Part V.

Blackburn Primary Care
Associates, PC
1990 Turquoise Drive
Blackburn, WI 54937

Phone: 608-459-8857
Fax: 608-459-8860
E-mail:
blackburnom@blackburnpca.com
www.blackburnpca.com

BLACKBURN PRIMARY CARE ASSOCIATES, P.C.

Supply Inventory List

Purpose:

Date:

Description and Item Number	Needed On Hand	Currently On Hand	Date Ordered	Price Per Unit	Total Price	Date Received

WORK PRODUCT 12-3

Name: _____

Equipment Inventory

Complete the form on the next page according to the instructions in Part VII.

EQUIPMENT INVENTORY LIST

Physical Condition

Asset or serial number	Item description (make and model)	Location	Condition	Vendor
82069279P	Laptop Computer	Dr. Lopez's Office	EXC	Toshiba

Financial Information

Years of service left	Initial value	Down payment	Date purchased or leased	Loan term in years	Loan rate	Monthly payment	Monthly operating costs	Total monthly cost
5	$1,695.00	n/a	9/15/2001	n/a	n/a	n/a	$27.00	$27.00

Maintenance Schedule

Maintenance Date	Condition of Equipment	Out of Service?	Maintenance Performed	Date in Service
9/25/2006	EXC	no	None needed	9/25/2006

Written Communications and Mail Processing

Vocabulary Review

Fill in the blanks with the correct vocabulary terms from this chapter.

1. Roberta has a(n) _____ tone in her voice when she speaks to the office staff, and this has caused friction between her and the employees.

2. Most of the mail that the Blackburn Clinic sends is classified as _____ mail, which means that it is sent within the boundaries of the United States.

3. Savannah asked Noble to _____ a memo among all of the employees.

4. Dr. Lupez suggested that the clinic sell or donate all of the _____ computer equipment once the new system arrived and was installed.

5. Jaci sometimes gets confused about subject and predicate _____ when she is writing.

6. Mrs. Abernathy reminded the students to make the margins _____ to the left when writing memorandums.

7. Dr. Lawler asked Roberta to order new stationery and specifically requested that the _____ be of a high quality.

8. All of the staff members enjoyed having Alicia as an intern because of her _____ personality with the patients.

9. The physicians considered rearranging the drug sample shelves _____ according to type of drug.

10. Dr. Hughes' _____ remark was out of character, and Suzanne was certain that he was simply stressed over a patient.

11. Ellen forgot to measure the _____ of the package before taking it to the post office to mail.

12. Jacqueline has a talent for writing _____ documents that are easy to understand.

Skills and Concepts

Part I: Correspondence and Envelopes

Label the parts of the letter in the figure below, and write in the number of lines required between each section.

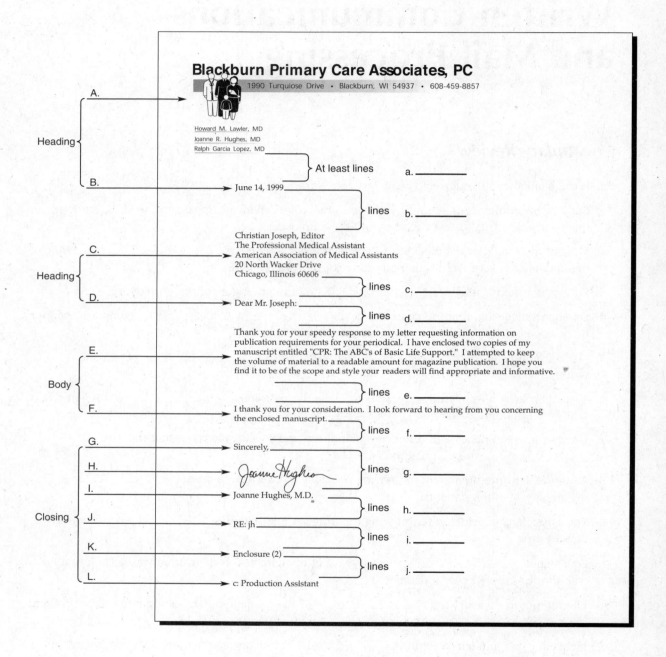

Complete Work Product 13-1 by writing the following addresses correctly according to OCR guidelines on the envelopes provided.

13. doctor john smith m.d. 301 west hughes street chicago illinois 54321

14. cindy johnson, physical therapist 1467 east green street suite 409b bayfield georgia 12345

15. jose kelley memorial lane number 321 west columbia florida 97654

Part II: Short Answer Questions

Provide short answers to the following questions.

16. What is a watermark?

_____

_____

_____

17. Why is a portfolio useful in the medical office?

_____

_____

_____

18. Explain how a ream of paper is determined.

_____

_____

_____

19. List several pieces of equipment used for written communications.

_____

_____

_____

20. List some of the supplies used for written correspondence.

_____

_____

_____

21. What is standard letter size paper?
_____

22. List the four parts of a letter.

    a. _____

    b. _____

    c. _____

    d. _____

23. Name three items that should be on a continuation page.

    a. _____

    b. _____

    c. _____

24. What is the difference between registered and certified mail?
_____
_____
_____

25. Name and briefly define the parts of speech.

    a. _____

    b. _____

    c. _____

    d. _____

    e. _____

    f. _____

    g. _____

    h. _____

26. List the four types of letter styles and the differences of each one.

    a. _____
    _____

    b. _____
    _____

    c. _____
    _____

    d. _____
    _____

27. List three things to do before answering a business letter.

a. _____

b. _____

c. _____

Part III: Letters and Memos

Using the letterhead form in Work Products 13-2 and 13-4, the memo form in Work Products 13-3 and 13-5, and the fax form in Work Product 13-6, complete the following activities. Write the documents using one of the four letter styles discussed in the chapter. If allowed by the instructor, use templates for added creativity and customization.

A. Initiate Correspondence—Complete Work Product 13-2.

Write a letter from Dr. Hughes to the President of the American Medical Association suggesting a topic for the next national convention. In the letter, indicate Dr. Hughes' interest in presenting the topic.

B. Initiate a Memo—Complete Work Product 13-3.

Write a memo to all employees, making a change in office policy. The new policy should state that the new budget for continuing education per employee will change from $300 annually to $500 annually. Be sure to set an effective date.

C. Respond to Correspondence—Complete Work Product 13-4.

Respond to an invitation to speak at a local Rotary Club meeting on the subject, "Health, Wellness, and Eating Well."

D. Respond to a Memo—Complete Work Product 13-5.

Respond to a memo from a supervisor who wants an update on the progress made toward arranging the drug sample area into categories as directed by the physician. Make certain to include an estimated date of completion of the project.

E. Initiate a Fax—Complete Work Product 13-6.

Design a coversheet for a fax message using the form in Work Product 13-6 or a template. On the coversheet, indicate that test results for a patient are attached. Be certain to address the issue of patient confidentiality.

Case Study

Read the case study and answer the questions that follow.

Barbara recently graduated as a medical assistant and obtained employment at a local physician's office. She and the office manager seemed to be at odds after Barbara redesigned several forms that had been in use at the clinic but had been copied over and over again and looked quite unprofessional. Barbara did not ask to redo the forms and was attempting to help and make a good impression. Since that incident the office manager has given Barbara two written reprimands for minor issues.

What should Barbara do?

_____

_____

_____

How could she have avoided this situation from the beginning?

_____

_____

_____

Is the office manager at fault? _____

_____

_____

_____

Workplace Applications

Collect several documents from various healthcare facilities. Compare the quality of the documents. Do they make a good first impression? Are they clearly copies that have been made over and over again? Grade the documents, and revise those that are graded below a B so that they present a positive, professional image of the facility.

Internet Activities

1. Compare the services offered by companies such as FedEx, UPS, DHL, and the USPS. Determine the lowest cost for sending an overnight letter or package.

2. Research reference books that would be valuable to the medical assistant's library. Find and compare costs, and make a list of several books that would be useful in the physician's office.

3. Go to the Microsoft Office home page and look for templates. Download several of the business templates, and customize them for the Blackburn Primary Care Associates.

Find a Word Puzzle

Find the words on the list in the following puzzle. Know the definition of each word on the list in relation to written communications and mail processing.

```
Z F C T Y L H U I X C I M C N D L I T T X J O Z Q A E M M A G Q Y L Y C L Y M Z
P D D P H I L H A L Z A W D D E W R Y V C C O X H Z L X U K D N F F Z Q B A J Q
P V K Y U N F R A Y V A T V F W G C R O G J J O T L M L D R I F C J J C R Y N B
R N H P S T J U E C E X R E M Y H P N M S S J G I L T V N O A M I I L G I T J G
E T D C O E Y Q O K Z B C X G Q B T H R Z F W O J E C O A F B I P D I N N P U W
V U C Q V R J Y K R P E B U B O I E T A N I M E S S I D R S E R B N A N Y N Y C
S A K F C N W W W E W R L V W N R R N K Y J P C A N X X O K Z S D F L A G A T Z
D H Q U N A T K R W P Z C A U B J I Y X E E T C J H H B M W X G A U V N F J A Q
H J N P C T B H Z B B B Z A R P L U C J F R H Q O H Z X E H F V S B Q X Y J W R
M P V A W I F X I K J I T O N X P T K A D G R Z N D A X M Z Y Y W G S W L Q Q K
O P E S D O O G W M D I Z N L Y S I K H L J H Y O B E V I J Z L U I G I H Y O K
J R K U P N L H Z R O D L Z N P L Z W U O L W R A T Q Q V R C Q Q A C Y B B O H
E M C J H A P U L N R M E N X P O I B U K V Y L B I A N N G U T Z H T Z E F V I
R G G Q I L B X X F I K S F Q W J L O L V J W O R H X O C E D G P P P Y L H W D
X Z X Z E G A Z B C H B M Y O I R Q F N B Z X I Z H I U J H K P Z J N M U E A P
V W S L R K A Z G P W F E F J F E K C Y B P J W M T G C F J C F A K R O E V Z J
T H K V L I Z C Q U V H H E C N U B I O L Y G I A Y S X U J W Q A P V O M Y R C
E N C L O S U R E O U Z C X I E C C X I F F Q T J D V K T Z I F Y Y Y A Z V R C
B W F U H K B V Q K D N W A T A H P M W J T U X B O L N U Z F F J T Q A W M A L
E K E I N M W V T C E L A M S C Y G V B D L L C W B C T Z I W J S I I W X B O J
E L E G F B C G I D C L E M E U T N R O A X X C T Y F M Z J R W O Q G I Z M Q N
Q B Q X U V R W N U P F S K M L A J P S T L A Y Z G Q L R Y M D E U E Y M G B N
X M W T O P C O R H M O I G O T O P E N I N G U T E T X H F D K Z R J X W Z O I
A R K M R N P S B U E B R K D W R O Z M E R X R X U U K P B W Q V A L Z X R D B
J M N V P S I S K S V O U T U B V K B F R G T U L P T V V T T G R P G I H P D J
K V Z L E Q A X G Q V K J Q F C B F D V H K B Y R R J W N F F E H A S L J D Q D
C U L R U I S Y R X V N L H F O B J I J O F E O F G B V E W M M L L Y C E X S S
X J R T N W N I V Y I W L S T Q L A C F E D O M N U H G W X V L E L T I Y G L H
H O U F W W I E P N G Z T Q T R O I J R J F S I U Q I J B F U R J X I L U F Y N
C D K U X R E P K U L K L K K P I I O G R K D E L E A I C C X E M Q O E T Z N C
A P M C N U D L R Y C R Y O G L I G L E Z A F G G A D M M Z O M A B P T X I Q N
K M H G I P Q O U I G P B F L B V R A S E Q M Y I A A A Q V E R G I Y T Z X V H
Q C D X M S Z O Z N C N C L T S J D C H B T O S S W S Y K K V E P O L E V N E F
C O M P L I M E N T A R Y N R O R B I S D S F O M O Z S F V D A E X H R R G W X
H E E B V U T H T R S L G X X T U E X V T U S W O W Y H E E R R P U E I J M M Q
I L I G D J V B X I I E M M O Z W L U L L S U N F N Q X E M O J R M X O H E R Z
H R R W I R T J R N L I A M E J P L W S G S O T E J X Z D R I X A R O S G D B V
I C A R P A G C M S E K Z C X V K Y H I B U J P I S G B G A A U H T U B B X E O
X N B F I G A T L I T F K B R I R S U V C G I D Q O U Q M C D C Q Z Q I G V L I
I P I H Q B T M V C L C J U A D C J L X F D W O R S R V X Y G L L T A U K V X D
```

Body	Enclosure	Memorandum
Categorically	Envelope	Messages
Complimentary	Girth	Opening
Continuation	Heading	Portfolio
Correspondence	International	Postscripts
Disseminate	Intrinsic	Proofread
Domestic	Letter	Salutation
Email	Margin	ZIP code

Chapter 13 Quiz

Name: _____

1. A durable formal paper used for office documents is called _____.

2. COD stands for _____ _____.

3. _____ mail is sent outside of U.S. borders.

4. Good _____ is essential to writing effective, professional business documents.

5. A(n) _____ of paper usually contains 500 sheets.

6. A(n) _____ is a marking in a paper that is visible when held up to the light.

7. The process of making notes of explanation is called _____.

8. Second and subsequent pages of a document are called _____ pages.

9. _____ provide high-resolution images of text and photos.

10. On standard letterhead, side margins are usually between _____ and _____ inches.

WORK PRODUCT 13-1

Name: _____

Addressing an Envelope

Complete the envelopes below according to the directions in Part I, Questions 13-15.

Blackburn Primary Care Associates, P.C.
1990 Turquoise Drive
Blackburn, WI 54937

Blackburn Primary Care Associates, P.C.
1990 Turquoise Drive
Blackburn, WI 54937

Blackburn Primary Care Associates, P.C.
1990 Turquoise Drive
Blackburn, WI 54937

WORK PRODUCT 13-2

Name: _____

Initiate Correspondence

Using the form below, write a letter according to the directions in Part III, Question A.

Blackburn Primary Care Associates
1990 Turquoise Drive
Blackburn, WI 54937
(555) 555-1234

WORK PRODUCT 13-3

Name: _____

Initiate a Memo

Using the form below, write a memo according to the directions in Part III, Question B.

MEMORANDUM

Date:

To:

From:

Subject:

- -

WORK PRODUCT 13-4

Name: _____

Respond to Correspondence

Using the form below, write a letter according to the directions in Part III, Question C.

Blackburn Primary Care Associates
1990 Turquoise Drive
Blackburn, WI 54937
(555) 555-1234

WORK PRODUCT 13-5

Name: _____

Respond to a Memo

Using the form below, write a memo according to the directions in Part III, Question D.

MEMORANDUM

Date:

To:

From:

Subject:

WORK PRODUCT 13-6

Initiate a Fax

Design a coversheet for a fax message using the form below according to the directions in Part III, Question E.

Blackburn Primary Care Associates
1990 Turquoise Drive
Blackburn, WI 54937
(555) 555-1234

CHAPTER **14**

Medical Records Management

Vocabulary Review

Fill in the blank with the correct vocabulary term from this chapter.

1. Veronica prefers a(n) _____ filing system, in which combinations of letters and numbers are used to identify a file.

2. Julia prefers a(n) _____ filing system, in which the letters of the alphabet are used to identify a file.

3. Paula Ann feels that only a(n) _____ filing system provides patient confidentiality.

4. Dr. Banford uses a _____ file to help him remember that a certain action must be taken on a certain date.

5. Teresa wants to _____ the current software library with programs for making brochures and designing websites.

6. The clinic physician records _____ information when questioning patients about their illness.

7. The clinic physician records _____ information when examining the patient.

8. When Mira files documents into medical records, she lays one report on top of another, with the most recent on top; this filing method is called _____.

9. The office manager is particular about the _____ under which documents are filed, because she wants to be able to access information quickly.

10. Dr. Lawler scheduled an appointment with his accountant to discuss the _____ of the office financial records.

11. Georgina avoids _____ by taking care of issues and documents as they are presented to her, rather than setting them aside for later.

12. Naomi has a _____ interest in the success of the new hospital, because she owns shares in its stock.

13. The medical assistant must never remove entries in a patient's record by _____.

14. Dr. Lupez's _____ _____ was irritable bowel syndrome, not colon cancer.

15. Jose read the memo about the new medical records _____ schedule with interest, because his job includes filing.

Skills and Concepts

Part I: Filing Medical Records

Place the following names in the correct order for filing in the right column.

Cassidy Kay Hale

Candace Cassidy LeGrand

Taylor Ann Jackson

Anton Douglas Conn

Beau Mitchell Gilbreath

Lorienda Gaye Robison

LaNelle Elva Crumley

Allison Gaile Yarbrough

Sarah Kay Haile

Marie Gracelia Stuart

Karry Madge Chapmann

Randi Ann Perez

Cecelia Gayle Raglan

Sarah Sue Ragland

Riley Americus Belk

Starr Ellen Beall

Charles Thomas Brown

George Scott Turner

Winston Roger Murchison

Sara Suzelle Montgomery

Tamika Noelle Frazier

Alisa Jordan Williams

Alisha Dawn Chapman

Bentley James Adams

Montana Skye Kizer

Dakota Marie LaRose

Robbie Sue Metzger

Thomas Charles Bruin

Butch John Adams

Carlos Perez Santos

Part II: Subjective and Objective Information

Note whether the following information is usually subjective or objective.

16. Patient address _____

17. Yellowed eyes _____

18. Patient email address _____

19. Insurance information _____

20. Elevated blood pressure _____

21. Bloated stomach _____

22. Complaint of headache _____

23. Weight of 143 lb _____

24. Bruises on upper arms _____

25. Patient phone number _____

Part III: Short Answer Questions

26. List four reasons that medical records exist.

    a. _____

    b. _____

    c. _____

    d. _____

27. Explain the concept of the ownership of medical records.

    _____

    _____

    _____

28. Why might color-coded files be more efficient than an alphabetic filing system?

    _____

    _____

    _____

29. What are the two major types of patient records found in a medical office?

    a. _____

    b. _____

30. What type of form should be completed if a patient no longer wishes to allow his or her medical records to be released to a person or organization?

    _____

Part IV: Releasing Medical Records

Complete an Authorization to Release Medical Records form using your name as the patient.

```
┌─────────────────────────────────────────────────────────────────┐
│                   RECORDS RELEASE AUTHORIZATION                   │
│                                                                   │
│  TO _____  │
│                         Doctor or Hospital                        │
│                                                                   │
│     _____  │
│                            Address                                │
│  I HEREBY AUTHORIZE AND REQUEST YOU TO RELEASE TO:                │
│                                                                   │
│                                                                   │
│                                                                   │
│  ALL RECORDS IN YOUR POSSESION CONCERNING _____ │
│                                                                   │
│  _____ILLNESS AND/OR   │
│                                                                   │
│  TREATMENT DURING THE PERIOD FROM _____TO _____.  │
│  NAME _____TEL. _____  │
│  ADDRESS_____   │
│  SIGNATURE _____DATE_____   │
│                    (If relative, state relationship)              │
│  WITNESS_____DATE_____  │
│           25-8104 © 1973 BIBBERO SYSTEMS, INC., PETALUMA,, CA.    │
└─────────────────────────────────────────────────────────────────┘
```

Part V: Changing or Correcting Medical Records

Correct the following medical record entries as noted as would be done in a medical chart. Then rewrite the entry correctly on the line provided.

31. The correct date of the appointment below was October 12, 20XX.

    10-21-20XX Patient did not arrive for scheduled appointment. *P. Smith, RMA*

    _____

32. The patient stated that the chest pain began 2 weeks ago.

    1-31-20XX   Patient complained of chest pain for the last 2 months. No pain noted in arms. No nausea. Desires ECG and blood work to check for heart problems. *R. Smithee, CMA*

    _____

    _____

    _____

33. The correct date for the last refill was 3-20-20XX.

   4-22-20XX   Patient requested that Rx for Vicodin be refilled. Last refill was 4-20-20XX.
   Dr. Lawton refused refill and requested patient schedule follow-up appointment. *S. Ragland, RMA*

   _____

   _____

   _____

   What additional follow-up might be needed in this situation?

   _____

   _____

   _____

34. A. Directions: Examine the file folder below. What information is available on the folder? What is the major advantage of this filing system?

   _____

   _____

   _____

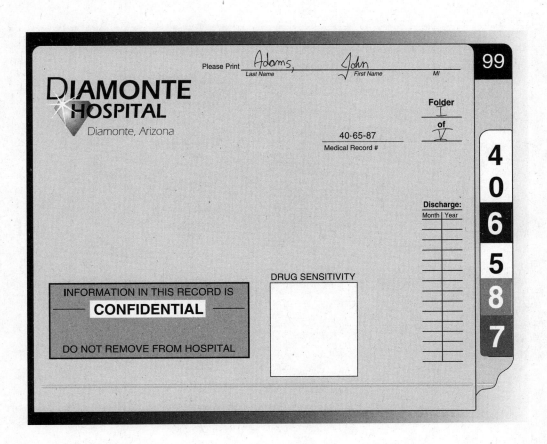

B. Directions: Label each type of filing system. What are some of the advantages and disadvantages?

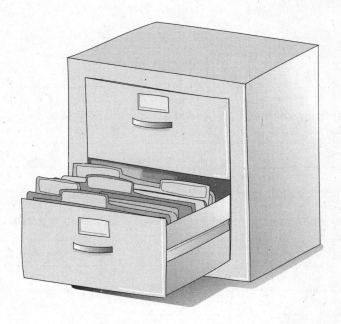

a. Type of system: _____

_____

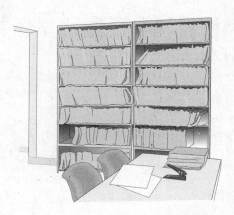

b. Type of system: _____

_____

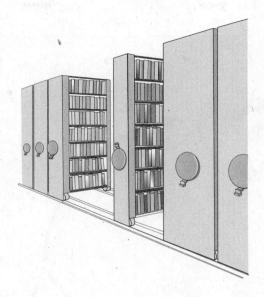

c. Type of system: _____

_____

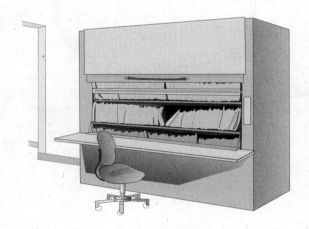

d. Type of system: _____

_____

35. A. Research various information storage systems. Describe the information storage systems shown in the following figures.

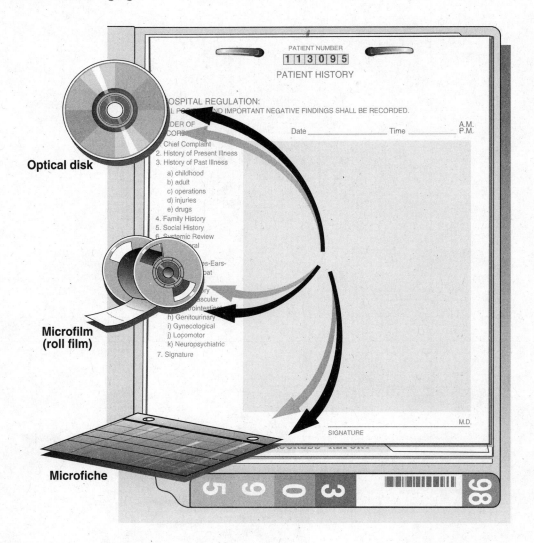

Optical disk

Microfilm (roll film)

Microfiche

Disk: _____

_____

_____

_____

Microfilm: _____

_____

_____

_____

Microfiche: _____

_____

_____

_____

B. Identify the item in the picture below. What are the advantages of using this item?

_____

_____

_____

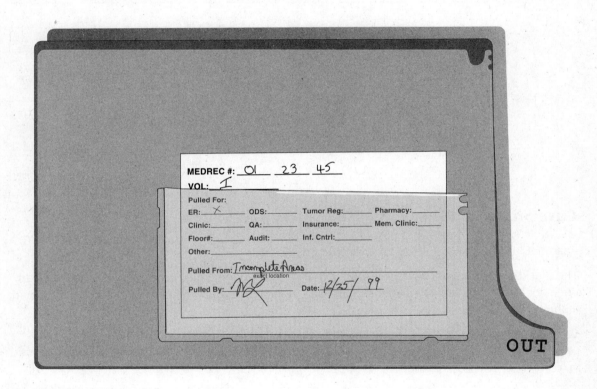

Part VI: Filing Procedures

36. List and explain the five basic filing steps.

a. _____

_____

_____

b. _____

_____

_____

c. _____

_____

_____

d. _____

_____

_____

e. _____

_____

_____

Case Study

Read the information below and answer the questions.

The Blackburn Clinic is considering the purchase of new filing equipment. They currently use an open-shelf method, with the patient's names in alphabetic order. They would like to change to an alphanumeric system.

What must they consider before making this change?

_____

_____

_____

How would the office implement this change so that it causes the least disruption to the patients and staff?

_____

_____

_____

Workplace Applications

Visit three medical offices and determine the type of filing system that each uses. Ask the receptionist what pros and cons exist for each filing system you encounter. Share this information with the class.

Internet Activities

1. Research filing systems on the Internet, and determine which system you would choose for a medical office. Cite three reasons for your choice.

2. Look for special color-coding systems on the Internet. How might these be used in a physician's office?

3. Look for filing tips on the Internet. See what helpful hints will assist you in filing faster and more efficiently in the medical office.

Chapter 14 Quiz

Name: _____

1. List three classifications of files.

   a. _____

   b. _____

   c. _____

2. The files of patients who are currently receiving treatment are called _____ files.

3. Arranging papers in filing sequence is called

   _____ .

   _____ .

   _____ .

4. Hyphenated elements of a name are treated as two separate units.

   a. True

   b. False

5. Numeric filing systems can be expanded without relocating all of the other files.

   a. True

   b. False

6. Who owns the patient's medical record?

   _____

   _____

   _____

7. When no restriction exists in a state for records retention, it is best to keep the records for _____ years.

8. Wall files offer less privacy and security than other systems.

   a. True

   b. False

9. POMR stands for _____

   _____

   _____

10. CBMR stands for _____

    _____

    _____

CHAPTER 15

Health Information Management

Vocabulary Review

Fill in the blanks with the correct vocabulary terms from this chapter.

1. Dr. Charles received a memo from Smith-Park Hospital that reminded him to _____ several of the medical records.

2. Janie records any _____ _____ that happens to a patient while he or she is in the hospital.

3. Chris asked if there was a way to _____ outgoing email messages so that they could not be altered before reaching their destination.

4. Anne knows that medical facilities must meet certain _____ to maintain accreditation.

5. After reviewing several hundred files, Alex was concerned about the _____ information in several patient records.

6. Bette reminded Joan to be careful not to _____ numbers or letters when entering information into the computer.

7. The _____ _____ office in a healthcare facility is concerned with providing the best and most efficient care possible to the patients.

8. Dr. Hughes knew that penicillin was a(n) _____ for Kathleen Schultz, so he ordered a different antibiotic.

9. Several _____ exist in the new user manual, and they must be corrected.

10. The medical assistant should never attempt to _____ the regulations that apply to medical records.

Skills and Concepts

Part I: Short Answer Questions

Answer the following questions briefly.

11. Define health information management in lay terms.

_____

_____

_____

12. List five ways in which healthcare data are used.

a. _____

b. _____

c. _____

d. _____

e. _____

13. Explain what is meant by the underuse of medical services.

_____

_____

_____

14. Explain what is meant by the overuse of medical services.

_____

_____

_____

15. List five of the statistics that are collected by NCHS.

a. _____

b. _____

c. _____

d. _____

e. _____

Part II: Characteristics of High-Quality Health Data

Determine which of the nine characteristics of high-quality health data is involved in the following scenarios. Use each quality only one time, and choose the one that best represents the facts contained in the scenario.

16. Janeen is concerned because the computer system did not upload the entries made during the previous day.

    _____

17. Suzanne found a notation inside the medical record that a patient was allergic to sulfa drugs, but she noticed that the sticker on the outside of the record was marked NKA.

    _____

18. Sabrina brought a chart to the physician's attention in which he had written to prescribe 200 mg of Imitrex to a patient. Sabrina had heard the physician tell the patient that he was prescribing 100 mg. The physician corrected the error before writing the prescription.

    _____

19. Steven was unfamiliar with an abbreviation used in the medical record. He asked the office manager about the abbreviation, and she explained its use in the physician's office. In previous facilities, Steve had seen the same abbreviation used a different way.

    _____

20. After an employee was terminated, Chris changed applicable passwords so that the individual could no longer access the system.

    _____

21. Patricia researched the HIPAA website to make certain she understood a portion of the privacy law.

    _____

22. The new patient database allows several staff members to access data at one time.

    _____

23. Joshua was reprimanded for not filing laboratory reports on a daily basis and allowing the documents to stack up over several days.

    _____

24. Dr. Adams realized that some information entered into the patient database was not being used for treatment purposes, so he sent a memo to the staff and confirmed that the information no longer needed to be collected.

    _____

Part III: Incident Reports

A medical assistant gives an injection of penicillin to a patient who reported an allergy to amoxicillin. The patient complains of itching and experiences shortness of breath and wheezing while sitting in the treatment room. The patient collapses to the floor and stops breathing. Cardiopulmonary resuscitation (CPR) is initiated, and an ambulance is called. The patient is transported on life support to the local emergency department. The patient dies 12 hours later. Complete an incident report for this sentinel event.

Incident Report
Do Not File in Medical Records

Confidential and privileged health care quality improvement information prepared in anticipation of litigation

Name: _____   Employee ☐ Patient ☐ Visitor ☐

Facility name: _____

Attending physician: _____
MR # _____ SS # _____
D.O.B. ___/___/___   Sex: M[ ] F[ ]
Admission date: ___/___/___
Primary diagnosis: _____
_____

Site (if applicable) _____
City _____
Facility ID# _____
State _____
Phone # _____

SECTION I: General Information

General Identification (circle one):
001 Inpatient
002 Outpatient
003 Nonpatient
004 Equipment only

Location (circle one):
005 Bathroom/toilet
006 Beauty shop
007 Cafeteria/dining room
008 Corridor/hall
009 During transport
010 Emergency department
011 Exterior grounds
012 ICU/SCU/CCU
013 Labor/delivery/birthing
014 Nursery
015 Outpatient clinic
016 Patient room
017 Radiology
018 Recovery room
019 Recreation area
020 Rehab
021 Shower room
022 Surgical suite
023 Treatment/exam room

Treatment Rendered (circle one):
024 Emergency room
025 First aid
026 None
026 Transfer to other facility
027 X-ray

SECTION II: Nature of Incident (Circle all that apply):

001 Adverse outcome after surgery or anesthetic
002 Anaphylactic shock
003 Anoxic event
004 Apgar score of 5 or less
005 Aspiration
006 Assault or altercation/combative event
007 Blood or IV variance
008 Blood/body fluid exposure
009 Code/arrest
010 Damage/loss of organ
011 Death
012 Dental-related complication
013 Dissatisfaction/noncompliance*
014 Equipment operation*
015 Fall with injury*
016 Fall without injury*
017 Handling of and/or exposure to hazardous waste
018 Informed consent issue
019 Injury to other
020 Injury to self
021 Loss of limb
022 Loss of vision
023 Medication variance*
024 Needle puncture/sharp injury
025 Paralysis
026 Patient-to-patient altercation
027 Perinatal complication*
028 Poisoning
029 Suspected nonstaff-to-patient abuse
030 Suspected staff-to-patient abuse
031 Thermal burn
032 Treatment/procedure issue
033 Ulcer: nosocomial stage III/IV

* Complete appropriate area in Section III

SECTION III: Type of Incident

If death, circle all that apply:
001 After medical equipment failure
002 After power equipment failure or damage
003 During surgery or postanesthesia
004 Within 24 hours of admission to facility
005 Within 1 week of fall in facility
006 Within 24 hours of medication error

Blood/IV Variance Issues (circle all that apply):
007 Additive
008 Administration consent
009 Contraindications/allergies
010 Equipment malfunction
011 Infusion rate
012 Labeling issue
013 Reaction
014 Solution/blood type
015 Transcription
016 Patient identification
017 Allergic/adverse reaction
018 Infiltration
019 Phlebitis

Dissatisfaction/Noncompliance (circle all that apply):
020 AMA
021 Elopement
022 Irate or angry (either family or patient)
023 Left without service
024 Noncompliant patient
025 Refused prescribed treatment

Falls (circle all that apply):*
001 Assisted fall
002 Found on floor
003 From bed
004 From chair
005 From commode/toilet
006 From exam table
007 From stretcher
008 From wheelchair
009 Patient states—unwitnessed
010 Unassisted fall
011 While ambulating
012 Witnessed fall

* For any marks in this field, Section V must be completed

Medication Variance Issues (circle all that apply):
013 Contraindication/allergies
014 Delay in dispensing
015 Incorrect dose
016 Expired drug
017 Medication identification
018 Narcotic log variance
019 Not ordered
020 Ordered, not given
021 Patient identification
022 Reaction
023 Route
024 Rx incorrectly dispensed
025 Time of dose
026 Transcription

Part IV: Confidentiality Statement

Evaluate the confidentiality statement for Diamonte Hospital below. Revise the statement to make it appropriate for a medical practice setting. Use proofreader marks to indicate your proposed changes on the confidentiality statement. Rewrite the completed, revised statement on the letterhead form on the next page.

DIAMONTE HOSPITAL

Diamonte, Arizona 89104 • TEL. 602-484-9991

CONFIDENTIALITY STATEMENT

I, _____ , understand that in the course of my activities/business at or for Diamonte Hospital, I am required to have access to and am involved in the viewing, reviewing, and/or processing of patient care data and/or health information.

I understand that I am obligated by State Law, Federal Law, and Diamonte Hospital to maintain the confidentiality of these data and information at all times.

I understand that a violation of these confidentiality considerations may result in punitive legal action against me.

I certify by my signature below that this Confidentiality Statement has been explained to me, and I agree to the principles contained herein as a condition of my activity/business at or for Diamonte Hospital.

_____
Signature/date

_____
Witness/date

Blackburn Primary Care Associates
1990 Turquoise Drive
Blackburn, WI 54937
(555) 555-1234

Case Study

Read the case study and answer the questions that follow.

Alberto discovered that three people accessed the medical records of one of the local professional football team's players, who had been brought to the physician's office to follow up on injuries sustained in a car accident. He realizes that the information accessed was the results of the player's blood alcohol level.

What should Alberto do?

_____

_____

_____

What type of penalty is appropriate for those who accessed the information, if any?

_____

_____

_____

Workplace Applications

Determine how total quality management ideas can be worked into a physician's office mission statement. Write a mission statement that stresses quality management. How does quality management affect patients in a medical office?

Internet Activities

1. Explore the NCHS website. Investigate one of the issues in the Vital Statistics area. Use information found there to write a report about any area of interest, and present it to the class.

2. Explore the JCAHO website. Peruse the sections of the site that refer to standards, patient safety, and sentinel events. Choose a fact, and write a brief report.

3. Research total quality management on the Internet, and write a two-page report on how quality management can improve efficiency in a physician's office.

Chapter 15 Quiz

Name: _____

1. The organization that promotes the field of health information management is

   _____ .

2. TQM stands for _____

   _____ .

3. What is JCAHO?

   _____

4. What is the NCHS?

   _____

5. What is a sentinel event?

   _____

   _____

   _____

6. What does HIPAA stand for?

   _____

7. Define risk management.

   _____

   _____

   _____

8. If information is available in a medical record when it is needed, it is said to be

   _____

9. Why are third-party payors interested in the information contained in the medical record?

   _____

   _____

   _____

10. The signature of the maker that indicates a medical record is accurate is called

   _____

CHAPTER 16

Privacy in the Physician's Office

Vocabulary Review

Fill in the blanks with the correct vocabulary terms from this chapter.

1. Dr. Lawton is considered a healthcare _____ because he provides services and treatments to patients.

2. The _____ against Dr. Rosales was one of his former patients, Risa Jackson, who felt his staff had violated her privacy.

3. Byron knows that he is not allowed to _____ any information about a patient without a release from the patient for that information.

4. Sarah could _____ from what the patient said that he was nervous about his upcoming surgery.

5. STAT Medical Billing provides services to the Blackburn Clinic, so they are considered to be a(n) _____ _____.

6. Julia has difficulty understanding the _____ in which many federal documents and regulations are written.

7. Janease knew that she could _____ two employees from guilt because they were both at lunch when the incident happened.

8. The _____ on the privacy statement was hard for a layperson to understand, so Annette decided to rewrite the document.

9. Roberta was assigned to be the temporary _____ _____ at the clinic while Maritza was on maternity leave.

10. The Office of _____ _____ investigates breaches of laws that pertain to HHS.

11. The Office of _____ _____ enforces privacy standards.

12. Dr. Hughes had to prove _____ _____ in that he made every attempt to notify the patient before mailing test results to her home.

13. The _____ _____ _____ _____ in a patient's record is private and must not be shared without a release from the patient.

14. Health information that is transmitted in electronic form is called _____ _____ _____.

15. The patient's information that pertains to his or her health is called _____ _____ _____.

Skills and Concepts

Part I: Health Insurance Portability and Accountability Act

Provide brief answers to the following questions.

16. List six benefits provided by the HIPAA Privacy Rule to patients and/or providers.

    a. _____

    b. _____

    c. _____

    d. _____

    e. _____

    f. _____

17. Briefly explain the Title I provision of HIPAA.

    _____

    _____

18. Briefly explain the Title II provision of HIPAA.

    _____

    _____

19. List six rights that HIPAA gives to patients.

    a. _____

    b. _____

    c. _____

    d. _____

    e. _____

    f. _____

20. List six items of information that a Notice of Privacy Policies must include the following.

    a. _____

    b. _____

    c. _____

    d. _____

    e. _____

    f. _____

Part II: Patient Rights under HIPAA

Determine which right under HIPAA applies to each of the following scenarios. Use each right only once.

21. Susan Enlow discovered that her date of birth was incorrect when she requested her medical records from the Blackburn Clinic. She was moving to another city and wished to take the records with her to her new provider. Susan surmised that the error might have been the reason that her insurance company rejected several claims. She contacted the Blackburn Clinic in writing and asked them to correct the error and to then determine if any claims were outstanding that might need to be resubmitted to her insurance carrier.

    Right to _____

22. Keiran requested that the clinic send a copy of his most recent physical examination and laboratory results to Dr. Ballard, who was seeing him about a long-standing problem with his knees.

    Right to _____

23. Louie requested that all communication from the physician's office be sent to his office address, because he was in the midst of a tense divorce.

    Right to _____

24. The Blackburn Clinic gives a copy of its Notice of Privacy Policy to all patients and makes certain that a signature is obtained or a note is attached to prove that the policy was offered to the patients.

    Right to _____

25. A few days after seeing Dr. Reynolds, Rita received an email from a company that offered multivitamins. Dr. Reynolds had suggested that she begin taking multivitamins and mentioned that a friend sold a vitamin drink that she might be interested in trying. Rita did not give permission for release of her email address at the visit. She called the clinic and asked if her email address had been distributed to anyone outside the clinic.

    Right to _____

26. Suyen made a written request to the Blackburn Clinic that no information regarding her treatment for drug dependency be released to anyone without her specific, written permission.

    Right to _____

Part III: Incidental Disclosures

Determine which of the following situations could be classified as an incidental disclosure.

Situation	Incidental Disclosure	
	Yes	No
27. Ms. Allen, a patient waiting in the x-ray department of a large clinic, overhears Dr. Smith mention that another patient has been diagnosed with testicular cancer, but she does not hear a patient's name during the discussion.		
28. Bob Mitchell, a patient at Mercy Hospital, overhears a physician telling his roommate that he needs surgery for carpal tunnel syndrome.		
29. As Zaria passes the nurses' station at a local hospital, she hears the nurses talking about the patient in room 2114. They mention that he has been diagnosed with terminal cancer. Zaria knows the patient's family and hears that the diagnosis has not been given to them yet.		
30. Paula Stanley signs in at the front desk of the medical clinic and notices that her college professor signed in to see the physician 30 minutes ago.		

Part IV: Notice of Privacy Practices

Read the Notice of Privacy Practices in Figure 16-2 of the textbook. Based on the information in that policy, answer the following questions.

31. Can the patient obtain a copy of his or her medical record?

❏ Yes   ❏ No

32. Can the patient request that certain information in his or her medical record not be released to certain persons or organizations?

❏ Yes   ❏ No

33. Can the patient have a copy of the Notice of Privacy Practices?

❏ Yes   ❏ No

34. Can the clinic use the information in the patient's medical record to compile statistics about certain diseases treated by the practice without additional permission from the patient?

❏ Yes   ❏ No

35. Does the clinic have to honor all requests from the patient regarding the release of his or her protected health information?

❏ Yes   ❏ No

Part V: Privacy in the Physician's Office

Find the words on the list in the puzzle.

```
P R O V I D E R V E G H E Y T Y G O C O T V G P S P N O F J F R L N O I L D K C
L D I S Q A T Q R S P N Z T Z M B X W A E D B R R D I X Y B R U U E E N Y O K T
Z L A T N E D I C N I L N I O H L C I R U T B O D O H F K S Y T D G G T O H Y F
X L E N V C H L R I A S E T U Z S L B Q Z M T C S T M P C F N S I Y U A R H O U
K C J X P E L C F I F A P N F V L I K P Q E L Q R H E O O E A H O W J M L L Y C
V E W J B L D G T I P B L E K Z A Y N B C S B P C B W U M R Y T Z V N C T E K N
A O K J C N G N C R N W P Z I G H W D T D S M M T N G E G L U V I D D N Q B S L
J W A S Q G E T O D R I C N E D B U E G I E V F E B L Q W G Y S P D B G N Z Z E
K T R D M D T V C V R S Y C N J N D E G S W Y U P P D A K R H M L P Z M H O R T
T V B G I A I Q O V T R X Q U H H E A V C D X Q M R K V Y S R E Q Q I B N Q K X
O X W F W S P L J K C Y H R J E E C W I L N M I P A R P D K A K Z B S Q W D K X
E X N M I Y P N J F C I D K A E F N G Y O G F S P L J J R K Y L G Q V L O W A H
W O V O Y U K M D O O B M L J O A A G Q S I H A X G M O A V B D P J V W O F S N
C A N V T H O T R F N T A T M O R P E U E U J V G P C P S I V U B S J A B Z I
F S N S W T I U M J E H W I S U K U T K R U M W I J V S L L J E Y I V L O R S B
W O A F J H D L U S I C R Z I F T S X W E O X X R F D F G F D C H T L M M Y X F
H S I B K P G T I N N A W M S N W C S W B A C S B T C O P N H E K Y A A Y E
Q K K H J K E C F B R L I W Z C X I S U Q R T B B A Z Q M G X E P Z Y Q H W O M
Z L F M N P V O W Y A R L P G M C R G C X S Y Z P S Z S Y H P G K W U H T M C M
K K F R C N R Q O P V T I S Q P Q B Z T Y H A K S U K A Y J A I E Q W E I S I A
Y F Z B J M U Q L O J P N I Q E P N V R B L I S O H C P H H L L Y X K V W G G S
F C M U A N S J I Q J R A U Z N B N U I Z Y E B E M Q K D Q K L S Q J U X F H E
T R A T N Y W V N P F F K A O W P L S M X G G J Y D T X U Y X I P Z R T Z C T O
W R I V U A F W H L K F W B N C Z I I X N W N H Y D M N M E M D W I X S D X F U
F O A B I R A Y F X C Z M B C Y C W N C U D N A P X T V E W N E U H B K Y R M M
N X I N E R H C I L W W C O M P L A I N A N T Y I K Z O S L S U V S L J R E J W
Q C K F S K P A C P X R D N Q C C D F D Z X G K E K R U L P A D J D O D G D Q W
P S N I S A K H R T J P V N P N H P F L H K Q R I K M A F H K V V D P P H P A O
C I R F E T C F J Q A Z P Q K C U L V G J Z O F C Z D B H S O D E A S A R R B Z
K J N D O L D T E H U M E F K W M D E A Y L T H L B S C X D F N F R V M C E Q E
V E J M X D G V I C B B U H S T K U M X P L B T N G V D O Y W X Y A P B J C M V
O H T F H W Y Z Y O B Z C D G R S Q X F E T A I C O S S A S S E N I S U B L Q H
W C E P M X X B I V N A N Z Z P V B G Q O P H P N Q W X R B G I E O Z P B U C B
L K L A V U Z N G X U D Q I Y I X G S L X V P E T J U O A J M N K V Q R Y D M A
V F F K A V R P F S T C X J C J L A N I Z D A J R E A K N U V X M Z K J V E R D
W S K F C X O A F Y E W S P C W N C D F I J P P J T Y Y F R B J Z W I F P M E V
Q B V Z Z V K Y E H D R R D V F N F R N I Y H H G W A F M J H M W X N I X I C F
P J Q U G M O P R Z R M M J K V V Z P L D X V G Q T H F U E N C N F A V C V Q
C G M G M O L X I Y U T I L B T A L A F U X R U Y X J S E O Q F A D R G B F K J
R J Y C W A V G L M Y P I G P Z L Q Q I C Q B I U V S W A Y J E I G Z B W M E E
```

Accountability	Insurance
Business associate	Legalese
Complainant	Preclude
Confidential	Prevalent
Disclosures	Privacy
Divulge	Protected health information
Due diligence	Provider
Entity	Provisions
Implement	Transaction
Incidental	Verbiage
Infer	

Case Study

Read the case study and answer the questions that follow.

Morgan was given a copy of the Privacy Law and told to write the Notice of Privacy Practices for their clinic. After she began reading the law, she became somewhat discouraged because of the legalese and the slow pace at which she had to read to make certain that she comprehended the message and requirements. She decided to attend a private training seminar on HIPAA compliance and found the instructor to be very knowledgeable.

How can such seminars be beneficial to the practice?

_____

_____

_____

How can the medical assistant determine if a seminar is worth attending?

_____

_____

_____

Research seminars in your area, and request information about them. Compare data with the information collected by the rest of the class.

Workplace Application

Determine what certifications are available that relate to HIPAA. What are the requirements for obtaining these special certifications? Why might these be beneficial for the medical assistant? Is there a particular certification you are interested in obtaining?

Internet Activities

1. Research the HIPAA website, and find information about complaints. Then write an office policy for patients that details how to make a complaint if the patient feels that his or her privacy has been violated.

2. Find the exact Public Law number that details the Health Insurance Portability and Accountability Act.

3. Research and write a report on HIPAA's Security Standard.

4. Find five additional links other than the HIPAA website that provide useful information on HIPAA compliance.

5. Determine misleading marketing ploys that are sometimes used in promoting HIPAA training.

6. Research programs that provide a specialized certificate in HIPAA proficiency.

Chapter 16 Quiz

Name: _____

1. Explain due diligence.

   _____

   _____

   _____

2. What does HIPAA stand for?

   _____

   _____

3. Explain the definition of individually identifiable health information.

   _____

   _____

4. On what date did HIPAA become effective?

   _____

5. Can sign-in sheets be HIPAA-compliant?

   _____

6. Is a Notice of Privacy Practices required during emergency treatment?

   _____

7. What agency hears complaints about breach of privacy policies?

   _____

8. If a patient sees another patient name when signing in, is this a breach of confidentiality or an incidental exposure?

   _____

9. What is a complainant?

   _____

10. What is a covered entity?

   _____

Basics of Diagnostic Coding

Vocabulary Review

Fill in the blanks with the correct vocabulary terms from this chapter.

1. Dr. Jurkoshek listed the _____, or the cause of the disorder, on the medical record.

2. _____ terms are always written in italics in the ICD-9 manual and may apply to a chapter, a section, a category, or a subcategory.

3. The initial identification of the condition or complaint that Perry Flowers expressed at the outpatient clinic is considered to be his _____ _____.

4. Julie noticed that the coding manual gave directions to look in another place. The notation she read was _____.

5. Angela knows that the word _____ can be interpreted as "and" or "or" in the ICD-9 manual.

6. Minnie enjoys _____, which is converting verbal or written descriptions into numeric and alphanumeric designations.

7. The signs and symptoms of a disease are its _____.

8. Alex noted that the coding manual listed a direction to see a specific category and knows that this direction must be followed when coding. That direction is _____ _____.

9. Services that support patient diagnoses are called _____ _____ _____.

10. Services that support patient treatment are called _____ _____ _____.

Coding Exercises

Code the following diagnoses to the highest level of specificity.

11. The Smith's newborn has a birthmark on his neck.

_____

12. Mr. Epstein suffers from Bruck's disease.

_____

13. Jenny developed bronchitis over spring break after inhaling gas fumes while sitting in a traffic jam.

_____

14. Carolyn has experienced dumping syndrome periodically since her gastric bypass surgery.

_____

15. Robert has experienced pain when he urinates for the past 3 weeks.

_____

16. Julia has been nauseated for about a week but has not complained of vomiting.

_____

17. Paul has trench foot, which is a condition of moist gangrene caused by freezing of wet skin.

_____

18. Benjamin was given a health examination the night he entered prison to serve a life sentence.

_____

19. Angela was classified as morbidly obese, so she qualified for gastric bypass surgery.

_____

20. Joseph was diagnosed with academic underachievement disorder and sent for counseling.

_____

21. Morgan Smith had an acute myocardial infarction, commonly referred to as a heart attack.

_____

22. Jessica was placed in the neonatal ICU because she was diagnosed with transient tachypnea at birth.

_____

23. Terri constantly struggles with her maxillary sinus, especially in the winter.

_____

24. The physician told Roger that he had epididymitis but it was not a result of a venereal disease.

_____

25. Judy has experienced neck pain for 1 week, but she does not know why the pain began.

_____

26. Kevin has suffered from low back pain for years.

27. Brad was bitten by a brown recluse spider.

28. The Abbotts' child died of sudden infant death syndrome.

29. Mitral stenosis was Mrs. Richland's final diagnosis.

30. Georgia went into anaphylactic shock after drinking milk.

31. Joey was taken to a psychologist because he was having recurrent nightmares.

32. Roger has benign essential hypertension.

33. Susan was having trouble breathing, and her physician told her that she had a nasopharyngeal polyp that needed to be removed.

34. Kristy's son, Christian, suffers with croup syndrome and has been hospitalized three times because of the disorder.

35. Ron saw Dr. Jarrett because of an anal fissure, which resulted from a nontraumatic tear of his anus.

36. Griffin saw Dr. Redford for treatment of a common head cold.

37. A tetanus toxoid vaccination was administered to a child who stepped on a rusty nail.

38. Mrs. Garrett developed a decubitus ulcer on her buttocks while she was a patient in a nursing home.

39. Paige has a migraine headache, and the physician did not mention intractable migraine in the medical record.

_____

40. Pat has Graves' disease, and the physician did not mention thyrotoxic crisis or storm on the medical record.

_____

41. Mary is in rehabilitation for episodic cocaine dependence.

_____

42. Jonathan has been diagnosed with attention deficit disorder, without mention of hyperactivity.

_____

43. Angelica has had chronic cystic mastitis for years.

_____

44. Mr. Robertson had a TIA at home and was rushed to the hospital.

_____

45. Ray noticed a ringing in his ears after working for 6 months on a construction site.

_____

46. Raul has been diagnosed with iron-deficient anemia because he is not getting enough iron in his diet.

_____

47. Camille has had recurrent earaches in the 2 years since her birth, and the physician diagnosed chronic purulent otitis media.

_____

48. Sally's newborn was diagnosed with pyloric stenosis and required surgery.

_____

49. Stephanie has a urinary tract infection, but the physician does not yet know what organism caused the illness.

_____

50. Don has insomnia, which the physician thinks is a result of drug abuse.

_____

51. Mabel Johnson has rheumatoid arthritis and takes daily medication to control the pain.

_____

52. Cynthia has a plantar wart but does not want to have it removed yet.

_____

53. Sebastian fractured his clavicle at the sternal end during a football game. The fracture was closed.

_____

54. Peggy contracted herpes simplex with herpetic vulvovaginitis.

_____

55. Eric noticed blood in his semen, and the physician diagnosed hematospermia.

_____

56. Kayla had a sore throat and fever and was diagnosed with infectious mononucleosis.

_____

57. Gerald has osteoarthritis in his shoulder region and is scheduled to begin physical therapy next week.

_____

58. Tray has had three headaches, not diagnosed as migraines, in the past week.

_____

59. Amanda was diagnosed with multiple sclerosis.

_____

60. Jeffrey has a personal history of alcoholism.

_____

61. Butch had four back surgeries and developed a continuous dependence on hydrocodone.

_____

62. Jake went to an ophthalmologist to have a splinter removed from his cornea.

_____

63. Tammy suffered from severe pain in the temporomandibular joint area.

_____

64. Josephine was struck by lightning during a thunderstorm.

_____

65. Barry's alcoholism has caused cirrhosis of the liver.

_____

66. The Wickers' newborn had a skin condition called *cradle cap*.

_____

67. Adam has been a paraplegic since a car wreck 2 years ago.

_____

68. Hudson suffered a ruptured abdominal aneurysm and had emergency surgery.

_____

69. Mr. Emmett had atherosclerosis of the extremities with gangrene just before his death.

_____

70. The woman with Munchausen syndrome had three children die before law enforcement grew suspicious.

_____

71. Ginger experienced dermatitis as a result of using a tanning bed.

_____

72. The Lewis' first child was born with Down syndrome.

_____

73. Lee Anna has experienced painful menstruation during her last three cycles.

_____

74. James had one testicle removed because of seminoma. The tumor was the primary site and incident of his cancer.

_____

75. Jacqueline has uncontrolled type II diabetes mellitus with ketoacidosis.

_____

76. Mrs. Julius died last week from congestive heart failure.

_____

77. Gary saw the physician to follow up on his previous diagnosis of cardiomegaly.

_____

78. Dr. Albertez thinks that Mr. Tidwell's Parkinson's disease was drug-induced.

_____

79. Jerry developed Kaposi's sarcoma during the final stages of AIDS. The sarcoma was present in his lymph nodes.

_____

80. Sally developed a postoperative fever because of an infection (code infection only).

_____

81. Terri attempted suicide by ingesting a handful of lithium.

_____

82. Beaumont's divorce affected every aspect of his life.

_____

83. Mr. Maxwell's physician knew that his patient would have to be hospitalized once he diagnosed diverticulitis of the colon with hemorrhaging. Mr. Maxwell, at age 95, could not risk staying at home and allowing the bleeding to continue.

_____

84. Susan was stung by a jellyfish while swimming off the coast of Mexico.

_____

85. Alaydra has tunnel vision, which makes it difficult to drive safely.

_____

86. The escaped criminal was cornered by the police and shot because he raised his gun and pointed it at a policeman.

_____

87. Riley has acute myocarditis and was admitted to the hospital.

_____

88. Alisha underwent artificial insemination in an effort to have a child.

_____

89. Jackie's baby was breech and was delivered using forceps.

_____

90. Ordell has acute esophagitis and complained that he had been sick for 3 days.

_____

91. Robert dislocated his shoulder while playing baseball. This was a closed anterior dislocation of the humerus.

_____

92. Betty has allergic gastroenteritis.

_____

93. Mrs. Ralphy was diagnosed with systemic lupus erythematosus.

_____

94. Winston has synovitis of the knee.

_____

95. Mrs. Radson had a skin condition known as *bullous pemphigoid,* in which blisters formed in patches all over her skin.

_____

96. Osteomalacia made it impossible for Robbie to walk.

_____

97. Henry has oral leukoplakia, which may have been caused by smoking a pipe.

_____

98. Ricky was diagnosed with acute lymphocytic leukemia.

_____

99. The Smithsons' 4-year-old daughter has Hurler's syndrome, which was diagnosed a few months after she was born.

_____

100. Patricia has had uterine endometriosis for several years and may require a hysterectomy in the future.

_____

Case Study

Dr. Rogers saw Mrs. Arrant in the office this morning. Mrs. Arrant has been diagnosed in the past with congestive heart failure, diabetes mellitus type II, and chronic myelocytic leukemia. She comes to the clinic today complaining of chest pain and has a fever of 101.8°. Code all of these conditions. In which order would they be written on an encounter form?

_____

_____

_____

Workplace Application

Determine what certifications are available that relate to coding. What are the requirements for obtaining these special certifications? Why might these be beneficial for the medical assistant? Is there a particular certification you are interested in obtaining?

Internet Activities

1. Research the AHIMA website, and explore opportunities for a career in coding.

2. Locate a job description for a medical billing and coding specialist, and determine the daily duties that coders perform in medical offices and/or large clinics.

3. Write a report on the importance of coding accurately. Share the information with the class.

4. Find five additional links other than the AHIMA website that provide useful information on billing and coding.

5. Research programs that provide a specialized certificate in billing and/or coding proficiency.

Chapter 17 Quiz

1. The cause of disorders is called the
   _____ .

2. The signs and symptoms of disease are
   called its _____ .

3. ICD-9 codes consist of _____
   primary digits and up to _____
   additional digits.

4. A non-malignant cancerous growth is said to
   be _____ .

5. A diagnosis that is questionable, probably, or
   likely is a _____ condition.

6. The medical term for a stroke is
   _____ .

7. The medical assistant should begin the
   search for a code in the _____
   index.

8. Codes that describe the circumstances
   of an accident or injury are called
   _____ codes.

9. Codes that explain the reason why a patient
   came into contact with a healthcare professional, even if no injury or illness exists, are
   called _____ codes.

10. The medical assistant should never code
    directly from the _____ .

Basics of Procedural Coding

Vocabulary Review

Fill in the blanks with the correct vocabulary terms from this chapter.

1. The primary procedure or service code selected when performing insurance billing or statistical research is a category _____ code.

2. Jerri sometimes has difficulty with _____ codes, which designate procedures or services that are grouped together and paid for as one procedure or service.

3. Jules prepared a(n) _____ or summary of the diagnostic statements on Mr. Ford's medical record.

4. _____ are found at the beginning of each of the six sections of the CPT-4 manual, and Rebecca refers to them often when coding procedures.

5. Category _____ codes are for new or experimental procedures.

6. A procedure, service, or diagnosis named after a person is called a(n) _____.

7. Codes in which the components of a procedure are separated and reported separately are called _____ codes.

8. Code additions that explain circumstances that alter a provided service or provide additional clarification or detail are called _____.

9. The main divisions of the CPT-4 manual are called _____.

10. Abbreviations are also called _____.

Coding Exercises

Code the following procedures.

11. Dr. Smith visits Eula Fairbanks, a patient with dementia, in the nursing home for less than 30 minutes.

_____

12. Jessica Lundy, a newborn, was admitted to the pediatric critical care unit after her birth, where Dr. Williams provided her initial care.

_____

13. Because Lucille Westerman had multiple health problems, she was admitted for observation after a fainting spell. Dr. Adams took a comprehensive history and performed a thorough examination, then made medical decisions of high complexity regarding her care.

_____

14. Dr. Wray saw Tammy Luttrell in the office as a new patient. He took a detailed history and performed a detailed examination, then made medical decisions of low complexity.

_____

15. Sylvia Julius saw Dr. Bridges for her allergies. The physician took a problem-focused history, performed a problem-focused examination, and made straightforward decisions regarding her care.

_____

16. Bonnie Sadler comes to the office to have blood work drawn for an obstetric panel. What is the code for the obstetric panel only?

_____

17. The office charges Bonnie Sadler, a college student, for drawing a blood specimen. What is the code for venipuncture?

_____

18. Terri Smithson had laparoscopic gastric bypass surgery using the Roux-en-Y procedure.

_____

19. Kim Errant had an outpatient kidney imaging with vascular flow to make certain that her kidneys were functioning normally.

_____

20. Georgie Ebersol had blood drawn for a total bilirubin. Code the blood test only.

_____

21. Roy Messing's urine was tested for total protein.

_____

22. Jerry Orchard was tested for his blood alcohol level.

_____

23. Andrea Adams has a bleeding disorder and has to undergo regular coagulation time tests. Her physician uses the Lee and White method.

_____

24. Dr. Airheart sent Roberto's specimen to the microbiology laboratory to check for *Cryptosporidium*.

_____

25. The body was sent to the county medical examiner's office for a forensic autopsy, which was performed by Dr. Stein.

_____

26. Jonathan Boyd was required to have a polio vaccine by his school. He received an oral dose.

_____

27. Julia Anderson has a lithium level drawn to make certain that her dosage was accurate and appropriate.

_____

28. Cynthia Hernandez was exposed to hepatitis, so her physician ordered an acute hepatitis panel.

_____

29. Sam Livingston, a baby in the neonatal unit, had total bilirubin tests drawn each morning.

_____

30. Susan's husband has blood drawn regularly to measure his quinidine levels.

_____

31. Bobby had to undergo treatment of a clavicular fracture, without manipulation, after his injury during a football game.

_____

32. Betty received anesthesia for the vaginal delivery of her child.

_____

33. Anesthesia was provided to Ron Smith, a brain-dead patient whose organs were being harvested for donation.

_____

34. Dr. Partridge participated in a complex, lengthy telephone call regarding a patient who was scheduled for multiple surgeries.

_____

35. When Terri Anderson was involved in a major car accident, the ER physician took a comprehensive history and performed a thorough examination, and made highly complex decisions.

_____

36. Tim Taylor is a new patient with a small cyst on his back. Dr. Young took a problem-focused history and performed a problem-focused examination, then made straightforward medical decisions.

_____

37. Jim Angelo, an established patient, saw the physician for a minor cut on the back of his hand. The physician spent approximately 10 minutes with Jim.

_____

38. Vera Carpenter was admitted to the hospital for diabetes mellitus, congestive heart failure, and an infection of unknown origin. Dr. Antonetti performed a consultation that took about an hour, including the time spent writing orders in her medical record.

_____

39. Carla had a nasal polyp removed that was hindering her ability to breathe. The excision was a simple one and was performed in Dr. Wilson's office.

_____

40. Darla's son, Andy, was examined for pinworms.

_____

41. The police asked the laboratory technician to perform an arsenic test on a tube of blood.

_____

42. An incision was made into the newborn's pyloric sphincter to allow food to travel through his digestive system.

_____

43. Ben, a 6-year-old, had his tonsils and adenoids removed after recurrent infections.

_____

44. Edward had one testicle removed because of a growing tumor attached to it. An inguinal approach was used, and during the surgery the physician explored the abdominal area to look for other growths.

_____

45. Alex's mother insisted that she have her ears pierced by a physician so that the procedure would be as clean as possible.

_____

46. Fonda was diagnosed with an abdominal ectopic pregnancy, which Dr. Tomlinson removed surgically.

_____

47. The medical assistant performed a simple urinalysis, using a dipstick and a microscope to examine the specimen.

_____

48. Wayne had blood drawn for a CBC with an automated WBC.

_____

49. Paula had an inflammation somewhere inside her body, as evidenced by her sedimentation rate. The test was automated.

_____

50. Jimmie's physician ordered computed tomography of his abdomen with contrast material.

_____

51. Joan had a laparoscopic biopsy of her left ovary.

_____

52. Craig had to undergo a direct repair of a ruptured aneurysm of the carotid artery, which was performed by neck incision.

_____

53. Emma was given a urine pregnancy test in the clinic before receiving x-ray examinations to diagnose her back disorder, using a color comparison test kit.

_____

54. Jennifer's child was tested for serum albumin.

_____

55. Angela had a qualitative lactose test using a urine specimen.

_____

56. Sarah was required to have a blood chemistry test for methadone by her probation officer.

_____

57. The two children that had been lost in the woods were tested for Rocky Mountain spotted fever.

_____

58. Marcus has a total T-cell count every month.

_____

59. After her needlestick injury, Felicia was tested for the hepatitis B surface antibody.

_____

60. Dr. Torrid felt that Katrina might have the Epstein-Barr virus, so he tested for the early antigen.

_____

61. Dr. Battson performed a chlamydia culture on the vaginal specimen.

_____

62. Juan was given a test for herpes simplex, type 2.

_____

63. Mr. Albertson was given a blood test for uric acid.

_____

64. Derrick had a Western blot test last week. The interpretation and report are due back to the physician by tomorrow.

_____

65. Roy had a urine test for total protein.

_____

66. The emergency physician ordered a lead test on the small child, thinking that she had perhaps ingested some paint chips.

_____

67. Joy has monthly blood tests to evaluate her iron-binding capacity.

_____

68. Andi was tested for chromium yesterday and has a return appointment next week.

_____

69. All gastric bypass patients are required to have a basic metabolic panel before surgery is scheduled.

_____

70. June had an obstetric panel run on her second appointment with the physician.

_____

71. Royce had a chest x-ray, single frontal view, to check for pneumonia.

_____

72. Dr. True suspected that Joey had fractured his sternum, so he ordered an x-ray that would show two views of the bone.

_____

73. Jessalyn had an MRI of her spinal canal and its contents.

_____

74. Dr. Tompkins visited a new patient at her home and spent about 20 minutes diagnosing and treating her for the flu.

_____

75. Dr. Revy was on standby for about 20 minutes while the decision was made as to whether the patient would have a cesarean section.

_____

76. Judge Jordan has his blood checked for potassium levels monthly.

_____

77. Steven Pauly needs a chest x-ray examination, and the physician has requested four views.

_____

78. Linda Ellis had a complete hip x-ray examination with two views because her physician was considering hip replacement surgery.

_____

79. Judy had a theophylline level drawn during her last office visit.

_____

80. Joy had a closed treatment of a coccygeal fracture.

_____

81. Mrs. Dickson went to see Dr. Donner for a complete radiologic examination of the scapula.

_____

82. Bobbie returned to the physician's office to have a short leg walking cast applied after wearing the larger cast for 4 weeks.

_____

83. Dr. Angell ordered a radiologic examination of Sylvia's mastoids, requesting two views.

_____

84. Sammy had a uric acid test during his last office visit.

_____

85. Peter asked his physician to repeat his CPK total because it had been slightly high on his last visit.

_____

86. Bryce has a digoxin level drawn every 3 months.

_____

87. The pathologist prepared tissue for drug analysis.

_____

88. Julie was quite dehydrated for a week, so her physician ran an electrolyte panel.

   _____

89. Frank asked the physician how a magnesium level related to his illness.

   _____

90. Joel's physician felt that he had an adrenal insufficiency, so he ordered an ACTH stimulation panel.

   _____

91. All three children who lived in the condemned home were subjected to a quantitative carbon monoxide test.

   _____

92. When Ariel turned 50, her physician recommended that she have an occult blood test annually.

   _____

93. Most diabetics periodically have a blood glucose test performed at the physician's office in addition to the test strip checks that they perform at home.

   _____

94. Selenium can be detected with a blood test.

   _____

95. Sarah's infant returned to the physician's office to have a PKU test a few weeks after she was born.

   _____

96. Van Stephens had blood work done on Monday to check his triglycerides.

   _____

97. Karry has been to the physician for several days in a row to have ovulation tests, which are done by visual color comparison.

   _____

98. Samuel's vitamin K test results were slightly below normal.

   _____

99. Dr. Grant runs a spun microhematocrit on each of his pregnant patients at every prenatal visit.

   _____

100. Trent had a serum folic acid test run this morning at his physician's office.

   _____

Case Study

Find all procedures that need to be coded for billing purposes in the following text.

Roberta Sleether is a new patient who saw Dr. Morganstern, complaining of feeling tired all of the time. She stated that she was exhausted even after a full 8 hours of sleep at night. Roberta said that she did not have much of an appetite and that she had been eating mostly salads and chicken, with a bowl of fruit as snacks. She is not overweight and her blood pressure and other vital signs were normal. Dr. Morganstern decided to perform a CBC, an electrolyte panel, and a lipid panel. He also ordered a urinalysis, an iron-binding capacity, and a vitamin B_{12} test. The physician asked if she had noticed any blood in her urine or stool, and she denied blood in the urine but did mention she had several episodes of diarrhea. Dr. Morganstern added an occult blood test as well as a stool culture to check for pathogens. The physician placed Roberta on multivitamin therapy and told her to return in 1 week to discuss her laboratory test results. He spent approximately 30 minutes with Roberta, taking a detailed history and performing a detailed examination, making low complexity medical decisions. Roberta scheduled her appointment for the following week and left the clinic.

_____
_____
_____
_____

Workplace Applications

1. Select a medical specialty, and research the procedure codes that would be commonly used within that practice.

2. Contact a practice and make an appointment to meet the person(s) who perform coding tasks. Discuss the challenges and rewards of the job. Prepare a report for the class based on the interview with the coders.

3. Design an encounter form for a fictional medical practice. Choose the specialty, and make certain that the codes chosen for the form are applicable to the specialty practice.

Internet Activities

1. Research job postings on the Internet that relate to billing and coding.

2. Working in groups, prepare a report on the sections of the CPT-4 manual. Discuss the most common codes within each section.

3. Search for coding hints and tips online. Prepare a report for the class, and discuss the tips and how to use them to code more effectively.

Chapter 18 Quiz

Name: _____

1. The physical condition of the patient is called the physical _____.

2. The medical assistant should never code from the _____.

3. _____ provides additional clarification or detail about a procedure or service.

4. The CPT-4 contains _____ sections.

5. The _____ & _____ section is the location of codes for office visits.

6. Procedure codes that are grouped together and paid as one service are called _____ codes.

7. The appendixes of the CPT-4 are rarely used in everyday coding.

   a. True

   b. False

8. The physician's office uses which group of codes most frequently?

   a. Category I codes

   b. Category II codes

   c. Category III codes

9. To create an outline or summary of information from a text or medical record is to compile a(n) _____.

10. The patient's status tells the medical assistant whether the patient is new or _____.

CHAPTER 19

Basics of Health Insurance

Vocabulary Review

Fill in the blanks with the correct vocabulary terms from this chapter.

1. United Healthcare is the insurance _____ that the Blackburn Clinic contracted for health coverage that is offered to employees for $85 per paycheck.

2. Anna called the human resources department to make certain that Roberto had met the _____ requirements for health insurance coverage, because he was only a part-time employee.

3. Barbara requested quotes from several insurance companies for a(n) _____ _____, because she and her daughter needed insurance coverage and Barbara was self-employed.

4. Ms. Anderson requested information about a _____ policy to supplement her Medicare insurance benefits.

5. Georgia suggested that the college establish a(n) _____ _____ plan because of its growth and its ability to fund its own insurance program.

6. Sgt. Smithson's family is covered for healthcare benefits through the military's _____ program.

7. The maximum amount of money that Blue Cross will pay for a certain benefit is its

   _____ _____.

8. Randy is covered under an entitlement program called a _____ plan, because he works for the Federal Bureau of Investigation.

9. Sharon makes a $20 _____ each time she visits the physician's office.

10. The office manager reviewed the _____ _____, which explained the benefits paid by Medicaid on the referenced claims.

11. John Ford is the _____ coordinator in human resources, and he constantly compares policies and other perks to make certain that his company offers a competitive package to employees.

12. Most managed care policies require that patients obtain _____ for surgery and many other treatments and procedures.

13. The medical assistant must check the _____ date on insurance cards to make certain that the policy is in force and has not expired.

14. Traditional health insurance plans, or _____ plans, pay for all or a share of the cost of covered services regardless of which provider is used.

15. Beatrice pays the premium to her insurance company, which makes her the _____.

16. The _____ process is required by some insurers and forces the provider to obtain permission to perform certain procedures and services.

17. Janna's _____ amount is $500, which she must pay before her insurance will cover services and procedures.

18. Private insurance is sometimes called _____ insurance.

19. Joy established a _____ _____ account, which is tax-deferred and designed for individuals and families who choose to fund their own healthcare expenses.

20. Dr. Saxton is a _____ provider and has entered into a contract with Aetna, agreeing to provide medical services to its members and abide by the rules and regulations set forth by the company.

21. Dr. Abbott made a _____ to Dr. Breckenridge because the patient needed surgery.

22. Jaynie is covered by both of her parents' insurance policies, so the _____ rule determines which policy is considered the primary one.

23. A _____ _____ contracts with the government to handle and mediate insurance claims from medical facilities, home health agencies, or providers of medical services.

24. Limitations on an insurance contract for which benefits are not payable are called _____.

25. Bob's children are considered to be his _____ on his insurance policy.

26. Jarrod is the _____ and is responsible for paying his wife's medical bills.

27. The payment made to keep an insurance company in force is called a _____.

28. The process of going to a specialist without being required to obtain permission from the primary care provider is called a _____ _____.

29. The business decided on an insurance policy that contained a _____ that had a provision for obstetric care.

30. _____ is a payment method wherein a fixed amount of money is reimbursed to the provider for patients enrolled during a specific time period, regardless of the services rendered or number of times that the provider was visited.

Skills and Concepts

Part I: Cycle of Health Insurance

Place the following tasks related to the health insurance cycle in the proper order. Place the number of the task (1, 2, 3, etc.) in the blank next to the question number.

31. _____ Calculate insurance deductibles and co-insurance amounts and provide the patient with a statement showing out-of-pocket expenses that the patient will owe.

32. _____ Post payments and adjustments on the patient ledger or account and examine the EOB, ROMB, or RA to identify what was paid, reduced, or denied.

33. _____ Obtain information from the patient and insured.

34. _____ Bill the patient for any outstanding balance.

35. _____ Perform diagnostic and procedural coding and review the encounter form for completeness once the patient is seen by the provider.

36. _____ Complete an insurance claim form and submit it to the insurance company.

37. _____ Follow up on any rejected or unpaid claims and requests for more information from the insurance company.

38. _____ Verify the patient's eligibility for insurance payment and benefits available, exclusions, and whether special authorizations are needed for any services or procedures.

39. _____ Obtain preauthorization or permission, if applicable, for referrals or special services and procedures.

Part II: Types of Health Insurance

Place the name of the type of insurance described in the blank.

40. Insurance type that is often purchased when a person does not qualify for inclusion in a group or government-sponsored plan; is often more expensive than group policies

_____

41. Provides healthcare coverage for dependents of military personnel

_____

42. Federal health insurance program that provides healthcare coverage for individuals age 65 and older

_____

43. Type of insurance in which the employer pays employee healthcare costs from the employer's own funds

_____

44. A type of self-insurance in which small companies, the self-employed, and uninsured persons can purchase health insurance policies and/or make tax-free deposits to an account; the money is used to pay medical expenses when they occur

_____

45. Federal government program that provides healthcare coverage for medically indigent people

_____

46. Covers a number of people under a single master contract issued to their employer or to an association with which the people are affiliated

_____

47. Protects wage earners against the loss of wages and the cost of medical care resulting from an occupational accident or disease

_____

Part III: Types of Insurance Benefits

Match the types of insurance benefits with their description.

48. Hospitalization   _____

49. Surgical   _____

50. Basic medical   _____

51. Major medical   _____

52. Disability   _____

53. Dental care   _____

54. Vision care   _____

55. Medicare supplement   _____

56. Special risk insurance   _____

57. Liability insurance   _____

58. Life insurance   _____

59. Long-term care insurance   _____

    a. Pays all or part of a surgeon's and/or assistant surgeon's fees

    b. Protects a person in the event of a certain type of accident, such as an airplane crash

    c. Covers a continuum of broad-ranged maintenance and health services to chronically ill, disabled, or mentally retarded persons

    d. Provides protection against especially large medical bills resulting from catastrophic or prolonged illnesses

    e. Provides payment of a specified amount on an insured's death

    f. Pays all or part of a physician's fee for nonsurgical services, including hospital, home, and office visits

    g. Provides reimbursement for all or a percentage of the cost for refraction, lenses, and frames

    h. Pays the cost of all or part of the insured person's hospital room and board and specific hospital services

    i. Often includes benefits for medical expenses payable to individuals who are injured in the insured person's home or during an automobile accident

    j. Policy purchased to help defray medical costs not covered by Medicare

    k. Pays expenses involved with care of teeth and gums

    l. Weekly or monthly cash benefits provided to employed policyholders who become unable to work as a result of an accident or illness

Part IV: Short Answer Questions

Answer the following short answer questions.

60. List four ways that insurance benefits are determined.

    a. _____

    b. _____

    c. _____

    d. _____

61. Define *usual, customary*, and *reasonable*.

    a. usual _____

    b. customary _____

    c. reasonable _____

62. Define *managed care*.

    _____

    _____

    _____

63. List three advantages and three disadvantages to the managed care concept.

    Advantages

    _____

    _____

    _____

    Disadvantages

    _____

    _____

    _____

64. What are the two basic models of managed care?

    a. _____

    b. _____

65. Does the physician have a choice as to whether he or she accepts Medicaid patients?

    _____

66. List three types of persons who would qualify for Medicare.

    a. _____

    b. _____

    c. _____

67. List three types of persons who would qualify for Medicaid.

a. _____

b. _____

c. _____

68. List 10 items of information that the medical assistant should obtain from the patient before calling the insurance company for preauthorization or precertification.

a. _____

b. _____

c. _____

d. _____

e. _____

f. _____

g. _____

h. _____

i. _____

j. _____

69. What is the *Federal Register?*

_____

_____

_____

70. Define *referral*.

_____

_____

_____

Case Study

Survey all class members and determine the various types of insurance coverage that are represented by the students. Assign each student a different insurance company, and have them call to verify benefits. Choose a medical procedure and have the students call and verify the amounts of coverage for that particular procedure. If students are uncomfortable in exchanging health insurance information, allow them to verify and obtain amounts of coverage for their own insurance.

_____

_____

_____

Workplace Applications

1. Working in small groups, obtain a quote for health insurance coverage for a small group. Use the Internet to research companies and choose three or four from which to obtain quotes.

2. Design a document that provides information as to what should be placed in each box of the health insurance claim form. Place the document into a report cover with sheet protectors, and turn it in for a special project grade.

3. Obtain encounter forms from several different physicians' offices. Use them to create mock patients, listing a diagnosis and several procedures. Complete an insurance claim form for each patient and encounter form. As an option, work in groups and present the patient to the class.

Internet Activities

1. Research the various individual policies that are available. Obtain a quote for healthcare coverage from one company. Share the information with the class, and compare the cost of individual policies with those of group policies. Discuss the differences.

2. Investigate medical savings accounts, and determine how these accounts work, as well as how benefits for healthcare expenses are paid.

3. Conduct a survey of 25 physicians, and ask them what insurance plans they see in the office most frequently. Research these companies on the Internet and determine their benefits and costs. Prepare a report that compares the five most frequently mentioned companies.

Chapter 19 Quiz

Name: _____

1. Medicare and Medicaid serve essentially the same type of person.
   a. True
   b. False

2. Indemnity plans are never used now that most patients have a managed care plan.
   a. True
   b. False

3. An independent practice association is a type of health maintenance organization.
   a. True
   b. False

4. TRICARE is used only by individuals over the age of 65.
   a. True
   b. False

5. Managed care plans and regulations seldom ever change.
   a. True
   b. False

6. The RVS was developed to help physicians establish rational, relative fees.
   a. True
   b. False

7. The limit that is placed on the amount that will be reimbursed for a particular service or procedure is called the *allowable*.
   a. True
   b. False

8. Utilization review committees review individual cases to make certain that medical services are necessary.
   a. True
   b. False

9. Third party payors do not have much influence on what healthcare providers can charge.
   a. True
   b. False

10. Many patients, especially older individuals, believe that their healthcare insurance pays for all charges.
    a. True
    b. False

The Health Insurance Claim Form

Vocabulary Review

Fill in the blanks with the correct vocabulary terms from this chapter.

1. Suzanne is adamant about sending _____ to insurance companies so that there are no delays in receiving reimbursements.

2. A hard copy of an insurance claim that has been completed and sent by surface mail is called a(n) _____.

3. Dr. Dexter was assigned a(n) _____, which is his lifetime 10-digit number that replaces the PIN and UPIN.

4. _____ separate, check, and redistribute claims electronically to various insurance carriers and often offer additional services to physicians.

5. Jules referenced the _____ when she researched the Johnson records.

6. Paula received a _____ claim and must clarify the questions raised by the insurance company before resubmitting the claim.

7. Dr. Rosen has patients sign a(n) _____ so that insurance companies will pay claims directly to the physician.

8. _____ claims have errors or omissions that must be corrected and resubmitted if reimbursement is to be received.

9. A(n) _____ or _____ signature is scanned and accepted as proof of approval for the content of an electronic document.

10. The electronic scanning of printed items as images and the use of special software to recognize these images is called _____.

Skills and Concepts

Part I: Completing Insurance Claim Forms

Complete a claim form using the patient information in each of the following scenarios. Use the claim forms in Work Products 20-1 through 20-5.

11. Complete Claim Form #1 (Work Product 20-1) using the information below.

Today's Date: 9-29-20XX

Mr. Jackson, an established patient, has suffered from situational depression since his wife of 47 years died last winter. He has a history of congestive heart failure and intermittent high blood pressure. He comes to the office on July 23, 20XX, for treatment of his depression. Dr. Swakoski sees Mr. Jackson and counsels him about medication for his condition. He is with the patient for about 25 minutes. He gives Mr. Jackson a week's worth of samples of Cymbalta and writes a prescription for the drug that is refillable for 3 months. The charge for the office visit is $85.00. File this claim with BC/BS.

Donald W. Jackson (patient and insured)
77834 High Road Way
Los Angeles, CA 90010
818-665-0098 (home)
SS# 567-99-0067
Insurance: BC/BS and Medicare
ID# 567990067
Employer: Retired
DOB: 3-8-1940
Diagnosis: Depression, CHF, HTN
Procedures: Office visit
Account Number: JAD0067

Family Health Center
120 E. Northwest Highway
Los Angeles, CA 90010
818-624-0112
Federal Tax ID# 75-6102034

BC/BS
11001 Spring Way, Suite 200
Sacramento, CA 90012
800-443-0033

Theodore Swakoski, MD
NPI# 6170421616
BS Provider# 621604211

12. Complete Claim Form #2 (Work Product 20-2) using the information below.

Today's Date: 9-29-20XX

Mr. Adams, an established, married patient, comes to the office because of an episode of bronchitis. He states that he has felt poorly for about 1 week and that he now is having trouble getting a full breath of air. He has had moderate pain on coughing and admits that the cough has kept him awake or has awakened him. He says he has bronchitis about once per year in the fall months. Dr. Abbott sees Mr. Adams for about 15 minutes in the office. He prescribes an antibiotic, a cough syrup, and Hycodan. Dr. Abbott knows that Mr. Adams is also diabetic, so he draws blood for a glucose test to make certain that the levels are normal. He suggests that Mr. Adams refrain from work for the 2 days leading into the weekend and return to work on Monday. Dr. Abbott asks if Mr. Adams is still having trouble sleeping, as reported on his last office visit. He admits that he is still suffering from insomnia even apart from the bronchitis. Mr. Adams also admits that his marriage is failing, and suggests that the stress may be contributing to the insomnia. Dr. Abbott gives him a prescription for Ambien CR along with the other prescriptions. Mr. Adams is to return to the clinic in 1 week if he is not feeling better. The charge for the office visit is $77, and the blood sugar test is $12. Mr. Adams pays his $20 copay.

Benjamin C. Adams
55180 Grand Avenue Parkway
Austin, Texas 78706
512-998-1354 (home)
SS# 445-74-8363
Insurance: Humana PPO
ID# 445748363
Employer: Texas Department of Public Safety
DOB: 7-2-1954
Diagnosis: Acute bronchitis; diabetes mellitus type II, controlled; insomnia
Procedures: Office visit, blood glucose test
Account Number: ADB8363

Family Medical Clinic
1216 E. Lamar Blvd.
Austin, Texas 78704
512-624-0112
Federal Tax ID# 75-8210612

Humana
PO Box 3031103
Chicago, IL 60068
800-611-1216

Barnabas Abbott, MD
NPI 4712678920

13. Complete Claim Form #3 (Work Product 20-3) using the information below.

Today's Date: 9-29-20XX

Suanne Snell comes to the office complaining of severe pain in her lower left quadrant. She states that the pain came on suddenly and that she has a history of ovarian cysts. Ms. Snell is clearly in severe pain, so Dr. Jackman gives her an injection of Toradol. Once the medication has taken effect, he performs a pelvic examination and determines that the most likely cause of her pain is a ruptured ovarian cyst. Dr. Jackman sends Ms. Snell to the hospital for an ultrasound examination and will see her in the emergency room later in the afternoon. Ms. Snell has no other significant health problems. Her office visit is $85.00 and, plus $25 for the injection. Dr. Jackman spends about 40 minutes with Suanne.

Suanne L. Snell
4545 Rustic
Los Angeles, CA 90002
818-445-9970 (home)
SS# 665-76-5568
Insurance: Aetna HMO
ID# 665765568
Employer: Marriott Hotels International
DOB: 9-3-1964
Diagnosis: Ruptured ovarian cyst
Procedures: Office visit, injection
Account Number: SNS5568

Medical Surgical Clinic
4800 S. Broadway Blvd.
Los Angeles, CA 90012
818-261-1122
Federal Tax ID# 75-6120662

James Jackman, DO
NPI 8216740292

Aetna
PO Box 310661
Sacramento, CA 90121
800-996-8445

14. Complete Claim Form #4 (Work Product 20-4) using the information below.

Today's Date: 9-29-20XX

Celeste Huntington, a single female, arrives at the clinic today as a new patient. Celeste was referred to Dr. Tyler by Dr. William R. Curry, a friend of Dr. Tyler's from medical school. She has been diagnosed with systemic lupus erythematosus and periodically experiences a great deal of pain. She arranged to forward her medical records to Dr. Tyler several weeks ago, and she made today's appointment before her move to Annapolis. Dr. Tyler has worked with numerous patients who have lupus and is understanding about their needs and the challenges they face in living a normal life. Celeste states that she needs to refill her medications, and Dr. Tyler reviews them with her, agreeing to refill her prescription Motrin (800 mg), Lortab (10 mg) and Phenergan suppositories (50 mg). She says that she uses the Motrin every day or so but rarely uses the Lortab, although she prefers to keep a supply on hand for those times that the disease strikes her aggressively. She mentions that she has not had a well-woman examination in 2 years because of the sale of her home and the purchase of their new one in Annapolis. Dr. Tyler performs the well-woman examination and writes Celeste an order to have a mammogram. He also performs a breast examination, which is included in the well-woman examination. He spends about 45 minutes with Celeste. She leaves with her prescriptions and is ordered to return in 3 months if she does not feel the need to return before that time. She is charged $179 for the new patient office visit and $55 for the Pap smear and well-woman examination.

Celeste C. Huntington
554 Georgetown Way
New Rochelle, NY 10801
914-889-6675 (home)
SS# 433-99-2364
Insurance: United Health Care PPO
ID# 433992364
Employer: Loist and Earnest Law Firm
DOB: 9-3-1960
Diagnosis: Systemic lupus erythematosus
Procedures: Office visit, Pap smear
Account Number: HUC2364

New Rochelle Family Medicine
2002 Front Street, Suite 600
New Rochelle, NY 10800
914-661-0001
Federal Tax ID# 75-6234710

United Healthcare
PO Box 292928
New York, NY 10021
212-660-1100

Richard Tyler, MD
NPI 6779354390

William R. Curry, MD
NPI 4619907217

15. Complete Claim Form #5 (Work Product 20-5) using the information below.

Today's Date: 9-29-20XX

Patricia Saxton, a married female, has several health problems and is a frequent visitor to Dr. Handley's office. She is insured through her own policy with Unicare and is also insured on her husband's policy through Assurant Health. She has Graves' disease, malignant HTN, bursitis of the right knee, and carpel tunnel syndrome. She arrives at the office today to have her blood pressure checked. While she is in the waiting area, she develops mild chest pains, so the medical assistant brings her to the back office immediately and performs an ECG. Dr. Handley looks at the strip and feels that Patricia may have recently had a mild heart attack, so he refers her to Dr. Stern, a cardiologist. The office sets up an afternoon appointment for Ms. Saxton, and she leaves the clinic with her husband with instructions to drive directly to Dr. Stern's office. They promise to do so.

Ms. Saxton is charged for the office visit ($165.00) and an EKG ($45.00). She is with Dr. Handley for approximately 50 minutes.

Patricia N. Saxton
13104 Highway 798 South
Tyler, TX 75701
903-882-4453 (home)
SS# 334-88-9907
Insurance: Unicare PPO
ID# 334889907
Employer: Self-employed
Husband: Levern R. Saxton
Employer: Kelly Tires
SS# 621-12-6701
ID# 621126701
DOB: 7-8-1953
Diagnosis: Malignant HTN, Graves' disease, bursitis, carpel tunnel syndrome
Procedures: Office visit, ECG
Account Number: SAP9907

South Tyler Health Clinic
120 E. West Street
Tyler, Texas 75703
903-566-1112
Federal Tax ID# 75-2162704

Wendell Handley, DO
NPI 5682103541

Unicare
12000 Walker Blvd., St. 100
Dallas, Texas 75225
800-921-0091

Assurant Health
PO Box 704
Dallas, Texas 75229
800-621-1000

Part II: Determining Diagnosis and Procedure Codes

Determine the proper diagnosis and procedure codes as indicated below.

16. Diagnosis: Lou Gehrig's disease; hydrocodone dependence

_____

_____

Procedures: Office visit, new patient (10 minutes)

_____

17. Diagnosis: Generalized osteoarthritis in upper arm

_____

Procedures: Office visit, established patient (10 minutes); basic metabolic panel; lipid panel

_____

_____

18. Diagnosis: Foreign body in ear

_____

Procedures: Office visit, established patient (10 minutes)

_____

19. Diagnosis: Burn over 40% of body surface because of car accident with another vehicle while a passenger in the car

_____

_____

Procedures: Hospital admission, new patient, physician spends approximately 50 minutes treating patient

_____

20. Diagnosis: Rosacea

_____

Procedure: Office visit, established patient (15 minutes)

_____

21. Diagnosis: Sunburn, third degree

_____

Procedures: Office visit, established patient (10 minutes)

_____

22. Diagnosis: Tachycardia, neonatal

_____

Procedures: Hospital visit, 2 days, inpatient subsequent care (25 minutes)

_____

23. Diagnosis: Pernicious anemia

_____

Procedures: Office visit, established patient, (25 minutes); sedimentation rate, automated; CBC, automated

_____

_____

_____

24. Diagnosis: Attention deficit disorder with hyperactivity; acute cystitis

_____

_____

Procedures: Office visit, established patient (15 minutes); urinalysis

_____

_____

25. Diagnosis: Mastitis after delivery of baby

_____

Procedures: Office visit, established patient (5 minutes)

_____

Case Study

Research the history of the CMS-1500 claim form. Determine when it was first used and the changes that the form has undergone since its inception. Prepare a report that details these changes, including the most recent modifications to the CMS-1500 (08/05). Present the report to the class.

Workplace Application

Collect several blank encounter forms from various medical specialties. Distribute the forms to classmates, sharing and trading the various forms. Mark several procedures on the forms and at least two diagnoses codes. Prepare a CMS-1500 claim based on information on the encounter forms. Share the information in class, and explain the coding choices that were made on each claim.

Internet Activities

1. Review the National Uniform Claim Committee website. Find the User Manual for the CMS-1500 Claim Form (08/05).

2. Find three companies that sell the CMS-1500 claim form. Compare costs and determine the least expensive place to order the form.

3. Research software applications that are available for completing CMS-1500 forms. Determine which of those applications that are available for purchase would be good investments for a physician's office.

Chapter 20 Quiz

Name: _____

1. ICD-9-CM codes are not needed on the CMS-1500.

   a. True

   b. False

2. OCR stands for _____
   _____.

3. A claim filed without any errors or omissions is called a _____ claim.

4. The place of service code for a physician's office is _____.

5. The NPI is the _____
   _____.

6. The current CMS-1500 form used for filing claims was revised in _____ of
   _____.

7. _____ of _____ means that the patient has authorized the payment of benefits directly to the provider.

8. SOF stands for _____
   _____.

9. Block 24E of the CMS-1500 claim form refers back to the _____
   codes that are listed in Block 21.

10. The patient account number must be noted on the CMS-1500 claim form.

    a. True

    b. False

WORK PRODUCT 20-1

Name: _____

Complete a CMS-1500 Claim Form

Complete Claim Form #1 using the information in Part I, Question 11.

1500

HEALTH INSURANCE CLAIM FORM

APPROVED BY NATIONAL UNIFORM CLAIM COMMITTEE 08/05

PICA		PICA

CARRIER

1. MEDICARE MEDICAID TRICARE CHAMPUS CHAMPVA GROUP HEALTH PLAN FECA BLK LUNG OTHER	1a. INSURED'S I.D. NUMBER (For Program in Item 1)

(Medicare #)   (Medicaid #)   (Sponsor's SSN)   (Member ID#)   (SSN or ID)   (SSN)   (ID)

2. PATIENT'S NAME (Last Name, First Name, Middle Initial)	3. PATIENT'S BIRTH DATE MM DD YY SEX M F	4. INSURED'S NAME (Last Name, First Name, Middle Initial)

5. PATIENT'S ADDRESS (No., Street)	6. PATIENT RELATIONSHIP TO INSURED Self Spouse Child Other	7. INSURED'S ADDRESS (No., Street)

CITY	STATE	8. PATIENT STATUS Single Married Other	CITY	STATE

ZIP CODE	TELEPHONE (Include Area Code) ( )	Employed Full-Time Student Part-Time Student	ZIP CODE	TELEPHONE (Include Area Code) ( )

PATIENT AND INSURED INFORMATION

9. OTHER INSURED'S NAME (Last Name, First Name, Middle Initial)	10. IS PATIENT'S CONDITION RELATED TO:	11. INSURED'S POLICY GROUP OR FECA NUMBER

a. OTHER INSURED'S POLICY OR GROUP NUMBER	a. EMPLOYMENT? (Current or Previous) YES NO	a. INSURED'S DATE OF BIRTH MM DD YY SEX M F

b. OTHER INSURED'S DATE OF BIRTH MM DD YY SEX M F	b. AUTO ACCIDENT? PLACE (State) YES NO	b. EMPLOYER'S NAME OR SCHOOL NAME

c. EMPLOYER'S NAME OR SCHOOL NAME	c. OTHER ACCIDENT? YES NO	c. INSURANCE PLAN NAME OR PROGRAM NAME

d. INSURANCE PLAN NAME OR PROGRAM NAME	10d. RESERVED FOR LOCAL USE	d. IS THERE ANOTHER HEALTH BENEFIT PLAN? YES NO If yes, return to and complete item 9 a-d.

READ BACK OF FORM BEFORE COMPLETING & SIGNING THIS FORM

12. PATIENT'S OR AUTHORIZED PERSON'S SIGNATURE I authorize the release of any medical or other information necessary to process this claim. I also request payment of government benefits either to myself or to the party who accepts assignment below. SIGNED _____ DATE _____	13. INSURED'S OR AUTHORIZED PERSON'S SIGNATURE I authorize payment of medical benefits to the undersigned physician or supplier for services described below. SIGNED _____

14. DATE OF CURRENT: MM DD YY ILLNESS (First symptom) OR INJURY (Accident) OR PREGNANCY(LMP)	15. IF PATIENT HAS HAD SAME OR SIMILAR ILLNESS. GIVE FIRST DATE MM DD YY	16. DATES PATIENT UNABLE TO WORK IN CURRENT OCCUPATION MM DD YY FROM TO MM DD YY

17. NAME OF REFERRING PROVIDER OR OTHER SOURCE	17a. 17b. NPI	18. HOSPITALIZATION DATES RELATED TO CURRENT SERVICES MM DD YY FROM TO MM DD YY

19. RESERVED FOR LOCAL USE	20. OUTSIDE LAB? YES NO $ CHARGES

21. DIAGNOSIS OR NATURE OF ILLNESS OR INJURY (Relate Items 1, 2, 3 or 4 to Item 24E by Line) 1. 2. 3. 4.	22. MEDICAID RESUBMISSION CODE ORIGINAL REF. NO. 23. PRIOR AUTHORIZATION NUMBER

24. A. DATE(S) OF SERVICE From To MM DD YY MM DD YY	B. PLACE OF SERVICE	C. EMG	D. PROCEDURES, SERVICES, OR SUPPLIES (Explain Unusual Circumstances) CPT/HCPCS MODIFIER	E. DIAGNOSIS POINTER	F. $ CHARGES	G. DAYS OR UNITS	H. EPSDT Family Plan	I. ID. QUAL.	J. RENDERING PROVIDER ID. #
1								NPI	
2								NPI	
3								NPI	
4								NPI	
5								NPI	
6								NPI	

PHYSICIAN OR SUPPLIER INFORMATION

25. FEDERAL TAX I.D. NUMBER SSN EIN	26. PATIENT'S ACCOUNT NO.	27. ACCEPT ASSIGNMENT? (For govt. claims, see back) YES NO	28. TOTAL CHARGE $	29. AMOUNT PAID $	30. BALANCE DUE $

31. SIGNATURE OF PHYSICIAN OR SUPPLIER INCLUDING DEGREES OR CREDENTIALS (I certify that the statements on the reverse apply to this bill and are made a part thereof.) SIGNED _____ DATE _____	32. SERVICE FACILITY LOCATION INFORMATION a. NPI b.	33. BILLING PROVIDER INFO & PH # ( ) a. NPI b.

WORK PRODUCT 20-2

Name: _____

Complete a CMS-1500 Claim Form

Complete Claim Form #2 using the information in Part I, Question 12.

WORK PRODUCT 20-3

Name: _____

Complete a CMS-1500 Claim Form

Complete Claim Form #3 using the information in Part I, Question 13.

WORK PRODUCT 20-4

Name: _____

Complete a CMS-1500 Claim Form

Complete Claim Form #4 using the information in Part I, Question 14.

1500

HEALTH INSURANCE CLAIM FORM

APPROVED BY NATIONAL UNIFORM CLAIM COMMITTEE 08/05

| | PICA | | | | | | | | PICA | | |

1. MEDICARE ☐ (Medicare #)   MEDICAID ☐ (Medicaid #)   TRICARE CHAMPUS ☐ (Sponsor's SSN)   CHAMPVA ☐ (Member ID#)   GROUP HEALTH PLAN ☐ (SSN or ID)   FECA BLK LUNG ☐ (SSN)   OTHER ☐ (ID)   **1a.** INSURED'S I.D. NUMBER   (For Program in Item 1)

2. PATIENT'S NAME (Last Name, First Name, Middle Initial)

3. PATIENT'S BIRTH DATE   MM   DD   YY   SEX   M ☐   F ☐

4. INSURED'S NAME (Last Name, First Name, Middle Initial)

5. PATIENT'S ADDRESS (No., Street)

6. PATIENT RELATIONSHIP TO INSURED   Self ☐   Spouse ☐   Child ☐   Other ☐

7. INSURED'S ADDRESS (No., Street)

CITY   STATE

8. PATIENT STATUS   Single ☐   Married ☐   Other ☐   Employed ☐   Full-Time Student ☐   Part-Time Student ☐

CITY   STATE

ZIP CODE   TELEPHONE (Include Area Code) ( )

ZIP CODE   TELEPHONE (Include Area Code) ( )

9. OTHER INSURED'S NAME (Last Name, First Name, Middle Initial)

10. IS PATIENT'S CONDITION RELATED TO:

11. INSURED'S POLICY GROUP OR FECA NUMBER

a. OTHER INSURED'S POLICY OR GROUP NUMBER

a. EMPLOYMENT? (Current or Previous)   YES ☐   NO ☐

a. INSURED'S DATE OF BIRTH   MM   DD   YY   SEX   M ☐   F ☐

b. OTHER INSURED'S DATE OF BIRTH   MM   DD   YY   SEX   M ☐   F ☐

b. AUTO ACCIDENT?   PLACE (State)   YES ☐   NO ☐

b. EMPLOYER'S NAME OR SCHOOL NAME

c. EMPLOYER'S NAME OR SCHOOL NAME

c. OTHER ACCIDENT?   YES ☐   NO ☐

c. INSURANCE PLAN NAME OR PROGRAM NAME

d. INSURANCE PLAN NAME OR PROGRAM NAME

10d. RESERVED FOR LOCAL USE

d. IS THERE ANOTHER HEALTH BENEFIT PLAN?   YES ☐   NO ☐   *If yes,* return to and complete item 9 a-d.

READ BACK OF FORM BEFORE COMPLETING & SIGNING THIS FORM

12. PATIENT'S OR AUTHORIZED PERSON'S SIGNATURE I authorize the release of any medical or other information necessary to process this claim. I also request payment of government benefits either to myself or to the party who accepts assignment below.

SIGNED _____ DATE _____

13. INSURED'S OR AUTHORIZED PERSON'S SIGNATURE I authorize payment of medical benefits to the undersigned physician or supplier for services described below.

SIGNED _____

14. DATE OF CURRENT: MM   DD   YY   ◄ ILLNESS (First symptom) OR INJURY (Accident) OR PREGNANCY(LMP)

15. IF PATIENT HAS HAD SAME OR SIMILAR ILLNESS. GIVE FIRST DATE   MM   DD   YY

16. DATES PATIENT UNABLE TO WORK IN CURRENT OCCUPATION   MM   DD   YY   FROM   TO   MM   DD   YY

17. NAME OF REFERRING PROVIDER OR OTHER SOURCE   17a.   17b. NPI

18. HOSPITALIZATION DATES RELATED TO CURRENT SERVICES   MM   DD   YY   FROM   TO   MM   DD   YY

19. RESERVED FOR LOCAL USE

20. OUTSIDE LAB?   YES ☐   NO ☐ $ CHARGES

21. DIAGNOSIS OR NATURE OF ILLNESS OR INJURY (Relate Items 1, 2, 3 or 4 to Item 24E by Line)

1. |___.___
2. |___.___
3. |___.___
4. |___.___

22. MEDICAID RESUBMISSION CODE   ORIGINAL REF. NO.

23. PRIOR AUTHORIZATION NUMBER

24. A. DATE(S) OF SERVICE						B. PLACE OF SERVICE	C. EMG	D. PROCEDURES, SERVICES, OR SUPPLIES (Explain Unusual Circumstances)		E. DIAGNOSIS POINTER	F. $ CHARGES	G. DAYS OR UNITS	H. EPSDT Family Plan	I. ID. QUAL.	J. RENDERING PROVIDER ID. #
From			To					CPT/HCPCS	MODIFIER						
MM	DD	YY	MM	DD	YY										
1															NPI
2															NPI
3															NPI
4															NPI
5															NPI
6															NPI

25. FEDERAL TAX I.D. NUMBER   SSN ☐ EIN ☐

26. PATIENT'S ACCOUNT NO.

27. ACCEPT ASSIGNMENT? (For govt. claims, see back)   YES ☐   NO ☐

28. TOTAL CHARGE $

29. AMOUNT PAID $

30. BALANCE DUE

31. SIGNATURE OF PHYSICIAN OR SUPPLIER INCLUDING DEGREES OR CREDENTIALS (I certify that the statements on the reverse apply to this bill and are made a part thereof.)

SIGNED _____ DATE _____

32. SERVICE FACILITY LOCATION INFORMATION

a. **NPI**   b.

33. BILLING PROVIDER INFO & PH # ( )

a. **NPI**   b.

NUCC Instruction Manual available at: www.nucc.org

APPROVED OMB-0938-0999 FORM CMS-1500 (08/05)

249

WORK PRODUCT 20-5

Name: _____

Complete a CMS-1500 Claim Form

Complete Claim Form #5 using the information in Part I, Question 15.

CHAPTER 21

Professional Fees, Billing, and Collecting

Vocabulary Review

Fill in the blanks with the correct vocabulary terms from this chapter.

1. Jesse has a(n) _____ _____ of $464.00, which represents the total amount she owes after her insurance paid a portion of her bill.

2. Mrs. Ramone has a(n) _____ on her account for an overpayment, so the office manager sent her a check for that amount.

3. Robert's mother is the _____ of his bill because she promised to pay the full amount for her son.

4. Julia had to _____ collections proceedings on several accounts last month because the patients had not made payments as promised.

5. One of the tasks that Pamela enjoys is _____ payments that arrive in the mail to patient accounts.

6. _____ _____ are used more and more often for payments in the physician's office.

7. An organization under contract to the government to handle insurance claims from providers is called a(n) _____ _____.

8. Mrs. Richland called the office to get the balance on her _____.

9. The office staff has been debating as to whether they should continue to offer _____ _____ to other healthcare providers and their staff members.

10. A business _____, which is any exchange or transfer of goods, services, or funds, must always be recorded.

11. Anna made several _____ for various bills that were due last week.

12. Dr. Taylor's fee _____ is a compilation of the fees he has charged over the past fiscal year.

13. The Peete family was considered _____ _____ because they could not afford medical care, even though they were able to pay basic living expenses.

14. Deb sometimes confuses a credit with a(n) _____, which is a deduction from a revenue, net worth, or liability account.

15. Jessica totaled the _____ for the day, which came from patient and insurance payments.

16. State Farm is considered a(n) _____ _____ _____, because Bethany's injuries were sustained in a car accident and State Farm will pay her medical bills.

17. Dr. Martin reviewed his fee _____, which is a compilation of preestablished fee allowances for given services or procedures.

18. Suzy sent a statement of _____ to all patients who had a balance over $5.00.

19. The Blackburn Clinic uses a computer to determine patient account balances, but June remembers when they used a manual _____ _____.

20. When Madelyn received the denial from Mr. Paul's insurance company, she wondered if he had paid his _____.

Skills and Concepts

Part I: Fee Schedules and Billing Forms

21. Examine the fee schedule on the next page, and answer the following questions.

    a. What is the charge for this consultation?

    b. What is the charge for a 99203?

    c. Why is the charge different for a 99213?

    d. What is the most expensive procedure on the list? CPT code _____

    e. Which injection is more expensive, insulin or vitamin B_{12}?

22. Use the same fee schedule to complete the billing forms in Work Products 21-1, 21-2, and 21-3. Circle the codes and fill in the charges for each patient. Assume that all of the patients have a previous balance of zero.

Work Product 21-1: Marilyn Westmoreland, established patient, straightforward, penicillin injections (75 mg), diagnosis—tonsillitis.

Work Product 21-2: Jane Wells, consultation, high complexity, ECG, diagnosis—chest pain.

Work Product 21-3: Paula Johnson, new patient, detailed, epinephrine injection (0.3 mL), diagnosis—rash.

FEE SCHEDULE

BLACKBURN PRIMARY CARE ASSOCIATES, PC
1990 Turquiose Drive
Blackburn, WI 54937
608-459-8857

Federal Tax ID Number: 00-0000000

BCBS Group Number: 14982
Medicare Group Number: 14982

OFFICE VISIT, NEW PATIENT

Focused, 99201	$45.00
Expanded, 99202	$55.00
Intermediate, 99203	$60.00
Extended, 99204	$95.00
Comprehensive, 99205	$195.00
Consultation, 99245	$250.00

OFFICE VISIT, ESTABLISHED PATIENT

Minimal, 99211	$40.00
Focused, 99212	$48.00
Intermediate, 99213	$55.00
Extended, 99214	$65.00
Comprehensive, 99215	$195.00

OFFICE PROCEDURES

EKG, 12 lead, 93000	$55.00
Stress EKG, Treadmill, 93015	$295.00
Sigmoidoscopy, Flex; 45330	$145.00
Spirometry, 94010	$50.00
Cerumen Removal, 69210	$40.00
Collection & Handling	
Lab Specimen, 99000	$9.00
Venipuncture, 35415	$9.00
Urinalysis, 81000	$20.00
Urinalysis, 81002 (Dip Only)	$12.00
Influenza Injection, 90724	$20.00
Pneumococcal Injection, 90732	$20.00
Oral Polio, 90712	$15.00
DTaP, 90700	$20.00
Tetanus Toxoid, 90703	$15.00
MMR, 90707	$25.00
HIB, 90737	$20.00
Hepatitis B, newborn to age 11 years, 90744	$60.00
Hepatitis B, 11-19 years, 90745	$60.00
Hepatitis B, 20 years and above 90746	$60.00
Intramuscular Injection, 90788	
Penicillin	$30.00
Cephtriaxone	$25.00
Solu-Medrol	$23.00
Vitamin B-12	$13.00
Subcutaneous Injection, 90782	
Epinephrine	$18.00
Susphrine	$25.00
Insulin, U-100	$15.00

COMMON DIAGNOSTIC CODES

Ischemic Heart Disease	414.9
w/o myocardial infarction	411.89
w/coronary occlusion	411.81
Hypertension, Malignant	401.0
Benign	401.1
Unspecified	401.9
w/congest. heart failure	402.91
Asthma, Bronchial	493.9
w/COPD	493.2
allergic, w/S.A.	493.91
allergic, w/o S.A.	493.90
Kyphosis	737.10
w/osteoporosis	733.0
Osteoporosis	733.00
Otitis Media, Acute	382.9
Chronic	382.9

Part II: Ledgers and Computing Patient Balances

Work through the following information, and record it on the ledger cards presented in the corresponding work product pages. Use one ledger for each exercise.

Ledger 1—Work Product 21-4:

Meagan Joy Reynolds
5534 Joe Pool Lake Road #233
Cedar Hill, Texas 75884
972-334-0423 (home)
972-331-0934 (cell)
meaganjoy@internet4.com
MR# REYM3341

Entry #	Transaction
1.	Meagan comes to the Blackburn Primary Care Clinic on April 12 as a new patient. Her initial charge is $375 because she had a series of x-ray examinations, which were used to diagnose a blockage in her small intestine. Dr. Lupez recommends that she have surgery to correct the blockage as soon as possible. Meagan pays her bill in full with check #7110, although she has insurance coverage through her own policy with Prudential and her husband's policy through Southwest United Healthcare.
2.	Meagan checks into Mercy Hospital and has surgery on April 21. Dr. Lupez charges $7500 for the surgery and aftercare, which will take approximately 6 weeks. This charge will be filed with Meagan's insurances.
3.	Meagan returns to the clinic on April 30 for a follow-up office visit. The charge is $150, which she pays in full with check #7261. Dr. Lupez says that she is doing very well since her surgery and asks her to return in mid May for another checkup.
4.	On May 2 the clinic receives an insurance payment from Prudential in the amount of $6200. This money is applied to Meagan's account. The check number is 617761.
5.	On May 3 the clinic receives check #7313 in the mail from Meagan for $300, which is applied to her account.
6.	Meagan returns to the clinic on May 14 for an office visit. The charge is $75, and she pays $50 with check #7512.
7.	Southwest United sends a check to the clinic for $800 on May 27, which is applied to her account. The check number is 8710.
8.	Meagan sends a check for $125 to be put toward her account. The check, #7915, is posted on June 2.
9.	Meagan returns to the clinic for an office visit and laboratory work on June 17. Her charges total $352, and she pays $150 with check #8116.
10.	On June 20 the clinic receives Meagan's check toward her account for $100. Her check number is 8411.
11.	Meagan visits the clinic for treatment of a migraine headache on June 26. Her charge is $85, and she pays $50 with check #8626. She schedules a follow-up visit with Dr. Lupez for June 30.
12.	When Meagan returns for her follow-up visit on June 30, her office visit is $85, but she is unable to make a payment.
13.	On July 5 the clinic receives a payment from Prudential on behalf of Meagan for $276. The Prudential check number is 721146.
14.	On July 18 the clinic receives a check #9210 from Southwest United on behalf of Meagan for $124.
15.	On July 31 the clinic refunds Meagan's credit balance to her using clinic check #9425.
16.	The previous transaction brings Meagan's account to zero.

Ledger 2—Work Product 21-5:

Zachary Paul Staley
2324 Hill Avenue Plaza
Grosse Pointe, MI 48230
313-445-9987 (home)
313-565-6623 (cell)
zachattack@aol.com
MR# STAZ9823

Entry #	Transaction
1.	Zachary Staley visited the clinic on June 6 as a new patient and was diagnosed as having diabetes. His charge was $215. He paid his $15 copay with check #126.
2.	On June 12, a check arrived from Permian Health for $180 on Zachary's account. The check number was 21617.
3.	Zachary returned to the clinic on June 15 for an office visit and laboratory work. The total charge was $128, and Zachary paid his $15 copay with check #214.
4.	On June 16 Zachary returned to the clinic without an appointment because he felt extremely dizzy and nauseated. He was seen by Dr. Hughes, who determined that his blood sugar had dropped substantially. After his condition was stabilized, his wife picked him up and took him home. She paid his $15 copay with check #217 and the total charge for the visit was $70.
5.	On July 7, check #36171 arrived from Permian Health on Zachary's account in the amount of $142.
6.	Bethany, an insurance biller, realized that a $7 charge was not allowed for a laboratory test on Zachary's account. The office policy allows disallowed charges under $10 to be written off, so Bethany adjusts his account by $7.
7.	Zachary returns to the clinic for a routine visit on July 26 and has laboratory work done. The total charge is $156, and Zachary pays his $15 copay with check #310.
8.	On August 1 Zachary has a brief office visit and is charged $70. Zachary forgot his checkbook, so he did not pay his copay.
9.	On August 16 Permian sends check #41217 in the amount of $102 toward Zachary's account.
10.	On August 21 Permian sends check #42168 in the amount of $55 toward Zachary's account.
11.	On August 30 the clinic receives check #561 from Zachary in the amount of $40 to be placed against his account.
12.	September 6 is Zachary's next office visit, and he is charged $70. He pays his $15 copay with check #587.
13.	Zachary sends $40 toward his account, which is received by the clinic on September 9. His check number is 620.
14.	Permian Health sends check #53121 in the amount of $98 to the clinic to be applied to Zachary's account.
15.	On October 3 the clinic receives check #681 from Zachary, who remembers that he did not pay his copay on August 1. He guesses that he owes about $40 total, but is unsure, so he sends $20.
16.	The clinic realizes that Zachary has overpaid on his account and sends him a refund for his credit balance.

Ledger 3—Work Product 21-6:

Lynn Annette Wilson
755 South Wheeley #4A
Sacramento, CA 94203
209-552-5437 (home)
209-553-7789 (cell)
lynnannw@yahoo.com
MR# WILL8845

Entry #	Transaction
1.	Lynn Annette is a single mother of four who has had a difficult year. She lost a job after contracting infectious mononucleosis and missing 3 weeks of work. She had barely recovered from that illness when she was diagnosed with ulcerative colitis. Her medical bills have become increasingly difficult to pay, although she did secure a new job and recently became eligible for coverage through Aetna. She is a determined woman with the best of intentions but often must put rent, utilities, and food costs before the payment of her medical bills. She comes to the clinic for a regular office visit on July 7. Her charges are $125 and she is able to pay the entire bill, since she has been saving the money for several weeks. She pays with check #1205.
2.	On July 12, Lynn Annette returns to the office and has laboratory work. Her charges are $89, and she pays her $20 copay with check #1314.
3.	Bethany in the insurance office notices that Lynn Annette was charged $9 for a single laboratory chemistry test that is not covered by her insurance. Because Bethany knows that Lynn Annette has faced financial difficulties this year, she adjusts the bill so that Lynn Annette will not be responsible for the charge. She also makes a note for the physicians that Lynn Annette's insurance does not cover that particular laboratory test and explains that an alternate chemistry test that will produce the same results is covered. The adjustment is made on July 19.
4.	Aetna sends an insurance payment (check #7611493) toward Lynn Annette's account that is received on July 23. The payment is for $85.
5.	Bethany processes a refund for Lynn Annette and sends her check #5612 from the clinic account. This brings her balance to zero.
6.	Lynn Annette comes to the office for a regular visit on August 1. Her charges are $284, and she pays her copay of $20 with check #1517.
7.	On August 18 the clinic receives a check from Aetna for $200 toward Lynn Annette's account. The check number is 8267484.
8.	Lynn Annette sends check #1622 in the amount of $64 to clear her account on August 31.
9.	On September 12 Lynn Annette's recent check payment is returned by her bank for insufficient funds. The clinic adds a charge of $30 to her account as a returned check fee.
10.	Lynn Annette comes to the clinic and apologizes for her recent returned check. She explains that she missed getting her paycheck into the bank in time to cover the payment. She brings a cashier's check to cover the check and the fee. The date is September 20.
11.	Lynn Annette has minor surgery in the office on October 15. The charge is $750, and she pays a copay of $20 in cash.
12.	On February 12 Lynn Annette sends a $20 payment on her account, using check #2612. She encloses a note that says she is still having financial difficulties and will send another payment as soon as she can.
13.	On April 10, Lynn Annette sends a payment of $5 using check #2711.
14.	On May 12, the clinic receives a payment from Lynn Annette in the amount of $5, using check #2781.
15.	In accordance with the clinic policy of reporting accounts to a collection agency after 3 months of nonpayment, Bethany reluctantly reports Lynn Annette's account to Smith Collections. The full balance is written off.
16.	On September 12 a payment of $100 is received from Lynn Annette. Bethany forwards the payment to the collection agency.

Complete a Day Sheet

23. Complete the proofs in Work Product 21-7 using the figures given.

Part III: Short Answer Questions

Provide the answers to the questions in the blanks below.

24. Define the following terms.

a. Usual

_____

_____

b. Customary

_____

_____

c. Reasonable

_____

_____

25. List four billing methods commonly used in the physician's office.

a. _____

b. _____

c. _____

d. _____

26. What notation should be made under the return address on statement envelopes?

_____

27. Briefly explain cycle billing.

_____

_____

28. What are the pitfalls of fee adjustments?

_____

_____

_____

29. What three values are considered when determining professional fees?

a. _____

b. _____

c. _____

30. Why are estimates useful in patient treatment?

_____

_____

31. List five general rules to follow when telephone collecting.

a. _____

b. _____

c. _____

d. _____

e. _____

32. List four ways that payment for medical services is accomplished.

a. _____

b. _____

c. _____

d. _____

33. Explain why patients sometimes fail to pay their accounts.

_____

_____

_____

34. What is professional courtesy, and why is it less common now than in years past?

_____

_____

_____

35. Briefly explain how "skips" can be traced.

_____

_____

_____

Case Study

Read back through the information about Lynn Annette Wilson on Ledger 3. How could the medical assistant help Lynn Annette to keep her account out of collections? What could be said to her during a friendly phone call to encourage her to be regular with her payments? Write two collection letters to Lynn Annette. Make the first letter a gentle reminder. The second letter should express that the account will be placed for collection if regular payments are not forthcoming. Use the stationery provided in Work Products 21-8 and 21-9 to write the collection letters.

Workplace Applications

Mr. Sanchez comes to the desk to check out after seeing the physician. When Sarah tells him that his bill is $95, he complains that he only saw the physician for 10 minutes. The fee is in accordance with the evaluation and management guidelines. Explain the fees to Mr. Sanchez. Use the space below to write what you would say to him as an explanation of his fees.

_____
_____
_____
_____
_____
_____

Use the space below to write a dialogue that can be used to ask a patient for payment as he or she is checking out.

_____
_____
_____
_____
_____
_____

Internet Activities

1. Research medical billing companies on the Internet, and compare the costs of the various services that they offer. Prepare a report or presentation for the class.

2. Search for patient accounting software, and explore the options available for the physician's office. Write a brief report on one software product, and present it to the class.

Chapter 21 Quiz

Name: _____

1. A statement that shows finance charges is called a(n) _____.

2. What is a "skip"?

   _____

   _____

3. Name an advantage of small claims court.

   _____

   _____

4. Collection agencies can charge 40% to 60%.

   a. True

   b. False

5. The total of all account balances that are due to the physician is called _____.

6. The pegboard is also called a(n)

   _____ _____ .

   _____ system.

7. What kind of balance occurs when an account is overpaid?

   _____

8. What is the term for the person who is responsible for a bill?

   _____

9. What is the name of the form that is attached to a medical record and on which the physician notes the charges and diagnosis?

   _____

10. UCR stands for _____ ,

    _____ , and _____ .

WORK PRODUCT 21-1

Name: _____

Complete the billing form below page using the information in Part I, Question 22.

Blackburn Primary Care Associates, PC
1990 Turquoise Drive
Blackburn, WI 54937
(608) 459-8857

Howard M. Lawler, MD   11
Joanne R. Hughes, MD   21
Ralph Garcia Lopez, MD   31
TAX ID NO. 00-00000000

GUARANTOR NAME AND ADDRESS	PATIENT NO.	PATIENT NAME	DOCTOR NO.	DATE
	DATE OF BIRTH	TELEPHONE NO.	INSURANCE	

INSURANCE: CODE | DESCRIPTION | CERTIFICATE NO.

OFFICE - NEW

X	CPT	SERVICE	FEE
	99201	Prob Foc/Straight	
	99202	Exp Prob/Straight	
	99203	Detailed/Low	
	99204	Compre/Moderate	
	99205	Compre/High	

OFFICE - ESTABLISHED

X	CPT	SERVICE	FEE
	99211	Nurse/Minimal	
	99212	Prob Foc/Straight	
	99213	Exp Prob/Low	
	99214	Detailed/Moderate	
	99215	Compre/High	

OFFICE - CONSULT

X	CPT	SERVICE	FEE
	99241	Prob/Foc/Straight	
	99242	Exp Prob/Straight	
	99243	Detailed/Low	
	99244	Compre/Moderate	
	99245	Compre/High	

PREVENTIVE CARE - ADULT

X	CPT	SERVICE	FEE
	99385	18-39 Initial	
	99386	40-64 Initial	
	99387	65+ Initial	
	99395	18-39 Periodic	
	99396	40-64 Periodic	
	99397	65+ Periodic	

GASTROENEROLOGY

X	CPT	SERVICE	FEE
	45300	Sigmoidoscopy Rig	
	45305	Sigmoid Rig w/bx	
	45330	Sigmoidoscopy Flex	
	45331	Sigmoid Flex w/bx	
	45378	Colonoscopy Diag	
	45380	Colonoscopy w/bx	
	46600	Anoscopy	

CARDIOLOGY & HEARING

X	CPT	SERVICE	FEE
	93000	EKG (Global)	
	93015	Stress Test (Global)	
	93224	Holter (Global)	
	93225	Holter Hook Up	
	93227	Holter Interpretation	
	94010	Pulm Function Test	
	92551	Audiometry Screen	

INJECTIONS & IMMUNIZATION

X	CPT	SERVICE	FEE
	86585	TB Skin Test	
	90716	Varicella Vaccine	
	90724	Flu Vaccine	
	90732	Pneumovax	
	90718	TD Immunization	
	90782	Injection IM*	
	90788	Injection IM Antibiot*	
		Injection joint*	

REPAIR & DERMATOLOGY

X	CPT	SERVICE	FEE
	17110	Warts: #	
		Tags: #	
		Lesion Excis	
		Lesion Destruct	

SIZE CM: SITE:
MALIG: PREMAL/BEN:
(Check One Above)
Simple Closure
Intermed Closure
SIZE CM: SITE:

| | 10060 | I&D Abscess | |
| | 10080 | I&D Cyst | |

OTHER

SUPPLIES/DRUGS*

DRUG NAME:
UNIT/MEASURE:
QUANTITY

SM   MED   MAJOR
(circle one)
FOR ALL INJECTIONS, SUPPLY DRUG
INFORMATION

DIAGNOSTIC CODES: ICD-9-CM

- [ ] 789.0 Abdominal Pain
- [ ] 795.0 Abnormal Pap Smear
- [ ] 706.1 Acne Vulgaris
- [ ] 477.0 Allergic Rhinitis
- [ ] 285.9 Anemia, NOS
- [ ] 281.0 Pernicious
- [ ] 411.1 Angina, Unstable
- [ ] 427.9 Arythmia, NOS
- [ ] 440.9 Arteriosclerosis
- [ ] 714.0 Arthritis, Rheumatoid
- [ ] 414.0 ASHD
- [ ] 493.90 Asthma, Bronchial W/O Status Ast.
- [ ] 493.91 Asthma, Bronchial W/Status Ast.
- [ ] 466.1 Bronchiolitis, Acute
- [ ] 466.0 Bronchitis, Acute
- [ ] 727.3 Bursitis
- [ ] 786.50 Chest Pain
- [ ] 574.20 Cholelithiasis
- [ ] 372.30 Conjunctivitis, Unspecified
- [ ] 564.0 Constipation
- [ ] 496 COPD
- [ ] 692.9 Dermatitis, Allergic
- [ ] 250.01 Diabetes Mellitus, ID
- [ ] 250.00 Diabetes Mellitus, NID
- [ ] 558.9 Diarrhea
- [ ] 562.11 Diverticulitis
- [ ] 562.10 Diverticulosis

- [ ] 782.3 Edema
- [ ] 492.8 Emphysema
- [ ] V16.0 Family History Of Diabetes
- [ ] 780.6 Fever of Undetermined Origin
- [ ] 578.9 G.I. Bleeding, Unspecified
- [ ] 727.41 Ganglion of Joint
- [ ] 535.0 Gastritis, Acute
- [ ] V72.3 Arythmia, NOS
- [ ] 748.0 Headache
- [ ] 550.90 Hernia, Inguinal, NOS
- [ ] 054.9 Herpes Simplex
- [ ] 053.9 Herpes Zoster
- [ ] 708.9 Hives/Urticaria
- [ ] 401.1 Hypertension, Benign
- [ ] 401.0 Hypertension, Malignant
- [ ] 402.90 Hypertension, W/O CHF
- [ ] 244.9 Hypothyroidism, Primary
- [ ] 380.4 Impacted Cerumen
- [ ] 487.1 Influenza
- [ ] 564.1 Irritable Bowel Syndrome
- [ ] 464.0 Laryngitis, Acute
- [ ] 454.9 Leg Varicose Veins
- [ ] 424.0 Mitral Valve Prolapse
- [ ] 412 Myocardial Infarction, Old
- [ ] 715.90 Osteoarthritis, Unspec. Site
- [ ] 620.2 Ovarian Cyst

- [ ] 614.9 Pelvic Inflammatory Disease
- [ ] 685.1 Pilonidal Cyst
- [ ] 462 Pharyngitis, Acute
- [ ] 627.2 Postmenopausal Bleeding
- [ ] 625.4 Premenstrual Tension
- [ ] 782.1 Rash
- [ ] 569.3 Rectal Bleeding
- [ ] 398.90 Rheumatic Heart Disease, NOS
- [ ] 431.9 Sinusitis, Acute, NOS
- [ ] 782.1 Skin Eruption, Rash
- [ ] 845.00 Sprain, Ankle
- [ ] 848.9 Sprain, Muscle, Unspec. Site
- [ ] 785.6 Swollen Glands
- [ ] 246.9 Thyroid Disease, Unspecified
- [ ] 463 Tonsillitis, Acute

- [ ] 474.0 Tonsillitis, Chronic
- [ ] 465.9 Upper Respiratory Infection, Acute
- [ ] 599.0 Urinary Tract Infection
- [ ] V03.9 Vaccination/Bacterial Dis.
- [ ] V06.8 Vaccination/Combination
- [ ] V04.8 Vaccination, Influenza
- [ ] 616.10 Vaginitis, Vulvitis, NOS
- [ ] 780.4 Vertigo
- [ ] 787.0 Vomiting, Nausea
- [ ] _____
- [ ] _____
- [ ] _____

RETURN APPOINTMENT

_____ Days
_____ Weeks
_____ Months

Authorization Number:
▶ _____

Place of Service:
( ) Office
( ) Emergency Room
( ) Inpatient Hospital
( ) Outpatient Hospital
( ) Nursing Home

BALANCE DUE

DATE OF SERVICE	CPT CODE	DIAGNOSIS CODE(S)	CHARGE

TOTAL CHARGE	$
AMOUNT PAID	$
PREVIOUS BAL	$
BALANCE DUE	$

Check #: _____
(Circle Method of Payment)
CASH   CHECK   MC   VISA

Physician's Signature
▶ _____

WORK PRODUCT 21-2

Name: _____

Complete the billing form below using the information in Part I, Question 22.

Blackburn Primary Care Associates, PC
1990 Turquoise Drive
Blackburn, WI 54937
(608) 459-8857

Howard M. Lawler, MD   11
Joanne R. Hughes, MD   21
Ralph Garcia Lopez, MD   31
TAX ID NO. 00-00000000

GUARANTOR NAME AND ADDRESS	PATIENT NO.	PATIENT NAME		DOCTOR NO.	DATE

	DATE OF BIRTH	TELEPHONE NO.	INSURANCE		
			CODE	DESCRIPTION	CERTIFICATE NO.

OFFICE - NEW

X	CPT	SERVICE	FEE
	99201	Prob Foc/Straight	
	99202	Exp Prob/Straight	
	99203	Detailed/Low	
	99204	Compre/Moderate	
	99205	Compre/High	

OFFICE - ESTABLISHED

X	CPT	SERVICE	FEE
	99211	Nurse/Minimal	
	99212	Prob Foc/Straight	
	99213	Exp Prob/Low	
	99214	Detailed/Moderate	
	99215	Compre/High	

OFFICE - CONSULT

X	CPT	SERVICE	FEE
	99241	Prob Foc/Straight	
	99242	Exp Prob/Straight	
	99243	Detailed/Low	
	99244	Compre/Moderate	
	99245	Compre/High	

PREVENTIVE CARE - ADULT

X	CPT	SERVICE	FEE
	99385	18-39 Initial	
	99386	40-64 Initial	
	99387	65+ Initial	
	99395	18-39 Periodic	
	99396	40-64 Periodic	
	99397	65+ Periodic	

GASTROENEROLOGY

X	CPT	SERVICE	FEE
	45300	Sigmoidoscopy Rig	
	45305	Sigmoid Rig w/bx	
	45330	Sigmoidoscopy Flex	
	45331	Sigmoid Flex w/bx	
	45378	Colonoscopy Diag	
	45380	Colonoscopy w/bx	
	46600	Anoscopy	

CARDIOLOGY & HEARING

X	CPT	SERVICE	FEE
	93000	EKG (Global)	
	93015	Stress Test (Global)	
	93224	Holter (Global)	
	93225	Holter Hook Up	
	93227	Holter Interpretation	
	94010	Pulm Function Test	
	92551	Audiometry Screen	

INJECTIONS & IMMUNIZATION

X	CPT	SERVICE	FEE
	86585	TB Skin Test	
	90716	Varicella Vaccine	
	90724	Flu Vaccine	
	90732	Pneumovax	
	90718	TD Immunization	
	90782	Injection IM*	
	90788	Injection IM Antibiot*	
		Injection joint*	

REPAIR & DERMATOLOGY

X	CPT	SERVICE	FEE
	17110	Warts: #	
		Tags: #	
		Lesion Excis	
		Lesion Destruct	
SIZE CM:		SITE:	
MALIG:		PREMAL/BEN:	
		(Check One Above)	
		Simple Closure	
		Intermed Closure	
SIZE CM:		SITE:	
	10060	I&D Abscess	
	10080	I&D Cyst	

OTHER / SUPPLIES/DRUGS*

DRUG NAME:
UNIT/MEASURE:
QUANTITY

SM   MED   MAJOR
(circle one)

FOR ALL INJECTIONS, SUPPLY DRUG
INFORMATION

DIAGNOSTIC CODES: ICD-9-CM

- ☐ 789.0 Abdominal Pain
- ☐ 795.0 Abnormal Pap Smear
- ☐ 706.1 Acne Vulgaris
- ☐ 477.0 Allergic Rhinitis
- ☐ 285.9 Anemia, NOS
- ☐ 281.0 Pernicious
- ☐ 411.1 Angina, Unstable
- ☐ 427.9 Arythmia, NOS
- ☐ 440.9 Arteriosclerosis
- ☐ 714.0 Arthritis, Rheumatoid
- ☐ 414.0 ASHD
- ☐ 493.90 Asthma, Bronchial W/O Status Ast.
- ☐ 493.91 Asthma, Bronchial W/Status Ast.
- ☐ 466.1 Bronchiolitis, Acute
- ☐ 466.0 Bronchitis, Acute
- ☐ 727.3 Bursitis
- ☐ 786.50 Chest Pain
- ☐ 574.20 Cholelithiasis
- ☐ 372.30 Conjunctivitis, Unspecified
- ☐ 564.0 Constipation
- ☐ 496 COPD
- ☐ 692.9 Dermatitis, Allergic
- ☐ 250.01 Diabetes Mellitus, ID
- ☐ 250.00 Diabetes Mellitus, NID
- ☐ 558.9 Diarrhea
- ☐ 562.11 Diverticulitis
- ☐ 562.10 Diverticulosis

- ☐ 782.3 Edema
- ☐ 492.8 Emphysema
- ☐ V16.0 Family History Of Diabetes
- ☐ 780.6 Fever of Undetermined Origin
- ☐ 578.9 G.I. Bleeding, Unspecified
- ☐ 727.41 Ganglion of Joint
- ☐ 535.0 Gastritis, Acute
- ☐ V72.3 Arythmia, NOS
- ☐ 748.0 Headache
- ☐ 550.90 Hernia, Inguinal, NOS
- ☐ 054.9 Herpes Simplex
- ☐ 053.9 Herpes Zoster
- ☐ 708.9 Hives/Urticaria
- ☐ 401.1 Hypertension, Benign
- ☐ 401.0 Hypertension, Malignant
- ☐ 402.90 Hypertension, W/O CHF
- ☐ 244.9 Hypothyroidism, Primary
- ☐ 380.4 Impacted Cerumen
- ☐ 487.1 Influenza
- ☐ 564.1 Irritable Bowel Syndrome
- ☐ 464.0 Laryngitis, Acute
- ☐ 454.9 Leg Varicose Veins
- ☐ 424.0 Mitral Valve Prolapse
- ☐ 412 Myocardial Infarction, Old
- ☐ 715.90 Osteoarthritis, Unspec. Site
- ☐ 620.2 Ovarian Cyst

- ☐ 614.9 Pelvic Inflammatory Disease
- ☐ 685.1 Pilonidal Cyst
- ☐ 462 Pharyngitis, Acute
- ☐ 627.1 Postmenopausal Bleeding
- ☐ 625.4 Premenstrual Tension
- ☐ 782.1 Rash
- ☐ 569.3 Rectal Bleeding
- ☐ 398.90 Rheumatic Heart Disease, NOS
- ☐ 431.9 Sinusitis, Acute, NOS
- ☐ 782.1 Skin Eruption, Rash
- ☐ 845.00 Sprain, Ankle
- ☐ 848.9 Sprain, Muscle, Unspec. Site
- ☐ 785.6 Swollen Glands
- ☐ 246.9 Thyroid Disease, Unspecified
- ☐ 463 Tonsillitis, Acute

- ☐ 474.0 Tonsillitis, Chronic
- ☐ 465.9 Upper Respiratory Infection, Acute
- ☐ 599.0 Urinary Tract Infection
- ☐ V03.9 Vaccination/Bacterial Dis.
- ☐ V06.8 Vaccination/Combination
- ☐ V04.8 Vaccination, Influenza
- ☐ 616.10 Vaginitis, Vulvitis, NOS
- ☐ 780.4 Vertigo
- ☐ 787.0 Vomiting, Nausea
- ☐ ___ _____
- ☐ ___ _____
- ☐ ___ _____
- ☐ ___ _____

RETURN APPOINTMENT

_____ Days
_____ Weeks
_____ Months

Authorization Number:
▶ _____

BALANCE DUE

DATE OF SERVICE	CPT CODE	DIAGNOSIS CODE(S)	CHARGE

Place of Service:
( ) Office
( ) Emergency Room
( ) Inpatient Hospital
( ) Outpatient Hospital
( ) Nursing Home

TOTAL CHARGE	$
AMOUNT PAID	$
PREVIOUS BAL	$
BALANCE DUE	$

Check #: _____

(Circle Method of Payment)
CASH   CHECK   MC   VISA

Physician's Signature
▶ _____

WORK PRODUCT 21-3

Name: _____

Complete the billing form below using the information in Part I, Question 22.

Blackburn Primary Care Associates, PC
1990 Turquoise Drive
Blackburn, WI 54937
(608) 459-8857

Howard M. Lawler, MD   11
Joanne R. Hughes, MD   21
Ralph Garcia Lopez, MD   31
TAX ID NO. 00-00000000

GUARANTOR NAME AND ADDRESS	PATIENT NO.	PATIENT NAME	DOCTOR NO.	DATE
	DATE OF BIRTH	TELEPHONE NO.	INSURANCE	

INSURANCE: CODE | DESCRIPTION | CERTIFICATE NO.

OFFICE - NEW

X	CPT	SERVICE	FEE
	99201	Prob Foc/Straight	
	99202	Exp Prob/Straight	
	99203	Detailed/Low	
	99204	Compre/Moderate	
	99205	Compre/High	

OFFICE - ESTABLISHED

X	CPT	SERVICE	FEE
	99211	Nurse/Minimal	
	99212	Prob Foc/Straight	
	99213	Exp Prob/Low	
	99214	Detailed/Moderate	
	99215	Compre/High	

OFFICE - CONSULT

X	CPT	SERVICE	FEE
	99241	Prob/Foc/Straight	
	99242	Exp Prob/Straight	
	99243	Detailed/Low	
	99244	Compre/Moderate	
	99245	Compre/High	

PREVENTIVE CARE - ADULT

X	CPT	SERVICE	FEE
	99385	18-39 Initial	
	99386	40-64 Initial	
	99387	65+ Initial	
	99395	18-39 Periodic	
	99396	40-64 Periodic	
	99397	65+ Periodic	

GASTROENEROLOGY

X	CPT	SERVICE	FEE
	45300	Sigmoidoscopy Rig	
	45305	Sigmoid Rig w/bx	
	45330	Sigmoidoscopy Flex	
	45331	Sigmoid Flex w/bx	
	45378	Colonoscopy Diag	
	45380	Colonoscopy w/bx	
	46600	Anoscopy	

CARDIOLOGY & HEARING

X	CPT	SERVICE	FEE
	93000	EKG (Global)	
	93015	Stress Test (Global)	
	93224	Holter (Global)	
	93225	Holter Hook Up	
	93227	Holter Interpretation	
	94010	Pulm Function Test	
	92551	Audiometry Screen	

INJECTIONS & IMMUNIZATION

X	CPT	SERVICE	FEE
	86585	TB Skin Test	
	90716	Varicella Vaccine	
	90724	Flu Vaccine	
	90732	Pneumovax	
	90718	TD Immunization	
	90782	Injection IM*	
	90788	Injection IM Antibiot*	
		Injection joint*	

REPAIR & DERMATOLOGY

X	CPT	SERVICE	FEE
	17110	Warts: #	
		Tags: #	
		Lesion Excis	
		Lesion Destruct	

SIZE CM: SITE: _____
MALIG: PREMAL/BEN:
(Check One Above)
Simple Closure
Intermed Closure

OTHER

SUPPLIES/DRUGS*

DRUG NAME:
UNIT/MEASURE:
QUANTITY

SM   MED   MAJOR
(circle one)

FOR ALL INJECTIONS, SUPPLY DRUG
INFORMATION

| 10060 | I&D Abscess |
| 10080 | I&D Cyst |

SIZE CM: SITE:

DIAGNOSTIC CODES: ICD-9-CM

☐ 789.0	Abdominal Pain	☐ 782.3	Edema	☐ 614.9	Pelvic Inflammatory Disease	☐ 474.0	Tonsillitis, Chronic
☐ 795.0	Abnormal Pap Smear	☐ 492.8	Emphysema	☐ 685.1	Pilonidal Cyst	☐ 465.9	Upper Respiratory Infection, Acute
☐ 706.1	Acne Vulgaris	☐ V16.0	Family History Of Diabetes	☐ 462	Pharyngitis, Acute	☐ 599.0	Urinary Tract Infection
☐ 477.0	Allergic Rhinitis	☐ 780.6	Fever of Undetermined Origin	☐ 627.1	Postmenopausal Bleeding	☐ V03.9	Vaccination/Bacterial Dis.
☐ 285.9	Anemia, NOS	☐ 578.9	G.I. Bleeding, Unspecified	☐ 625.4	Premenstrual Tension	☐ V06.8	Vaccination/Combination
☐ 281.0	Pernicious	☐ 727.41	Ganglion of Joint	☐ 782.1	Rash	☐ V04.8	Vaccination, Influenza
☐ 411.1	Angina, Unstable	☐ 535.0	Gastritis, Acute	☐ 569.3	Rectal Bleeding	☐ 616.10	Vaginitis, Vulvitis, NOS
☐ 427.9	Arythmia, NOS	☐ V72.3	Arythmia, NOS	☐ 398.90	Rheumatic Heart Disease, NOS	☐ 780.4	Vertigo
☐ 440.9	Arteriosclerosis	☐ 748.0	Headache	☐ 431.9	Sinusitis, Acute, NOS	☐ 787.0	Vomiting, Nausea
☐ 714.0	Arthritis, Rheumatoid	☐ 550.90	Hernia, Inguinal, NOS	☐ 782.1	Skin Eruption, Rash	☐ ____	_____
☐ 414.0	ASHD	☐ 054.9	Herpes Simplex	☐ 845.00	Sprain, Ankle	☐ ____	_____
☐ 493.90	Asthma, Bronchial W/O Status Ast.	☐ 053.9	Herpes Zoster	☐ 848.9	Sprain, Muscle, Unspec. Site	☐ ____	_____
☐ 493.91	Asthma, Bronchial W/Status Ast.	☐ 708.9	Hives/Urticaria	☐ 785.6	Swollen Glands	☐ ____	_____
☐ 466.1	Bronchiolitis, Acute	☐ 401.1	Hypertension, Benign	☐ 246.9	Thyroid Disease, Unspecified		
☐ 466.0	Bronchitis, Acute	☐ 401.0	Hypertension, Malignant	☐ 463	Tonsillitis, Acute		
☐ 727.3	Bursitis	☐ 402.90	Hypertension, W/O CHF				
☐ 786.50	Chest Pain	☐ 244.9	Hypothyroidism, Primary				
☐ 574.20	Cholelithiasis	☐ 380.4	Impacted Cerumen				
☐ 372.30	Conjunctivitis, Unspecified	☐ 487.1	Influenza				
☐ 564.0	Constipation	☐ 564.1	Irritable Bowel Syndrome				
☐ 496	COPD	☐ 464.0	Laryngitis, Acute				
☐ 692.9	Dermatitis, Allergic	☐ 454.9	Leg Varicose Veins				
☐ 250.01	Diabetes Mellitus, ID	☐ 424.0	Mitral Valve Prolapse				
☐ 250.00	Diabetes Mellitus, NID	☐ 412	Myocardial Infarction, Old				
☐ 558.9	Diarrhea	☐ 715.90	Osteoarthritis, Unspec. Site				
☐ 562.11	Diverticulitis	☐ 620.2	Ovarian Cyst				
☐ 562.10	Diverticulosis						

RETURN APPOINTMENT

_____ Days
_____ Weeks
_____ Months

Authorization Number:
▶ _____

BALANCE DUE

DATE OF SERVICE	CPT CODE	DIAGNOSIS CODE(S)	CHARGE

Place of Service:
( ) Office
( ) Emergency Room
( ) Inpatient Hospital
( ) Outpatient Hospital
( ) Nursing Home

TOTAL CHARGE	$
AMOUNT PAID	$
PREVIOUS BAL	$
BALANCE DUE	$

Check #: _____
(Circle Method of Payment)
CASH   CHECK   MC   VISA

Physician's Signature
▶ _____

WORK PRODUCT 21-4

Name: _____

Fill out the ledger using the information in Part II, Ledger 1.

Blackburn Primary Care Associates, PC
1990 Turquoise Drive
Blackburn, WI 54937
Phone: 608-459-8857
Fax: 608-459-8860
E-mail: blackburnom@blackburnpca.com
www.blackburnpca.com

Patient Name _____

Address _____

City _____ State _____ Zip _____

Home Phone _____ Cell Phone _____

Email _____ MR# _____

Account Ledger							
Entry #	Date	Reference	Service	Charge	Payment	Adj	Current Balance
1							
2							
3							
4							
5							
6							
7							
8							
9							
10							
11							
12							
13							
14							
15							
16							

WORK PRODUCT 21-5

Name: _____

Fill out the ledger using the information in Part II, Ledger 2.

Blackburn Primary Care Associates, PC
1990 Turquoise Drive
Blackburn, WI 54937
Phone: 608-459-8857
Fax: 608-459-8860
E-mail: blackburnom@blackburnpca.com
www.blackburnpca.com

Patient Name _____

Address _____

City _____ State _____ Zip _____

Home Phone _____ Cell Phone _____

Email _____ MR# _____

			Account Ledger				
Entry #	Date	Reference	Service	Charge	Payment	Adj	Current Balance
1							
2							
3							
4							
5							
6							
7							
8							
9							
10							
11							
12							
13							
14							
15							
16							

WORK PRODUCT 21-6

Name: _____

Fill out the ledger using the information in Part II, Ledger 3.

Blackburn Primary Care Associates, PC
1990 Turquoise Drive
Blackburn, WI 54937
Phone: 608-459-8857
Fax: 608-459-8860
E-mail: blackburnom@blackburnpca.com
www.blackburnpca.com

Patient Name _____

Address _____

City _____ State _____ Zip_____

Home Phone _____ Cell Phone _____

Email _____ MR# _____

			Account Ledger				
Entry #	Date	Reference	Service	Charge	Payment	Adj	Current Balance
1							
2							
3							
4							
5							
6							
7							
8							
9							
10							
11							
12							
13							
14							
15							
16							

WORK PRODUCT 21-7

Name: _____

Complete the proofs below using the figures given.

Make certain that the final totals in Boxes 2 and 3 match exactly.

Today's Totals

Column A	Fees/Charges	$896.00
Column B	Payments	$1643.00
Column C	Adjustments	$36.00
Column D	New Balance	$3526.00
Column E	Old Balance	$4309.00

Daily Proof - Box One
Arithmetic Posting Proof

Column E	
Plus Column A	
Subtotal	
Minus Column B	
Subtotal	
Minus Column C	
Equals Column D	

Accounts Receivable
Beginning of Month $9071.00
Column A MTD $6589.00
Column B MTD $8226.00
Column C MTD $294.00
Year to Date – Box Three
Accounts Receivable Proof

Accounts Receivable
Previous Day 7923.00
Month to Date – Box Two
Accounts Receivable Proof

Accounts Receivable Previous Day	
Plus Column A	
Subtotal	
Minus Column B	
Subtotal	
Minus Column C	
Accounts Receivable End of Day	

Accounts Receivable Beginning of Month	
Plus Column A Month to Date	
Subtotal	
Minus Column B Month to Date	
Subtotal	
Minus Column C Month to Date	
Accounts Receivable Month to Date	

↑———— TOTALS MUST EQUAL ————↑

WORK PRODUCT 21-8

Name: _____

Blackburn Primary Care Associates
1990 Turquoise Drive
Blackburn, WI 54937
(555) 555-1234

WORK PRODUCT 21-9

Name: _____

Blackburn Primary Care Associates
1990 Turquoise Drive
Blackburn, WI 54937
(555) 555-1234

CHAPTER **22**

Banking Services and Procedures

Vocabulary Review

Fill in the blanks with the correct vocabulary terms from this chapter.

1. Judy was unaware that checks were processed through _____ before they arrived at her bank.

2. Because Alicia was the person who wrote the check, she was considered to be the _____.

3. When the Blackburn Clinic purchased the ultrasound machine, they paid $10,000 toward the _____ so that they would be charged less interest.

4. Pamela wrote a check to Samantha, so Pamela is the _____ and Samantha is the _____.

5. The _____ of a check is the person who is presenting it for payment and may not be the person named as the payee.

6. Grace studied the _____ _____ _____, which is a series of laws that regulates sales of goods, commercial paper, secured transactions in personal property, and many aspects of banking.

7. First National Bank is considered the _____ for Dr. Lupez' business checking accounts.

8. Instruments that are legally transferable to another party are considered _____.

9. Rhonda made several _____ from the clinic checking account to pay monthly bills and order supplies.

10. As soon as the monthly bank statement arrives, Rhonda does a _____ _____ to make certain that the statement and checkbook balance are in agreement.

Skills and Concepts

Part I: Short Answer Questions

Provide the answers to the questions in the blanks below.

11. List the four requirements of a negotiable instrument.

    a. _____

    b. _____

    c. _____

    d. _____

12. Name several advantages to online banking.

    _____

    _____

    _____

13. Why is customer service such an important aspect of today's medical offices?

    _____

    _____

    _____

14. List seven types of checks.

    a. _____

    b. _____

    c. _____

    d. _____

    e. _____

    f. _____

    g. _____

15. Describe each type of endorsement.

    a. blank

    _____

    b. restrictive

    _____

    c. special

    _____

    d. qualified

    _____

16. List five reasons that checks should be deposited promptly.

   a. _____

   b. _____

   c. _____

   d. _____

   e. _____

17. Provide five guidelines for check acceptance.

   a. _____

   b. _____

   c. _____

   d. _____

   e. _____

18. List three reasons that an individual might stop payment on a check.

   a. _____

   b. _____

   c. _____

19. Explain the ABA number and what each part of the number means.

   _____

   _____

   _____

20. List the three basic steps for preparing a deposit slip.

   a. _____

   b. _____

   c. _____

Part II: Writing Checks for Disbursement of Funds

Write checks to pay the following bills. The beginning balance in the checkbook is $4562.79. Use the checks numbered 5648 to 5651 on p. 287.

21. Write check #5648 to the American Medical Association for $356.00 for new coding books.

22. Write check #5649 to the Blackburn Utility Company for $46.90 to pay the water bill.

23. Write a check for the office mortgage payment to First National Bank, in the amount of $1,700.00. Use check #5650.

24. Write check #5651 to pay a pharmacy bill of $98.34.

25. Determine the balance of the account after the funds in questions 21 to 24 have been deducted.

Part III: Writing Refund Checks

Write checks for the following refunds. Use the ending balance from question 25 to determine the final balance in the checking account. Use the checks numbered 5652 to 5655 on page 288.

26. Ms. Patty Bailey should receive a refund in the amount of $34.55 for an overpayment. Use check #5652.

27. Write a check for Julie Smithy for $224.12. Her insurance company paid more than expected, so she is entitled to a refund. Use check #5653.

28. Cindy Chan paid $10 more than she owed when she was seeing Dr. Hughes. Refund her money using check #5654.

29. Carter Graves decided to postpone his knee surgery when his wife suddenly became ill. Use check #5655 to refund his $500 deposit.

30. Determine the balance of the checking account after the funds in questions 26 to 29 have been deducted.

Part IV: Prepare a Bank Deposit

Prepare a bank deposit detail for a $2230.00 deposit. Use the information in questions 31 to 34. Record your answers on the figure in Work Product 22-1.

31. Cash receipts total $646.68; $2.68 was in coins.

32. Check payments were #2387 for $67.00 from Sue Patrick and #460 for $50.00 from Ronald Rodriguez.

33. Credit card payments were $25.00 and $67.00. Pam Adtkins paid the $25.00 payment, and Brad Wilson paid the $67.00 payment.

34. An insurance payment for Alejandro Sanchez arrived in the amount of $1374.32. The payment was from Aetna and was check #309.

Part V: Reconcile a Bank Statement

Reconcile the bank statement using the facts and figure that follow. Use the figure on page 289 to show your work.

35. The checkbook balance is $4616.96.

36. The statement balance is $6792.79 (this amount includes the deposit of $2230.00—do not add that amount in again).

37. Three checks are outstanding: check #5648 for $356.00; check #5649 for $46.90; and check #5650 for $1770.00.

38. Does the checkbook reconcile with the statement?

Check 5648

5648

DATE _____

TO _____

FOR _____

BALANCE BROUGHT FORWARD		
DEPOSITS		
BALANCE		
AMT THIS CK		
BALANCE CARRIED FORWARD		

BLACKBURN PRIMARY CARE ASSOCIATES, PC
1990 Turquoise Drive
Blackburn, WI 54937
608-459-8857

5648

94-72/1224

DATE _____

PAY TO THE ORDER OF _____ $ _____

_____ DOLLARS

DERBYSHIRE SAVINGS
Member FDIC
P.O. BOX 8923
Blackburn, WI 54937

FOR _____

⑈055003⑈ 446782011⑈ 678800470

Check 5649

5649

DATE _____

TO _____

FOR _____

BALANCE BROUGHT FORWARD		
DEPOSITS		
BALANCE		
AMT THIS CK		
BALANCE CARRIED FORWARD		

BLACKBURN PRIMARY CARE ASSOCIATES, PC
1990 Turquoise Drive
Blackburn, WI 54937
608-459-8857

5649

94-72/1224

DATE _____

PAY TO THE ORDER OF _____ $ _____

_____ DOLLARS

DERBYSHIRE SAVINGS
Member FDIC
P.O. BOX 8923
Blackburn, WI 54937

FOR _____

⑈055003⑈ 446782011⑈ 678800470

Check 5650

5650

DATE _____

TO _____

FOR _____

BALANCE BROUGHT FORWARD		
DEPOSITS		
BALANCE		
AMT THIS CK		
BALANCE CARRIED FORWARD		

BLACKBURN PRIMARY CARE ASSOCIATES, PC
1990 Turquoise Drive
Blackburn, WI 54937
608-459-8857

5650

94-72/1224

DATE _____

PAY TO THE ORDER OF _____ $ _____

_____ DOLLARS

DERBYSHIRE SAVINGS
Member FDIC
P.O. BOX 8923
Blackburn, WI 54937

FOR _____

⑈055003⑈ 446782011⑈ 678800470

Check 5651

5651

DATE _____

TO _____

FOR _____

BALANCE BROUGHT FORWARD		
DEPOSITS		
BALANCE		
AMT THIS CK		
BALANCE CARRIED FORWARD		

BLACKBURN PRIMARY CARE ASSOCIATES, PC
1990 Turquoise Drive
Blackburn, WI 54937
608-459-8857

5651

94-72/1224

DATE _____

PAY TO THE ORDER OF _____ $ _____

_____ DOLLARS

DERBYSHIRE SAVINGS
Member FDIC
P.O. BOX 8923
Blackburn, WI 54937

FOR _____

⑈055003⑈ 446782011⑈ 678800470

5652

DATE _____
TO _____
FOR _____

BALANCE BROUGHT FORWARD		
DEPOSITS		
BALANCE		
AMT THIS CK		
BALANCE CARRIED FORWARD		

BLACKBURN PRIMARY CARE ASSOCIATES, PC
1990 Turquoise Drive
Blackburn, WI 54937
608-459-8857

5652
94-72/1224

DATE _____

PAY TO THE ORDER OF _____ $ _____

_____ DOLLARS

DERBYSHIRE SAVINGS Member FDIC
P.O. BOX 8923
Blackburn, WI 54937

FOR _____

⑈055003⑈ 446782011⑈ 678800470

5653

DATE _____
TO _____
FOR _____

BALANCE BROUGHT FORWARD		
DEPOSITS		
BALANCE		
AMT THIS CK		
BALANCE CARRIED FORWARD		

BLACKBURN PRIMARY CARE ASSOCIATES, PC
1990 Turquoise Drive
Blackburn, WI 54937
608-459-8857

5653
94-72/1224

DATE _____

PAY TO THE ORDER OF _____ $ _____

_____ DOLLARS

DERBYSHIRE SAVINGS Member FDIC
P.O. BOX 8923
Blackburn, WI 54937

FOR _____

⑈055003⑈ 446782011⑈ 678800470

5654

DATE _____
TO _____
FOR _____

BALANCE BROUGHT FORWARD		
DEPOSITS		
BALANCE		
AMT THIS CK		
BALANCE CARRIED FORWARD		

BLACKBURN PRIMARY CARE ASSOCIATES, PC
1990 Turquoise Drive
Blackburn, WI 54937
608-459-8857

5654
94-72/1224

DATE _____

PAY TO THE ORDER OF _____ $ _____

_____ DOLLARS

DERBYSHIRE SAVINGS Member FDIC
P.O. BOX 8923
Blackburn, WI 54937

FOR _____

⑈055003⑈ 446782011⑈ 678800470

5655

DATE _____
TO _____
FOR _____

BALANCE BROUGHT FORWARD		
DEPOSITS		
BALANCE		
AMT THIS CK		
BALANCE CARRIED FORWARD		

BLACKBURN PRIMARY CARE ASSOCIATES, PC
1990 Turquoise Drive
Blackburn, WI 54937
608-459-8857

5655
94-72/1224

DATE _____

PAY TO THE ORDER OF _____ $ _____

_____ DOLLARS

DERBYSHIRE SAVINGS Member FDIC
P.O. BOX 8923
Blackburn, WI 54937

FOR _____

⑈055003⑈ 446782011⑈ 678800470

THIS WORKSHEET IS PROVIDED TO HELP YOU BALANCE YOUR ACCOUNT

1. Go through your register and mark each check, withdrawal, Express ATM transaction, payment, deposit, or other credit listed on this statement. Be sure that your register shows any interest paid into your account, and any service charges, automatic payments, or Express Transfers withdrawn from your account during this statement period.

2. Using the chart below, list any outstanding checks, Express ATM withdrawals, payments, or any other withdrawals (including any from previous months) that are listed in your register but are not shown on this statement.

3. Balance your account by filling in the spaces below.

ITEMS OUTSTANDING		
NUMBER	**AMOUNT**	
TOTAL	$	

ENTER

The NEW BALANCE shown on
this statement_____$

ADD

Any deposits listed in your register $
or transfers into your account $
which are not shown on this $
statement.   +$ _____

TOTAL

CALCULATE THE SUBTOTAL_____$

SUBTRACT

The total outstanding checks and
withdrawals from the chart at left_____-$

CALCULATE THE ENDING BALANCE

This amount should be the same
as the current balance shown in
your check register_____$

Case Study

The Internet has changed the way that business is conducted, both in the United States and beyond the U.S. borders. Some individuals are quite comfortable in making purchases and paying bills on the computer. How safe are these practices? How can the medical assistant know that online bill-pay services are safe and secure? Research this information, and prepare a report for the class.

Workplace Application

The more versatile the medical assistant is, the more valuable he or she will be to the physician-employer. Often, new graduates hesitate in asking patients to pay their accounts. However, the MA who is able to collect patient accounts increases the cash flow in the office. How might the medical assistant gain useful skills in the area of collections?

Internet Activities

1. Explore several types of billing software. Determine which seems to be the best option for a medium-sized family practice clinic. Pay special attention to software that has banking features.

2. Investigate the history of banking, and prepare a report for the class.

3. Research safety measures that are designed to keep confidential banking information private. How do privacy policies affect Internet banking? How can the medical assistant ensure that private information remains private? Prepare a paper or report for the class on this subject.

Chapter 22 Quiz

Name: _____

1. The ABA number is on the bottom of a check.

   a. True

   b. False

2. Always write the check stub

   _____

3. A(n) _____ check has an itemized stub.

4. Why might an individual stop payment on a check?

5. Check washing is a type of

   _____

6. The person presenting a check for payment is the _____.

7. The person who writes a check is the

   _____

8. The person named on a check as the recipient of the amount shown is the

   _____

9. Funds paid out are called _____

10. M-banking is banking by _____

WORK PRODUCT 22-1

Name: _____

Fill in the bank deposit figure on the next page using the information in Part IV, Questions 31-34.

BANK DEPOSIT DETAIL

BANK NUMBER	PAYMENTS			CREDIT CARD
	BY CHECK OR PMO	BY COIN OR CURRENCY		

TOTALS

CURRENCY

COIN

CHECKS

CREDIT CARDS

TOTAL RECEIPTS

LESS CREDIT CARD $

TOTAL DEPOSITS

DEPOSIT DATE: _____ FIRM: _____

Management of Practice Finances

Vocabulary Review

Fill in the blanks with the correct vocabulary terms from this chapter.

1. Jenna told Andrea that a(n) _____ year is often different from a calendar year.

2. Julia works with the accounts _____, which are monies that are owed to the physicians.

3. Anna works with the accounts _____, which are monies that the physicians owe to others.

4. Once per year Dr. Medina has his accountant total his _____, which include the entire properties that are subject to the payment of debts.

5. Larry is the supervisor of the _____ department, which records all business and accounting transactions.

6. The _____ in question was sent last month, but the equipment never arrived, so Julia questions whether she should pay the entire balance due.

7. The Rosales Clinic uses the _____ basis of accounting, in which income is recorded when received and expenses are recorded when paid.

8. When the total ending balance of patient ledgers equals the total of accounts receivable control, the two are said to be _____ _____.

9. The accountant prepared a(n) _____ sheet for December 31, which showed the total assets, liabilities, and capital for the clinic.

10. The Tyler Clinic uses the _____ basis of accounting, in which income is recorded when earned and expenses are recorded when incurred.

11. Alice keeps a(n) _____ _____ in her desk that summarizes accounts paid out.

12. Each patient receives a(n) _____ every month if the balance on his or her account is more than $5.00.

13. Running a(n) _____ _____ is one method of checking the accuracy of accounts.

14. Joy takes minor expenses, such as those for sodas and small donations, from the _____ _____ fund.

15. Dr. Lupez asked his accountant to prepare a statement of _____ and _____ for the previous fiscal year.

16. To determine whether the journal and the ledger are in balance, Julia runs an accounts receivable _____ _____.

17. A(n) _____ _____ _____ is a summary for a specific time period that shows a beginning balance, an ending balance, and all of the expenditures during that particular period.

18. Angelique keeps a record of all accounts paid out in a(n) _____ _____.

19. Something that is owed, or a debt, is called a(n) _____.

20. The monetary value of a property or of an interest in a property in excess of claims or liens against it is called _____.

Skills and Concepts

Part I: Short Answer Questions

Provide the answers to the questions in the blanks below.

21. The financial records of any business should show the following at all times:

   a. _____

   b. _____

   c. _____

   d. _____

22. When writing numbers, keep the columns straight and write _____ _____ _____.

23. The manual disbursement journal must show the following:

   a. _____

   b. _____

   c. _____

24. The three most common accounting systems found in medical offices are:

   a. _____

   b. _____

   c. _____

25. Differentiate between accounting and bookkeeping.

_____

_____

_____

26. List three cardinal rules of bookkeeping.

   a. _____

   b. _____

   c. _____

27. List two disadvantages of a single-entry system.

   a. _____

   b. _____

28. The IRS requires that complete records be kept on all employees, including the following:

   a. _____

   b. _____

   c. _____

   d. _____

29. What is Form 940 used for, and when must it be filed?

_____

_____

_____

30. List seven expense categories often found in a physician's office budget.

   a. _____

   b. _____

   c. _____

   d. _____

   e. _____

   f. _____

   g. _____

Part II: Bookkeeping Systems

Briefly explain the three types of bookkeeping systems.

31. Single-entry system

_____

_____

_____

32. Double-entry system

_____

_____

_____

33. Pegboard/write-it-once system

_____

_____

_____

34. Which of the three systems do you think would be the easiest to work with in the medical office? Why?

_____

_____

_____

Part III: Forms

Write a brief description of what each of the following forms is used for.

35. SS-5

_____

_____

_____

36. W-2

_____

_____

_____

37. W-3

_____

_____

_____

38. W-4

_____

_____

_____

Case Study

Read the case study and complete the exercise following it.

Kristy Stephens works for Dr. Mitchell, who has a small office in a suburban area just outside of Birmingham, Alabama. The longer that Kristy works for Dr. Mitchell, the more she learns about accounting and the business side of running a successful medical practice. Kristy is a very organized person and wants to make certain that she follows the right procedures and understands why a certain task must be done a certain way. She wants to establish a calendar that shows what duties should be done at what times.

Determine when all of the forms in Part III must be turned in or filed. Add tax day to the calendar. Print the calendar, showing all filing dates on it. If a template will help, use one from the Microsoft Office homepage.

Workplace Applications

Complete the following math review test. Turn it in to your instructor to grade, or grade it in class.

Solve the following addition problems:

1. $99 + 104$ = _____
2. $78 + 57$ = _____
3. $98 + 128$ = _____
4. $187 + 233$ = _____
5. $284 + 440$ = _____
6. $306 + 291$ = _____
7. $204 + 278$ = _____
8. $409 + 246$ = _____

9. 15 + 74   = _____

10. 181 + 369 = _____

Solve the following subtraction problems:

11. 290 − 303 = _____

12. 231 − 263 = _____

13. 453 − 156 = _____

14. 459 − 325 = _____

15. 318 − 105 = _____

16. 398 − 294 = _____

Solve the following multiplication problems:

17. 46 × 24 = _____

18. 11 × 49 = _____

19. 48 × 17 = _____

20. 26 × 24 = _____

21. 42 × 15 = _____

22. 5 × 49 = _____

23. 47 × 12 = _____

24. 26 × 34 = _____

25. 45 × 21 = _____

Solve the following division problems:

26. 1950 ÷ 13 = _____

27. 50350 ÷ 53 = _____

28. 12105 ÷ 15 = _____

29. 9712 ÷ 16 = _____

30. 13500 ÷ 20 = _____

Internet Activities

1. Investigate bookkeeping software on the Internet, and use any tutorials or trial software available. Determine a good program for use in the medical office, and be able to defend your decision in a class presentation.

2. Look for math worksheet sites, and work through some of them for practice.

Chapter 23 Quiz

Name: _____

1. A document inside a package that lists the package's contents is a(n)

   _____

   _____ .

2. A bill sent to a patient on a monthly basis is also called a(n)

   _____ .

3. For how many years should payroll records be kept?

   _____

4. What is a W-4 form?

   _____

   _____

5. What is FUTA? _____

6. Define *bookkeeping*.

   _____

   _____

7. Name two bases of accounting.

   _____

   _____

8. What is a disbursement?

   _____

   _____

9. What type of fund is used for minor expenses?

   _____

10. Name two types of bookkeeping systems.

    _____

    _____

CHAPTER 24

Medical Practice Management and Human Resources

Vocabulary Review

Fill in the blanks with the correct vocabulary terms from this chapter.

1. Dr. Hughes enjoys offering _____ to employees who perform over and above the call of duty.

2. Lucia told a(n) _____ lie to her supervisor, which almost resulted in termination of her employment.

3. The staff enjoys _____ talks and recently traveled to North Dallas to hear Zig Ziglar speak.

4. Employee _____ can indicate the working conditions at a facility; when the staff members are happy with their jobs, they tend to remain in their positions for a number of years.

5. Mrs. Gordon has always been a great promoter of employee _____, never failing to offer her smile and a kind word to others.

6. Ruth Ann was written up for _____ after she and Sue Lynn, her supervisor, had a rather loud and tense discussion last week.

7. The marketers _____ young women in their latest advertisements to promote the hospital expansion in the labor and delivery department.

8. New employees may find it helpful to be assigned a(n) _____, who will assist them as they learn the office routines and responsibilities.

9. The office manager assigned several new duties to Ann, including development of meeting _____.

10. Sandy had 17 performance _____ to give over the course of the week.

11. People in the medical field sometimes experience _____ and feel a need to separate themselves from the profession for a period of time.

12. Paul was charged with _____ after he took money from the physical therapy clinic where he formerly worked.

13. The physicians and management personnel have worked hard to develop such a(n) _____ team.

14. A(n) _____ of _____ is necessary in any organization, even the smaller ones.

15. Barbara is _____ with her paperwork and very seldom makes an error.

Skills and Concepts

Part I: Office Managers

Provide brief answers to the following questions.

16. Why is it a good idea to have one person in charge of office operations?

_____

_____

_____

17. Most management problems can be avoided by carefully defining the areas of:

    a. _____

    b. _____

18. What usually happens if a manager helps employees get what they want and need from a job?

_____

_____

_____

19. Managers who have a group of outstanding employees are usually looked on as

    _____ _____.

20. List the three basic types of leaders.

    a. _____

    b. _____

    c. _____

21. List and explain three types of power.

    a. _____

    b. _____

    c. _____

22. The office manager must always have enough written _____ when terminating an employee.

23. List five ways to motivate employees.

    a. _____

    b. _____

    c. _____

    d. _____

    e. _____

24. What is a "yes" person?

_____

25. What is one of the most effective ways to improve employee morale?

_____

Part II: Hiring and Terminating Employees

Fill in the blanks with the best answers.

26. One of the most effective methods of finding new employees is through word of _____.

27. Calling a job candidate to schedule an interview presents an opportunity to judge how well he or she speaks on the _____.

28. Have the job candidate fill out the application at the office by hand so that the applicant's _____ can be evaluated.

29. If the job candidate feels at _____, he or she will be able to share strengths and will communicate better during the interview.

30. Relationships with those who work in the medical office should above all else be _____.

31. Candidates may be required to submit to a _____ check, especially if they will be handling office finances.

32. One of the most critical errors in bringing a new staff member to the team is not providing fair and adequate _____ and _____.

33. Well-written job _____ list the essential functions of the job and reveal the chain of command that should be followed in the office.

34. A dismissed employee should never be left in the office _____.

35. Always check at least _____ references when hiring a new employee.

Part III: Leading during Transitions and Change

Add the appropriate word to the following sentences about change.

36. Change _____.

37. _____ with the change.

38. _____ change.

39. _____ to change quickly.

40. _____ change.

41. Anticipate _____.

Part IV: Meeting Agendas

Place the following activities in the correct numeric order for a staff meeting.

_____ Discussion of unfinished business

_____ Adjournment

_____ Discussion of problems in administrative area

_____ Discussion of new business

_____ Reading of last meeting's minutes

_____ Discussion of problems in clinical area

_____ Discussion of problems in common areas

Part V: Medical Practice Management

Find the words on the list in the puzzle.

```
R I P B U T S S M E N T O R T Y M X H U E J I S P Z G L A M
E N C O S T Q D U V M Z P C U R M W I X H Y A E Q N A D E Y
T S K J F U I M N B N B W U O A A A O Q D M Z D J I S N T Q F
E U U B C K P L N A O V V Q N L V M N C A D J G I E I M C J
N B O K G P A U I I M R T W R L D S O I E Q A A G C N J V M
T O R Z F Z M X Q M W I D I U I A M M R X R R A U Z O N C W
I R N O I T A V I T O M R I B C A I M G A P R L U U U X Q C
O D X N P B G W M V B P I P N N H Q M P P L O L X F F B H E
N I V I T J L E G R I K I E E A L Q S A W U E V O G H A E L
X N F T A Z M R E A Y W N F G R T I L A S D L I I O I N Z B
U A Y V L B O A F F A F C A X V D E H H R Z T T F N A Y G A
S T U X U X W C B U R S E R C O U H T K F N P D O I L M X R
D I E L B A F F A Y K B N V R G U F D H R T Z F J T S P D T
S O L Z N F D S O U N I T K Q J Y L Y L B B C E N R G A Z E
L N Q D F L T K T A P K I E R K F S N M C O R X U A Q D E N
X C P E X T R I N S I C V H J O B P R K M I M A M A A X Q E
P O U Q T U E J A A U C E N Q W H B Z M B H O G H Q L V Z P
K R U N I V Q Q Y C Q J S V S K Q P A R V M Y H F V N X N M
R W E X J N S T I P Y H Z Z D B W N W E W Z F F V D T S B I
L G J E G R T X N J H W P P A L D N A L S O P S C H G M Q F
Y G Z K D A H R C E K B P Y R G N A B H Y O Q L B N X K Y T
X M V F J V D N I A M G M P Q D A V Q I A G M W Q B B H D L
L U B O S G X T K N P E V E S M Z J H G C O P T G W M T H N
H F F D Y O P E U P S C L A J O J V I O B Z Z Z N T E W G J
N O I T N E V M U C R I C Z C C B X H C M Q Z O E A N R P W
L L G K N F Y R B Y A Q C X Z K S E P X X H Z S R J T X U G
P L S G Q M I C R O M A N A G E S V N D B D V S C C J A J W
B T S Q L M U T J H B B G N Z I B P B B P K S D Q U K U L O
O S H D V K Y A T B B W U I V G L M A C X V F B F T E F V B
R K X C E F X E D X D T U E B S C Q E C E G Z D Z I P B G L
```

Affable

Agenda

Ancillary

Appraisal

Blatant

Burnout

Chain of command

Circumvention

Cohesive

Disparaging

Embezzlement

Extrinsic

Impenetrable

Incentives

Insubordination

Intrinsic

Mentor

Meticulous

Micromanage

Morale

Motivation

Reprimands

Retention

Subordinate

Targeted

Case Study

Read the case study and perform the exercise following it.

Belinda is a single mother with two children. She recently was divorced from her husband and is in the process of rebuilding her life. She enrolled in medical assisting school 8 months ago and is now preparing for graduation. Throughout her time in classes she has researched medical facilities on the Internet and has found several that are close to her apartment complex.

Belinda has several goals in life, and the most important ones involve her family. She wants to secure a job that will allow her to take care of her children, assure them a good education, and save for their college tuition. She knows that she needs to find a job that offers health benefits. Belinda is a loyal employee and has a good work history, so she is hopeful that her positions from graduation forward will be such that she is able to make steady progress toward reaching her goals.

What goals do you have for your life after graduation? Assess your personal situation, and determine five long-term (life) goals, five short-term (1 year or more away) goals, and 10 immediate goals for the next six months. Write the goals down. For the long- and short-term goals, include a few sentences that explain why the goal is important to you. Make certain that all of the immediate goals are attainable in a 6-month period.

Once completed, look over your list daily. Write down all of the progress made toward the goals, and celebrate when each one is attained. It may be beneficial to keep a journal that details the progress made toward your goals and set new ones as the original ones are met.

Workplace Applications

Section I

Revise or write a new patient information booklet, and split into groups of classmates to work on different sections of the booklet. Plan a staff meeting, sending a memo to each classmate who should attend. Write an agenda for the meeting, set a time limit, and determine a general subject to discuss. Each group should discuss its portion of the booklet during the meeting.

Section II

Compose a rough draft of your resume. Allow three different classmates to proofread the document and make suggestions. Draft a final copy, and turn it in to the instructor for a grade.

Internet Activities

1. Perform a job search for medical assisting positions in the local geographic area. Look for the 15 most interesting opportunities, and print the job descriptions. Compare the job requirements with the skills learned. If appropriate, apply for the positions.

2. Use the Internet to research a person whom you consider a leader. Read material about this person's life, and write a report about his or her ability as a leader. Share the report with the class.

3. Investigate budgeting ideas by doing research on the Internet. Determine what items must be included in the budget, then list all of the bills and payments that must be made each month. A budget template may be available on the Microsoft website and can be downloaded for use. Make the estimates as close as possible to your actual income and expenses. Turn the budget in to the instructor.

Chapter 24 Quiz

Name: _____

1. Name three types of leaders.

   a. _____

   b. _____

   c. _____

2. Name three types of managers.

   a. _____

   b. _____

   c. _____

3. Stealing from an employer is called

   _____.

4. Refusing to obey authority is called

   _____.

5. _____ evaluations involve other staff members and their input with regard to a co-worker's performance.

6. _____ is a part of every person's life and happens in every business, so the ability to adapt and be flexible is a valuable skill.

7. Having a(n) _____ of personality types usually works better in an office than having several employees with the same type of personality.

8. The medical assistant should always follow up an interview with a(n) _____
   _____.

9. By sharpening _____ skills, the medical assistant may obtain a higher salary than the physician's first offer.

10. A(n) _____ is a listing of the items for discussion during a staff meeting.

Medical Practice Marketing and Customer Service

Vocabulary Review

Fill in the blanks with the correct vocabulary terms from this chapter.

1. Drs. Julie and Robert Todd truly enjoy _____, because it provides an opportunity to reach and involve diverse audiences using key messages and effective programs.

2. Monica has identified several _____ _____ and has a strong plan for marketing efforts that she plans to implement over the next year.

3. When developing a marketing plan, clearly establish _____ and think about the long- and short-term goals for the practice.

4. Monica wants to develop a(n) _____ business plan that is workable and will be flexible if changes become necessary.

5. One area that Monica hopes to improve is the _____ laboratory, because much of the equipment is outdated and needs to be replaced.

Skills and Concepts

Part I: Short Answer Questions

Provide a brief answer to the following questions.

6. List the three steps that are generally followed when preparing to implement or change medical marketing strategies.

   a. _____

   b. _____

   c. _____

7. What is meant by "reaching the target market"?

   _____

   _____

   _____

8. List five specific planning steps that are effective when developing marketing strategies.

   a. _____

   b. _____

   c. _____

   d. _____

   e. _____

9. List several phrases that should never be used with patients, especially when attempting to provide exceptional customer service.

   a. _____

   b. _____

   c. _____

   d. _____

10. Explain the concept that good customer service is a commitment.

   _____

   _____

   _____

11. What are the four P's of marketing?

   a. _____

   b. _____

   c. _____

   d. _____

12. How does the provider determine what services to offer at the practice?

   _____

   _____

   _____

   _____

13. Provide five examples of community involvement that may help a medical practice to grow.

   a. _____

   b. _____

   c. _____

   d. _____

   e. _____

14. What is the difference between advertising and public relations?

_____

_____

_____

15. List the four basic steps used to create a website.

a. _____

b. _____

c. _____

d. _____

Part II: Website Evaluation

Research various websites for healthcare organizations, preferably in your geographic area. Rate the websites from 1 to 10 (10 being the best), and provide comments about the most outstanding portions of the site.

Website Name

1. _____

2. _____

3. _____

4. _____

5. _____

Website Name

6. _____

7. _____

8. _____

9. _____

10. _____

Website	Overall Appeal	Content	Ease of Navigation	Fonts	Consistency	Comments

Part III: Customers in the Physician's Office

Provide brief answers to the questions below.

16. Who are some of the customers who visit the medical office?

_____

_____

_____

17. Explain how to provide patients and other guests in the office with exceptional customer service.

_____

_____

_____

_____

Case Study

Read the case study and answer the question at the end.

Lorendia has worked for Dr. Johnson for over 15 years, but recently she has been forced to cut her hours from 40 per week to 35 per week. She was diagnosed with chronic fatigue syndrome, and she struggles toward the end of the week because of the symptoms of the disease. Lorendia has become more and more impatient with the people who come to the physician's office, and it is common for her to make a snippy remark when she is behind in her duties. Her attitude has alienated her from most of the employees. Although her job performance is not acceptable now, for the majority of her career at the clinic her work has been above reproach.

How can this situation be resolved so that Lorendia can keep her job yet improve her performance?

_____

_____

_____

Workplace Application

Providing exceptional customer service can actually interfere with job duties. Some workers use customer service as an excuse to chat with patients and avoid other duties. How can the medical assistant strike a balance between providing the customer service that patients deserve and completing all of the tasks that are required each day?

Internet Activities

1. Research customer service, and develop your own, original definition of the concept of customer service. Present your thoughts to the class by creating a professional presentation.

2. Research public relations, and make a list of the various "free" ways that publicity can be generated for the office. Choose five ideas that you feel are the best. Email these ideas to each of your classmates. If the entire class participates, everyone will have numerous fresh ideas to use once they begin their career. Write the ideas on index cards and keep them in a box, or develop a port-folio of ideas.

3. Design a fictional website using free software on the Internet. If appropriate, share the site with classmates and compare ideas.

Chapter 25 Quiz

Name: _____

1. Name the four P's of marketing.

   a. _____

   b. _____

   c. _____

   d. _____

2. List several free marketing or public relations resources.

   _____

   _____

3. What is a hyperlink?

   _____

4. What is the final stage of implementing a marketing plan?

   _____

5. Staff members are internal customers.

   a. True

   b. False

6. Define *marketing*.

   _____

   _____

   _____

7. What is the first step of marketing?

   _____

8. A URL is a(n) _____.

9. A group of individuals to whom marketing is focused is called a(n)

   _____

   _____

10. An ISP is a(n) _____

    _____.

CHAPTER 26

Infection Control

Vocabulary Review

Define the following terms.

1. Anaphylaxis

_____

2. Antibody

_____

3. Antigen

_____

4. Antiseptic

_____

5. Autoimmune

_____

6. Contaminated

_____

7. Germicides

_____

8. Pathogenic

_____

9. Permeable

_____

10. Relapse

_____

11. Remission

_____

12. Vector

_____

Match the following terms with their definitions.

13. _____ Disinfection

14. _____ Medical asepsis

15. _____ Surgical asepsis

16. _____ Sanitization

17. _____ Sterilization

a. Removal or destruction of disease-causing organisms after they leave the body

b. Destruction of all microorganisms

c. Destruction of organisms before they enter the body

d. Cleansing process that decreases the number of microorganisms to a safe level as dictated in public health guidelines

e. Process of killing pathogenic organisms or rendering them inactive

Define the following terms related to disease processes.

18. Chronic

_____

19. Latent

_____

20. Acute

_____

Skills and Concepts

21. List five groups of infectious organisms.

a. _____

b. _____

c. _____

d. _____

e. _____

22. Label the diagram with the following terms.

a. Reservoir host _____

b. Entry (any body opening) _____

c. Transmission mode (air, food, hand, insects, body fluid) _____

d. Exit mode (mouth, skin, rectum, body fluid) _____

e. Susceptible host _____

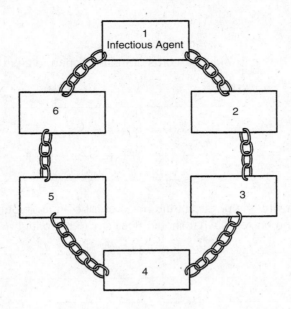

23. Describe the impact of the inflammatory response on the body's ability to defend itself against infection.

_____

_____

_____

24. Explain the difference between cell-mediated and humoral immunity.

_____

_____

_____

25. List six common errors of disinfection.

a. _____

b. _____

c. _____

d. _____

e. _____

f. _____

26. Explain the five major areas included in the OSHA Compliance Guidelines.

a. _____

b. _____

c. _____

d. _____

e. _____

Case Studies

1. Rosa is explaining the signs and symptoms of inflammation to a patient. List the four classic symptoms.

   _____

   _____

   _____

   _____

2. A patient asks Rosa why the physician did not prescribe an antibiotic for her viral illness. Knowing about viruses and bacteria, what should Rosa say to the patient?

   _____

   _____

   _____

3. While performing venipuncture, Rosa experienced an accidental needlestick. Describe the post-exposure instructions and follow-up procedures.

   _____

   _____

   _____

   _____

4. Rosa identifies the need to educate her patient about proper asepsis. However, in a busy office, there is not a lot of extra time. What can Rosa do during her time with the patient to properly educate them on aseptic techniques?

   _____

   _____

   _____

5. Rosa is setting up a sterile field for a mole removal the physician is about to perform. During her preparation, a piece of sterile gauze falls into the sink. The sink was cleaned earlier in the day. Can Rosa use the gauze? Why or why not? What should she do?

   _____

   _____

   _____

Workplace Applications

1. Employers with workers who are at risk for occupational exposure to blood or other infectious materials must implement an Occupational Safety and Health Administration (OSHA) Exposure Control Plan that details employee protection procedures. List seven items that should be included in the plan.

a. _____   e. _____

b. _____   f. _____

c. _____   g. _____

d. _____

2. Rosa is concerned she may have an allergy to latex gloves. What signs and symptoms should she look for? Is Rosa's employer required to supply Rosa with latex-free gloves if she does indeed have a latex allergy? Why or why not?

_____

_____

_____

3. Rosa is helping to update the OSHA Exposure Control Plan in her office. She wants to include a policy for wearing gloves. List six different times gloves should be worn.

a. _____

b. _____

c. _____

d. _____

e. _____

f. _____

4. Review Procedure 26-2: Perform Medical Aseptic Hand Washing in your textbook. What did you learn? Practice proper hand washing for the next 24 hours. Note any new habits you have formed. Do you see any improvement? Have you noticed the hand-washing behaviors of others?

_____

_____

_____

Internet Activity

Visit www.osha.gov. View the OSHA Bloodborne Pathogens Standards. What can you do within your workplace to prevent accidental exposure to blood-borne pathogens? Did you find anything surprising within the guidelines or the website? Prepare to discuss your answers in class.

Chapter 26 Quiz

Name: _____

1. Viruses may be treated with antibiotics.

   a. True

   b. False

2. List the signs and symptoms of
   inflammation.

   a. _____

   b. _____

   c. _____

   d. _____

3. Describe the procedure for proper
   handwashing.

4. Define nosocomial.

5. _____ is the cleansing
   process that decreases the number of
   microorganisms to a safe level as dictated in public health guidelines.

6. List three potentially infectious fluids.

   a. _____

   b. _____

   c. _____

7. Describe three things the medical
   assistant can do for the environmental
   protection of the office.

   a. _____

   b. _____

   c. _____

8. Define the two factors needed for
   proper handwashing.

   a. _____

   b. _____

9. Handwashing must be performed after
   gloves are taken off.

   a. True

   b. False

10. Define *antibody*.

   _____

CHAPTER **28**

Patient Education

Vocabulary Review

Fill in the blanks with the correct vocabulary terms from this chapter.

1. The holistic model suggests that _____ should take into consideration all aspects of patient life including patients' _____, _____, _____, _____, and _____ needs.

Skills and Concepts

2. List six guidelines for patient education.

   a. _____

   b. _____

   c. _____

   d. _____

   e. _____

   f. _____

3. List seven factors that influence learning.

   a. _____

   b. _____

   c. _____

   d. _____

   e. _____

   f. _____

   g. _____

4. Identify eight approaches to language barriers.

a. _____

b. _____

c. _____

d. _____

e. _____

f. _____

g. _____

h. _____

Fill in the blanks with the appropriate terms.

5. One of the most important aspects of patient teaching is to be _____ and provide information about _____ patients want to know _____ patients want to know it.

6. List 10 barriers to patient learning.

a. _____

b. _____

c. _____

d. _____

e. _____

f. _____

g. _____

h. _____

i. _____

j. _____

7. Identify five guidelines for ordering educational materials.

a. _____

b. _____

c. _____

d. _____

e. _____

Complete the following statement.

8. The role of the medical assistant educator includes:

a. _____

b. _____

c. _____

d. _____

e. _____

f. _____

g. _____

h. _____

Fill in the blanks with the appropriate terms.

9. Teaching methods that are effective include use of _____ materials, videos, and approved _____ sites to gather information; referral to community _____ and experts; _____ demonstration of medical skills; examination of patients' records of events; and involving _____ in the education process.

Teaching Plan Checklist

10. Use the following checklist to design and present a program for a patient during your externship, or role-play with a fellow classmate.

A. Conduct patient assessment.

- Consider pertinent patient factors.
- Identify barriers to learning.
- Prioritize patient information.
- Determine immediate and long-term needs.
- Decide on appropriate teaching materials and methods.
  Complete _____

B. Prepare the teaching area, and assemble necessary equipment and materials.

- Use supplies and equipment the patient will use at home.
- Provide positive feedback for correct display of skills.
  Complete _____

C. Maintain adequate, not too fast, pace.

Complete _____

D. Repeatedly ask for patient feedback to confirm understanding.

- Eliminate barriers to learning.
- Address immediate learning needs.
- Use repetition and rephrasing to promote understanding.
  Complete _____

E. Summarize the material learned or the skill mastered at the end of each teaching interaction.

Complete _____

F. Outline a plan for the next meeting.

Complete _____

G. Evaluate the teaching plan.

- Was there enough time to complete the lesson?
- Was the patient physically and psychologically ready for the information?
- Were the goals for the session reached?
Complete _____

H. Document the teaching intervention.

- Material covered.
- Patient response or level of skill performance.
- Plans for next session.
- Community referrals.
Complete _____

Case Studies

1. MaryAnn has recently been diagnosed with hypercholesterolemia. As Taylor is discussing diet and exercise recommendations, MaryAnn replies that she doesn't think the cholesterol is something she should be concerned with, and with working two jobs she is "forced" to dine out and eat "on the run" most days. What type of barriers will Taylor need to overcome? What type of patient education material should Taylor provide to her?

_____
_____
_____

2. Describe how patient age and development age will result in the need to adapt the teaching plan of the following patients. What changes will you make to the methods of delivery? Are there any learning barriers to overcome? What types of patient information will you provide to each?

a. A 74-year-old woman who has been recently diagnosed with type 2 diabetes. Before her diagnosis, she had not seen a doctor in 20 years. She loves to cook for her large family but complains of difficulty reading recipes as the diabetes has resulted in diabetic retinopathy.

_____
_____
_____

b. An 11-year-old boy, recently diagnosed with type 1 diabetes. He loves to play sports and is very active. His father complains that he plays so much that it is difficult to get him to eat properly. He is afraid of needles, and the doctor has ordered him to begin using insulin and a glucometer immediately.

_____

_____

_____

Workplace Applications

1. Gather a list of community resources for the patient in the area of which you live. What population are the resources geared to? What is the contact information? What services do they offer?

2. Taylor, a medical assistant for a family practice office, has been asked by Dr. Norberger to create patient education files for each examination room. The file should contain handouts on chronic disease, nutrition, exercise and healthy lifestyle. Create a list of 15 topics that should definitely be included in this file. Why did you choose them? How may they be helpful to the doctor and the patients?

3. As Taylor begins to obtain and develop educational supplies for the patient education files, what are some guidelines she should follow as she reviews the information available? What other teaching materials should she consider using in addition to the handouts?

Chapter 28 Quiz

Name: _____

1. Describe the holistic model of patient education.

2. List some areas on which patient education might focus.

3. The sixth- to eighth-grade level is recommended for brochures for the general public.
   a. True
   b. False

4. List some examples of teaching materials.
   a. _____
   b. _____
   c. _____

5. A quiet area is recommended for patient education.
   a. True
   b. False

6. Include _____ and significant others in education.

7. Emotional state can affect patient learning.
   a. True
   b. False

8. Name two physical barriers to learning.
   a. _____
   b. _____

9. What is the first step in developing a teaching plan?

10. List ways to evaluate learning.

CHAPTER 29

Nutrition and Health Promotion

Vocabulary Review

Describe the dietary imbalances that contribute to each of the following health problems.

1. Anemia

   _____

   _____

2. Cancer

   _____

   _____

3. Constipation

   _____

   _____

4. Diabetes

   _____

   _____

5. Hypercholesterolemia

   _____

   _____

6. Hypertension

   _____

   _____

7. Osteoporosis

   _____

   _____

Fill in the blanks with the appropriate terms.

8. A(n) _____ nutrient, such as cholesterol, can be created within the body and does not need to be included in the diet.

9. _____ are chemical organic compounds composed of carbon, hydrogen, and oxygen and are primarily plant products in origin. They are divided into three groups based on the complexity of their molecules: simple sugars, complex carbohydrates (starch), and dietary fiber.

10. _____ is a storage form of fuel that is used to supplement carbohydrates as an available energy source.

11. _____ is produced by the liver and is found in animal foods; can produce athero-sclerotic plaque deposits in arteries.

12. _____ are composed of units known as *amino acids*, which are the materials that our bodies use to build and repair tissues.

13. Vitamins are divided into two groups: _____-soluble vitamins (A, D, E, and K) and _____-soluble vitamins (B complex and C).

14. The _____ is the amount of energy needed by fasting, resting individuals to maintain vital function.

15. Dietary fiber is commonly called _____.

Define the following terms.

16. Metabolism

_____

17. Anabolism

_____

18. Catabolism

_____

Skills and Concepts

19. How does culture influence our dietary choices? Why is this important to note when providing nutrition education to patients?

_____

_____

_____

_____

Examine the nomogram below and answer the following questions.

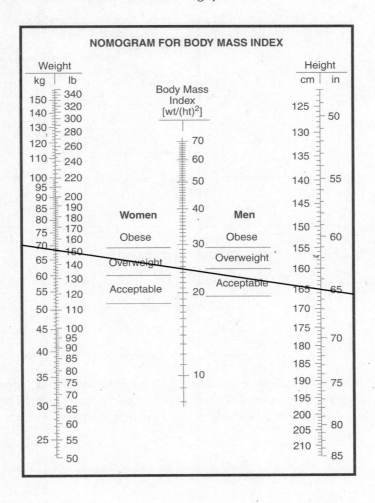

NOMOGRAM FOR BODY MASS INDEX

20. What is the purpose of the nomogram?

_____

_____

21. How much does this patient weigh in pounds? In kilograms?

_____

22. What is the height in inches? In centimeters?

_____

23. What is the body mass index (BMI)?

_____

24. Use the nomogram to calculate your own BMI.

_____

25. List four functions of water.

   a. _____

   b. _____

   c. _____

   d. _____

26. List four functions of proteins.

   a. _____

   b. _____

   c. _____

   d. _____

27. What is the glycemic index? How is it used to manage blood sugar levels?

   _____

   _____

   _____

   _____

28. Examine the figure that shows the anatomy of Mypyramid on the next page. Label the different sections. How does this pyramid differ from the traditional food guide pyramid? Do you think these changes will persuade individuals to lead healthier lifestyles?

   _____

   _____

   _____

   _____

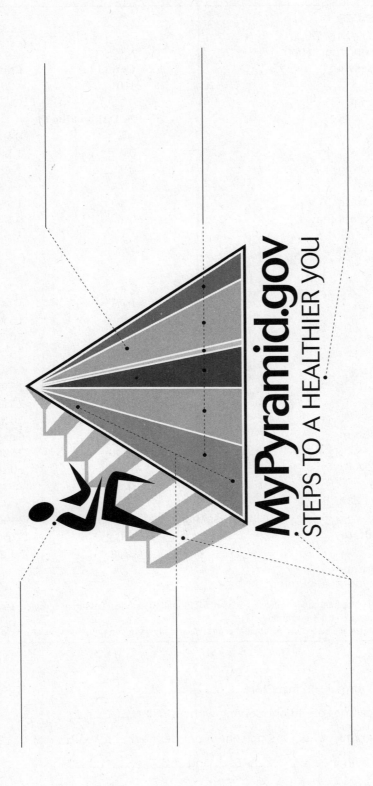

Examine the nutrition facts label that follows, and answer the next questions.

NUTRITION FACTS
Serving size: 1 ¼ cups (30 g)
Servings per container: about 16

Amount per serving		Cereal	Cereal with ½ cup skim milk
Calories		110	190
Calories from fat		0	0
		% Daily value**	
Total fat 9 g*		0%	0%
Saturated fat 0 g		0%	1%
Cholesterol 0 mg		0%	1%
Sodium 270 mg		11%	14%
Total carbohydrate 26 g		9%	11%
Dietary fiber less than 1 g		0%	0%
Sugars 3 g			
Other carbohydrate 22 g			
Protein 2 g			
Vitamin A		0%	6%
Vitamin C		10%	10%
Calcium		0%	15%
Iron		50%	50%
Thiamin		25%	25%
Niacin		25%	25%
Vitamin B$_6$		25%	25%
Folate		25%	25%
Vitamin B$_{12}$		25%	30%
Amount per serving		Cereal	Cereal with ½ cup skim milk
Calories		2000	2500
Total fat	Less than	65 g	60 g
Saturated fat	Less than	20 g	25 g
Cholesterol	Less than	300 mg	300 mg
Sodium	Less than	2400 mg	2400 mg
Total carbohydrate		300 g	375 g
Dietary fiber		25 g	30 g

Calories per gram:
Fat 9 ● Carbohydrate 4 ● Protein 4

*Amount in cereal. One half cup skim milk adds an additional 40 calories. Less than 5 mg cholesterol, 65 mg sodium, 6 g total carbohydrate (6 g sugars), and 4 g protein.
**Percent daily values are based on 2000-calorie diet. Your daily values may be higher or lower depending on your calorie needs.

29. What is the normal serving size? _____

30. How many calories are in one serving without milk? _____

31. How many grams of fiber are present in one serving? _____

32. This food is high in _____ and _____.

33. What is the total number of carbohydrate for 2½ cups of cereal? _____

34. If one serving of CHO equals 15 g, then how many servings of CHO are in 1¼ cups of cereal?

Case Studies

1. Mrs. Barton has been recently diagnosed with type 2 DM. At her office visit today she reports that her glucometer readings 2 hours after eating breakfast have been running on average 230 to 300. Below is Mrs. Barton's food diary for breakfast:

Monday Breakfast	Tuesday Breakfast	Wednesday Breakfast
1½ c cereal 4 oz OJ	2 pancakes 2 Tbsp syrup 4 oz OJ	1 blueberry muffin 1 banana 1 cup of tea

What should Marcia notice from the food diary? What conclusions can Marcia draw from Mrs. Barton's breakfast choices and the resulting blood glucose readings?

_____

_____

_____

Mrs. Barton has asked Marcia to create a sample breakfast menu for the next 3 days. Create the menu in the following chart. Why do you think this will better regulate Mrs. Barton's blood glucose?

Thursday Breakfast	Friday Breakfast	Saturday Breakfast

2. Suzie's recent blood work results show an LDL of 176 and a total cholesterol of 256. Suzie does not seem concerned with these results and wonders why the physician wants her to follow a low-cholesterol diet. What can Marcia tell Suzie about the risks of hyperlipidemia? What are the recommended ranges for total cholesterol and LDL? Document the teaching intervention in the patient's chart.

_____

_____

_____

Workplace Applications

1. Marcia is gathering material for a patient education brochure describing the importance of fiber consumption. What is the function of fiber in the diet? Include the difference between soluble and insoluble fiber. What is the daily dietary recommendation for fiber intake? Create a list of foods high in fiber for Marcia to include in her brochure.

2. Marcia has been asked to assist the physician with research for a journal article. The article is titled "The Importance of Antioxidants." Prepare a list of foods high in antioxidants to be included in the article.

3. The internal medicine clinic where Marcia works frequently sees patients with hypertension. The recommended treatment for lowering blood pressure is the Dietary Approaches to Stop Hypertension (DASH) diet. Describe the guidelines included in the DASH diet.

Internet Activities

1. The "5 A Day for Better Health" Program is one of the nation's largest initiatives for nutrition. The goal of the program is to increase the national fruit and vegetable consumption to five per day by 2010. Visit the program's website at www.5aday.org. Why is the consumption of fruits and vegetables so important? Keep a food diary for 1 week. Have you met the goal of "5 A Day"? If not, how do you plan to add more fruits and vegetables to your diet?

2. Visit www.mypyramid.gov. Go to the "My Pyramid Plan" and insert your age, gender, and level of physical activity. View and print your personalized pyramid to answer the following questions.

   a. The results are based on a calorie pattern of how many calories?

   b. What is the recommended amount of grains?

   c. What tips do you find will enable you to fulfill these requirements?

   d. What is your daily recommendation for physical activity?

   e. Do your current eating habits support the results found on your personalized pyramid?

   f. What areas in your own diet need modification?

Chapter 29 Quiz

Name: _____

1. Name two functions of protein.

   a. _____

   b. _____

2. Name the two types of lipoproteins.

   a. _____

   b. _____

3. What is the benefit of omega-3 fatty acids?

4. Name two eating disorders.

   a. _____

   b. _____

5. What types of oil are monounsaturated?

   a. _____

   b. _____

6. Obesity is caused by excessive
   _____ intake.

7. _____ includes sugars and starches.

8. Fiber is also called _____.

9. List three studies included in the health screening process.

   a. _____

   b. _____

   c. _____

10. Antioxidants include vitamins
    _____ and _____.

CHAPTER 32

Principles of Pharmacology

Vocabulary Review

Match the following terms with their definitions.

1. _____ Drugs that are used to treat the disorder and cure it; for example, antibiotics cure bacterial infections

2. _____ Drugs that do not cure but provide relief from pain or symptoms related to the disorder; an example is the use of an antihistamine for allergic symptoms

3. _____ Drugs that prevent the occurrence of a condition; for example, vaccines prevent the occurrence of specific infectious diseases

4. _____ Drugs that help determine the cause of a particular health problem; an example is injection of antigen serum for allergy testing

5. _____ Drugs that provide patients with substances needed to maintain heath; examples are estrogen replacement therapy for menopausal women and administration of insulin to patients with diabetes

6. _____ Medications sold without prescription

7. _____ Drugs that are not protected by trademark

8. _____ Pertaining to a gluelike substance

9. _____ Denoting any medication route other than the gastrointestinal route

10. _____ Space within a vessel or tube

11. _____ Drug formulation in which tablets are coated with a special compound that does not dissolve until the tablet is exposed to the fluids of the small intestine.

a. Prophylactic

b. Therapeutic

c. Replacement

d. Palliative

e. Diagnostic

f. Parenteral

g. Colloidal

h. Generic

i. Enteric-coated

j. Over-the-counter

k. Lumen

For each of the following terms, define the type of drug action and give an example.

12. Analgesic

_____

13. Anesthetic

_____

14. Antibiotic

_____

15. Antidepressant

_____

16. Antihistamine

_____

17. Antihypertensive

_____

18. Antiinflammatory

_____

19. Antineoplastic

_____

20. Antitussive

_____

Skills and Concepts

Fill in the blank with DEA, FDA, or FTC.

21. The _____ regulates over-the-counter drug advertising.

22. The _____, a division of the Department of Health and Human Services, was created in 1936 to regulate the development and sale of all prescription and over-the-counter drugs.

23. The _____ was established in 1973 as part of the Department of Justice to enforce federal laws regarding the use of illegal drugs.

24. Every medical practice should have a copy of the controlled substances regulations. The medical assistant may secure this list from a regional office of the _____.

25. In addition to approving new drugs for the marketplace, the _____ is also responsible for establishing standards for their purity and strength during the manufacturing process and for ensuring that generic brands are effective and safe.

26. Each physician who prescribes or who has controlled substances on site must register with the _____ for a Controlled Substance Registration Certificate and will receive a specific registration number that must be included on all controlled substance prescriptions.

27. List five specific guidelines for prescription orders of controlled substances.

a. _____

b. _____

c. _____

d. _____

e. _____

Indicate which statements are true (T) and which statements are false (F).

28. _____ The chemical name represents the drug's exact formula.

29. _____ The generic drug name is assigned by the manufacturer and is protected by copyright.

30. _____ Brand names are capitalized.

31. _____ The PDR is the most commonly used drug reference book.

32. _____ A prescription is an order written by the physician for the compounding or dispensing and administration of drugs to a particular patient.

33. List six of the factors that can affect drug action.

a. _____

b. _____

c. _____

d. _____

e. _____

f. _____

Case Studies

1. Martha's first patient of the day has some prescriptions that need to be refilled. Look up each drug in the PDR to become familiar with the drug's indications and possible side effects, then prepare the following prescriptions for the physician's signature:

   a. Crestor 10 mg; take one pill daily. Dispense 90 tablets with three refills.

   b. Atenolol 50 mg; take one and a half pills by mouth every morning. Dispense 1-month supply with one refill.

   c. Xanax 0.5 mg; take one to two tablets at bedtime as needed. Dispense 30 tablets with no refills.

2. Mrs. Jones calls the office and states that she wants to discontinue her Diovan 80 mg because she has no prescription coverage. She states, "I feel fine and don't even know why I'm taking this medication!" What patient education can Martha provide to Mrs. Jones to make her understand the importance of continuing her current medication? Is there anything Martha can do to help Mrs. Jones' drug coverage? Document your conversation for the physician's review and recommendations.

3. A patient comes to the office today for a refill of Vicodin ES 7.5/500 mg, one pill every 8 hours as needed with food. After checking the medical record, you notice the patient had a prescription written 5 days ago for the same drug and was dispensed 30 pills at that time. Is it too early for this drug to be refilled? Provide your documentation to the physician. What type of information should you include?

4. The physician has recommended OTC medication for treatment of symptoms of the common cold. What types of things should Martha encourage her patients to do when they are choosing an OTC?

5. What types of medication should be considered when obtaining a medical history. What information about these medications should be documented in the patient's chart?

Workplace Applications

1. Martha has noticed that the other medical assistants in the office are unsure of the drug classifications for controlled substances. Prepare an educational handout for the office to use as a resource. The handout should include a definition of "controlled substance," an explanation of each schedule (I to V), the potential for abuse and/or addiction, and some examples of drugs in each schedule. Note whether the prescription can be written or oral.

2. The route of administration used will depend on the intended use of the drug. What route of administration would Martha expect to see for each of the illnesses or medications listed below (oral, topical, inhaled, sublingual, mucous membrane, or parenteral route)? Why?

   a. Annual flu vaccination

   b. Bronchodilator for treatment of an acute asthma attack

   c. Hyperlipidemia

   d. Nitroglycerin used for angina

   e. Dermatitis

   f. Allergic rhinitis

   g. Insulin

   h. Tinea pedis

   i. Conjunctivitis

Internet Activity

Search the Internet for articles on prescription drug abuse. What types of things can the medical assistant do to aid in preventing the abuse of prescription drugs?

Chapter 32 Quiz

Name: _____

1. List three factors that affect drug action.

   a. _____

   b. _____

   c. _____

2. A _____ increases peristaltic activity of the large intestine.

3. Pharmacology is the broad science that deals with the origin, nature, chemistry, effects, and uses of drugs.

   a. True

   b. False

4. Pharmaceutical companies developing new medications must first gain DEA approval before the drugs can be sold to consumers.

   a. True

   b. False

5. A diuretic increases urinary output and decreases blood pressure.

   a. True

   b. False

6. Schedule II drugs are closely monitored and controlled.

   a. True

   b. False

7. List three types of drug classifications.

   a. _____

   b. _____

   c. _____

8. PDR stands for _____.

CHAPTER 33

Pharmacology Math

Vocabulary Review

Define the following terms:

1. Dispense

   _____

2. Stat

   _____

3. Unit dose

   _____

4. Nomogram

   _____

5. Surface area

   _____

6. Route

   _____

Fill in the blanks with basic drug label terms.

7. The size or amount of the drug available in the drug package is the _____.

8. _____ is the potency of the drug.

9. A(n) _____ is the pure drug that is dissolved in a liquid to form a solution.

10. Usually sterile water or saline, the _____ is the liquid that dissolves the solute.

Skills and Concepts

11. What are the three basic steps the medical assistant must complete for accurate calculation of a prescribed dose?

    a. _____

    b. _____

    c. _____

Part I: Metric System

Consider the following fundamental units of the metric system:

Mass or weight: gram (g) *always lowercase*

Volume: liter (L) *always capitalized*

Length: meter (m) *always lowercase*

Consider the following equivalents:

Mass and Weight	Volume
1 kg = 1000 g	1 kL = 1000 liters
1 g = 1000 mg	1 L = 1000 mL (or cc)
1 mg = 1000 μg	1 mL (or 1 cc) = 1000 μL
1 dg = 0.1 g or $^1/_{10}$ g	1 dL = 0.1 L or $^1/_{10}$ L
1 cg = 0.01 g or $^1/_{100}$ g	1 cL = 0.01 L or $^1/_{100}$ L
1 mg = 0.001 g or $^1/_{1000}$ g	1 mL (or 1 cc) = 0.001 L or $^1/_{1000}$ L

Write the prefix for the following (remember to write the prefixes in lowercase).

12. _____ $^1/_{100}$ of a unit

13. _____ $^1/_{10}$ of a unit

14. _____ $^1/_{1000}$ of a unit

15. _____ $^1/_{1,000,000}$ of a unit

16. _____ 10 units

17. _____ 100 units

18. _____ 1000 units

Convert the following by moving the decimals, by multiplication, or by division. Show your work in the space to the right of the questions.

19. 1.5 L = _____ mL

20. 500 mg = _____ g

21. 3 g = _____ mg

22. 2000 mg = _____ g

23. 2.5 g = _____ mg

24. 0.5 g = _____ mg

25. 500 mL = _____ L

26. 0.75 g = _____ mg

27. 1 kg = _____ g

28. 1000 mg = _____ g

Part II: Apothecary System and Household Measurements

29. The basic unit of weight in the apothecary system for a solid measurement is the _____.

30. The basic unit of volume in the apothecary system for a liquid measurement is _____.

31. Household measurements are not precisely accurate, so they should never be used in the medical setting.

    a. True

    b. False

32. The household measurement for weight is _____.

33. In household measurements, liquid oral medications are taken by the drop, teaspoon, or tablespoon and are supplied in bottles labeled in ounces or pints.

    a. True

    b. False

34. Supply the abbreviations or symbols for these metric, apothecary system, and common household units.

    a. ounce _____

    b. teaspoon _____

    c. milligram _____

    d. grain _____

    e. pint _____

    f. dram _____

    g. tablespoon _____

Use the conversions to complete the questions that follow.

Mass and Weight	Volume
1 cup = 8 oz	1 tsp = 5 mL (cc)
1 oz = 2 Tbsp	1 Tbsp = 15 mL (cc)
1 Tbsp = 3 tsp	1 fl oz = 30 mL (cc)
1 tsp = 60 drops	1 grain = 60 mg

35. A standard teaspoon equals 5 mL. If a liquid drug has 100 mg/teaspoon, how many milligrams are in each milliliter? _____

    a. How did you determine your answer?

    _____

    _____

    _____

36. You are asked to give 2 teaspoons of cough medicine to a child. How many milliliters will you give?

_____

37. How many teaspoons are in 1 oz? _____

38. Now that you know that 5 mL is the same as 1 tsp, how many milliliters are in 1 oz?

_____

Part III: Conversions between Systems of Measurement

Conversions between units of measurements can also be done by using the following formula:

$$\text{Have} \times \frac{\text{Wanted}}{\text{Have (conversion)}} = \text{Unit Wanted in New System}$$

Convert pounds to kilograms. The conversion factor is 1 kg = 2.2 lb. Show your work in the space to the right of the questions.

39. 150 lb = _____ kg

40. 78 lb = _____ kg

41. 18 kg = _____ lb

42. 210 lb = _____ kg

43. 71 kg = _____ lb

44. 198 lb = _____ kg

45. 112 lb = _____ kg

46. 163 lb = _____ kg

47. 21 kg = _____ lb

48. 4.4 lb = _____ kg

Convert inches to centimeters. There are 2.5 cm/inch. Show your work in the space to the right of the questions.

49. 62 inches = _____ cm

50. 34 inches = _____ cm

51. 97 inches = _____ cm

52. 5′0″ = _____ inches = _____ cm

53. 6′2″ = _____ inches = _____ cm

Part IV: Decimals and Percents

The act of dividing a fraction results in a decimal number. Decimal numbers can then be converted to percentages by moving the decimal two spaces to the right, as follows:

$0.25 = 25.0\%$, commonly written 25%

Convert the following decimals to percentages. Show your work in the space to the right of the questions.

54. $0.75 = $ _____ %

55. $0.33 = $ _____ %

56. $0.25 = $ _____ %

57. $1.0\ \ = $ _____ %

58. $0.50 = $ _____ %

Part V: Ratio and Proportion

A proportion is written as follows:

$$\frac{4}{16} = \frac{1}{4} \quad \text{or} \quad 4:16::1:4$$

Use *cross-multiplication* to solve for x. Show your work in the space to the right of the questions.

59. $3:4 = x:12$

60. $1:2 = x:6$

61. $2:5 = x:100$

62. $2:6 = x:12$

63. $1:3 = x:75$

Case Studies

Calculate the following doses of medication. Remember the following standard formula:

$$\frac{\text{Available strength}}{\text{Ordered strength}} = \frac{\text{Available amount}}{\text{Amount to give}}$$

Physician's Order	Label Reads	Amount to Give	Practice Charting
Keflex 500 mg	250 mg capsule		
Lasix 40 mg	20 mg tablet		
Zoloft 75 mg	25 mg tablet		
Claritin 30 mg	10 mg tablet		
Prilosec 40 mg	10 mg capsule		
Celebrex 200 mg	100 mg capsule		
Vioxx 12.5 mg	25 mg		
Lanoxin 0.125 mg	0.25 mg tablet		
Coumadin 20 mg	5 mg tablet		
Augmentin 250 mg	500 mg per 5 mL		
Prednisone 40 mg	5 mg tablet		
Prozac 20 mg	10 mg capsule		
Synthroid 0.44 mg	88 µg per tablet		
Zocor 60 mg	20 mg tablet		
Glucophage 1 g	500 mg tablet		
Zestril 2.5 mg	5 mg tablet		
Norvasc 10 mg	2.5 mg tablet		
Cipro 750 mg	250 mg tablet		
Zyrtec syrup 4 mg	5 mg/5 mL		
Zovirax 200 mg	400 mg tablet		

Pediatric Dosages

Clark's Rule

Clark's rule is based on the weight of the child. It uses 150 lb (70 kg) as the average adult weight and assumes that the child's dose is proportionately less. The formula is as follows:

$$\text{Pediatric dose} = \frac{\text{Child's weight in pounds}}{150 \text{ lb}} \times \text{Adult dose}$$

Order	Adult Dose	Child's Weight	Amount to Give
Penicillin	100,000 U	22 lb	
Benadryl	50 mg	13 lb	
Tylenol	500 mg	54 lb	
Sudafed	60 mg	37 lb	

West's Nomogram

West's nomogram uses a calculation of the body surface area (BSA) of infants and young children to determine the pediatric dose.

$$\text{Pediatric dose} = \frac{\text{(BSA) of child in m}^2}{1.7 \text{ m}^2 \text{ (average adult BSA)}} \times \text{Adult dose}$$

Order	Adult Dose	Child's BSA	Amount to Give
Penicillin	100,000 U	0.5 m^2	
Benadryl	50 mg	0.3 m^2	
Tylenol	500 mg	0.6 m^2	
Sudafed	60 mg	0.7 m^2	

Workplace Applications

Use Clark's rule, West's nomogram, or the body weight method to answer the following questions:

1. A child weighs 42 lb. The physician orders 1 mg of medication per kilogram. How many kilograms does the child weigh? How many milligrams of medication do you need to give?

2. An infant weighs 14 lb. The adult dose is 100 mg. When Clark's rule is used, how much is the pediatric dose?

3. The physician orders 5 mg of medication per kilogram of body weight. The patient weighs 145 lb. How many milligrams do you give?

4. The child has a BSA of 0.9 m^2, and the adult dose is 200 mg. According to West's nomogram, what is the pediatric dose?

5. The nurse practitioner orders 250 mg of Rocephin to be given by injection. The vial contains Rocephin at a concentration of 500 mg/mL. How much medication will the medical assistant draw into the syringe?

6. The patient takes 5000 U of heparin by injection each day. The vial contains heparin, 10,000 U/mL. How much heparin does the home health nurse need to draw up into the syringe?

7. The patient weighs 163 lb. The order is for 2 mg/kg. How much medicine does the patient need?

8. The physician orders Phenergan 12.5 mg by mouth. You have Phenergan syrup that has a concentration of 25 mg/5 mL. How many milliliters will you give?

9. You need to give a 500-unit injection of vitamin B$_{12}$. You have on hand vitamin B$_{12}$ at a concentration unit of 1000 units/mL. How much will you measure in the syringe?

10. An infant who weighs 11 lbs is ordered amoxil q6hr. The label reads 250 mg in 5 cc of suspension. The recommended range of the medication for an infant is 15 mg/kg/day. How much should the child receive per dose?

11. An infant who weighs 12 lbs 5 ounces is ordered Diflucan qid for the treatment of thrush. The label reads 150 mg in 3 cc of suspension. The recommended range of the medication is 3 mg/kg/day. How much should the child receive per dose?

12. An infant is ordered Zantac bid. The infant weighs 35 lbs. The label reads 300 mg in 5 cc of suspension. The recommended range of the medication is 10 mg/kg/day. How much should the child receive per dose?

Internet Activity

Use the Internet or a drug reference book to collect information and make index cards for 20 commonly used drugs. Include the following information:

Brand name:	
Generic name:	
Type of drug:	
Usual dose:	
Uses:	

Chapter 33 Quiz

Name: _____

1. One cup equals _____ oz.

2. One teaspoon equals _____ mL.

3. 16.4 kg = _____ lb

4. A grain is part of the _____ system.
   a. metric
   b. household
   c. apothecary

5. A liter is a unit of
   a. weight
   b. volume
   c. length

6. Milliliters are sometimes called
   _____.

7. It is acceptable to administer a medication you did not prepare.
   a. True
   b. False

8. There are _____ lb in 1 kg.

9. Clark's rule uses a child's age to calculate dosage.
   a. True
   b. False

10. To prepare a drug for administration:
    _____.

CHAPTER 34

Administering Medications

Vocabulary Review

Match the following terms with their definitions.

1. _____ Angled tip of a needle

2. _____ Narrowing of the bronchiole tubes

3. _____ Abnormal accumulation of fluid in the interstitial spaces of tissues

4. _____ A coating added to an oral medication that resists the effects of stomach juices; designed so medicine is absorbed in the small intestine

5. _____ Sealed so that no air is allowed to enter

6. _____ Low blood pressure

7. _____ Administering repeated injections of diluted extracts of the substance that causes an allergy; also called *desensitization*

8. _____ An abnormally hard, inflamed area

9. _____ Administering a double dose for the first dose of the medication; usually done with antibiotic therapy to reach therapeutic blood levels quickly

10. _____ Surgical removal of the breast; usually includes excision of lymph nodes in the axillary region

11. _____ The curved formation of liquids in a container

12. _____ Excretion of an unusually large amount of urine

a. Bevel

b. Scored tablet

c. Hypotension

d. Polyuria

e. Volatile

f. Wheal

g. Viscosity

h. Vasodilation

i. Immunotherapy

j. Loading dose

k. Edema

l. Meniscus

m. Bronchoconstriction

n. Induration

o. Enteric-coated

p. Mastectomy

q. Hermetically sealed

13. _____ Drug in pill form manufactured with an indentation for division through the center

14. _____ Increase in the diameter of a blood vessel

15. _____ The quality of being thick; property of resistance to flow in a fluid

16. _____ Referring to an explosive substance's capacity to vaporize at a low temperature

17. _____ Localized area of edema or a raised lesion

Solid Oral Forms

Define the following.

18. Scored

_____

19. Tablet

_____

20. Buffered

_____

21. Capsule

_____

22. Caplet

_____

23. Time-released

_____

Liquid Oral Forms

Define the following.

24. Syrup

_____

25. Aromatic waters

_____

26. Liquors

_____

27. Suspension

_____

28. Emulsion

_____

29. Gel or magma

_____

30. Tinctures

_____

31. Elixirs

_____

Mucous Membrane Forms

List the site of absorption for the following.

32. Buccal

_____

33. Sublingual

_____

34. Inhalation

_____

Topical Forms

Describe the following.

35. Lotion

_____

36. Liniment

_____

37. Ointment

_____

38. Transdermal

_____

Parenteral Forms

Define the following.

39. Vial

_____

40. Ampule

_____

41. Multiuse

_____

42. Prefilled

_____

43. Cartridge system

_____

Skills and Concepts

44. List the seven rights of drug administration.

    a. _____
    b. _____
    c. _____
    d. _____
    e. _____
    f. _____
    g. _____

45. When should the medical assistant check the drug label?

    _____

    _____

    _____

46. List four things the medical assistant can do to ensure safety of medication administration.

    a. _____
    b. _____
    c. _____
    d. _____

Label the following statements as either "ampule" or "vial."

47. Has a rubber stopper _____

48. Has sharp edges after it is opened _____

49. Is always single-use _____

50. Must have air injected into it before medicine can be removed _____

51. Can be multiuse _____

52. A filtered needle is required to avoid getting glass in the syringe _____

53. Has a vacuum after it is opened _____

54. Extra care is required to avoid contamination _____

55. Always disposed of in a sharps container _____

56. Gauze or an unopened alcohol prep should be used to prevent injury as the neck breaks away _____

57. List four routes of parenteral administration. Include approved abbreviations.

   a. _____

   b. _____

   c. _____

   d. _____

Parenteral Medication Equipment

Indicate which statements about needles are true (T) and which statements are false (F).

58. _____ Needles may be purchased separately or as part of a needle-syringe unit.

59. _____ The diameter or lumen size of a needle is called its gauge.

60. _____ The larger the gauge number is, the smaller the diameter of the needle.

61. _____ Gauges 25 and 26 are commonly used for subcutaneous injections.

62. _____ Gauges 20 to 23 are usually necessary for intramuscular injections when the medication is thick (e.g., penicillin).

63. _____ Needles that are ½ or ⅝ inch long are used for intramuscular injections.

64. _____ Needles that are ½ or ⅝ inch long are used for subcutaneous injections.

65. _____ A contaminated needle should be immediately placed in a sharps container.

66. _____ The parts of the needle are the barrel, calibrated scale(s), plunger, and tip.

67. _____ Longer needles are necessary for depositing drugs intradermally.

68. Label the syringes in the figure below.

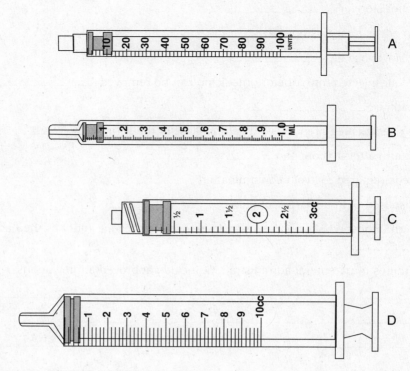

a. On the insulin syringe, draw a line at 62 units.

b. On the tuberculin syringe, draw a line at 0.3 mL.

c. On the 3-cc Luer-Lok syringe, draw a line at ½ cc.

d. On the 10-cc slip-tip syringe, draw a line at 4.8 cc.

Injection Sites

69. Label the intramuscular, intradermal, and subcutaneous injection sites correctly on the following figure.

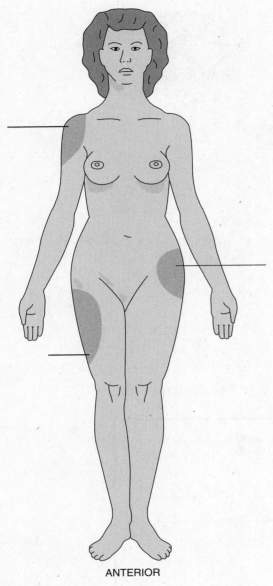

ANTERIOR

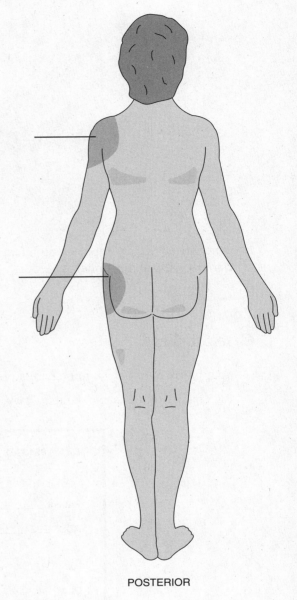

POSTERIOR

a. Deltoid

b. Ventrogluteal

c. Vastus lateralis

d. Gluteal (dorsogluteal)

Pediatric Sites

70. On the following figure, label and name the appropriate injection site for a small child who is too young to walk.

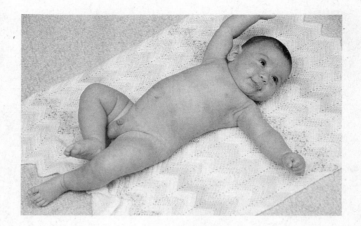

71. When instilling ear drops into an infant's ear, you must straighten the ear canal. In what direction do you pull the pinna? _____

Case Studies

1. Your physician asks you to prepare a prescription for his signature. Prepare the following:

   RF: Lipitor 10 mg, take one tablet daily. Dispense 30 tablets with three refills.

DEA#: 8543201   John Jones, M.D.   Tel: 544-8976
                     108 N. Main St.
                     City, State

Patient _____ DATE _____

ADDRESS _____

Rx:

Disp:

Sig:

Refill _____ Times
Please label ☑ _____

RF: Ativan 1 mg, take one to two tablets as needed at bedtime. Dispense 30 tablets with no refills.

```
DEA#: 8543201      John Jones, M.D.   Tel: 544-8976
                   108 N. Main St.
                   City, State

Patient _____   DATE _____

ADDRESS _____


Rx:

Disp:

Sig:



Refill _____ Times
Please label ☑   _____
```

2. Dorothy is administering DTaP 0.5 mL intramuscularly to a 5-year-old patient. What site should she use? Document the procedure.

3. You have just administered allergy injections to a patient. As you are informing the patient that he must wait in the office for 20 minutes to monitor any reactions, the patient informs you that he is unable to remain in the office. What should you do? Document your answer.

4. Dorothy is providing instruction on the use of an Epipen to a patient with an allergy to bee stings. Provide step-by-step instructions for the patient. Using your knowledge of patient education, what are some points to remember with demonstration? What types of materials should you give the patient to take home? Document your session with the patient in the medical record.

5. Amanda is very nervous about receiving her kindergarten vaccinations today. What can Dorothy do to calm her fears?

6. You are gathering a new patient history for Dr. Thau. What types of questions should you ask the patient with regard to his or her medication usage? Role-play with a partner, interviewing each other about medication use. Document your findings.

Workplace Applications

1. Dorothy has been asked by Dr. Thau to update the medication abbreviation list to be included as part of the policies and procedures manual. Use the list below to spell out each.

   a. q4h _____

   b. tid _____

   c. qid _____

   d. bid _____

   e. q3h _____

   f. HS _____

   g. AC _____

   h. PC _____

   i. PRN _____

   j. PO _____

   k. NPO _____

   l. PR _____

   m. IV _____

   n. SC (SQ) _____

   o. IM _____

   p. SL _____

   q. QD _____

   r. QOD _____

   s. QAM _____

   t. QPM _____

Dorothy is in charge of organizing a newly constructed examination room. The room will be used for medication administration, and Dorothy wants to make sure it is fully equipped. What supplies must Dorothy order to fulfill OSHA guidelines? What are some other items she may want to ensure are in the room to make patients as comfortable as possible?

Chapter 34 Quiz

Name: _____

1. An 18-gauge needle is larger than a 23-gauge needle.

   a. True

   b. False

2. A tuberculin syringe holds _____ mL (cc).

3. An ampule is multiuse.

   a. True

   b. False

4. One site for subcutaneous injection is the:

   a. vastus lateralis

   b. deltoid

   c. gluteal (dorsogluteal)

   d. abdomen

5. The safest site for an intramuscular injection on a small child is the:

   a. vastus lateralis.

   b. deltoid.

   c. gluteal (dorsogluteal).

6. Milliliters are sometimes called _____ on syringes.

7. The _____ is the slanted part of a needle.

8. _____ is the route for heparin and insulin.

9. Z-track is used for an intramuscular injection of an irritating substance.

   a. True

   b. False

10. Intradermal medication is usually given at a 90-degree angle.

    a. True

    b. False

Assisting with Medical Emergencies

Vocabulary Review

Define the following.

1. Cyanosis _____

2. Dyspnea _____

3. Ecchymosis _____

4. Emetic _____

5. Fibrillation _____

6. Hematuria _____

7. Mediastinum _____

8. Myocardium _____

9. Necrosis _____

10. Photophobia _____

11. Polydipsia _____

12. Polyuria _____

13. Transient ischemic attack _____

Fill in the blanks with the correct terms.

14. _____ is defined as the immediate care given to a person who has been injured or has suddenly become ill.

15. AED stands for _____.

16. CPR stands for _____.

17. CVA stands for _____.

18. TIA stands for _____.

19. MI stands for _____.

20. _____ is the most dangerous form of heat-related injury and results in a shutdown of body systems.

21. _____ are the initial signs of a heat-related emergency.

22. Patients with _____ appear flushed and report headaches, nausea, vertigo, and weakness.

Skills and Concepts

23. List five classic symptoms of a heart attack.

    a. _____

    b. _____

    c. _____

    d. _____

    e. _____

24. List seven types of shock.

    a. _____

    b. _____

    c. _____

    d. _____

    e. _____

    f. _____

    g. _____

25. Sprains and strains are treated with:

    a. _____

    b. _____

    c. _____

    d. _____

26. Give five examples of situations in which patients with abdominal pain should be seen by a healthcare provider immediately.

    a. _____

    b. _____

    c. _____

    d. _____

    e. _____

Case Studies

1. Sally calls the office complaining of lumbar pain that has been present for the past 2 weeks. What type of triage questions should you ask the patient? When should the patient be seen in the office? Provide the appropriate documentation.

2. Mr. Walker, a 64-year-old patient of Dr. Bendt, calls the office complaining of shortness of breath, pressure in the chest, and sweating for the last hour. As you examine the patient's chart, you see that Mr. Walker is a smoker and obese. What advice should you give the patient? Show your documentation.

    After you refer Mr. Walker to the emergency room, he refuses to go, stating "I don't feel well enough to drive to the hospital." What advice would you provide the patient? Document your conversation.

3. A patient calls, stating that she has found a tick on her left forearm. Explain the proper technique for removal of the tick. What signs and symptoms should the patient watch for? Document your conversation.

Workplace Applications

1. At a recent office meeting, triage difficulties were addressed. You have been assigned the duty of streamlining the triage questions as the patients call in. In addition, the physician would like you to make a list of "home care advice" to go along with the symptoms. The work should also include "if" and "how soon" the patient should be seen in the office or under what circumstances he or she should be referred to the emergency room. Include the following situations in your project.

Asthma	Insect bites and stings
Wounds	Head injuries
Burns	Chest pain
Back pain	Dysuria
URI	Syncope
Hyperglycemia	High blood pressure

2. As a medical assistant you understand that there are many different signs and symptoms of medical emergencies. In order to educate the patients about the importance of early detection and treatment, Dr. Bendt has asked you to create an informative brochure for them. The brochure should include the following:

   a. Definition of illness

   b. Importance of early detection

   c. Signs and symptoms

   d. Risk factors

   e. Prevention recommendations

   f. What should be done if you think you are experiencing this condition

3. Cheryl is in charge of establishing the office crash cart. What type of supplies should be included in the cart? What medications should be included? How should the cart and supplies be maintained? Where should the cart be kept?

Internet Activities

1. You notice that your CPR certification is about to expire. Search for a list of certification sites in your area. Make a list of the contact information, and share the locations with your classmates.

2. Perform a search for the Poison Control Center in your area. Search for and create a list of ideas for ways to prevent poisoning. Create an informative poster to display in your physician's office.

Chapter 35 Quiz

Name: _____

1. AED stands for _____.

2. A _____ seizure involves uncontrolled muscular contractions.

3. List three symptoms of a heart attack.

   a. _____

   b. _____

   c. _____

4. Explain the difference between strains and sprains.

5. Explain how the Rule of Nines pertains to burns.

6. Define *epistaxis*. _____

7. When assessing an open wound, the first thing the medical assistant should do is put on gloves.

   a. True

   b. False

8. An effective way to lower the victim's temperature is to _____.

9. Describe some common symptoms of dehydration.

10. Insulin shock is a type of hyperglycemia.

    a. True

    b. False

CHAPTER 36

Assisting in Ophthalmology and Otolaryngology

Vocabulary Review

Match the following terms with their definitions.

1. _____ Adjustment of the eye for seeing various sizes of objects at different distances

2. _____ Reduction or dimness of vision with no apparent organic cause; often referred to as *lazy eye syndrome*

3. _____ An allied healthcare professional specializing in evaluation of hearing function, detection of hearing impairment, and determination of the anatomic site of impairment

4. _____ Structures found in the retina that make the perception of color possible

5. _____ A small pit in the center of the retina that is considered the center of clearest vision

6. _____ Any substance or medication that causes constriction of the pupil

7. _____ Region at the back of the eye where the optic nerve meets the retina; considered the blind spot of the eye because it contains only nerve fibers and no rods or cones and therefore is insensitive to light

8. _____ Second cranial nerve, which carries impulses for the sense of sight

a. Cones

b. Accommodation

c. Seborrhea

d. Psoriasis

e. Rods

f. Audiologist

g. Amblyopia

h. Photophobia

i. Optic nerve

j. Otosclerosis

k. Ototoxic

l. Fovea centralis

m. Optic disc

n. Miotic

9. _____ Formation of spongy bone in the labyrinth of the ear, often causing the auditory ossicles to become fixed and unable to vibrate when sound enters the ear

10. _____ A substance or medication that damages the eighth cranial nerve or the organs of hearing and balance

11. _____ Abnormal sensitivity to light

12. _____ Usually chronic, recurrent skin disease marked by bright red patches covered with silvery scales

13. _____ Structures located in the retina of the eye and forming the light-sensitive elements

14. _____ Excessive discharge of sebum from the sebaceous glands, forming greasy scales or cheesy plugs on the body

Fill in the blanks with the correct terms.

15. A(n) _____ is a licensed medical physician who can diagnose eye disorders, prescribe medication, conduct eye screenings, prescribe glasses or contact lenses, and perform otic surgery.

16. _____ are trained to fill prescriptions written for corrective lenses by grinding the lenses and dispensing eyewear.

17. A _____ can conduct eye examinations, diagnose vision problems and eye diseases, and treat visual defects through corrective lenses and eye exercises.

Skills and Concepts

18. On the following figure, label the structures of the outer eye.

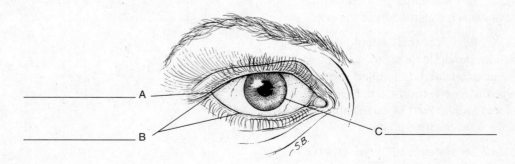

19. Name the two disorders of the outer eye that are pictured in the following figures.

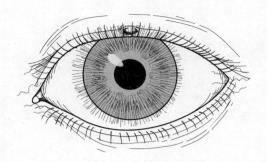

a. _____

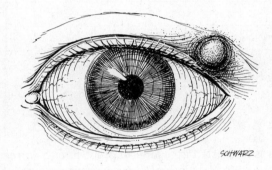

b. _____

20. List and define three refractive errors.

a. _____
   _____

b. _____
   _____

c. _____
   _____

21. List three signs and symptoms of refractive errors.

   a. _____

   b. _____

   c. _____

22. Compare and contrast strabismus and amblyopia.

   _____

   _____

   _____

   _____

23. Differentiate between otitis media and otitis externa.

   _____

   _____

   _____

   _____

Case Studies

1. One of Amy's patients is interested in a surgical procedure to correct her myopia. What can Amy tell her patient about the different types of correction procedures?

2. Joe, a 5-year-old patient, is brought to the office today with itchy, watery eyes with a purulent discharge. His mother states that Joe's older brother was recently seen in the office with the same symptoms. What type of problem do you think Joe has? Is it contagious? What education can Amy provide to Joe and his mother to stop the spread of infection? Document the patient education intervention.

3. A patient comes to the office today complaining of pain and swelling in the left eye. As Amy obtains a history, she finds that the patient may have wood chips in her eye. The physician orders an eye irrigation to be performed on the patient. Amy administers 10 cc of sterile saline into the patient's left eye. Document the case and the procedure using the SOAPE format.

   S: _____

   _____

   O: _____

   _____

Refer to the charts in the following figure while answering the next group of questions.

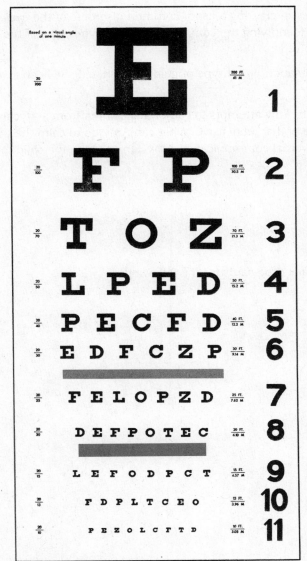
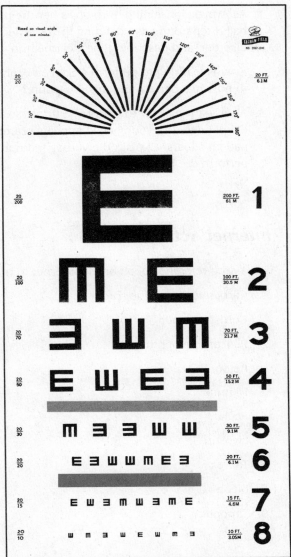

4. Your patient can read line number 8 with the right eye, number 9 with the left eye, and number 8 with both eyes on the Snellen chart. Document your findings. Use appropriate abbreviations. Be sure to include the date and your signature.

_____

_____

5. Your patient cannot read English. He indicates that he can see line number 6 with the right eye, number 5 with the left eye, and number 6 with both eyes on the E chart. How will you have your patient respond so that you know your findings are accurate? Document your findings below.

_____

_____

Workplace Applications

1. As Amy is in training, Kim gives her the task of creating a list of common disorders of the eyeball. Prepare the list, defining the disorder, identifying the common signs and symptoms of the disorder, and describing the treatment involved.

2. Amy is learning to perform a Snellen examination. What type of guidelines should she keep in mind while performing this procedure?

3. After learning how to perform a throat swab, Amy attempts to gather a specimen from a 4-year-old patient. The young child appears scared and apprehensive. What can Amy do to calm the patient's fears? Explain the verbal and nonverbal communication Amy can use with the child to perform the procedure.

Internet Activities

Use a drug reference book or the Internet to make drug cards for the following.

1. Carbamide peroxide (Debrox)

2. Cortisporin otic

3. Pilocarpine ophthalmic

4. Betoptic

5. Diamox

6. Acular

7. Livostin

8. Tobrex

9. Bleph-10

10. Timoptic

Chapter 36 Quiz

Name: _____

1. Nearsightedness is called _____.

2. OD means _____.

3. What is the name of the test for color blind-
   ness? _____

4. AS means _____.

5. List two types of glaucoma:
   a. _____
   b. _____

6. PERRLA means _____.

7. Describe the functions of the middle ear.

8. The pinna is part of the inner ear.
   a. True
   b. False

9. Describe the proper technique for ear
   irrigation.
   _____
   _____

Assisting in Dermatology

Vocabulary Review

Define the following terms.

1. Alopecia

_____

2. Cryosurgery

_____

3. Debridement

_____

4. Ecchymosis

_____

5. Electrodesiccation

_____

6. Exacerbation

_____

7. Hyperplasia

_____

8. Jaundice

_____

9. Keratin

_____

10. Leukoderma

_____

11. Opaque

_____

12. Remission

_____

Fill in the blanks with the correct terms.

13. Sebaceous glands release _____, an oily substance that lubricates the skin.

14. The epidermis is the thin uppermost layer, and the _____ is the thicker layer beneath.

15. A variety of microorganisms called normal or resident _____ are found on the skin and may increase the risk for integumentary system infections.

16. _____ is a common contagious, superficial infection caused by streptococci or Staphylococcus aureus.

17. _____ is a disorder of the hair follicle and sebaceous gland unit.

18. _____ is characterized by a vesicular rash located on the face, neck, elbows, posterior knees and behind the ears.

19. _____ is an inherited recessive trait, where patients are unable to produce melanin, so they have white hair and skin and lack pigment in the iris.

Skills and Concepts

20. Describe the major functions of the skin.

_____

_____

_____

21. Label the three layers of the skin in the following drawing.

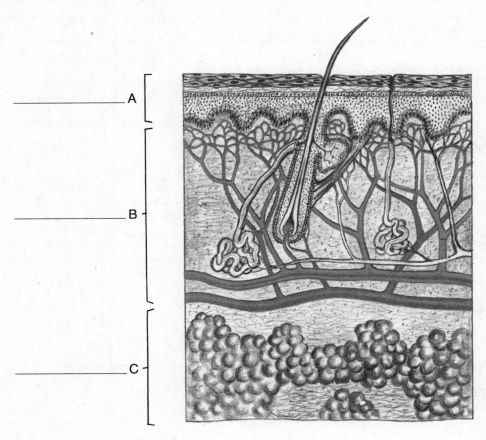

_____ A

_____ B

_____ C

Define and give an example of the following.

22. Macule

_____

_____

23. Papule

_____

_____

24. Plaque

_____

_____

25. Fissure

_____

_____

26. Pustule

_____

_____

27. Vesicle

_____

_____

28. Bulla

_____

_____

29. Cyst

_____

_____

30. Ulcer

_____

_____

31. Wheal

_____

_____

32. List and describe four types of inflammatory skin disorders.

    a. _____

    b. _____

    c. _____

    d. _____

33. List and describe two types of autoimmune disorders.

    a. _____

    b. _____

34. List and describe the three different types of burns.

    a. _____

    b. _____

    c. _____

35. Discuss the differences between benign and malignant tumors. Provide examples of each.

_____

_____

_____

_____

36. List the seven warning signs of cancer.

   a. C _____

   b. A _____

   c. U _____

   d. T _____

   e. I _____

   f. O _____

   g. N _____

37. List the early warning signs of malignant melanoma.

   a. _____

   b. _____

   c. _____

   d. _____

38. List and describe three ways to perform allergy testing.

   a. _____

   b. _____

   c. _____

39. List three procedures for appearance modification.

   a. _____

   b. _____

   c. _____

Case Studies

1. A patient complains of a red, flat rash with intense itching. What types of triage questions should you ask this patient? Use the correct medical terminology to chart your findings. Use appropriate abbreviations. Be sure to include the date and your signature.

2. A patient comes to the office with a red, raised rash with small blisters. What type of triage questions should you ask this patient? Use the correct medical terminology to chart your findings. Use appropriate abbreviations. Be sure to include the date and your signature.

3. A patient calls and states there is redness on her upper arm. What questions do you need to ask before scheduling the appointment? What vital signs should be obtained for the patient? Why? With a partner, role-play the case; document your findings.

4. A 6-year-old patient comes to the office today with a red, raised area around the mouth and nose. As Melissa examines the area she notices it is moist, inflamed, and crusted. What type of infection do these symptoms represent? With your knowledge of this infection, what patient education can you provide the patient and parents with regard to stopping the spread of infection? What types of medications are used to treat this infection? Document the case.

5. A 15-year-old patient comes to the office today complaining of acne over the face and neck. What types of treatment options are available? Are there any contraindications to the different types of treatment? Document your patient education session.

Workplace Applications

1. Patient education is an important part of Melissa's job. Often patients are not aware of the medical terms given to common infections. Examine the following list of mycotic infections, and provide the common name for each.

   a. Tinea pedis

   b. Tinea cruris

   c. Tinea corporis

   d. Tinea unguium

What type of medication is used to treat mycotic infections?

2. Scabies (itch mite) and pediculosis (lice) are the two most common parasites to infest individuals. Dr. Lee has asked Melissa to develop a patient education handout on how to prevent the spread of these infestations. Include common medications used for treatment, as well as how they are taken. What can patients do around the house to eliminate mites or lice? Who should be treated?

3. One of Melissa's duties is to assist the physician during tissue biopsies. What types of things should she do to prepare for such procedures?

Internet Activities

1. Search the Internet for a list of sun safety recommendations. How can you reduce the risk of skin cancer? Create a list of ideas, and compare it with those of your classmates.

2. Locate an article online regarding the treatment and management of different types of burns. Summarize the article, and be prepared to share your findings in class.

Chapter 37 Quiz

Name: _____

Match the following terms with their definitions.

1. _____ Shingles
2. _____ Pustule
3. _____ Fissure
4. _____ Allegra
5. _____ Varicella
6. _____ Nevi
7. _____ Scabies
8. _____ Sebum
9. _____ Bilirubin
10. _____ Resident flora

a. An oily substance that lubricates the skin.

b. Moles

c. An oral medication used to treat allergic reactions

d. A variety of microorganisms found on the skin

e. Chicken pox

f. Herpes zoster

g. Orange-colored pigment in bile, which when it accumulates leads to jaundice

h. Itch mite

i. Small elevation on the skin containing pus

j. Cracklike sore

CHAPTER 38

Assisting in Gastroenterology

Vocabulary Review

Supply the correct term for each definition.

1. _____ The surgical joining together of two normally distinct organs

2. _____ A hard, impacted mass of feces in the colon

3. _____ Narrow slits or clefts in the abdominal wall

4. _____ Gas expelled through the anus

5. _____ Abnormal enlargement of the liver

6. _____ Valve guarding the opening between the ileum and cecum

7. _____ Surgical formation of an opening of the ileum on the surface of the abdomen through which fecal material is emptied

8. _____ Black, tarry stool containing digested blood; usually caused by bleeding in the upper gastrointestinal tract

9. _____ Tumors on stems frequently found in the mucosal lining of the colon

10. _____ Physicians who are concerned with the diseases and disorders involving the stomach, small intestine, large intestine (colon), appendix, and the accessory organs of the liver, gallbladder, and pancreas

Define the following terms.

11. Peritoneum

_____

12. Mesentery

_____

13. Omentum

_____

14. Adhesions

_____

15. Ascites

_____

16. Examine the following case. Rewrite the case using medical terminology and the proper abbreviations.

Ms. Pullman comes to the office today complaining of pain in the upper right area of her abdomen. Her symptoms include a lack of appetite, profuse sweating, and a yellowish hue to her skin. On examination Dr. Sahani finds an abnormal enlargement of the liver. The blood tests reveal a decrease in the volume percentage of red blood cells in the whole blood.

_____

_____

_____

_____

_____

_____

Skills and Concepts

17. Describe the three primary functions of the digestive system.

a. _____

b. _____

c. _____

18. Label the structures of the upper abdominal cavity on the following figure.

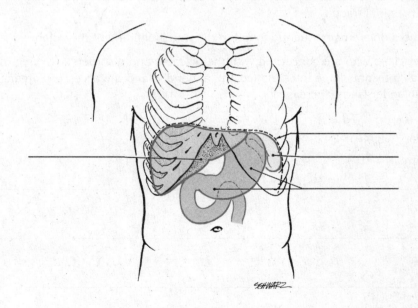

Abdominal Regions

19. List the nine regions of the abdomen in the grid below.

Fill in the blanks.

20. The gallbladder is located in the _____ quadrant of the abdomen.

21. The appendix is located in the _____ quadrant of the abdomen.

22. The stomach is located in the _____ quadrant of the abdomen.

23. The liver is located in the _____ quadrant of the abdomen.

24. The pancreas is located in the _____ quadrant of the abdomen.

25. List the seven parts of the large intestine; start with the vermiform appendix.

 a. _____

 b. _____

 c. _____

 d. _____

 e. _____

 f. _____

 g. _____

Complete the following sentences.

26. The _____ delivers bile from the liver to the duodenum where digestion is completed.

27. The _____ intestine is made up of the duodenum, jejunum, and ileum.

28. The small intestine is lined with transverse folds of tissue called _____.

29. List three disorders of the esophagus and stomach.

 a. _____

 b. _____

 c. _____

30. List 10 disorders of the intestines.

a. _____

b. _____

c. _____

d. _____

e. _____

f. _____

g. _____

h. _____

i. _____

j. _____

31. List two disorders of the liver and gallbladder.

a. _____

b. _____

32. List four tests performed for patients with ulcers.

a. _____

b. _____

c. _____

d. _____

33. Complete the following chart, describing the mode of transmission and patients at risk for developing different types of hepatitis.

Hepatitis Type	Mode of Transmission	Persons at Risk
A (infectious hepatitis)		
B (serum hepatitis)		
C (non-A, non-B)		

Case Studies

1. Joan's first patient of the day is complaining of pain in the RUQ. What kinds of questions should Joan ask the patient? In what position should the patient be placed? How should the patient be gowned and/or draped? What type of vital signs should Joan measure? Document your case.

2. Rita was recently diagnosed with a hiatal hernia. Dr. Sahani has prescribed Prilosec 20 mg once daily for the patient and has asked Joan to provide education on the drug (using the PDR), as well as any dietary modifications. Document the case.

3. Dr. Sahani has ordered a screening hemoccult kit for a patient. Explain the test to the patient and why it is necessary. What collection instructions should Joan provide the patient?

4. While you are answering the telephone, a patient calls complaining of right upper quadrant pain. She is concerned about her appendix. Using your knowledge of acute appendicitis, what are the common signs? What questions should Joan ask the patient? What instructions should Joan provide the patient? Include the documentation for the patient's chart. What tests can be done to confirm the diagnosis?

5. Charles is scheduled for a barium swallow tomorrow. Explain the purpose of the procedure as well as any patient preparation involved.

6. Anna is going to have a colonoscopy next week. She calls the office and asks Joan if she will be able to drive herself home after the test. What is Joan's response? Anna is also confused about the patient preparation for the test. What preparation should Joan give Anna with regard to the test?

7. A patient is suspected of having cholelithiasis. The patient is at 24 weeks' gestation. What test should be ordered for this patient? Why?

Workplace Applications

1. Many of Joan's patients are unsure of the risk factors for developing certain types of cancer. List and describe some of the most common risk factors.

2. Dr. Sahani has asked Joan to create a patient education handout describing the definition, cause, signs, symptoms, diagnosis, and treatment options for GERD. Be sure to use terminology patients will understand.

3. Food poisoning is a disorder resulting from the ingestion of food that contains bacterial or toxic material. Create a chart for Joan to use as a resource when identifying the common sources, signs, and symptoms of different microorganisms.

Microorganism	Source	Signs and Symptoms
Staphylococcus aureus		
Escherichia coli		
Salmonella		
Campylobacter jejuni		
Clostridium botulinum		

Internet Activity

Use a drug reference book or the Internet to make drug cards for the following. Include drug classification, generic name, usual dose for an adult, and drug form.

1. Imodium

2. Lomotil

3. Phenergan

4. Tigan

5. Anzemet

6. Zofran

7. Biaxin

8. Bentyl

9. Levsin

10. Axid

11. Prevacid

12. Prilosec

13. Tagamet

14. Zantac

15. Nexium

16. Protonix

Chapter 38 Quiz

Name: _____

1. The liver is located in the _____ region.

2. Biaxin and Zithromax are antibiotics used to treat ulcers.

   a. True

   b. False

3. _____, which is the narrowing and hardening of the pyloric sphincter at the distal end of the stomach, is typically seen as a congenital defect in infants.

4. Define *diverticulosis*.

5. List two foods to avoid before an occult blood screening.

   a. _____

   b. _____

6. Hepatitis _____ is food-borne, whereas hepatitis _____ is blood-borne.

7. List two causes of ulcers.

   a. _____

   b. _____

8. During colonoscopy, the patient should be in the _____ position.

9. _____ is a food-borne illness caused by eating raw eggs, poultry, or shellfish.

10. Nexium is used to treat _____.

CHAPTER **39**

Assisting in Urology and Male Reproduction

Vocabulary Review

Define the following terms.

1. Albuminuria

   _____

2. Azotemia

   _____

3. Casts

   _____

4. Copulation

   _____

5. Erythropoietin

   _____

6. Urgency

   _____

7. Urology

   _____

Supply the terms for four types of urinary tract infections.

8. Inflammation of the urethra

   _____

9. Infection of the urinary bladder

   _____

10. An inflammation of the renal pelvis and kidney

    _____

11. Degenerative inflammation of the glomeruli

    _____

Define the following terms.

12. Creatinine

_____

13. BUN

_____

14. UA

_____

15. PSA

_____

Match the following terms with their definitions.

16. _____ Epididymis

17. _____ Balanitis

18. _____ Impotence

19. _____ Prostatitis

20. _____ BPH

21. _____ Cryptorchidism

22. _____ Hydrocele

23. _____ Enuresis

24. _____ Renal calculi

a. Long, coiled tube that rests on the top and lateral side of each testis

b. Bed wetting

c. Kidney stones

d. Signs and symptoms include urinary urgency and frequency; difficulty starting urination; hematuria; and repeated UTIs

e. Undescended testicles

f. Inflammation of the prostate

g. Inflammation of the glans penis

h. A form of erectile dysfunction

i. Sac of clear fluid in the scrotum

Skills and Concepts

25. List and describe the three processes of urine formation.

   a. _____

   b. _____

   c. _____

26. Explain the pathway of urine from the renal pelvis to the outside of the body.

_____

_____

_____

_____

27. List the general signs and symptoms of a urinary tract infection.

a. _____

b. _____

c. _____

d. _____

28. Label the structures of the scrotum on the following figure.

29. Describe three of the different types of treatments for prostate cancer.

a. _____

b. _____

c. _____

Case Studies

1. A patient comes to the office today complaining of severe lumbar pain and dysuria. The patient has a history of kidney stones. What diagnostic procedure would be best recommended for the patient? Why? What type of patient preparation will Sara need to provide the patient? If the patient had allergies to dye, what test would then be recommended?

_____

_____

_____

2. A 29-year-old male patient comes to the office complaining of discharge of pus, an itching sensation at the opening of the urethra, and burning on urination. What type of questions should Sara ask the patient? How should the patient disrobe and be positioned? What do you think is the likely diagnosis? How might this diagnosis be confirmed? What type of patient education should Sara provide? Document the case.

_____

_____

_____

3. You collected a clean-catch urine specimen from a male patient. The urine is dark orange but clear. The amount of urine was 460 cc. The patient appeared to be comfortable during the procedure. Document your findings. Use appropriate abbreviations. Be sure to include the date and your signature.

_____

_____

_____

Workplace Applications

1. Sara is updating the policies and procedures manual for her office. She notices that the manual lacks instructions for a clean-catch urine collection. Provide the steps for instructing a patient about how to gather a clean-catch specimen. Describe the importance of this type of collection process.

2. Sara deals with many patients with renal failure. She must be proficient in explaining the differences between peritoneal dialysis and hemodialysis. What are the advantages and disadvantages of each?

3. The physician is examining a male patient for the presence of a hernia. What region of the abdomen is typically examined?

   a. Why are males at risk for developing an inguinal hernia?

4. Design a handout explaining the details and instructions for a testicular self-examination.

   a. What is the importance of this exam? How often should it be done? Who should be performing it?

   b. What are the different approaches Sara could take to educate her male patients about testicular self-examinations? What types of resources could she provide?

Internet Activities

1. Use a drug reference book or the Internet to make drug cards for the following. Include the drug classification, generic name, usual dose, and drug form.

   a. Keflex

   b. Bactrim

   c. Viagra

   d. Flomax

   e. Hytrin

   f. Detrol

   g. Ditropan

   h. Xylocaine

2. Use the Internet to search for conferences and training sessions in your area that would aid your continuing education.

   a. Why is it important to attend these conferences?

   b. Do the conferences you found offer continuing education units?

   c. Share your findings with the rest of the class.

Chapter 39 Quiz

Name: _____

1. Renin regulates _____.

2. Erythropoietin controls the formation of
   _____

3. Cryptorchidism means
   _____

4. KUB stands for _____
   _____

5. List two drugs used to treat UTIs.
   a. _____
   b. _____

6. The urethra connects the kidneys to the
   bladder.
   a. True
   b. False

7. Enuresis means _____.

8. List two types of dialysis.
   a. _____
   b. _____

9. IVP stands for _____ and is used
   to diagnosis _____.

10. The _____ is the functional unit
    of the kidney.

CHAPTER 40

Assisting in Obstetrics and Gynecology

Vocabulary Review

Define the following terms.

1. Rectocele

_____

2. Uterine prolapse

_____

3. Cystocele

_____

4. PID

_____

5. Endometriosis

_____

6. Dilation and curettage

_____

7. Abruptio placenta

_____

8. Placenta previa

_____

9. Hysterectomy

_____

10. Ultrasonography

_____

11. Chorionic villus sampling

_____

12. Amniocentesis

_____

13. Alpha-fetoprotein (AFP)

_____

14. Mammography

_____

15. Colposcopy

_____

16. Cryosurgery

_____

Fill in the blanks with the correct terms.

17. Term pertaining to women who have had two or more pregnancies

_____

18. Thin, yellow, milky fluid secreted by the mammary glands a few days before and after delivery

_____

19. An x-ray procedure to guide the insertion of a needle into a specific area of the breast

_____

20. Spotting or bleeding between menstrual cycles

_____

21. Excessive menstrual blood loss, such as a menses lasting longer than 7 days

_____

22. Absence of menstruation for a minimum of 6 months

_____

23. Absence of menstruation for a period of 35 days to 6 months

_____

Skills and Concepts

24. Label the structures in the following figure.

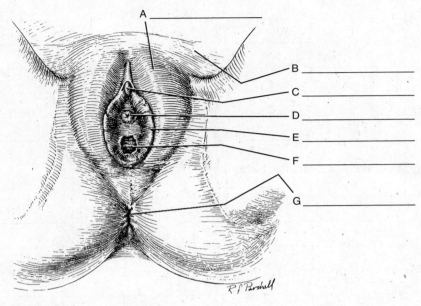

25. List and describe the three phases of menstruation.

a. _____
_____

b. _____
_____

c. _____
_____

26. Name three bacterial STDs.

a. _____
_____

b. _____
_____

c. _____
_____

27. Name three benign gynecologic tumors.

a. _____

b. _____

c. _____

28. List and describe four gynecologic cancers.

a. _____
   _____

b. _____
   _____

c. _____
   _____

d. _____
   _____

29. List five types of naturally occurring abortions.

a. _____

b. _____

c. _____

d. _____

e. _____

30. List and describe two different types of placental abnormalities.

a. _____
   _____

b. _____
   _____

31. Labor is the physiologic process by which the uterus expels the fetus and the placenta. It is divided into three stages. Define each stage of labor.

a. Stage I: _____
   _____

b. Stage II: _____
   _____

c. Stage III: _____
   _____

Case Studies

1. A 20-year-old patient arrives today for her annual Pap smear. She has questions regarding the different types of birth control available. What are some of the factors involved with choosing a type of contraception? Using the following chart, create a resource for the different types of contraception.

Type	Failure Rate	Characteristics	Contraindications	Side effects
Condom (barrier method)				
Diaphragm or cervical cap (barrier method)				
Intrauterine device (IUD)				
Depo Provera				
Oral contraceptives				
Hormonal patch				
Vaginal ring				

2. You receive a telephone call from a female patient who is experiencing side effects from oral contraceptives. What symptoms will you ask about?

   a. A _____

   b. C _____

   c. H _____

   d. E _____

   e. S _____

3. Carly comes to the office today for a prenatal check up. She states she has been experiencing some pelvic pain and burning on urination for 5 days. She has also recently stopped taking her prenatal vitamins because she states they cause her nausea. This is her first pregnancy, and she is very nervous about the examination. How can Betsy calm her fears? What test results and information should be gathered before the physician's examination? Is there any advice Betsy could provide with regard to the prenatal vitamins and any other patient education? After Betsy has finished measuring the necessary vital signs and gathering the laboratory specimens, how should Carly be robed and draped? Once the physician begins the internal examination, how should she be positioned? Document the case.

4. The physician has asked you to prepare the patient for a bimanual examination. How should the patient be robed and draped? How should you position the patient? What type of supplies will Dr. Beck need to complete the examination?

5. Mary has been ordered to have a baseline mammogram done. What patient preparation should Betsy be sure to tell Mary before her examination?

Workplace Applications

1. Dr. Beck has asked Betsy to create a patient education handout for patients with fibrocystic breast disease. Include the disease definition, possible causes, and signs and symptoms. Are there any dietary restrictions?

2. One of Betsy's duties includes instructing patients on how to perform a breast self-examination. With a partner, explain the steps of this procedure. When should it be performed? What should the patient be feeling for? Why are breast self-examinations important?

3. Betsy has been instructed to gather a health history on a patient. What type of questions should she ask? Include both open-ended and closed-ended questions. Practice your interviewing technique with a partner. What did you find most difficult about the interview?

Internet Activities

1. Use a drug reference book or the Internet to make drug cards for the following. Include drug classification, generic name, usual dose, and drug form.

   a. Tamoxifen

   b. Premarin

   c. Prempro

   d. Methotrexate (for use in ectopic pregnancies)

   e. Evista

   f. Effexor

2. Osteoporosis is a loss of bone tissue and a decrease in the bone's density. However, osteoporosis may be prevented and/or controlled with proper calcium intake. Search the internet for public health programs or patient education programs available in your area that deal with osteoporosis prevention. What do the programs consist of? How do they increase awareness for this disease? How are the programs monitored? Is there a cost? Which program would you most recommend to someone you know? Share your research with your classmates.

Chapter 40 Quiz

Name: _____

1. Define *AFP*.

   _____

   _____

2. What type of equipment should be prepared in the examination room for an annual Pap examination?

   _____

   _____

   _____

3. Define *multiparous*

   _____

   _____

4. What are some common causes of PID?

   _____

   _____

5. Fosamax is used to treat _____ .

6. Define *menorrhagia*.

   _____

   _____

7. Name the typical position used for female pelvic examinations.

   _____

8. What are some of the common side effects of oral birth control pills?

   _____

   _____

9. Define *rectocele*.

   _____

   _____

10. Describe the function of HCG.

    _____

    _____

CHAPTER 41

Assisting in Pediatrics

Vocabulary Review

Match the following terms with their definitions.

1. _____ Microcephaly

2. _____ Serous

3. _____ Hydrocephaly

4. _____ Stridor

5. _____ Rhonchi

6. _____ Attenuated

7. _____ Suppurative

8. _____ Laryngoscopy

   a. Weakened virulence or change in virulence of a pathogenic microorganism

   b. Enlargement of the cranium caused by abnormal accumulation of cerebrospinal fluid within the cerebral system

   c. Visual examination of the voice box area through an endoscope equipped with a light and mirrors for illumination

   d. Small size of the head in relation to the rest of the body

   e. Continuous dry rattling in the throat or bronchial tube caused by partial obstruction

   f. Thin, watery, serum-like drainage

   g. Shrill, harsh respiratory sound heard during inhalation in laryngeal obstruction

   h. Formation and/or discharge of pus

9. Describe the difference between growth and development.

_____

_____

_____

Skills and Concepts

The Denver II Developmental Screening Test is a standardized tool that is given to children between 1 month and 6 years of age to screen healthy infants for developmental delays, to validate concerns about an infant's development, or to monitor high-risk children for potential problems.

10. When should the test be administered?

    _____

11. The assessment focuses on the following four areas. Describe each of the following tools, and provide examples of each.

    a. Gross motor skills

    _____

    _____

    b. Language skills

    _____

    _____

    c. Fine motor-adaptive skills

    _____

    _____

    d. Personal skills

    _____

    _____

The following chart describes different growth and development theories. Fill in the missing theories to complete the chart.

Age Group	Freud—Psychosexual Theory	Piaget—Cognitive Theory	Erickson—Psychosocial Theory	Kohlberg—Moral Reasoning
Infant	Oral stage; child operates with the pleasure principle and the id develops	12.	Building basic trust vs. mistrust; learning drive and hope	Avoids punishment and obeys for obedience's sake
Toddler	Passes through oral aggressive stage to anal stage; elimination is used to control and inhibit	Coordinates more than one thought at a time; uses thought to create new solutions	13.	Avoids punishment and the power of authority figures
Preschool to early school years	From phallic stage, in which the ego (conscious reality) develops, to the latent stage, in which the superego (morality) develops	Intuitive-preoperational; preschooler is egocentric and has magical thinking; early school years, begins to develop understanding of cause and effect; functions symbolically using language; develops understanding of life events and relationships	Preschool processing initiative vs. guilt and attempting to develop direction and purpose; mimics others and is more purposeful in establishing goals	14.
School age	15.	Concrete operations: uses mental reasoning to solve problems; attempts to reach logical solutions; tests beliefs to establish values	Industry vs. inferiority; establishing methods for solving problems and a feeling of competence; is mastering tasks and using hands to create things	Conventional morality; doing what is expected is important; needs to be good in own eyes as well as according to what he or she perceives others expect of him or her; wants to please others
Adolescence	Genital stage	16.	Identity vs. role confusion; developing self-identity that will determine devotion and fidelity in future relationships	Postconventional morality; developing a respect for the laws of society; considers the greatest good for the greatest number; values are related to one's group; behavior controlled internally

Fill in the blanks in the following statements.

17. Infection or inflammation of the middle ear is called _____.

18. _____ is viral inflammation of the larynx and the trachea just beneath it that causes edema and spasm of the vocal cords.

19. During an _____ _____, the bronchial tubes begin to spasm, thereby decreasing the amount of air that can pass through them, while at the same time tissue lining the bronchioles becomes edematous and secretes mucus.

20. _____ is a viral infection of the small bronchi and bronchioles that usually affects children under 3 years of age. The infection varies in severity and is seen in children with a family history of asthma and children exposed to cigarette smoke.

21. Common treatments for _____ include zanamivir (Relenza), which is inhaled every 12 hours, and oseltamivir (Tamiflu), which is available in pill form.

22. _____ can be caused by a bacterial or viral infection that produces a white or yellowish pus that may cause the eyelids to stick shut in the morning.

23. _____, or "slapped cheek disease," is an infection caused by parvovirus B19.

24. _____ is caused by a member of the herpesvirus group and is transmitted by direct or indirect droplets from the respiratory tract of an infected person. The incubation period is 14 to 21 days.

25. _____ is an inflammation of the membranes that cover the brain and spinal cord.

26. _____ is the best prevention for Reye's syndrome.

27. List and discuss the five stages of Reye's syndrome.

a. _____
b. _____
c. _____
d. _____
e. _____

28. List 10 safety guidelines for parents with small children.

a. _____
b. _____
c. _____
d. _____
e. _____
f. _____
g. _____
h. _____
i. _____
j. _____

Case Studies

1. Susie is concerned about approaching young children and how and when to involve the parents. Examine the following age groups. Provide tips for approaching children within each specific group.

   a. Infants (0-12 months)

   b. Toddlers and preschoolers (2-6 years)

   c. School-aged children (7-11 years)

   d. Adolescents (12-18 years)

2. A mother comes to the office today complaining that her 4-week-old baby has experienced crying episodes lasting 3 to 4 hours four times during the last week. What type of questions should Susie ask the mother? Role-play this case with a partner, and document your findings. The physician diagnoses the baby as having colic. What type of patient education should Susie provide to the parent?

3. The physician instructs a patient complaining of diarrhea to consume a "BRAT" diet. Define this dietary recommendation.

4. A patient has recently been diagnosed with asthma. The physician has asked Susie to educate the patient and parents on the common triggers of asthma attacks. Document the conversation.

5. Susie is trying to obtain vital signs from a 4-year-old child who is refusing to stand on the scale or cooperate while her temperature is taken. What can Susie do to try and make the child cooperate? What is the best way to take this patient's temperature?

Workplace Applications

1. Childhood obesity is a growing epidemic in the United States. The clinic for which you work is providing an in-service presentation to provide staff education about this growing problem. Susie and the other staff members are asked to create a list of possible reasons for this growing trend. List these potential causes, and describe some solutions to be discussed during the in-service presentation.

2. At a recent office meeting, the staff concluded that a patient education handout regarding the common cold would benefit the patients in the office. Susie has decided to take on this responsibility.

   a. Creatively design an informative handout for the patients of the office.

   b. Be sure to include the definition of the common cold.

   c. How is the infection spread to others? Describe ways to eliminate the spread of infection.

   d. What are the common signs and symptoms? When should the patient be seen in the office?

   e. What are some common OTC medications the physician would recommend?

   f. Include instructions for use of a bulb syringe.

3. Susie is reorganizing the patient waiting room and wants to include some helpful and educational resources for the patients to view. Create a list of possible items Susie could place in the waiting room.

Internet Activities

1. Use a drug reference book or the Internet to make drug cards for the following. Include drug classification, generic name, usual pediatric dose, and drug form.

   a. Amoxicillin

   b. Ceclor

   c. Cipro

   d. Augmentin

   e. EryPed

   f. Septra

   g. Singulair

   h. Albuterol

2. Search the CDC website for VIS (vaccination information sheets). Print a copy for each of the immunizations recommended in the immunization schedule. Why are these education handouts important to use in the office?

3. Flu vaccinations are recommended for children over 6 months of age. Search the CDC website for dosage instructions. Describe dosage instructions for children who have not had the vaccination before and for those who have had the injection before. When should a patient *not* receive the flu vaccination?

Chapter 41 Quiz

Name: _____

1. _____ is a respiratory condition with bronchospasms and inflammation.

2. _____ is a viral disorder with cough and stridor.

3. Chickenpox is another name for

   _____.

4. Inflammation of the brain and spinal cord is called _____.

5. MMR stands for _____,
   _____, and _____.

6. The medical specialty that deals with children is _____.

7. Average birth weight is _____.

8. By age _____, a child has reached 50% of his or her adult height and weight.

9. _____ is a disorder that is characterized by abdominal pain during infancy.

10. Define *growth and development*.

    _____

    _____

WORK PRODUCT 41-1

Name: _____

Maintaining Immunization Records

Using the CDC-recommended immunization schedule in Figure 41-6 of the text, answer the following questions.

A patient comes to the office today for her 15-month-old child's checkup. The parents bring in a copy of the child's immunization record (listed later). Using the CDC's recommended immunization schedule, which immunizations should the patient expect to receive today?

After the physician is finished with the examination, the following immunizations are ordered. Gather the necessary VIS from the CDC website. Document the patient education and administration of the vaccines in the chart. Record the immunizations in the patient's immunization record, which follows.

Physician orders:

1. DTaP: Lot# 23155

    Expiration Date: October 2008

    Dose 0.5 mL administered IM

    Manufacturer: Overtus Pharmaceuticals

    Site: right proximal vastus lateralis

2. Poliovirus: Lot# 54633

    Expiration Date: May 2007

    Dose: 0.5 mL IM

    Manufacturer: Parker

    Site: right distal vastus lateralis

3. MMR: Lot# 99332

    Expiration Date: Dec. 2008

    Dose: 0.5 mL SQ

    Manufacturer: Parker

    Site: left vastus lateralis

4. Document in the chart record: Patient had chickenpox disease in August 2005.

Documentation:

Immunization	Dose	Date Given	Health Professional/Clinic	Signature of Administering Personnel
Hepatitis B	0.5 mL	1. 05/01/2005 2. 06/01/2005 3. 11/12/2005	North Hills Ped. North Hills Ped. Dept. of Health	S Kwong S Kwong AH
Diphtheria, tetanus, and pertussis	0.5 mL	1. 05/01/2005 2. 07/01/2005 3. 09/01/2005 4. 5.	North Hills Ped. North Hills Ped. North Hills Ped.	S Kwong S Kwong S Kwong
Hib	0.5 mL	1. 05/01/2005 2. 07/01/2005 3. 09/01/2005 4.	North Hills Ped. North Hills Ped. North Hills Ped.	S Kwong S Kwong S Kwong
Inactivated poliovirus	0.5 mL	1. 05/01/2005 2. 07/01/2005 3. 4.	North Hills Ped. North Hills Ped.	S Kwong S Kwong
Measles, mumps, rubella varicella		1. 2.		
Meningococcal				
Pneumococcal	0.5 mL	1. 05/01/2005 2. 07/01/2005 3. 4. 5.	North Hills Ped. North Hills Ped.	S Kwong S Kwong
Influenza	0.25 mL 0.25 mL	10/28/2005 11/28/2005	Dept. of Health Dept. of Health	AH AH
Hepatitis A		1. 2.		

CHAPTER 42

Assisting in Orthopedic Medicine

Vocabulary Review

Define the following terms.

1. Kyphosis

   _____

2. Lordosis

   _____

3. Luxation

   _____

4. Subluxation

   _____

5. Thoracic

   _____

6. Tendon

   _____

7. Ligament

   _____

Skills and Concepts

8. List five general functions of the musculoskeletal system.

   a. _____

   b. _____

   c. _____

   d. _____

   e. _____

9. In the figure below, label the bones of the extremities.

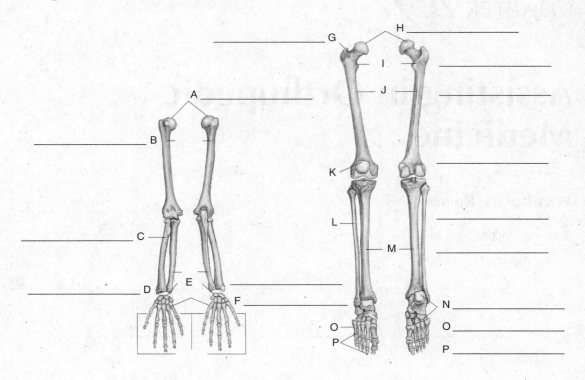

10. Label the following drawing with muscle, tendons, insertion, and origin.

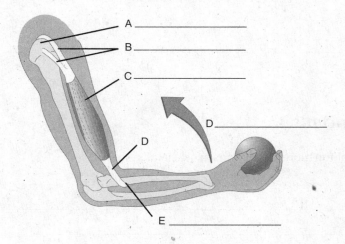

11. Label the three types of muscles shown in the following figure.

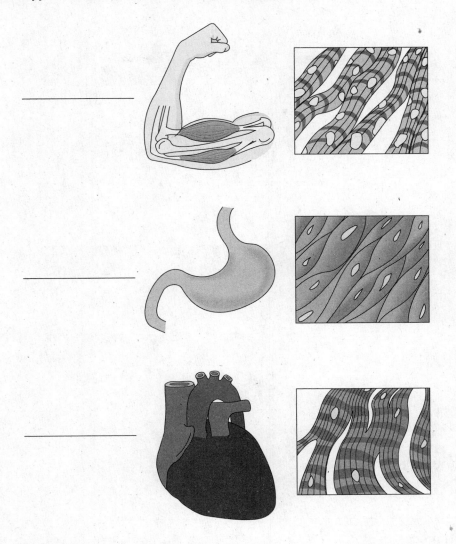

Identify the correct types of joints in the following descriptions.

12. _____ permit the skull to grow with the child but have very limited flexibility.

13. _____ allow for the greatest range of motion by permitting the joint to rotate in a complete circle.

14. The _____ joints of the elbow and knee allow for movement in one plane, such as bending up and down.

Indicate which statements are true (T) and which statements are false (F).

15. _____ The tibia is distal to the femur.

16. _____ The patella is superior to the metacarpals.

17. _____ The radius is lateral to the ulna.

18. _____ The tibia is medial to the fibula.

19. _____ The metatarsals are inferior to the tarsals.

20. Label each type of range of motion.

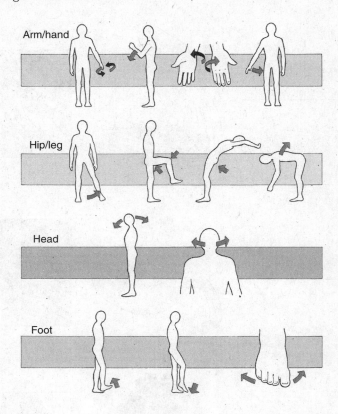

Define the following.

21. Gout

_____

22. Osteoarthritis

_____

23. Rheumatoid arthritis

_____

24. Review and label the fractures shown in the following figure. Match the name of the fracture with the letter corresponding to the illustration of the fracture in the figure in the list on the next page.

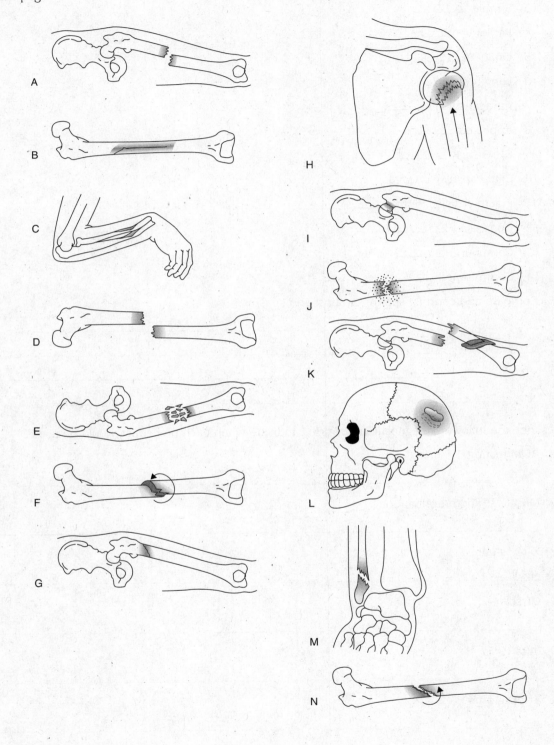

1. Transverse _____

2. Spiral _____

3. Simple _____

4. Pathologic _____

5. Oblique _____

6. Longitudinal _____

7. Intracapsular _____

8. Impacted _____

9. Greenstick _____

10. Extracapsular _____

11. Fracture/dislocation _____

12. Depressed _____

13. Compound _____

14. Comminuted _____

25. Compare and contrast sprains, strains, and spasms.

_____

_____

_____

_____

Describe the following diagnostic procedures. Indicate when each procedure would be used.

26. ROM testing

_____

27. Muscle strength evaluation

_____

28. X-ray studies

_____

29. CT scans

_____

30. MRI

_____

31. Arthrograms

_____

32. Bone scans

_____

33. EMG/NCS

_____

34. Biopsy

_____

35. Myelogram

_____

Case Studies

1. A patient comes to the office with pain, tenderness, and deformity of the fingers. What questions should you ask? What medications will you ask about? Document the case.

2. A patient calls the office asking about fibromyalgia. She heard about the disease on a TV commercial and would like some information regarding the disorder. What can you tell her regarding signs, symptoms, associated disorders, diagnosis, and treatment?

3. A patient on crutches comes to the office for a recheck of an ankle sprain. What should the medical assistant be aware of when obtaining the patient's weight, height, and vital signs? How should the patient be prepared for the examination? Document the case.

4. A patient calls the office explaining that he has just fallen and twisted his ankle. What instructions should the medical assistant give the patient regarding applying an ice pack? Remember to document the instructions in the patient's chart.

5. The physician has ordered crutches for a patient with a knee injury. It is the duty of the medical assistant to properly fit the patient. How should Kaiwan fit the patient? What patient education should Kaiwan provide the patient?

Workplace Applications

1. The office manager has asked you to develop an Osteoporosis Awareness Prevention Program for the office staff. Together with a partner, brainstorm ideas for the development of this program.

   a. Many of the staff are young women. Why should they be concerned with osteoporosis?

   b. What are common risk factors for osteoporosis?

   c. What can individuals do to reduce their risk?

   d. What are common treatments?

   e. Using your knowledge of the disease, what type of activities can you implement into this program?

2. A patient calls the office and requests the results of her recent MRI study. After finding the patient's chart, you notice that the physician has not yet reviewed the results. The impression states: HNP of L3 and L4. What should Kaiwan tell the patient? Why? Document a message in the patient's chart.

Internet Activities

1. Use a drug reference book or the Internet to make drug cards for the following. Include drug classification, generic name, usual adult dose, and drug form.

   a. Aspirin

   b. Motrin

   c. Prednisone

   d. Zyloprim

   e. Colchicine

   f. Anaprox

   g. Cataflam

   h. Relafen

   i. Toradol

   j. Voltaren

   k. Naprosyn

   l. Orudis

   m. Celebrex

   n. Acetaminophen

2. Search the Internet for information describing proper lifting and patient transfer techniques. Why are proper mechanics important? Make notes of different techniques, and demonstrate your findings to the class.

Chapter 42 Quiz

Name: _____

1. The _____ is the large bone of the upper leg.

2. There are _____ bones in the thoracic spine.

3. A(n) _____ fracture is one in which the skin is broken.

4. SLE stands for _____ _____.

5. _____ arthritis is an autoimmune disease that attacks the synovial fluid and results in deformity.

6. The long part of the bone is the _____.

7. Inflammation of the joint is called _____.

8. _____ connect muscle to bone.

9. _____ connect bones at a joint.

10. The elbow joints flex and _____.

Assisting in Neurology and Mental Health

Vocabulary Review

Define the following terms.

1. Anoxia

   _____

2. Ataxia

   _____

3. Atrophy

   _____

4. Coma

   _____

5. Diplopia

   _____

6. Gait

   _____

7. Aura

   _____

8. Contralateral

   _____

9. Paresthesia

   _____

10. Syncope

    _____

Define the following procedures.

11. MRI

_____

_____

12. CT

_____

_____

13. EEG

_____

_____

14. Lumbar puncture

_____

_____

Skills and Concepts

15. Label the functional structures and lobes of the brain on the following figure.

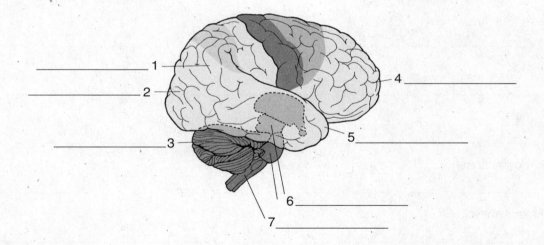

Describe the functions of each of the following.

16. CSF

_____

_____

17. Cerebellum

_____

_____

18. Brain stem

_____

_____

19. Hypothalamus

_____

_____

20. Cerebrum

_____

_____

21. Spinal nerves

_____

_____

22. Cranial nerves

_____

_____

23. Autonomic nerves

_____

_____

24. Label the cranial nerves on the following figure.

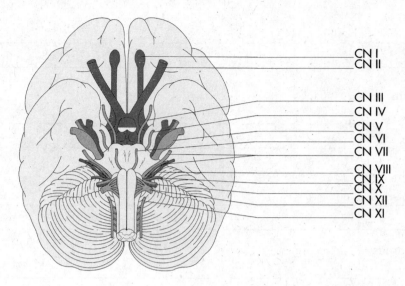

CN I _____

CN II _____

CN III _____

CN IV _____

CN V _____

CN VI _____

CN VII _____

CN VIII _____

CN IX _____

CN X _____

CN XI _____

CN XII _____

25. Differentiate between a thrombus and an embolus.

_____

_____

Fill in the blanks.

26. CVA is commonly referred to as _____ or brain attack.

27. This _____ often consists of some form of visual disturbance, such as dark lines across or spots within the visual field.

28. Absence or _____ seizures are a less serious form of seizure consisting of momentary clouding of consciousness and loss of contact with reality.

29. The typical presentation of _____ includes muscular rigidity, unilateral pill-rolling tremor of the hand, high-pitched monotone voice, and a _____-like facial expression. The patient has a bent-forward posture with the head bowed. Muscular tremors and _____ increase.

30. _____ results from the progressive inflammation and deterioration of the myelin sheaths, leaving the nerve fibers uncovered.

31. _____, or Lou Gehrig's disease, is a progressive, destructive neurologic disease that results in muscle atrophy.

32. _____ affects the seventh cranial nerve of the face. It occurs suddenly and usually subsides spontaneously over several weeks to several months.

33. Carpal tunnel syndrome results from a compression or entrapment of the _____ nerve as it courses past the carpal bones of the _____ toward the hand.

34. List nine signs and symptoms that suggest possible neurologic problems.

    a. _____

    b. _____

    c. _____

    d. _____

    e. _____

    f. _____

    g. _____

    h. _____

    i. _____

35. Describe a Brudzinski's sign. How is it performed, and what does it demonstrate?

    _____

    _____

    _____

    _____

36. Compare and contrast encephalitis and meningitis.

_____

_____

_____

_____

Case Studies

1. A patient comes to the office complaining of numbness in the left side of the face and difficulty walking. The patient is having difficulty with speech and is easily confused. With a partner, role-play this case. Measure vital signs. What questions should you ask the patient? Document your findings. What appears to be the preliminary diagnosis?

2. On discharge from the hospital, a patient is prescribed Coumadin. Inform the patient about the drug's actions, side effects, and precautions for taking the medication. Document your patient education session.

3. A mother calls and states that her son sustained a head injury at school today while playing football. She is concerned about the possibility of a concussion. What questions should the medical assistant ask the mother? Explain to the mother the signs and symptoms that might be of concern.

4. A patient comes to the office to discuss depression. She is crying and upset while you take her vital signs. What communication skills should the medical assistant remember to employ? What questions should you ask the patient? Describe some of the common signs and symptoms of depression.

Workplace Applications

1. The office has been asked to discuss depression at a community health seminar. What can you tell the audience about depression? What are some of the symptoms of depression?

2. Your office manager has asked you to create a patient education guide describing the common risk factors for CVA. What items should be included?

3. Patients on warfarin (Coumadin) must constantly be monitored. Blood work is ordered regularly. How might an office ensure that patients are following orders and getting their laboratory work done on a timely basis? Why is this close monitoring necessary?

Internet Activities

1. Use a drug reference book or the Internet to make drug cards for the following. Include drug classification, generic name, usual adult dose, and drug form.

   a. Coumadin

   b. Plavix

   c. Imitrex

   d. Heparin

   e. Maxalt

   f. Sumatriptan succinate

   g. Effexor

   h. Dilantin

   i. Phenobarbital

   j. Valproic acid

   k. Prozac

2. One of the duties of the medical assistant may be to administer a "mini-mental status examination." Search the Internet for different types of mini-mental status examinations. How are these tools used? What type of approach will the medical assistant want to use when administering this tool? Practice with a partner. Be prepared to discuss your findings in class.

Chapter 43 Quiz

Name: _____

1. Define *hemiplegia*.

2. Describe the lumbar puncture procedure.

3. List three signs and symptoms of depression.

   a. _____

   b. _____

   c. _____

4. Faulty development of the fetus resulting in deformities or deviations from normal is known as _____.

5. _____ specialize in the diagnosis and treatment of medical disorders and conditions of the nervous system.

6. The _____ system includes the brain and spinal cord.

7. Afferent nerves carry impulses to the brain.

   a. True

   b. False

8. _____ receive the nervous impulse from a preceding neuron and carry it into the cell body.

9. The gyri are separated by shallow grooves called _____.

CHAPTER **44**

Assisting in Endocrinology

Vocabulary Review

Match the following terms with their definitions.

1. Glycosuria

2. Glycogen

3. Glucagon

   a. _____ A hormone produced by the alpha cells of the pancreatic islets; stimulates the liver to convert glycogen into glucose.

   b. _____ The abnormal presence of glucose in the urine.

   c. _____ The sugar (starch) formed from glucose and stored mainly in the liver.

Fill in the blanks.

4. Excessive thirst is called _____.

5. _____ is a hormone that stimulates the production and secretion of glucocorticoids; it is released by the anterior pituitary gland.

6. _____ is a hormone secreted by the beta cells of the pancreatic islets in response to increased levels of glucose in the blood.

7. _____ means abnormal production of ketone bodies in the blood and tissue, resulting from fat catabolism in cells. Ketones accumulate in large quantities when fat instead of glucose is used as fuel for energy in cells.

8. _____ is a hormone secreted by the anterior lobe of the pituitary gland that stimulates the secretion of hormones produced by the thyroid gland.

9. _____ means increased appetite.

10. _____ is a hormone secreted by the posterior pituitary gland; it encourages fluid reabsorbsion in the renal tubules of the kidneys and a possible elevation in blood pressure. It is also known as *vasopressin*.

11. _____ is excessive urine production.

Skills and Concepts

12. Define negative feedback, and give an example of how it works in the body.

_____

_____

_____

13. The hormones released by the anterior pituitary gland are:

    a. _____

    b. _____

    c. _____

    d. _____

    e. _____

    f. _____

14. Three conditions related to alterations in growth hormone are:

    a. _____

    b. _____

    c. _____

15. Differentiate between type 1 and type 2 diabetes.

_____

_____

_____

_____

16. Differentiate between diabetic coma and insulin shock.

_____

_____

_____

17. Name and define the three "poly" conditions of diabetes mellitus.

    a. _____

    _____

    b. _____

    _____

    c. _____

    _____

18. Describe each of the following laboratory tests.

  a. Thyroid stimulating hormone (TSH)

  _____

  _____

  b. Sodium

  _____

  _____

  c. Potassium

  _____

  _____

  d. Glycohemoglobin or hemoglobin A_{1c}

  _____

  _____

Case Studies

1. A patient with diabetes has come to your office because of a sore on the right great toe. He states that he was trimming a corn a week ago and the area has become painful. You notice that the area is red and warm to the touch. The patient is wearing beach sandals. The patient's fasting blood sugar (FBS) is 348. Oral temperature is 100.9° F. His blood pressure is 182/110, and pulse is 88. Document the case.

2. A patient at the clinic was recently diagnosed with diabetes insipidus. The physician asked you to educate the patient on the common signs and symptoms. What information do you want to be sure to include?

3. A patient comes to the office today complaining of fatigue, loss of hair, muscle cramps, menorrhagia, and thick, dry, puffy skin. Her vital signs show a pulse of 56, a temperature of 97.7° F, and a weight gain of 25 lb over the last 3 months. What condition do these signs and symptoms suggest? What laboratory work will the physician most likely order? Document the case.

4. A patient calls the office today stating that she is 20 weeks pregnant and is concerned about her risk for gestational diabetes. What questions would you ask her? Educate the patient on the risk factors of gestational diabetes. Describe the counseling you give her.

5. Miguel has been providing diabetes nutritional education to Jerry for over 6 months now. Unfortunately, the effort seems to be unsuccessful. Jerry explains that he feels good and does not see why he should change his eating habits. Explain to Jerry the different types of long-term complications related to poorly controlled diabetes. Should Miguel provide any additional patient education? Why or why not?

6. A patient comes to the laboratory and states she is there for a blood test to screen for prediabetes. What tests could this include? What are the diagnostic criteria for prediabetes?

Workplace Applications

1. The medical assistant must have knowledge of the different medications prescribed for patients with endocrine abnormalities. Use the PDR to identify the indications for the following drugs:

    a. Synthroid

    b. Hydrocortisone

    c. Byetta

    d. DiaBeta

    e. Glucophage

    f. Prandin

    g. Micronase

    h. Glucovance

    i. Avandia

    j. Actos

2. Create a handout that describes the difference between hypoglycemic and hyperglycemic episodes.

3. Carrie has been using her glucometer for the past 4 months and states that she does not feel the routine controls need to be done. Explain to Carrie the importance of doing the controls and when they should be performed.

Internet Activities

1. Go to www.diabetes.org. Locate the diabetes risk assessment tool, and take the test. Are you surprised at the results? What lifestyle changes can you make to decrease your risk for diabetes?

2. Patients on a diabetic meal plan often feel they are limited with regard to the different foods they are allowed to eat. Search the Internet for different recipes and their nutritional exchanges for diabetes. Create a small collection of recipes you can share with your patients. Be sure your selections include a variety of foods so that your list appeals to a large population.

Chapter 44 Quiz

Name: _____

1. The posterior pituitary gland secretes:

   a. _____

   b. _____

2. Too much growth hormone causes

   _____.

3. Another term for hyperthyroidism is
   _____ disease.

4. Cortisol _____ blood
   glucose levels.

5. List two types of diabetes mellitus.

   a. _____

   b. _____

6. Insulin shock occurs when the blood glucose
   level is too low.

   a. True

   b. False

7. Diabetic coma occurs with a very
   _____ blood glucose level.

8. Older adults are at risk for

   _____.

   a. type 1 diabetes

   b. type 2 diabetes

9. A hemoglobin A_{1c} test can detect

   _____.

10. Iodine deficiency is related to simple goiter
    formation.

    a. True

    b. False

CHAPTER 45

Assisting in Pulmonary Medicine

Vocabulary Review

Define the following terms.

1. Apnea

_____

2. Atelectasis

_____

3. Dyspnea

_____

4. Empyema

_____

5. Hemoptysis

_____

6. Hemothorax

_____

7. Hypercapnia

_____

8. Hyperpnea

_____

9. Hypoxemia

_____

10. Orthopnea

_____

11. Pleurisy

_____

12. Pneumothorax

_____

13. Pyothorax

_____

14. Rhinoplasty

_____

15. Rhinorrhea

_____

16. Tachypnea

_____

17. Thoracotomy

_____

Skills and Concepts

18. Explain the process of ventilation. Include the action of the diaphragm and the intercostal muscles.

_____

_____

_____

_____

19. Label the following drawing with these anatomic landmarks: anterior, posterior, and midaxillary lines.

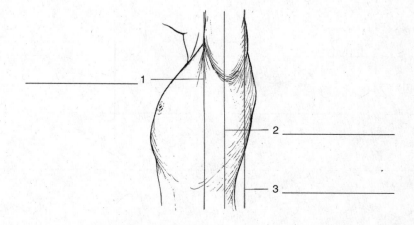

20. On the following figure, label the structures of the respiratory system, head, and chest.

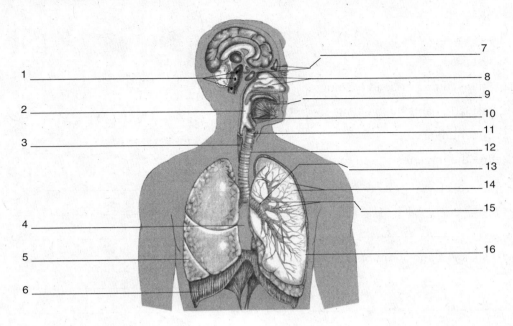

1 _____
2 _____
3 _____
4 _____
5 _____
6 _____

7 _____
8 _____
9 _____
10 _____
11 _____
12 _____
13 _____
14 _____
15 _____

16 _____

21. Label the lobes of the lungs on the following figure.

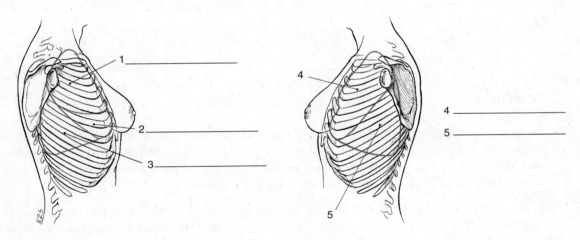

1 _____
2 _____
3 _____
4 _____
5 _____

4 _____
5 _____

Fill in the blanks.

22. _____ cancer is the leading cause of cancer-related deaths for both men and women in the United States.

23. A positive _____ reaction indicates the possibility of active or dormant tuberculosis or exposure to the disease.

24. _____ is a noninvasive method of evaluating the oxygen saturation of hemoglobin in arterial blood, as well as the pulse rate.

Match the following occupations with the associated lung diseases.

25. Anthracosis _____

26. Silicosis _____

27. Asbestosis _____

    a. Stone cutting or sand blasting

    b. Insulation and shipbuilding

    c. Coal mining

28. Define the three tests used to diagnose TB.

    a. _____

    b. _____

    c. _____

29. List six signs and symptoms of obstructive sleep apnea.

    a. _____

    b. _____

    c. _____

    d. _____

    e. _____

    f. _____

Case Studies

1. Dr. Samuelson orders a nebulizer treatment for a patient having an acute asthma attack. How should Michael prepare for this procedure? Describe the steps for administering a nebulizer treatment to a patient. What information should you provide for the patient? What should Michael watch for while the patient is undergoing the treatment?

2. Maura, a 10-year-old patient, has recently been diagnosed with asthma. To help her better understand how to recognize her symptoms, Dr. Samuelson has asked Michael to teach Maura how to use a peak flow meter. Role-play with a partner and document the case.

3. A patient calls the office and requests an antibiotic for chest congestion. The patient is busy working today and refuses an appointment. What should the medical assistant do in this situation? Why?

4. A patient arrives today complaining of high fever, chills, dyspnea, chest pain during inspiration, and general malaise. The patient is a smoker. Dr. Samuelson suspects pneumonia. What tests are done to confirm the diagnosis? How may the physician determine whether the pneumonia is viral or bacterial? What is the treatment for bacterial pneumonia? What is the treatment plan for viral pneumonia?

Workplace Applications

1. Create a handout outlining the use of a metered-dose inhaler.

2. Michael is getting ready to obtain a sputum sample. What universal precautions should Michael follow? What equipment will he need to use? Why?

3. What instruction should the medical assistant provide a patient while scheduling a bronchoscopy?

Internet Activity

One of the duties of a medical assistant is to serve as a resource for patients. Search the Internet for pulmonologists and respiratory durable medical equipment providers in your area. Create either a circular file or an address book with the names, addresses, phone numbers, and fax numbers for each resource. Include any additional information your patients may need (e.g., accepted insurance plans, services provided, hospital contacts).

Chapter 45 Quiz

Name: _____

1. Which of the following is *not* a risk factor for lung cancer?

   a. Genetic disposition

   b. Chronic exposure to asbestos

   c. Smoking

   d. Sinusitis

4. Which of the following is a part of the medical assistant's role in performing pulmonary function tests?

   a. Performing the procedure

   b. Ordering the procedure

   c. Positioning the patient

   d. Interpreting the results

2. Dilation of the bronchi and bronchioles associated with secondary infection or ciliary dysfunction.

   a. Hypercapnia

   b. Bronchiectasis

   c. Chronic bronchitis

   d. Asthma

5. A pulse oximeter is useful in assessing a patient with

   a. Pneumonia

   b. Bronchitis

   c. Emphysema

   d. All of the above

3. Discharge of nasal secretions.

   a. Rhinorrhea

   b. Rhinitis

   c. Clubbing

   d. Sinusitis

Assisting in Geriatrics

Vocabulary Review

Match the following terms with their definitions.

1. _____ The secretion or discharge of tears

2. _____ A sore or ulcer over a bony prominence that is a result of ischemia from prolonged pressure; a bedsore

3. _____ Protein that forms the inelastic fibers of tendons, ligaments, and fascia

4. _____ Pertaining to the ribs

5. _____ Essential part of elastic connective tissue that, when moist, is flexible and elastic

   a. Collagen

   b. Costal

   c. Decubitus ulcer

   d. Elastin

   e. Lacrimation

Skills and Concepts

6. List five myths and stereotypes about aging.

   a. _____

   b. _____

   c. _____

   d. _____

   e. _____

7. Describe the effects of aging on the cardiovascular system.

_____

_____

_____

_____

8. What can aging patients do to decrease the risk of cardiovascular disease?

_____

_____

_____

_____

9. List seven risk factors for cognitive decline.

a. _____

b. _____

c. _____

d. _____

e. _____

f. _____

g. _____

10. Describe the stages of Alzheimer's disease.

a. First Stage: _____

_____

b. Second Stage: _____

_____

c. Terminal Stage: _____

_____

11. List six suggestions for helping the elderly prevent and treat dry skin.

a. _____

b. _____

c. _____

d. _____

e. _____

f. _____

12. List six suggestions for helping the older adult with mobility, dexterity, and balance.

a. _____

b. _____

c. _____

d. _____

e. _____

f. _____

Case Studies

1. A patient is having difficulty staying steady on his feet and must use a walker to move. How can the medical assistant aid the patient? What approach will the MA want to take while preparing the patient for the physician?

2. A patient comes to the office today for a follow-up appointment because of orthostatic hypotension. What questions should Bill ask the patient? How should Bill measure the patient's vital signs? Document the case.

3. A patient has recently had a decline in diabetes treatment compliance. What factors should Bill be aware of that may factor into the patient's diabetes management? How can Bill help the patient overcome these factors?

4. A patient comes to the office today complaining of constipation. What questions should Bill ask the patient? What are the possible causes of constipation in an aging population? Document the case.

5. Mary is concerned about her risk for osteoporosis. What can Bill tell Mary about common risk factors for developing osteoporosis? Is there anything she can do to prevent the decrease of bone density? What tests are done to diagnosis osteoporosis?

6. A patient is having difficulty hearing Bill as he is obtaining the health history. What suggestions can you give Bill to help him communicate with this hearing-impaired patient?

Workplace Applications

1. You are asked to speak at a local community center about preventing injuries. What suggestions can you discuss for preventing falls?

2. Your office sees many geriatric patients daily. What are some common barriers for an aging population when they come into the office? What changes can you make to provide a safe and welcoming environment?

3. One of the duties of the medical assistant is to inform patients about living wills or advanced directives. What information should the medical assistant provide to the patient? Why is it important for a patient to have a living will?

4. Patient education is vital to the understanding of various disease processes and health maintenance. Describe some guidelines for effective patient education with older adults.

Internet Activities

1. Search the Internet for resources for the aging population. Create a list of resources in and around your area that might aid your patients (e.g., discounted meals, living arrangements, transportation services, social and support groups, home health aides).

2. One of the reasons patients do not comply with medication orders is the lack of prescription coverage. Search the Internet for programs that provide patient assistance for medications. What are the criteria for enrollment? Be prepared to discuss your finding in class.

Chapter 47 Quiz

Name: _____

1. Describe two skin changes in the elderly:

   a. _____

   b. _____

2. Define *alopecia*.

   _____

   _____

3. Older adults frequently have problems with
   _____.

   a. diarrhea

   b. constipation

   c. vomiting

4. Define *presbycusis*.

   _____

   _____

   _____

5. Describe *glaucoma*.

   _____

   _____

   _____

6. What is a cataract?

   _____

   _____

7. _____ cause the greatest
   number of injuries in the elderly.

8. DNR stands for _____.

9. _____ is used to treat
   impotence.

10. PLMD stands for _____.

    _____

    _____

Assisting with Diagnostic Imaging

Vocabulary Review

Match the following terms with their definitions.

1. Forward or front portion of the body or body part

2. Pertaining to the head; toward the head

3. Away from the head; the opposite of cephalad

4. Away from the source or point of origin

5. To the outside, at or near the surface of the body or a body part

6. Below, farther from the head

7. Deep, near the center of the body or a part; the opposite of external

8. Referring to the side; away from the center to the left or right

9. Toward the center of the body or of a body part; the opposite of lateral

10. Referring to the palm (anterior surface) of the hand

11. Referring to the sole of the foot

12. Backward or back portion of the body or body part; the opposite of anterior

13. Toward the source or point of origin; the opposite of distal

14. Above, toward the head; the opposite of inferior

a. distal

b. internal

c. plantar

d. medial or mesial

e. palmar

f. external

g. anterior

h. inferior

i. lateral

j. posterior

k. cephalic, cephalad

l. caudal, caudad

m. superior

n. proximal

Fill in the blanks with the correct terms.

15. _____ refers to the making of x-ray images called *radiographs*.

16. X-rays can penetrate most substances to some degree, but some substances, such as metals and bones, are more difficult to penetrate and are said to be _____.

17. _____ is a technique performed with special equipment that permits the radiologist to view x-ray images in motion.

18. The _____ scanner consists of a movable table with remote control, a circular gantry structure that supports the x-ray tube and detectors, an operator console with a monitor, and the supporting computer system.

19. _____ medicine scans do not provide clear images of anatomic structures. They are used to obtain information about the function of organs and tissues.

Fill in the blanks by choosing the correct terms from the following list.

Recumbent

Upright

Prone

Lateral recumbent

Supine

Dorsal recumbent

Ventral recumbent

20. Lying face down is known as the _____ position.

21. Lying down is referred to as _____.

22. Lying on the back with the knees bent and the feet flat on the table is called _____.

23. Lying on the side is _____.

24. Lying face down, prone, is called _____.

25. Lying face up is known as the _____ position.

26. Having an x-ray examination while standing or seated would be called a(n) _____ view.

Skills and Concepts

27. Name the directions and planes of the body shown in the following figure.

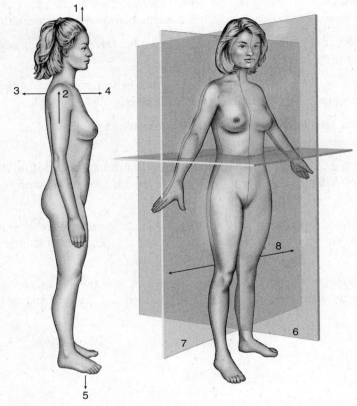

1. _____

2. _____

3. _____

4. _____

5. _____

6. _____

7. _____

8. _____

28. List and describe the four prime factors of exposure.

a. _____

b. _____

c. _____

d. _____

Indicate which statements are true (T) and which statements are false (F). For other statements, fill in the blanks.

29. T   F   Patients with cardiac pacemakers cannot have MRI examinations.

30. T   F   Radiation control regulations do not require that female patients of childbearing age be advised of potential radiation hazards before x-ray examination.

31. T   F   If the patient is supine facing the x-ray tube, the projection is said to be anteroposterior (AP).

32. T   F   X-rays do not linger in the room after the exposure, and they are not capable of making the objects in the room radioactive.

33. The radiographer selects the correct cassette and places a _____ marker on it to identify the patient's right or left side.

34. The _____ (R) is the conventional unit of radiation exposure that represents a measurement of radiation intensity and is determined by the interaction of the x-ray beam with air.

35. To measure both therapeutic radiation doses and specific tissue doses received in diagnostic applications, the conventional unit is the _____, which stands for "radiation absorbed dose."

36. To measure occupational dose or other exposure that may involve more than one type of radiation, the dose equivalent unit used is the _____ which stands for "roentgen equivalent in man."

49 ASSISTING WITH DIAGNOSTIC IMAGING 519

37. Identify each type of radiographic projection in the following pictures.

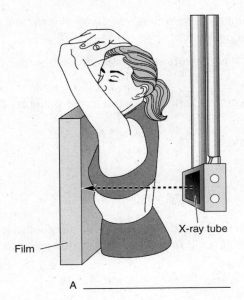

Film

X-ray tube

A _____

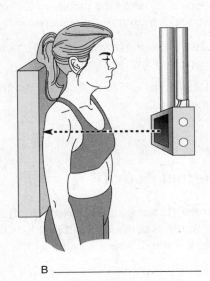

B _____

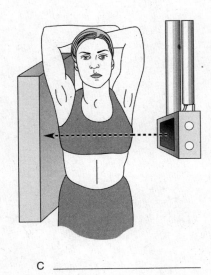

C _____

Case Studies

1. A patient with irritable bowel syndrome has been ordered to undergo a barium enema. What can Sara tell the patient about the examination? What is the patient preparation?

2. Sara is providing instruction to a patient for an MRI. Describe the procedure and any patient preparation.

3. Sara is assisting a patient during an x-ray examination. The patient asks, "What does the x-ray show? Is anything broken?" How should Sara respond to this patient?

Workplace Applications

1. Sara is assisting the radiology technician in moving the equipment. What safety precautions should Sara remember when moving the x-ray equipment?

2. Sara is putting away a recent shipment of films. What factors should she remember when handling and storing films?

3. What steps can Sara follow to minimize unnecessary radiation exposure to her patients? Describe these methods.

Internet Activity

Visit the Radiological Society of North America website. Explore the patient education section of the site. Become familiar with this site. Is it something you could find useful in a healthcare setting? What are the different features of the site?

Chapter 49 Quiz

Name: _____

1. An x-ray study taken in motion is
   _____.

2. Imaging of blood vessels is
   _____.

3. An AP view is when the patient is
   _____ the
   x-ray tube.

4. During _____ projection
   the sagittal plane of the body is parallel to the
   film.

5. The _____ plane divides the
   body into superior and inferior portions.

6. Devices for monitoring radiation exposure to
   personnel are called _____.

7. A _____ is a computerized
   image that pictures slices of the body.

8. An x-ray study of the breast is a
   _____.

9. An imaging technique that uses a large
   magnet is a _____.

10. A material that is used to fill in hollow organs
    for better visualization during a radiography
    procedure is called _____
    _____.

Assisting in the Clinical Laboratory

Vocabulary Review

Write the correct term in the space provided.

1. _____ A term used to describe a blood sample in which the red blood cells have ruptured.

2. _____ A cylindric glass or plastic tube used to deliver fluids.

3. _____ The substance or chemical being analyzed or detected in a specimen.

4. _____ A sample of body fluid, waste product, or tissue that is collected for analysis.

5. _____ A substance that is known to cause cancer.

6. _____ The ability of the eye to distinguish two objects that are very close together; the sharpness of an image.

7. _____ A portion of a well-mixed sample removed for testing.

8. _____ A substance that burns or destroys tissue by chemical action.

9. _____ A liquid used to dilute a specimen or reagent.

10. _____ A chemical added to the blood after collection to prevent clotting.

11. _____ An order found on a laboratory requisition indicating that the test must be done immediately (from the Latin word *statin,* meaning "at once").

12. _____ A substance that is known to cause birth defects.

13. _____ Fluids with a high concentration of protein and cellular debris that have escaped from the blood vessels and been deposited in tissues or on tissue surfaces.

14. _____ A sac filled with blood that may be the result of trauma.

15. _____ Fluid within the subarachnoid space, the central canal of the spinal cord, and the four ventricles of the brain.

16. _____ Substances added to a specimen to prevent deterioration of cells or chemicals.

17. _____ Private or hospital-based laboratories that perform a wide variety of tests, many of them specialized. Physicians often send specimens collected in the office to one of these for testing.

Skills and Concepts

18. Convert the following from Greenwich time to military time or from military time to Greenwich time

    a. 2:30 PM _____

    b. 12:00 PM _____

    c. 4:20 AM _____

    d. 1500 hours _____

    e. 1815 hours _____

19. Label the parts of a microscope in the following figure.

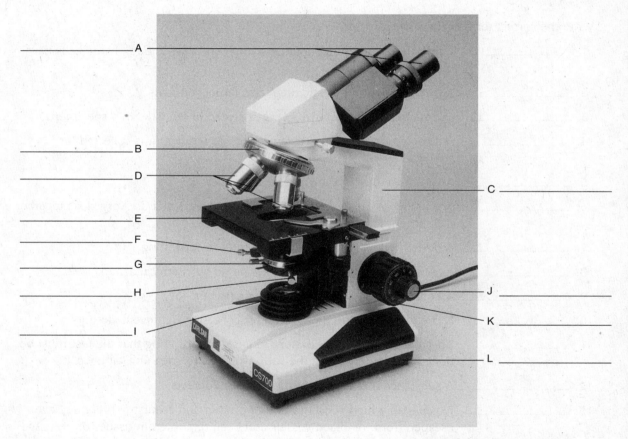

20. One blood glucose meter always reads 10% too high. Another meter reads anywhere from 5% to 9% too high. Which one is the more precise? Which one is the more accurate? How is accuracy different from precision?

    _____

    _____

    _____

    _____

21. List five times when it is absolutely necessary to wash your hands in the laboratory area.

    a. _____

    b. _____

    c. _____

    d. _____

    e. _____

22. Name three types of hazards in the laboratory setting.

    a. _____

    b. _____

    c. _____

23. Differentiate between qualitative and quantitative results. Give an example of each.

    _____

    _____

    _____

    _____

24. Name the four major divisions of the clinical laboratory.

    a. _____

    b. _____

    c. _____

    d. _____

25. Label each of the following according to its division.

    a. Hemoglobin _____

    b. Urine specific gravity _____

    c. Urine culture _____

    d. Blood glucose _____

    e. Throat culture _____

    f. White blood cell count _____

    g. Cholesterol _____

    h. Complete blood count _____

26. What is an MSDS? What type of information does it include?

    _____

    _____

    _____

    _____

27. What is the role of OSHA?

_____

_____

28. What is CLIA, and what are the three different levels of laboratory testing?

_____

_____

_____

_____

29. Describe the chain of custody. Why is it important? What steps must be followed?

_____

_____

_____

_____

Case Studies

1. Marsha is preparing to draw blood on a patient. What standard precautions should she take when doing the procedure?

2. Marsha has been asked to develop a safety manual for the office. What information should be included?

3. Marsha is in charge of performing the quality assurance in the office. Describe when QA testing should be done for the following tests.

   a. Urinalysis

   b. Pregnancy tests

   c. Glucometer test strips

   d. Automated chemistry analyses

   e. Temperature logs

Workplace Applications

1. Marsha is preparing a requisition form for a collected specimen. What information must be included?

2. On the thermometer drawings provided, mark the range of common laboratory temperatures for the following:

   a. Body and incubator temperature

   b. Room temperature

   c. Freezer temperature

   d. Refrigerator temperature

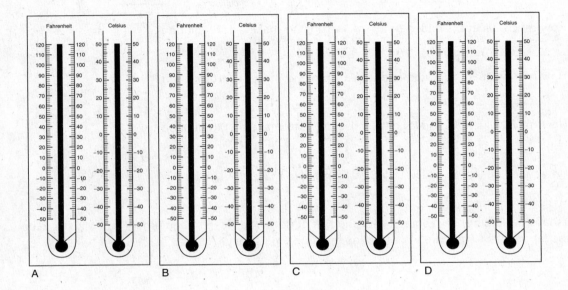

A   B   C   D

3. Your centrifuge starts to vibrate markedly while you are spinning a specimen. What should you check? What precautions should be taken while operating a centrifuge?

4. Record the volume in milliliters for the two cylinders pictured.

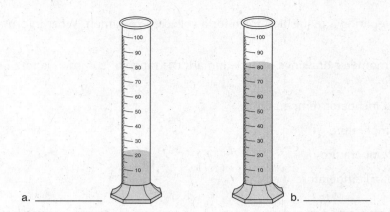

a. _____   b. _____

c. How much diluent is added to a 1-mL sample to make a 1:10 dilution?

_____ mL

d. How much diluent is added to a 2-mL sample to make a 1:10 dilution?

_____ mL

e. How much diluent is added to a 1-mL sample to make a 1:20 dilution?

_____ mL

f. How much diluent is added to a 2-mL sample to make a 1:10 dilution?

_____ mL

5. Marsha is evaluating the laboratory for the risk of fire. What type of equipment can Marsha keep in the laboratory to prepare in case of open flame emergency?

Internet Activity

Visit www.osha.gov, and locate the list of standard precautions. What tools does the website offer to healthcare workers?

Chapter 50 Quiz

Name: _____

1. A(n) _____ is a portion of a well-mixed sample removed for testing.

2. A(n) _____ specimen is one in which blood vessels have ruptured.

3. MSDS stands for _____.

4. When are laboratory assistants required to wash their hands?

5. What is the objective of quality control?

6. A simple laboratory test that can be performed at home is _____.

7. The FDA ensures quality of laboratory testing under what piece of legislation?

   _____

   _____

8. A(n) _____ laboratory test has numeric results.

9. A(n) _____ laboratory test has positive and negative results.

10. _____ is the government agency that deals with safety in the workplace.

11. Mouth-pipetting is forbidden in the laboratory setting.
    a. True
    b. False

12. If the eyepiece of the microscope is 10× and the high power is 40×, what is the total magnification?

    _____

13. The coarse adjustment should always be used with the oil emersion lens.
    a. True
    b. False

WORK PRODUCT 51-1

Name: _____

CLIA-Waived Tests: Perform Urinalysis

A 24-year-old patient comes to the office complaining of dysuria, burning on urination, and LBP for 3 days. The vital signs of the patient are as follows:

Wt: 145 lb

B/P: 112/66 mg/dL

T: 100.7F

P: 76

R: 16

Obtain a urine sample from the patient and perform a urinalysis. Record the results.

Color: _____

Clarity: _____

Glucose: _____

Ketones: _____

Specific gravity: _____

pH: _____

Blood: _____

Bilirubin: _____

Leukocytes: _____

Nitrates: _____

Protein: _____

Urobilinogen: _____

Using SOAPE format, document the case.

S: _____

_____

_____

O: _____

_____

_____

WORK PRODUCT 51-2

Name: _____

Screen Test Results and Follow-up

On completion of a urinalysis, the following results were noted:

Color: amber

Clarity: clear

Glucose: small

Ketones:positive

Specific gravity: 1.005

pH: 7.5

Blood: moderate

Bilirubin: negative

Leukocytes: negative

Nitrates: negative

Protein: small

Urobilinogen: 0.1

Using the table below, what can be noted from these test results?

Normal Urine Reference Range

Reference	Range
Color	Pale yellow to straw
Clarity	Clear to slightly turbid
Specific gravity	1.001-1.035
pH	4.6-8.0
Protein (mg/dL)	NEG
Glucose (mg/dL)	NEG
Ketone (mg/dL)	NEG
Bilirubin (mg/dL)	NEG
Blood (mg/dL)	NEG
Nitrite (mg/dL)	NEG
Urobilinogen (Ehrlich units)	0.1-1
White blood cells	NEG

Are there any questions the medical assistant should ask the patient regarding the findings?

_____

_____

_____

_____

Assisting in Microbiology and Immunology

Vocabulary Review

Fill in the blanks with the correct terms.

1. _____ Pertaining to or originating in the hospital; said of an infection not present or incubating before admission to the hospital

2. _____ An agent that causes disease, especially a living microorganism such as a bacterium or fungus

3. _____ A bacterial or fungal culture that contains a single organism

4. _____ A differentiated structure within a cell, such as a mitochondrion, vacuole, or chloroplast, which performs a specific function

5. _____ One billionth (10^{-9}) of a meter

6. _____ An organism of microscopic or submicroscopic size

7. _____ A single-celled or multicellular organism in which each cell contains a distinct membrane-bound nucleus

8. _____ Requiring specialized media or growth factors to grow

9. _____ A small capsule-like sac that encloses certain organisms in their dormant or larval stage

10. _____ A sample, as of tissue, blood, or urine, used for analysis and diagnosis

11. _____ A unicellular organism that lacks a membrane-bound nucleus

12. _____ A drug used to treat a broad range of infections

13. _____ Refers to conditions outside of a living body

14. _____ The process of removing pathogenic microorganisms or protecting against infection by such organisms

15. _____ The molecules needed for metabolism: carbohydrates, lipids, proteins, and nucleic acids

16. _____ The technique or process of keeping tissue alive and growing in a culture medium

17. _____ A drug that is used to treat infection

18. _____ A group of like or different atoms held together by chemical forces

19. _____ A medium used to keep an organism alive during transport to the laboratory

20. _____ Capable of living, developing, or germinating under favorable conditions

21. _____ A slide preparation in which a drop of liquid specimen or the like is covered with a coverslip and examined with a microscope

22. _____ Chemical released from cells that causes smooth muscle contraction and pain

23. _____ Glycoproteins produced by cells infected with a virus or another intracellular parasite that can be used medically as antiviral or anticancer therapeutics

24. _____ A protein produced by certain white blood cells that regulates immune responses by activating lymphocytes and initiating fever

Skills and Concepts

25. Identify the four shapes of bacteria shown in the figure.

a. _____

b. _____

c. _____

d. _____

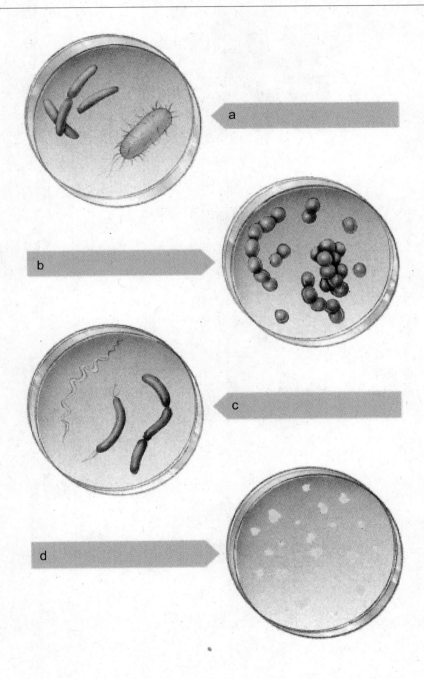

26. Identify the four types of disease-causing protozoa shown in the figure.

a. _____

b. _____

c. _____

d. _____

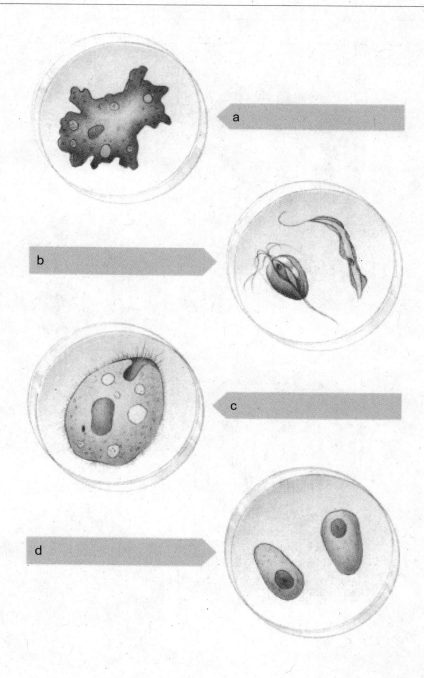

27. Identify the three pathogenic animals shown in the figure.

a. _____

b. _____

c. _____

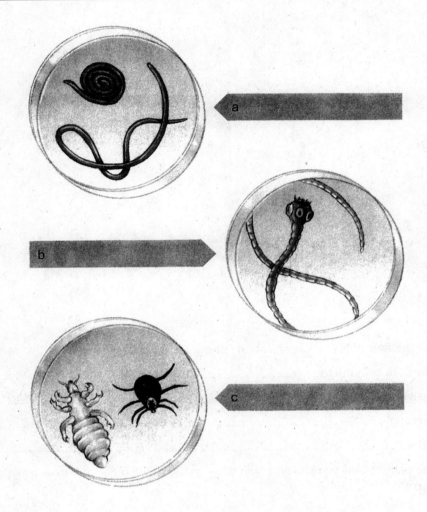

28. Identify the two fungi shown in the figure.

   a. _____

   b. _____

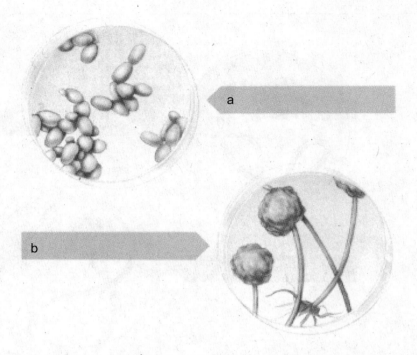

29. Describe the four different classifications of media.

   a. All-purpose or nutritive _____

   b. Selective _____

   c. Differential _____

   d. Enriched _____

30. Draw the pattern that you should make when you prepare a *Streptococcus pyogenes* culture on an agar plate.

31. Compare and contrast the throat culture for *Streptococcus pyogenes* with the rapid strep test.

_____

_____

_____

_____

Case Studies

1. A patient has been ordered to obtain a stool sample. What type of patient education should be included to ensure proper collection?

2. The office in which Anna works performs some rapid testing. Describe three microbiology tests that use a rapid identification technique.

3. A 5-year-old patient is brought to the office with pinworms. How do people usually become infected with the pinworm? Provide the patient education for specimen collection.

4. Anna is educating a patient on the importance of infection control. What factors should Anna be sure to cover?

Workplace Applications

1. Anna is preparing to obtain a sample for testing. What should she keep in mind as she is collecting the specimen? The specimen is an anaerobe. What elements are required for growth?

2. Describe some of the different equipment found in the microbiology laboratory.

3. What steps should Anna follow while performing a Gram stain? What reactions are seen with a gram-positive stain? What reactions are seen with a gram-negative stain?

4. List and describe the three CLIA-waived immunology tests that Anna may perform in the POL.

Internet Activity

Search the American Biological Safety Association website, www.absa.org. Become familiar with the site. What tools does the site have to help you maintain a safe laboratory environment?

Chapter 54 Quiz

Name: _____

1. Spheric bacteria are called

   _____ .

2. Rod-shaped bacteria are called

   _____ .

3. During a Gram stain,

   _____ is the

   decolorizing agent.

4. The organism that causes mononucleosis is

   _____

   _____ .

5. An organism that causes disease is a(n)

   _____ .

6. Bacteria requiring oxygen to live are called

   _____ ; those that will die in the

   presence of oxygen are called

   _____

7. _____ is the study of
   fungi and the diseases they cause.

8. _____ are transmitted
   through contaminated feces or drink and are
   present in moist environments and in bodies
   of water such as lakes and ponds.

9. The medical assistant must be aware that
   patient confidentiality is of utmost importance, but certain infections, such as sexually
   transmitted diseases and tuberculosis, must
   be reported to the CDC and to the local board
   of health.

   a. True

   b. False

10. A medium used to keep an organism alive
    during transport to the laboratory is called

    _____ .

Surgical Supplies and Instruments

Vocabulary Review

Fill in the blanks with the appropriate terms.

1. _____ Act of scraping a body cavity with a surgical instrument, such as a curette

2. _____ Opening or widening the circumference of a body orifice with a dilating instrument

3. _____ Sheet or band of fibrous tissue located deep in the skin that covers muscles and body organs

4. _____ Abnormal, tubelike passage between internal organs or from an internal organ to the body surface

5. _____ Open space, such as within a blood vessel, the intestine, a needle, or an examining instrument

6. _____ Rigid tube that surrounds a blunt trocar or a sharp, pointed trocar inserted into the body; when withdrawn, fluid may escape from the body through it, depending on where it is inserted

7. _____ Metal rod with a smooth rounded tip that is placed into hollow instruments to decrease destruction of the body tissues during insertion

8. _____ Localized collection of pus that may be under the skin or deep within the body that causes tissue destruction

9. _____ Open condition of a body cavity or canal

10. _____ Tumors with stems, frequently found on mucous membranes

11. _____ Metal probe that is inserted into or passed through a catheter, needle, or tube used for clearing purposes or to facilitate passage into a body orifice

12. _____ To cut or separate tissue with a cutting instrument or scissors

Skills and Concepts

13. List two medications that help control bleeding.

    a. _____

    b. _____

14. List four groups of surgical instruments, and give an example of each.

    a. _____

    b. _____

    c. _____

    d. _____

Name the instruments pictured in the following figures.

15.

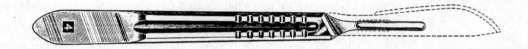

_____

16.

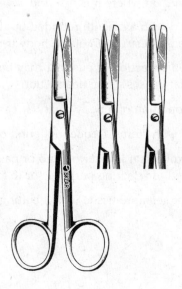

_____

17.

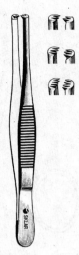

18.

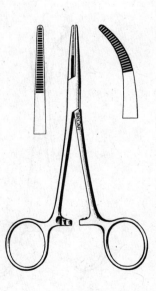

19.

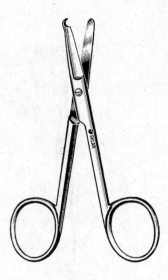

20.

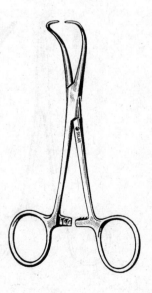

21.

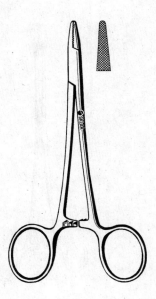

22.

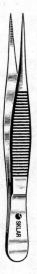

23.

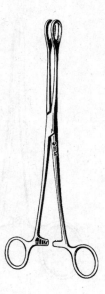

24.

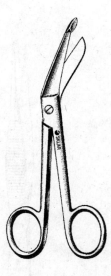

Indicate which statements are true (T) and which statements are false (F).

25. _____ Each instrument should always be unlocked before immersion in the chemical decontaminate to permit cleansing of the entire surface area.

26. _____ Instruments are always named after the person who designed them.

27. _____ Scissors have ratchets.

28. _____ A mosquito and Kelly are names of hemostats.

Match the following descriptions and instruments.

29. _____ Have a beak or hook to slide under sutures

30. _____ Jaws are shorter and look stronger than hemostat jaws

31. _____ Design and construction vary; have a fine tip for foreign object retrieval

32. _____ Have very sharp hooks

33. _____ Valves can be spread to facilitate viewing

34. _____ Probe tip is blunt

35. _____ Manufactured in different lengths; smooth-tipped; used to insert packing into or remove objects from nose and ear

   a. Bayonet forceps

   b. Towel forceps (towel clamp)

   c. Littauer stitch or suture scissors

   d. Needle holders

   e. Splinter forceps

   f. Nasal specula

   g. Bandage scissors

36. Describe some characteristics of ideal suture material.

   a. _____

   b. _____

   c. _____

   d. _____

37. Explain the difference between absorbable and nonabsorbable sutures. When would each type of suture be used?

   _____

   _____

   _____

   _____

Case Studies

1. You are assisting Dr. Samanski during a procedure. The physician has asked you to ensure there are three local anesthetics available in the room. List them.

2. Tom is preparing an instrument and supply pack for a cervical biopsy. What instruments should be included for autoclave?

Workplace Applications

1. Tom is in charge of establishing a room for minor office surgery. What features should be included in this examination room?

2. Tom is stocking the supplies in the surgery room. List four types of surgical solution commonly used.

3. Tom is showing a new employee the various instruments in the office. What should Tom tell the new employee about the care and inspection of the instruments?

Internet Activity

Search the Internet for surgical instruments. Review the names of instruments that you find on the Internet. Print the instruments and bring to class. Compare your findings with a classmate.

Chapter 55 Quiz

Name: _____

1. Metzenbaum, Mayo, and Iris are names of
_____ .

2. The primary purpose of a(n)
_____ is to hold the edges of a
wound together until natural healing occurs.

3. Allis, Bayonet, and Adson are
_____ .

4. Hemostats are a type of forceps or
_____ .

5. Normal physiologic sterile saline is
_____ % .

6. Local anesthetics have the
_____ suffix.

7. _____ is the scraping of a
body cavity with a surgical instrument.

8. A(n) _____ is a metal rod
with a smooth rounded tip that is placed in
hollow instruments to prevent injury during
insertion.

9. Betadine and Hibiclens are examples of
_____ .

10. Iodoform is used as a
_____ .

CHAPTER 56

Surgical Asepsis and Assisting with Surgical Procedures

Vocabulary Review

Match the following terms with their definitions.

1. Permeable

2. Contamination

3. Disease

4. Infection

5. Antiseptic

6. Edema

7. Spores

8. Pathogens

9. Sterilization

10. Disinfection

11. Microorganisms

12. Sanitization

a. Invasion of body tissues by microorganisms, which then proliferate and damage tissues

b. Living organisms that can be seen only with a light microscope

c. Disease-causing microorganisms

d. Allowing a substance to pass or soak through

e. Reducing the number of microorganisms to a relatively safe level

f. Thick-walled dormant form of bacteria, very resistant to disinfection measures

g. Complete destruction of all forms of microbial life

h. Substance that kills microorganisms

i. Becoming nonsterile by contact with any nonsterile material

j. Pathologic process having a descriptive set of signs and symptoms

k. Destruction of pathogens by physical or chemical means

l. Swelling between layers of tissue

Skills and Concepts

13. Describe the differences among sanitization, disinfection, and sterilization.

_____

_____

_____

_____

14. Describe the following types of sterilization indicators.

    a. Chemical _____

    _____

    b. Biologic _____

    _____

15. Describe the following common surgical procedures done in the physician's office.

    a. Cryosurgery _____

    _____

    b. Microsurgery _____

    _____

    c. Endoscopic procedures _____

    _____

    d. Electrosurgery _____

    _____

    e. Laser _____

    _____

16. Describe the importance of skin preparation. Explain the method of skin preparation.

_____

_____

_____

_____

Indicate which statements are true (T) and which statements are false (F).

17. _____ Air currents carry bacteria, so body motions over a sterile field and talking should be kept to a minimum.

18. _____ Infection can cause death in some circumstances.

19. _____ A sterile field can get wet but remain microorganism free.

20. _____ Sterile team members should always face each other.

21. _____ You should always keep the sterile field in your view.

22. _____ You should never turn your back on a sterile field or wander away from it.

23. _____ When autoclaving, you should place a gauze sponge around the tips of sharp instruments to prevent them from piercing the wrapping material.

24. _____ Nonsterile persons should never reach over a sterile field.

25. _____ All hinged instruments are wrapped in the closed position to allow full steam penetration of the joint.

26. _____ When using sterilizing bags, you should insert the grasping end of the instruments first.

27. Describe the three phases of wound healing

a. _____

b. _____

c. _____

28. What are the reasons for applying a sterile dressing?

a. _____

b. _____

c. _____

d. _____

Case Studies

1. Melissa is preparing instruments for the autoclave. What rules must Melissa follow when wrapping instruments for the autoclave?

2. Minor office procedures like mole removals are commonly done in Melissa's office. What is Melissa's role in these procedures?

3. As Melissa is preparing a patient for a procedure, the patient seems very anxious and worried. What can Melissa do to support the patient?

4. After a procedure is complete the medical assistant should provide the patient with postoperative instructions. Describe five reasons a patient should call the office postoperatively.

5. A patient comes to the office for a suture removal. The area—the left forearm—is covered with bandages. How should the patient be prepared for the procedure? What setup is required for this procedure? Document the case. Include the vital signs of the patient.

Workplace Applications

1. One of Melissa's job duties includes maintaining the autoclave. What types of PPE should be worn when loading, operating, and unloading the autoclave? Why?

2. What guidelines should be followed when unloading the autoclave?

3. A patient is scheduled for a surgical procedure in the office; what details should Melissa complete before the appointment?

4. The physician has ordered an open wound healing. What are some of the advantages of this type of healing process?

Internet Activity

One of your job duties is to purchase supplies for the minor office procedures. Search the internet for equipment and supplies typically needed in performing minor office procedures. Print a list of materials and prices. Share the information with your classmates. Did you find anything surprising?

Chapter 56 Quiz

Name: _____

1. Using electrocautery requires the patient to be connected to a _____.

2. Laser surgery requires sterile water to be available.

   a. True

   b. False

3. Describe the importance of informed consent.

   _____

   _____

   _____

4. Cryosurgery is _____ the tissue.

5. What are the 2 greatest sources of contamination when setting up the sterile field?

   a. _____

   b. _____

6. Name three types of sterilization.

   a. _____

   b. _____

   c. _____

7. A machine that uses steam and pressure to kill pathogens and spores is an

   _____

8. What is the purpose of autoclave tape?

   _____

   _____

9. What should be written on the outside of instruments after they are wrapped?

   _____

   _____

10. Sterile supplies expire after _____ days to _____ months depending on the packaging.

Career Development and Life Skills

Vocabulary Review

Fill in the blanks with the correct vocabulary terms from this chapter.

1. Jerri wrote a(n) _____ of the facts that she knew related to the theft of petty cash.

2. June found Daniel's attitude to be _____ and finally made a complaint to the office manager.

3. Because Allen was continuing his studies at night and was taking 12 credit hours, he was able to place his student loan in _____.

4. Medical assisting is one of the most versatile _____ that one can enter.

5. The physician asked Merri to _____ the documents for grammar and spelling.

6. Andrea found that _____ provided her with many more job leads than simply looking in the newspaper.

7. Ms. Moore, the office manager, attempted to get the employees to bring up only the _____ facts related to the conflict.

8. Joel tried to _____ his error by placing an amendment in the medical record.

9. Dr. Donat gave the information to Selinda to rewrite, because she could take the regulations and convert them into a(n) _____, clear document.

10. Mack called his lender to report that he had returned to school full-time so that he would not _____ on his loan.

Skills and Concepts

Part I: Short Answer Questions

11. List three ways that job search training helps the newly graduated medical assistant.

   a. _____

   b. _____

   c. _____

12. What are employers' three basic desires when looking for a new employee?

   a. _____

   b. _____

   c. _____

13. Define *job skills*, and give two examples.

   _____

   _____

   _____

14. Define *self-management skills*, and give two examples.

   _____

   _____

   _____

15. Define *transferable skills*, and give two examples.

   _____

   _____

   _____

16. What is meant when it is said that a medical assistant knows his or her personal needs?

   _____

   _____

   _____

17. List and define the two best job search methods.

   a. _____

   _____

   b. _____

   _____

18. Explain at least three ways that the Internet can be of help when searching for a job.

a. _____

_____

b. _____

_____

_____

c. _____

_____

_____

19. List five items that should be on a resume.

a. _____

b. _____

c. _____

d. _____

e. _____

20. List two things that should never be included on a resume.

a. _____

b. _____

Part II: Cover Letters

Write a professional cover letter following the suggestions in the textbook. Turn the cover letter in to the instructor, along with the assignment in Part III.

Part III: Job Applications

22. Complete the job application found on the following pages. Make certain that it is legible, accurate, and complete.

DIAMONTE
HOSPITAL

APPLICATION FOR EMPLOYMENT

This application is not a contract. It is intended to provide information for evaluating your suitability for employment. Please read each question carefully and give an honest and complete answer. Qualified applicants receive consideration for employment without unlawful discrimination because of sex, religion, race, color, national origin, age, disability, or other classification protected by law. Applications will remain active for three months.

PLEASE TYPE OR PRINT ALL INFORMATION

Date: _____

Position(s) applying for: _____

How did you learn about us? ☐ Walk-in ☐ Friend ☐ Relative ☐ Job hotline ☐ Employee ☐ Other
☐ Advertisement (Please state name of publication) _____ Referred by: _____

Name: _____
        Last   First   Middle initial

Mailing address: _____
                    City   State   Zip code

Phone: (____) _____ (____) _____ Social Security #: _____
        Home   Message

If related to anyone in our employ, state name and department: _____

If you have been employed under another name, please list here: _____

Are you under 18 years of age?.. ☐ Yes   ☐ No

Are you currently employed?.. ☐ Yes   ☐ No

May we contact your present employer?...................................... ☐ Yes   ☐ No

Do you have legal rights to work in this country?
  (Proof of legal rights to work in this country will be required upon employment)..... ☐ Yes   ☐ No

Have you ever been employed with us before?............................. ☐ Yes   ☐ No If "yes," give date(s): _____

Are you available to work: _____ ☐ Full-time ☐ Part-time ☐ Shift work ☐ Temporary

Are you available to work overtime if required?........................... ☐ Yes   ☐ No

How flexible are you in accepting varying scheduled hours?.................. ☐ Very flexible ☐ Somewhat flexible
                                                                          ☐ Need set schedule

Minimum salary desired: _____

Have you ever been discharged from a job or forced to resign?............. ☐ Yes   ☐ No
  Explain: _____

Have you ever been convicted of a felony?
  If "yes," please explain: _____   ☐ Yes   ☐ No
  Criminal convictions are not an absolute bar to _____
  employment but will be considered with respect _____
  to the specific requirements of the job for which _____
  you are applying. _____

EDUCATION

High school: _____   High school graduate/GED: ☐ Yes ☐ No
_____   Date:_____

College:_____   Graduated: ☐ Yes ☐ No

Major/field(s) of study: _____   Degree: _____
Date:_____

College:_____   Graduated: ☐ Yes ☐ No

Major/field(s) of study: _____   Degree:_____
Date:_____

Technical, business, or
correspondence school: _____   Graduated: ☐ Yes ☐ No

Major/field(s) of study: _____   Degree: _____
Date:_____

Describe any specialized training, apprenticeship, and skills such as computer,
office equipment, etc. _____
_____
_____
_____
_____
_____

LICENSES AND CERTIFICATIONS

Type of license(s)/certification(s): _____   Expiration date: _____

Type of license(s)/certification(s): _____   Expiration date: _____

Type of license(s)/certification(s): _____   Expiration date: _____

Verified by: _____

Date:_____

REFERENCES

(Give name, address, and telephone number of three references that you have known for at least one year who are not
related to you.)

Name: _____   Phone:_____   Years acquainted:_____

Address: _____   Business: _____

Name: _____   Phone:_____   Years acquainted:_____

Address: _____   Business: _____

Name: _____   Phone:_____   Years acquainted:_____

Address: _____   Business: _____

EMPLOYMENT EXPERIENCE

(Please list all employment experience, with most recent employment first. If more space is needed, please use the Additional Employment form.)

Employer: _____   Duties and skills performed: _____
Address: _____   _____
Phone number(s) _____   _____
Job title: _____   _____
Supervisor's name/title: _____   _____
Reason for leaving: _____   _____
Salary received: _____ *hourly / weekly / monthly* _____
Employed from: _____ to _____
                month / year   *month / year*

Employer: _____   Duties and skills performed: _____
Address: _____   _____
Phone number(s) _____   _____
Job title: _____   _____
Supervisor's name/title: _____   _____
Reason for leaving: _____   _____
Salary received: _____ *hourly / weekly / monthly* _____
Employed from: _____ to _____
                month / year   *month / year*

Employer: _____   Duties and skills performed: _____
Address: _____   _____
Phone number(s) _____   _____
Job title: _____   _____
Supervisor's name/title: _____   _____
Reason for leaving: _____   _____
Salary received: _____ *hourly / weekly / monthly* _____
Employed from: _____ to _____
                month / year   *month / year*

Do you expect any of the employers listed above to give you a poor reference? ☐ Yes ☐ No
If yes, explain: _____
_____

APPLICANT'S STATEMENT

I hereby certify that the statements and information provided are true, and I understand that any false statements or omissions are cause for termination. I agree to submit to a drug test and physical following any conditional offer of employment, and I grant permission to Diamonte Hospital to investigate my criminal history, education, prior employment history, and references, and hereby release all persons or agencies from all liability or any damage for issuing this information.

I understand that this application is current for only **three months**. At the end of that time, if I do not hear from Diamonte Hospital and still wish to be considered for employment, it will be necessary to update my application.

_____   _____
Signature of Applicant   *Date*

_____
Print Name

DIAMONTE
HOSPITAL

Part IV: Resumes

23. Write a professional resume following the suggestions in the textbook. Turn the resume and cover letter in to the instructor.

Part V: Interviews

24. Set up an interview with a physician's office. Perhaps the interview can lead to an externship or a position after graduation. Use the *Record of a Job Lead* form and the *Record of an Interview Form* to record pertinent information.

Part VI: Follow-up Activities

25. Write a thank-you card to the person with whom you interviewed. If a job opportunity exists, continue follow-up activities with the clinic.

Part VII: Goals

26. Set some realistic goals for your career in medical assisting by answering the following questions.

1. Where am I today?

_____
_____
_____
_____

2. Where will I be in 5 years?

_____
_____
_____
_____

3. Where will I be in 10 years?

_____
_____
_____
_____

4. What additional skills do I need to get to where I want to be?

_____
_____
_____
_____

Part VIII: Budgeting

27. Plan a budget for yourself using your actual living expenses.

The Guideline Budget

MONTHLY INCOME	AMOUNT
Net Income	
Spouse Net Income	
Child Support	
Other Income	

MONTHLY EXPENSES	AMOUNT
Rent	
Gas	
Electric	
Home/Renters Insurance	
Water/Sewage	
Trash	
Home Telephone	
Cell Telephone	
Pager	
Cable TV/Satellite	
Internet/DSL	
Child Care	
Lawn Care	
Clothing	
Food-Home	
Food-Work or School	
Food-Eating Out	
Laundry/Dry Cleaning	
Medical Expenses	
Dental Expenses	
Life Insurance	
Medical Insurance	
Dental Insurance	
Eyeglasses	
Prescriptions	
Automobile Payment	
Automobile Insurance	
Repairs	
Gas/Oil	
Furniture	
Beauty/Barber Shop	
Pet Expenses	
Student Loan	
Other Loans	
Credit Cards	
Church/Charities	
Birthdays	
Anniversaries	
Christmas	
Vacation Planning	
Entertainment	

Case Study

Monica was an exceptional student during school and graduated with a high GPA. After a successful externship and 1 month looking for employment, she has been unable to secure a job. She calls the placement officer at her school, who sends her on several interviews, which are also unsuccessful. The placement officer asks Monica to come to the school dressed for an interview and to bring her resume with her. As Monica is being interviewed, the placement officer is impressed with her appearance and her communications skills. Then she looks down at Monica's resume and realizes why Monica has not been hired. What problem did the placement officer probably discover? What can Monica do to be more likely to secure employment?

Workplace Activities

Make a list of 20 potential employers. Use the Internet to obtain information about the facilities. Make a list of five points about each potential employer that could be discussed in an interview. Also, find five ways that you qualify for a position in the facility. If appropriate, visit the facilities and make appointments for interviews. Obtain and complete a job application from each facility. Submit the application and a resume if you are close to the end of your training.

Internet Activities

1. Research potential employers in your geographic area. Find out as much information about the employers as possible. Keep a record of the information using the job lead forms provided in the text.

2. Use the job search sites mentioned in the text to locate potential job opportunities. Have your resume in electronic form ready to attach so that you can apply for the jobs that interest you.

3. Look for job search sites other than those in the textbook. Share the sites with your classmates.

4. Form a group on Yahoo! or another site that includes each classmate. Share emails and stay in touch with one another after graduation. Share leads that might lead to employment.

Chapter 57 Quiz

Name: _____

1. A fact sheet that summarizes an applicant's qualifications, education, and experience is called a _____.

2. Salary expectation should be clearly stated on the resume.

   a. True

   b. False

3. Name two of the most effective ways of job searching.

   a. _____

   b. _____

4. It is illegal for someone to ask about number of children, religion, and marital status during an interview.

   a. True

   b. False

5. Name the four phases of a job interview.

   a. _____

   b. _____

   c. _____

   d. _____

6. Name three traditional job search techniques.

   a. _____

   b. _____

   c. _____

7. What is the purpose of a cover letter?

   _____

   _____

8. When writing career objectives, what should you ask yourself?

   _____

   _____

   _____

   _____

9. List three things that employers want.

   a. _____

   b. _____

   c. _____

10. Describe three types of skills that could be included on a resume.

   a. _____

   b. _____

   c. _____

Student Name _____ Date _____ Score _____

Procedure 5-1 Recognize and Respond to Verbal Communications

Task: To be able to recognize verbal communication and respond to it in a professional manner.

Equipment and Supplies:
• Cards with various patient scenarios

Standards: Complete the procedure and all critical steps in _____ minutes with a minimum score of _____% within three attempts.

Scoring: Divide points earned by total possible points. Failure to perform a critical step that is indicated with an asterisk (*) will result in an unsatisfactory overall score.

Time began _____ **Time ended** _____

Steps	Possible Points	First Attempt	Second Attempt	Third Attempt
1. Choose a partner.	5	_____	_____	_____
2. Communicate the assigned message to the partner.*	20	_____	_____	_____
3. Allow the partner to respond.	10	_____	_____	_____
4. Restate the message from the partner.*	20	_____	_____	_____
5. Clarify unclear issues.	10	_____	_____	_____
6. Use professional wording.*	20	_____	_____	_____
7. Repeat three times, communicating each message clearly.	15	_____	_____	_____

Comments:

Total Points Earned _____ Divided by _____ Total Possible Points = _____ % Score

Instructor's Signature _____

Procedure 5-2 Recognize and Respond to Nonverbal Communications

Task: To be able to recognize nonverbal communication and respond to it in a professional way.

Equipment and Supplies:
• Cards with various statements that can be communicated in a nonverbal way

Standards: Complete the procedure and all critical steps in _____ minutes with a minimum score of _____% within three attempts.

Scoring: Divide points earned by total possible points. Failure to perform a critical step that is indicated with an asterisk (*) will result in an unsatisfactory overall score.

Time began _____ **Time ended** _____

Steps	Possible Points	First Attempt	Second Attempt	Third Attempt
1. Choose a partner.	5	_____	_____	_____
2. Communicate the assigned nonverbal message to the partner.*	20	_____	_____	_____
3. Allow the partner to respond.	10	_____	_____	_____
4. Restate the message from the partner verbally.*	20	_____	_____	_____
5. Clarify unclear issues.	10	_____	_____	_____
6. Use professional gestures and wording when interpreting the message.*	20	_____	_____	_____
7. Repeat three times, communicating each nonverbal message clearly.	15	_____	_____	_____

Comments:

Total Points Earned _____ Divided by _____ Total Possible Points = _____ % Score

Instructor's Signature _____

Student Name _____ Date _____ Score _____

Procedure 6-1 Perform Within Ethical Boundaries

Task: To enable the medical assistant to perform in an ethical manner in all situations.

Equipment and Supplies:
- Copy of the AAMA Code of Ethics
- Copy of the Medical Assistant Creed
- Copy of the Oath of Hippocrates

Standards: Complete the procedure and all critical steps in _____ minutes with a minimum score of _____% within three attempts.

Scoring: Divide points earned by total possible points. Failure to perform a critical step that is indicated with an asterisk (*) will result in an unsatisfactory overall score.

Time began _____ **Time ended** _____

Steps	Possible Points	First Attempt	Second Attempt	Third Attempt
1. Review the AAMA Code of Ethics.	10	_____	_____	_____
2. Review the Medical Assistant Creed.	20	_____	_____	_____
3. Review the Oath of Hippocrates.	10	_____	_____	_____
4. Briefly explain the Concepts in the AAMA Code of Ethics.*	10	_____	_____	_____
5. Repeat the Medical Assistant Creed from memory.*	30	_____	_____	_____
6. Briefly explain the Oath of Hippocrates.*	20	_____	_____	_____

Comments:

Total Points Earned _____ Divided by _____ Total Possible Points = _____ % Score

Instructor's Signature _____

Student Name _____ Date _____ Score _____

Procedure 7-1 Perform Within Legal Boundaries

Task: To perform duties within legal boundaries in the state where employed as a medical assistant.

Equipment and Supplies:
- Computer
- Text of various laws and regulations affecting the practice

Standards: Complete the procedure and all critical steps in _____ minutes with a minimum score of _____% within three attempts.

Scoring: Divide points earned by total possible points. Failure to perform a critical step that is indicated with an asterisk (*) will result in an unsatisfactory overall score.

Time began _____ **Time ended** _____

Steps	Possible Points	First Attempt	Second Attempt	Third Attempt
1. Research laws that apply to the medical offices in the state of residency.	10	_____	_____	_____
2. Prepare a report about the scope of practice of the medical assistant in the state of residency.	40	_____	_____	_____
3. Research the education and certification requirements for medical assistants.	10	_____	_____	_____
4. Complete an application for either the RMA or CMA examination.	20	_____	_____	_____
5. Identify options available to the medical assistant for maintaining his or her credentials.	20	_____	_____	_____

Comments:

Total Points Earned _____ Divided by _____ Total Possible Points = _____ % Score

Instructor's Signature _____

Student Name _____ Date _____ Score _____

Procedure 7-2 Demonstrate Knowledge of Federal and State Health Care Legislation and Regulations

Task: To be aware of federal and state legislation and regulations that apply to the employer's facility.

Equipment and Supplies:
- Computer
- Access to organizational websites that have established legislation and regulations that pertain to medical facilities
- Information about changes to and new federal and state legislation and regulations

Standards: Complete the procedure and all critical steps in _____ minutes with a minimum score of _____% within three attempts.

Scoring: Divide points earned by total possible points. Failure to perform a critical step that is indicated with an asterisk (*) will result in an unsatisfactory overall score.

Time began _____ **Time ended** _____

Steps	Possible Points	First Attempt	Second Attempt	Third Attempt
1. Review federal regulations that apply to healthcare workers.	25	_____	_____	_____
2. Review state regulations that apply to healthcare workers.	25	_____	_____	_____
3. Prepare a report on one of the laws that affects healthcare workers.	25	_____	_____	_____
4. Discuss the report in class focusing on compliance issues.	25	_____	_____	_____

Comments:

Total Points Earned _____ Divided by _____ Total Possible Points = _____ % Score

Instructor's Signature _____

Student Name _____ Date _____ Score _____

Procedure 8-1 Utilize Computer Software to Maintain Office Systems

Task: To use the office computer system at maximum capacity to run the various aspects of the physician's office.

Equipment and Supplies:
- Computer
- Computer software applications
- Software manuals
- Description of office systems
- Patient data
- Business data

Standards: Complete the procedure and all critical steps in _____ minutes with a minimum score of _____% within three attempts.

Scoring: Divide points earned by total possible points. Failure to perform a critical step that is indicated with an asterisk (*) will result in an unsatisfactory overall score.

Time began _____ Time ended _____

Steps	Possible Points	First Attempt	Second Attempt	Third Attempt
1. Determine the types of data that the physician's office needs to computerize.	10			
2. Discuss these needs with the physician and office manager.*	10			
3. Compile a budget for computer systems and/or upgrades.*	10			
4. Research computer systems that can handle the tasks designated by the physician.	10			
5. Invite sales representatives to present their options during a staff meeting.	10			
6. Compare benefits and drawbacks of each system.*	10			
7. Ask sales representatives any questions that arise during the comparison process.	10			
8. Discuss the final few choices with the physician and office manager.	10			

Steps	Possible Points	First Attempt	Second Attempt	Third Attempt
9. Decide on a computer system or upgrade that best fits the needs of the office.*	**10**			
10. Purchase or lease the computer system.	**10**			

Comments:

Total Points Earned _____ Divided by _____ Total Possible Points = _____ % Score

Instructor's Signature _____

Student Name _____ Date _____ Score _____

Procedure 9-1 Demonstrate Telephone Techniques: Answer the Telephone

Task: To answer the telephone in a professional manner and respond to a request for action.

Equipment and Supplies:
- Telephone
- Message pad
- Pen or pencil
- Appointment book
- Script for conversation

Standards: Complete the procedure and all critical steps in _____ minutes with a minimum score of _____% within three attempts.

Scoring: Divide points earned by total possible points. Failure to perform a critical step that is indicated with an asterisk (*) will result in an unsatisfactory overall score.

Time began _____ **Time ended** _____

Steps	Possible Points	First Attempt	Second Attempt	Third Attempt
1. Answer the phone after the first ring and before the third ring, speaking directly into the transmitter, with the mouthpiece 1 inch from the mouth.	20	_____	_____	_____
2. Speak distinctly with a pleasant tone and expression, at a moderate rate, and with sufficient volume. Remember to smile.	10	_____	_____	_____
3. Identify yourself and the office.*	20	_____	_____	_____
4. Verify the identity of the caller.	10	_____	_____	_____
5. Provide the caller with the requested information or service, if possible.	10	_____	_____	_____
6. Take a message for further action, if required.	20	_____	_____	_____
7. Terminate the call in a pleasant manner and replace the receiver gently.	10	_____	_____	_____

Documentation in the Medical Record

_____

_____

_____

_____

Comments:

Total Points Earned _____ Divided by _____ Total Possible Points = _____ % Score

Instructor's Signature _____

Student Name _____ Date _____ Score _____

Procedure 9-2 Demonstrate Telephone Techniques: Take a Telephone Message

Task: To take an accurate telephone message and follow up on the requests made by the caller.

Equipment and Supplies:
- Telephone
- Message pad
- Pen or pencil
- Notepad

Standards: Complete the procedure and all critical steps in _____ minutes with a minimum score of _____% within three attempts.

Scoring: Divide points earned by total possible points. Failure to perform a critical step that is indicated with an asterisk (*) will result in an unsatisfactory overall score.

Time began _____ **Time ended** _____

Steps	Possible Points	First Attempt	Second Attempt	Third Attempt
1. Answer the telephone using the guidelines in Procedure 9-1, Answering the Telephone.	10	_____	_____	_____

2. Using a message pad or notepad, take the phone message, obtaining the following information:
  a. The name of the person to whom the call is directed
  b. The name of the person calling
  c. The caller's daytime and/or current telephone number
  d. The reason for the call
  e. The action to be taken
  f. The date and time of the call
  g. The initials of the person taking the call
	20	_____	_____	_____

3. Repeat the information back to the caller after the message is recorded on the message pad.	10	_____	_____	_____
4. Provide the caller with an approximation of the time and date that he or she will be called back, if possible.	_____	_____	_____	_____
5. End the call, and wait for the caller to hang up first.	10	_____	_____	_____
6. Deliver the phone message to the appropriate person. Separate trays or slots for each staff member are helpful.	10	_____	_____	_____

Steps	Possible Points	First Attempt	Second Attempt	Third Attempt
7. Follow up on important messages.	10			
8. Keep old message books for future reference. Carbonless copies allow the facility to keep a permanent record of phone messages.	10			
9. File pertinent phone messages in the patient's chart.	10			

Comments:

Total Points Earned _____ Divided by _____ Total Possible Points = _____ % Score

Instructor's Signature _____

Procedure 9-3 Demonstrate Telephone Techniques: Call the Pharmacy with New or Refill Prescriptions

Task: To call in an accurate prescription to the pharmacy for a patient in the most efficient manner.

Equipment and Supplies:
- Prescription
- Notepad
- Patient chart
- Telephone

Standards: Complete the procedure and all critical steps in _____ minutes with a minimum score of _____% within three attempts.

Scoring: Divide points earned by total possible points. Failure to perform a critical step that is indicated with an asterisk (*) will result in an unsatisfactory overall score.

Time began _____ **Time ended** _____

Steps	Possible Points	First Attempt	Second Attempt	Third Attempt
1. Receive the call from the patient requesting a prescription. Use appropriate telephone technique.	10	_____	_____	_____
2. Obtain the following information from the patient: a. Patient's name b. Telephone number where he or she can be reached c. Patient's symptoms and current condition d. History of this condition e. Treatments the patient has tried f. Pharmacy name and telephone number	20	_____	_____	_____
3. Write in the patient's chart the prescription that the physician wishes the patient to have. Be very careful to transcribe the information correctly. Read it back to the physician.	10	_____	_____	_____
4. If the prescription is a refill, give the physician the patient's chart with the message requesting a refill attached, along with the information in step 2.	10	_____	_____	_____

Steps	Possible Points	First Attempt	Second Attempt	Third Attempt
5. Note the comments that the physician writes in the chart. If the prescription is written or a refill is approved, call the patient's pharmacy and ask to speak to a member of the pharmacy staff.	__10__	_____	_____	_____
6. Ask the pharmacy staff member to repeat the prescription back to you.	__10__	_____	_____	_____
7. Note in the chart the date and time that the prescription was called to the pharmacy.	__10__	_____	_____	_____
8. Call the patient to notify him or her that the prescription has been called in. Provide any information regarding the prescription doses, frequency, and so on, according to the physician's instructions. Tell the patient when to return to the office, if necessary. Ask the patient to write this information down.	__20__	_____	_____	_____

Comments:

Total Points Earned _____ Divided by _____ Total Possible Points = _____ % Score

Instructor's Signature _____

Student Name _____. Date _____ Score _____

Procedure 9-4 Demonstrate Telephone Techniques

Task: To project a professional image while handling telephone calls.

Equipment and Supplies:
- Telephone
- Message pad
- Phone cards from instructor
- Several telephones (not necessarily connected)

Standards: Complete the procedure and all critical steps in _____ minutes with a minimum score of _____% within three attempts.

Scoring: Divide points earned by total possible points. Failure to perform a critical step that is indicated with an asterisk (*) will result in an unsatisfactory overall score.

Time began _____ **Time ended** _____

Role-play answering a telephone using phone cards distributed by the instructor.

Steps	Possible Points	First Attempt	Second Attempt	Third Attempt
1. Greet the caller in a professional manner.*	5	_____	_____	_____
2. Identify the caller.*	10	_____	_____	_____
3. Determine to whom the caller wishes to speak.	5	_____	_____	_____
4. Ask to put the caller on hold.*	10	_____	_____	_____
5. Notify a fellow classmate that the call is for him or her, and prepare to do a mock transfer of the call.*	10	_____	_____	_____
6. Go back to the caller, and say that the call is now being transferred.	5	_____	_____	_____
7. Take a second call when on the phone with the first caller.	5	_____	_____	_____
8. Ask to place the first caller on hold.*	10	_____	_____	_____
9. Ask to put the second caller on hold.*	10	_____	_____	_____
10. Return to and complete the first call.	5	_____	_____	_____
11. Allow the caller to hang up first.*	10	_____	_____	_____

Steps	Possible Points	First Attempt	Second Attempt	Third Attempt
12. Return to and complete the second call.	5			
13. Allow the second caller to hang up first.*	10			

Comments:

Total Points Earned _____ Divided by _____ Total Possible Points = _____ % Score

Instructor's Signature _____

Student Name _____ Date _____ Score _____

Procedure 10-1 Schedule and Manage Appointments: Prepare Appointment Pages by Matrixing

Task: To establish the matrix of the appointment page, arrange appointments for 1 day, and enter information according to office policy.

Equipment and Supplies:
- Page from appointment book or computer program software
- Office policy for office hours and doctors' availability
- Clerical supplies
- Calendar
- Description of patients to be scheduled

Standards: Complete the procedure and all critical steps in _____ minutes with a minimum score of _____% within three attempts.

Scoring: Divide points earned by total possible points. Failure to perform a critical step that is indicated with an asterisk (*) will result in an unsatisfactory overall score.

Time began _____ **Time ended** _____

Steps	Possible Points	First Attempt	Second Attempt	Third Attempt
1. Mark the times that the physician will not be available to see patients to establish the matrix.*	20	_____	_____	_____
2. Peruse the list of patients who need appointments and their chief complaints.	10	_____	_____	_____
3. Consult guidelines to determine the length of time each patient needs with the physician.	15	_____	_____	_____
4. Allot appointment time according to the patient complaint and facilities available.	15	_____	_____	_____
5. Enter patient name and contact information in the appointment book or computer program.*	20	_____	_____	_____
6. Allow for buffer time in the morning and the afternoon for sick calls and emergencies.*	20	_____	_____	_____

Comments:

Total Points Earned _____ **Divided by** _____ **Total Possible Points** = _____ % **Score**

Instructor's Signature _____

Procedure 10-2 Schedule and Manage Appointments: Manage Appointments

Task: To manage appointments as they are cancelled, no showed, or rescheduled throughout the business day.

Equipment and Supplies:
- Appointment book or computer software
- Office procedure manual
- Appointment cards
- Clerical supplies
- Telephone (may role-play)

Standards: Complete the procedure and all critical steps in _____ minutes with a minimum score of _____% within three attempts.

Scoring: Divide points earned by total possible points. Failure to perform a critical step that is indicated with an asterisk (*) will result in an unsatisfactory overall score.

Time began _____ **Time ended** _____

Steps	Possible Points	First Attempt	Second Attempt	Third Attempt
1. Peruse the appointment schedule for the next day.	10	_____	_____	_____
2. Confirm all appointments.	10	_____	_____	_____
3. Document a patient's late arrival in the appointment book or on the computer.*	10	_____	_____	_____
4. Document a "no show" in the appointment book or on the computer.*	10	_____	_____	_____
5. Document a "no show" in the patient's medical record.*	10	_____	_____	_____
6. Attempt to call the patient who did not show for his or her appointment, and document the results of the call in the medical record.	10	_____	_____	_____
7. Set a new appointment if the patient is reached.	10	_____	_____	_____
8. Inform patients if the physician is running behind schedule by more than 30 minutes.	10	_____	_____	_____
9. Place a check in the appointment book as the patients arrive for their appointments.	10	_____	_____	_____
10. Have patients sign in, if applicable.	10	_____	_____	_____

Comments:

Total Points Earned _____ Divided by _____ Total Possible Points = _____ % Score

Instructor's Signature _____

Procedure 10-3 Schedule and Manage Appointments: Schedule New Patients

Task: To schedule a new patient for a first office visit.

Equipment and Supplies:
- Appointment book
- Scheduling guidelines
- Appointment card
- Telephone

Standards: Complete the procedure and all critical steps in _____ minutes with a minimum score of _____% within three attempts.

Scoring: Divide points earned by total possible points. Failure to perform a critical step that is indicated with an asterisk (*) will result in an unsatisfactory overall score.

Time began _____ **Time ended** _____

Steps	Possible Points	First Attempt	Second Attempt	Third Attempt
1. Obtain the patient's full name, birth date, address, and telephone number. *Note:* Verify the spelling of the name.	10	_____	_____	_____
2. Determine whether the patient was referred by another physician.	10	_____	_____	_____
3. Determine the patient's chief complaint and when the first symptoms occurred.*	20	_____	_____	_____
4. Search the appointment book for the first suit-able appointment time and an alternate time.	10	_____	_____	_____
5. Offer the patient a choice of these dates and times.	10	_____	_____	_____
6. Enter the mutually agreed-on time in the appointment book, followed by the patient's telephone number. *Note:* Indicate that the patient is new by adding the letters NP.	15	_____	_____	_____
7. If new patients are expected to pay at the time of the visit, explain this financial requirement when the appointment is made.	10	_____	_____	_____
8. Offer travel directions for reaching the office and parking instructions.	5	_____	_____	_____
9. Repeat the day and time of the appointment before saying goodbye to the patient.	10	_____	_____	_____

Comments:

Total Points Earned _____ Divided by _____ Total Possible Points = _____ % Score

Instructor's Signature _____

Student Name _____ Date _____ Score _____

Procedure 10-4 Schedule and Manage Appointments: Schedule Appointments with Established Patients or Visitors

Task: To schedule a general appointment either by telephone or in person.

Equipment and Supplies:
- Appointment book or computer software
- Office procedure manual
- Clerical supplies
- Appointment cards
- Telephone (may role-play)

Standards: Complete the procedure and all critical steps in _____ minutes with a minimum score of _____% within three attempts.

Scoring: Divide points earned by total possible points. Failure to perform a critical step that is indicated with an asterisk (*) will result in an unsatisfactory overall score.

Time began _____ Time ended _____

Steps	Possible Points	First Attempt	Second Attempt	Third Attempt
1. Consult the office policy manual to ensure that proper procedure is followed in scheduling appointments.	5	_____	_____	_____
2. Answer the phone by the third ring.*	10	_____	_____	_____
3. Identify the patient on the phone and obtain his or her telephone number.*	10	_____	_____	_____
4. Ask the reason for making the appointment.*	10	_____	_____	_____
5. Determine whether the appointment is for the person on the phone or a family member.	5	_____	_____	_____
6. Determine which provider or employee the person wishes to see.	5	_____	_____	_____
7. Give the caller a choice of 2 days of the week.*	10	_____	_____	_____
8. Give the caller a choice of morning or afternoon.*	10	_____	_____	_____
9. Give the caller a choice of times.*	10	_____	_____	_____
10. Write the appointment in the appointment book, or enter it into the computer.	5	_____	_____	_____

Steps	Possible Points	First Attempt	Second Attempt	Third Attempt
11. Repeat the appointment day, date, and time back to the caller, and thank him or her for calling.*	10	_____	_____	_____
12. Allow the caller to hang up the phone first.*	10	_____	_____	_____
13. If the appointment is made in person, complete an appointment card and give it to the patient.	n/a	_____	_____	_____

Comments:

Total Points Earned _____ Divided by _____ Total Possible Points = _____ % Score

Instructor's Signature _____

Student Name _____ Date _____ Score _____

Procedure 10-5 Schedule and Manage Appointments: Prepare an Appointment Card

Task: To provide a written notation of the appointment for the convenience of the patient (or other individual making the appointment) and to reduce missed appointments.

Equipment and Supplies:
- Appointment book or computer software
- Office procedure manual
- Appointment cards
- Clerical supplies
- Telephone (may role-play)

Standards: Complete the procedure and all critical steps in _____ minutes with a minimum score of _____% within three attempts.

Scoring: Divide points earned by total possible points. Failure to perform a critical step that is indicated with an asterisk (*) will result in an unsatisfactory overall score.

Time began _____ Time ended _____

Steps	Possible Points	First Attempt	Second Attempt	Third Attempt
1. Make an appointment according to previous procedures.	20	_____	_____	_____
2. Copy the appointment day, date, and time from the appointment book or computer screen.*	30	_____	_____	_____
3. Mention that 24-hour notice is appreciated when an appointment cannot be kept.	20	_____	_____	_____
4. Hand the appointment card to the patient or visitor, and wish him or her a pleasant day.*	30	_____	_____	_____

Comments:

Total Points Earned _____ Divided by _____ Total Possible Points = _____ % Score

Instructor's Signature _____

Student Name _____ Date _____ Score _____

Procedure 10-6 Schedule Outpatient Admissions and Procedures

Task: To schedule a patient for an outpatient diagnostic test ordered by a physician within the time frame needed by the physician, confirm the appointment with the patient, and issue all required instructions.

Equipment and Supplies:
- Diagnostic test order from physician
- Name, address, and telephone number of diagnostic facility
- Patient chart
- Test preparation instructions
- Telephone
- Patient demographic information
- Consent form

Standards: Complete the procedure and all critical steps in _____ minutes with a minimum score of _____% within three attempts.

Scoring: Divide points earned by total possible points. Failure to perform a critical step that is indicated with an asterisk (*) will result in an unsatisfactory overall score.

Time began _____ **Time ended** _____

Steps	Possible Points	First Attempt	Second Attempt	Third Attempt
1. Obtain an oral or written order from the physician for the exact procedure to be performed.	10	_____	_____	_____
2. Determine the patient's availability.	10	_____	_____	_____
3. Telephone the diagnostic facility. • Order the specific test needed. • Establish the date and time. • Give the name, age, address, and telephone number of the patient. • Determine any special instructions for the patient. • Notify the facility of any urgency for test results.	25	_____	_____	_____
4. Notify the patient of the arrangements, including: • Name, address, and telephone number of the diagnostic facility • Date and time to report for the test • Instructions concerning preparation for the test (e.g., eating restrictions, fluids, medications, enemas) Ask the patient to repeat the instructions.	25	_____	_____	_____

Steps	Possible Points	First Attempt	Second Attempt	Third Attempt
5. Note arrangements on the patient's chart.	20			
6. Place reminder in a "tickler" file or on a desk calendar.	10			

Documentation in the Medical Record

_____

_____

_____

_____

Comments:

Total Points Earned _____ Divided by _____ Total Possible Points = _____ % Score

Instructor's Signature _____

Procedure 10-7 Schedule Inpatient Admissions

Task: To schedule a patient for inpatient admission within the time frame needed by physician, confirm with the patient, and issue all required instructions.

Equipment and Supplies:
- Admission orders from physician
- Name, address, and telephone number of inpatient facility
- Patient demographic information
- Patient chart
- Any preparation instructions for the patient
- Telephone
- Admission packet for the patient

Standards: Complete the procedure and all critical steps in _____ minutes with a minimum score of _____% within three attempts.

Scoring: Divide points earned by total possible points. Failure to perform a critical step that is indicated with an asterisk (*) will result in an unsatisfactory overall score.

Time began _____ Time ended _____

Steps	Possible Points	First Attempt	Second Attempt	Third Attempt
1. Obtain an oral or written order from the physician for the admission.	10	_____	_____	_____
2. Precertify the admission with the patient's insurance company, if necessary.	20	_____	_____	_____
3. Determine the physician and patient availability if the admission is not an emergency.	10	_____	_____	_____

4. Telephone the diagnostic facility and schedule the admission.
  • Order any specific tests needed.
  • Provide the patient's admitting diagnosis.
  • Establish the date and time.
  • Convey the patient's room preferences.
  • Give the name, age, address, and telephone number of the patient.
  • Provide the demographic information for the patient, including insurance policy numbers and addresses for filing claims.
  • Determine any special instructions for the patient.
  • Notify the facility of any urgency for test results.
	20	_____	_____	_____

Steps	Possible Points	First Attempt	Second Attempt	Third Attempt
5. Notify the patient of the arrangements, including: • Name, address, and telephone number of the facility • Date and time to report for admission • Instructions concerning preparation for any procedures, if necessary (e.g., eating restrictions, fluids, medications, enemas) • What preadmission testing will be necessary, if any Ask the patient to repeat the instructions.	20			
6. Note arrangements and the admission on the patient's chart.	10			
7. Place reminder on the physician's tickler or desk calendar, if needed. Be sure the information is listed on the office schedule. If the physician keeps a list of all inpatients, add the patient's name to that list.	10			

Comments:

Total Points Earned _____ Divided by _____ Total Possible Points = _____ % Score

Instructor's Signature _____

Procedure 10-8 Schedule Inpatient Procedures

Task: To schedule a patient for inpatient surgery within the time frame needed by physician, confirm with the patient, and issue all required instructions.

Equipment and Supplies:
- Orders from physician
- Name, address, and telephone number of inpatient facility
- Patient demographic information
- Patient chart
- Any preparation instructions for the patient
- Telephone

Standards: Complete the procedure and all critical steps in _____ minutes with a minimum score of _____% within three attempts.

Scoring: Divide points earned by total possible points. Failure to perform a critical step that is indicated with an asterisk (*) will result in an unsatisfactory overall score.

Time began _____ **Time ended** _____

Steps	Possible Points	First Attempt	Second Attempt	Third Attempt
1. Obtain an oral or written order from the physician for the admission.	10	_____	_____	_____
2. Precertify the admission with the patient's insurance company, if necessary.	10	_____	_____	_____
3. Determine the physician availability if the surgery is not an emergency. Another physician may be the surgeon. If this is the case, the surgery will need to be coordinated with his or her office as well.	10	_____	_____	_____
4. Telephone the hospital surgical department, and schedule the procedure. • Order any specific tests needed. • Provide the patient's admitting diagnosis. • Establish the date and time. • Give the name, age, address, and telephone number of the patient. • Provide the demographic information for the patient, including insurance policy numbers and addresses for filing claims. • Determine any special instructions for the patient. • Notify the facility of any urgency of the surgery.	20	_____	_____	_____

Steps	Possible Points	First Attempt	Second Attempt	Third Attempt
5. Notify the patient of the arrangements, if the patient has not already been admitted to the hospital. Include the following: • Name, address, and telephone number of the facility • Date and time to report for admission • Instructions concerning preparation for any procedures, if necessary (e.g., eating restrictions, fluids, medications, enemas) • Tell what preadmission testing will be necessary, if any Ask the patient to repeat the instructions.	20			
6. The physician should review the consent form with the patient. Have the patient sign a consent for the surgical procedure. Keep the original consent in the patient's chart, and give a copy to the patient.	10			
7. Note arrangements on the patient's chart.	10			
8. Place reminder on the physician's tickler or desk calendar, if needed. Be sure the information is listed on the office schedule. If the physician keeps a list of all inpatients, add the patient's name to that list. Follow up with the hospital after the procedure regarding the patient's condition as required by the physician.	10			

Comments:

Total Points Earned _____ Divided by _____ Total Possible Points = _____ % Score

Instructor's Signature _____

Student Name _____ Date _____ Score _____

Procedure 11-1 Establish and Maintain the Medical Record: Organize a Patient's Medical Record

Task: To prepare patient charts for the daily appointment schedule and have them ready for the physician before the patients' arrival.

Equipment and Supplies:
- Appointment schedule for current date
- Patient files
- Clerical supplies (e.g., pen, tape, stapler)

Standards: Complete the procedure and all critical steps in _____ minutes with a minimum score of _____% within three attempts.

Scoring: Divide points earned by total possible points. Failure to perform a critical step that is indicated with an asterisk (*) will result in an unsatisfactory overall score.

Time began _____ Time ended _____

Steps	Possible Points	First Attempt	Second Attempt	Third Attempt
1. Review the list of appointments for the day.	5	_____	_____	_____
2. Identify each patient by name and/or medical record number.	5	_____	_____	_____
3. Pull the medical records for each established patient.	10	_____	_____	_____
4. Compare the records with the names on the list to make certain that the correct records have been pulled.*	20	_____	_____	_____
5. Make certain that all previously ordered tests are represented by the laboratory results in the record.	5	_____	_____	_____
6. Replenish forms in the records so that the physician will have adequate room to write notes and/or add information.*	20	_____	_____	_____
7. Annotate the appointment list with any special concerns.	5	_____	_____	_____
8. Arrange the medical records in the order that the patients will be seen.*	20	_____	_____	_____
9. Place the records in the designated place for easy retrieval once the patients begin to arrive.	10	_____	_____	_____

Comments:

Total Points Earned _____ Divided by _____ Total Possible Points = _____ % Score

Instructor's Signature _____

Student Name _____ Date _____ Score _____

Procedure 11-2 Establish and Maintain the Medical Record: Register a New Patient

Task: To complete a registration form for a new patient with information for credit and insurance claims and to inform and orient the patient to the facility.

Equipment and Supplies:
- Registration form
- Clerical supplies (pen, clipboard)
- Private conference area
- Materials and forms for building a new chart

Standards: Complete the procedure and all critical steps in _____ minutes with a minimum score of _____% within three attempts.

Scoring: Divide points earned by total possible points. Failure to perform a critical step that is indicated with an asterisk (*) will result in an unsatisfactory overall score.

Time began _____ Time ended _____

Steps	Possible Points	First Attempt	Second Attempt	Third Attempt
1. Determine whether the patient is new to the practice.	5			
2. Ask the patient to complete the patient information form.	5			
3. Enter the information from the form into the computer, or add the form to the patient's record in the prescribed place.	15			
4. Review the entire form to make certain that all information has been completed.*	15			
5. Make a copy of the insurance card, front and back.*	10			
6. Verify insurance coverage.*	15			
7. Construct the record using the materials prescribed by the medical office.	5			
8. Add progress notes so that the physician can document information in the patient record.*	15			
9. Attach an encounter form to the chart and give it to the clinical assistant for use during the patient's examination.*	15			

Comments:

Total Points Earned _____ Divided by _____ Total Possible Points = _____ % Score

Instructor's Signature _____

Student Name _____ Date _____ Score _____

Procedure 12-1 Explain General Office Policies

Task: To effectively communicate office policies and procedures to patients and visitors in the office.

Equipment and Supplies:
- Office policy manual
- Office procedure manual (if not included in policy manual)
- Patient information sheets (if needed)
- Office policy brochure

Standards: Complete the procedure and all critical steps in _____ minutes with a minimum score of _____% within three attempts.

Scoring: Divide points earned by total possible points. Failure to perform a critical step that is indicated with an asterisk (*) will result in an unsatisfactory overall score.

Time began _____ **Time ended** _____

Steps	Possible Points	First Attempt	Second Attempt	Third Attempt
1. Design an office policy brochure or website that contains general information for patients.* At a minimum, the brochure should contain the following: • Philosophy statement • Goals • Description of the medical practice • Location and/or map • Phone numbers • Pager numbers • Email and website addresses • Staff names and credentials • Services offered • Hours of operation • Appointment system • Cancellation policy • Prescription refill guidelines • Insurances accepted • Emergency procedures • Alternate physician coverage • Referral and records release policies • Special needs accommodations • Notice of privacy policies	30	_____	_____	_____
2. Offer the brochure to a new patient.	5	_____	_____	_____
3. Sit with the patient and explain each section of the document to him or her.*	20	_____	_____	_____

Steps	Possible Points	First Attempt	Second Attempt	Third Attempt
4. While explaining the brochure, look for verifications from the patient that signal understanding, using both body language and verbal statements.*	30	_____	_____	_____
5. Ask the patient if he or she has any questions. *	10	_____	_____	_____
6. Document in the medical record that the patient received the brochure.	5	_____	_____	_____

Comments:

Total Points Earned _____ Divided by _____ Total Possible Points = _____ % Score

Instructor's Signature _____

Student Name _____ Date _____ Score _____

Procedure 12-2 Instruct Individuals According to Their Needs

Task: To effectively communicate information to patients and visitors in the office so that they understand instructions from the physician.

Equipment and Supplies:
- Office policy manual
- Office procedure manual (if not included in policy manual)
- Patient information sheets
- Physician orders, if applicable
- Patient information brochure

Standards: Complete the procedure and all critical steps in _____ minutes with a minimum score of _____% within three attempts.

Scoring: Divide points earned by total possible points. Failure to perform a critical step that is indicated with an asterisk (*) will result in an unsatisfactory overall score.

Time began _____ **Time ended** _____

Steps	Possible Points	First Attempt	Second Attempt	Third Attempt
1. Determine the communication needs of the patient.	20	_____	_____	_____
2. Arrange for an interpreter, if applicable.	10	_____	_____	_____
3. If no employee speaks the language of the patient, make certain that he or she brings an interpreter to the appointment.	10	_____	_____	_____
4. Provide the given instructions to the patient.*	10	_____	_____	_____
5. While explaining the instructions, look for verifications from the patient—both body language and verbal statements—that signal understanding.*	20	_____	_____	_____
6. Have the patient restate the instructions to ensure complete understanding.*	20	_____	_____	_____
7. Provide the patient with any written documents that reiterate the given instructions and/or physician orders for tests, procedures, and/or hospital admission.	10	_____	_____	_____

Comments:

Student Name _____ Date _____ Score _____

Procedure 12-3 Perform an Inventory of Supplies and Equipment

Task: To establish an inventory of all expendable supplies in the physician's office and follow an efficient plan of order control using a card system.

Equipment and Supplies:
- File box
- Inventory and order control cards
- List of supplies on hand
- Metal tabs
- Reorder tabs
- Pen or pencil

Standards: Complete the procedure and all critical steps in _____ minutes with a minimum score of _____% within three attempts.

Scoring: Divide points earned by total possible points. Failure to perform a critical step that is indicated with an asterisk (*) will result in an unsatisfactory overall score.

Time began _____ Time ended _____

Steps	Possible Points	First Attempt	Second Attempt	Third Attempt
1. Write the name of each item on a separate card.	10	_____	_____	_____
2. Write the quantity of each item on hand in the space provided.	10	_____	_____	_____
3. Place a reorder tag at the point where the supply should be replenished.	20	_____	_____	_____
4. Place a metal tab over the order section of the card.	20	_____	_____	_____
5. When the order has been placed, note the date and quantity ordered and move the table to the on-order section of the card.	20	_____	_____	_____
6. When the order is received, note the date and quantity in the appropriate column, remove the tab, and refile the card. *Note:* If the order is only partially filled, let the tab remain until the order is complete.	20	_____	_____	_____

Comments:

Total Points Earned _____ Divided by _____ Total Possible Points = _____ % Score

Instructor's Signature _____

Student Name _____ Date _____ Score _____

Procedure 12-4 Prepare a Purchase Order

Task: To prepare an accurate purchase order for supplies or equipment.

Equipment and Supplies:
- List of current inventory
- Purchase order
- Pen
- Phone
- Fax machine

Standards: Complete the procedure and all critical steps in _____ minutes with a minimum score of _____% within three attempts.

Scoring: Divide points earned by total possible points. Failure to perform a critical step that is indicated with an asterisk (*) will result in an unsatisfactory overall score.

Time began _____ **Time ended** _____

Steps	Possible Points	First Attempt	Second Attempt	Third Attempt
1. Review the current inventory and determine what items need to be ordered.	10	_____	_____	_____
2. Complete the purchase order accurately, filling in all applicable spaces and blanks with the information requested.	15	_____	_____	_____
3. List the items to be ordered, including quantity, item numbers, size, color, price, and extended price. Be sure that all applicable information is included.	15	_____	_____	_____
4. Provide the physician's signature, DEA certificate, and medical license where needed.	15	_____	_____	_____
5. Call in, fax, mail, or submit the order electronically to the vendor. Keep a copy for your records. Keep any verification provided that the order was received.	15	_____	_____	_____
6. Note on the inventory which items are on order.	15	_____	_____	_____
7. Keep a copy of the order in the appropriate place in the office filing system.	15	_____	_____	_____

Comments:

Total Points Earned _____ Divided by _____ Total Possible Points = _____ % Score

Instructor's Signature _____

Student Name _____ Date _____ Score _____

Procedure 12-5 Perform Routine Maintenance of Administrative and Clinical Equipment

Task: To ensure that all office equipment is in good working order at all times.

Equipment and Supplies:
- Notecard or spreadsheet containing information on each piece of office equipment, including internal number and periods when the equipment needs servicing
- Pen or pencil
- Computer
- Access to all office equipment

Standards: Complete the procedure and all critical steps in _____ minutes with a minimum score of _____% within three attempts.

Scoring: Divide points earned by total possible points. Failure to perform a critical step that is indicated with an asterisk (*) will result in an unsatisfactory overall score.

Time began _____ **Time ended** _____

Steps	Possible Points	First Attempt	Second Attempt	Third Attempt
1. Gather information about each piece of equipment.* The following information is needed at a minimum: • Name of equipment • Type of equipment • Manufacturer's name • Address of manufacturer • Contact phone numbers for technical support • Contact phone numbers for manufacturer's main office • Date purchased • Cost of product • Original receipt showing where the item was purchased • Date warranty begins and ends • Addresses to send equipment if under warranty	20	_____	_____	_____
2. Enter information about each piece of equipment into a document or spreadsheet.*	20	_____	_____	_____
3. Design a document containing each month of the year.	5	_____	_____	_____
4. Mark which equipment needs servicing during which months.*	10	_____	_____	_____

Steps	Possible Points	First Attempt	Second Attempt	Third Attempt
5. Check which pieces of equipment need servicing this month.	10			
6. Schedule servicing and maintenance for the equipment on the list for the current month.	10			
7. Make certain servicing appointments are kept.*	20			
8. Record new information and scheduling needs on the document as needed.	5			

Comments:

Total Points Earned _____ Divided by _____ Total Possible Points = _____ % Score

Instructor's Signature _____

Student Name _____ Date _____ Score _____

Procedure 12-6 Locate Resources and Information for Patients and Employers: Make Travel Arrangements

Task: To make travel arrangements for the physician or another staff member.

Equipment and Supplies:
- Travel plan
- Telephone
- Telephone directory
- Typewriter or computer
- Typing paper

Standards: Complete the procedure and all critical steps in _____ minutes with a minimum score of _____% within three attempts.

Scoring: Divide points earned by total possible points. Failure to perform a critical step that is indicated with an asterisk (*) will result in an unsatisfactory overall score.

Time began _____ **Time ended** _____

Steps	Possible Points	First Attempt	Second Attempt	Third Attempt
1. Verify the dates of the planned trip. • Desired date and time of departure • Desired date and time of return • Preferred mode of transportation • Number in party • Preferred lodging and price range • Preferred ticketing method (electronic or paper)	20	_____	_____	_____
2. Telephone a trusted travel agency to arrange for transportation and lodging reservations.	10	_____	_____	_____
3. Arrange for traveler's checks, if desired.	10	_____	_____	_____
4. Pick up tickets or e-receipts or arrange for delivery.	10	_____	_____	_____
5. Check tickets to confirm conformance with the travel plan.	10	_____	_____	_____
6. Check to see that hotel and air reservations are confirmed.	10	_____	_____	_____

Steps	Possible Points	First Attempt	Second Attempt	Third Attempt
7. Prepare an itinerary, including all the necessary information • Date and time of departure • Flight numbers or identifying information of other modes of travel • Mode of transportation to hotel(s) • Name, address, and telephone number of hotel(s), with confirmation numbers if available • Name, address, and telephone number of travel agency • Date and time of return	10			
8. Place one copy of itinerary in the office file.	10			
9. Give several copies of the itinerary to the traveler.	10			

Comments:

Total Points Earned _____ Divided by _____ Total Possible Points = _____ % Score

Instructor's Signature _____

Student Name _____ Date _____ Score _____

Procedure 12-7 Identify Community Resources

Task: To help patients find organizations that can assist with their needs beyond the physician's office, and to establish a listing of community resources that can be used for referral purposes.

Equipment and Supplies:
- Phone book
- Internet access
- Library access
- Newspapers
- Local volunteer guides
- Computer
- Pen or pencil
- Notepad

Standards: Complete the procedure and all critical steps in _____ minutes with a minimum score of _____% within three attempts.

Scoring: Divide points earned by total possible points. Failure to perform a critical step that is indicated with an asterisk (*) will result in an unsatisfactory overall score.

Time began _____ **Time ended** _____

Steps	Possible Points	First Attempt	Second Attempt	Third Attempt
1. Research the resources available in the surrounding community.*	25	_____	_____	_____
2. Prepare a document or spreadsheet containing a list of the various resources.* Include the following information at a minimum: • Name of agency • Purpose or mission of agency • Physical address • Mailing address, if different • Phone numbers • Contact name • Hours of operation • Services offered or performed	25	_____	_____	_____
3. Update the information whenever a change is needed.	25	_____	_____	_____
4. Provide referrals to patients as needed.	25	_____	_____	_____

Comments:

Total Points Earned _____ Divided by _____ Total Possible Points = _____ % Score

Instructor's Signature _____

Student Name _____ Date _____ Score _____

Procedure 13-1 Respond to and Initiate Written Communications: Compose Business Correspondence

Task: To write documents that effectively communicate a professional message to the recipient.

Equipment and Supplies:
- Computer or word processor
- Word processing software
- Draft paper
- Letterhead
- Printer
- Pen or pencil
- Highlighter
- Envelope
- Other pertinent information needed to compose a letter
- Electronic or hard cover dictionary and thesaurus
- Writer's handbook
- Portfolio

Standards: Complete the procedure and all critical steps in _____ minutes with a minimum score of _____% within three attempts.

Scoring: Divide points earned by total possible points. Failure to perform a critical step that is indicated with an asterisk (*) will result in an unsatisfactory overall score.

Time began _____ **Time ended** _____

Steps	Possible Points	First Attempt	Second Attempt	Third Attempt
1. Determine the reason and goals for sending the correspondence.*	10	_____	_____	_____
2. Open a document on the computer and save it for easy reference.	10	_____	_____	_____
3. Date the letter.	10	_____	_____	_____
4. Type the inside address.	5	_____	_____	_____
5. Type a subject line and list the patient name or the subject of the correspondence.	5	_____	_____	_____
6. Type the body of the letter, paying strict attention to its goals.*	10	_____	_____	_____
7. Type the closing of the letter, and use the name of the person who will be considered the author.	10	_____	_____	_____

Steps	Possible Points	First Attempt	Second Attempt	Third Attempt
8. Proofread the document for accuracy and spelling.*	10			
9. Reread the letter to ensure that the goal of the letter has been met.*	10			
10. Address the envelope according to Postal Service OCR guidelines.*	10			
11. Affix the correct postage, and mail the letter.	10			

Comments:

Total Points Earned _____ Divided by _____ Total Possible Points = _____ % Score

Instructor's Signature _____

Student Name _____ Date _____ Score _____

Procedure 13-2 Respond to and Initiate Written Communications: Proofread Documents for Accuracy

Task: To compose a clearly written, grammatically correct business letter that is easily understandable by the reader and to eliminate spelling errors.

Equipment and Supplies:
• Stationery
• Computer or typewriter
• Correspondence to be answered or notes
• Proofreader's marks guide

Standards: Complete the procedure and all critical steps in _____ minutes with a minimum score of _____% within three attempts.

Scoring: Divide points earned by total possible points. Failure to perform a critical step that is indicated with an asterisk (*) will result in an unsatisfactory overall score.

Time began _____ Time ended _____

Steps	Possible Points	First Attempt	Second Attempt	Third Attempt
1. Place the stationery into the printer or type-writer.	10	_____	_____	_____
2. Read the letter to be answered or the notes about the correspondence to be written, and highlight any questions that should be answered or points to be made.	10	_____	_____	_____
3. Write the letter using good grammar.	10	_____	_____	_____
4. Print a draft copy of the letter. Read it carefully, and highlight changes to be made or note any additions to be made. Use proof-readers' marks.	20	_____	_____	_____
5. Revise the letter using the notes.	10	_____	_____	_____
6. Read the letter once again on the screen. Complete a spelling and grammar check if those tools are available on the computer.	10	_____	_____	_____
7. Print a final draft. Read the letter word for word, and check once again for errors.	10	_____	_____	_____
8. Have another person proofread especially important correspondence.	10	_____	_____	_____
9. Complete the final preparations for mailing the letter. Address the letter using guidelines for OCR and fast processing at the post office.	10	_____	_____	_____

Comments:

Total Points Earned _____ Divided by _____ Total Possible Points = _____ % Score

Instructor's Signature _____

Student Name _____ Date _____ Score _____

Procedure 13-3 Respond to and Initiate Written Communications: Prepare a Fax for Transmission

Task: To send a fax from the medical office and ensure that it arrives at its destination in a manner that protects confidentiality.

Equipment and Supplies:
• Fax machine
• Fax cover sheet
• Correspondence to be sent

Standards: Complete the procedure and all critical steps in _____ minutes with a minimum score of _____% within three attempts.

Scoring: Divide points earned by total possible points. Failure to perform a critical step that is indicated with an asterisk (*) will result in an unsatisfactory overall score.

Time began _____ **Time ended** _____

Steps	Possible Points	First Attempt	Second Attempt	Third Attempt
1. Fill out a fax cover sheet. Include the name of the person sending the fax and the person's phone number. List the name of the person to receive the fax and the fax number to which the document is being sent. Use cover sheets that contain a confidentiality statement.	20	_____	_____	_____
2. Note the number of pages that are being sent, including the cover page.	20	_____	_____	_____
3. Turn the last page upside down, and write the fax number on the top of the document. Many machines require the documents to be in place before the fax is started. This allows the user to see the number without having to memorize it and potentially making an error.	20	_____	_____	_____
4. Follow the instructions for individual fax machines.	20	_____	_____	_____
5. Be sure the machine is set to provide a verification that the fax went through. Print the verification and attach it to the fax. Verify the arrival of critical fax documents with a phone call. File the fax and verification sheet in the appropriate location.	20	_____	_____	_____

Comments:

Total Points Earned _____ Divided by _____ Total Possible Points = _____ % Score

Instructor's Signature _____

Student Name _____ Date _____ Score _____

Procedure 13-4 Respond to and Initiate Written Communications: Process Incoming Mail

Task: To efficiently sort through the mail that arrives in the medical office on a daily basis.

Equipment and Supplies:
- Computer or word processor
- Letterhead stationery
- Pen or pencil
- Highlighter
- Staple remover
- Paper clips
- Letter opener
- Date stamp
- Draft paper
- Stapler
- Transparent tape

Standards: Complete the procedure and all critical steps in _____ minutes with a minimum score of _____% within three attempts.

Scoring: Divide points earned by total possible points. Failure to perform a critical step that is indicated with an asterisk (*) will result in an unsatisfactory overall score.

Time began _____ **Time ended** _____

Steps	Possible Points	First Attempt	Second Attempt	Third Attempt
1. Sort the mail according to importance and urgency: • Physician's personal mail • Ordinary first class mail • Checks from patients • Periodicals and newspapers • All other pieces, including drug samples	10	_____	_____	_____
2. Open the mail neatly and in an organized manner.	10	_____	_____	_____
3. Stack the envelopes so that they are all facing in the same direction.	10	_____	_____	_____
4. Pick up the top one and tap the envelope so that when you open it you will not cut the contents.	10	_____	_____	_____
5. Open all envelopes along the top edge for easiest removal of contents.	10	_____	_____	_____

Steps	Possible Points	First Attempt	Second Attempt	Third Attempt
6. Remove the contents of each envelope and hold the envelope to the light to see that nothing remains inside.	10			
7. Make a note of the postmark when this is important.	10			
8. Discard the envelope after you have checked to see that there is a return address on the message contained inside. Some offices make it a policy to attach the envelope to each piece of correspondence until it has received attention.	10			
9. Date stamp the letter and attach any enclosures.	10			
10. If there is an enclosure notation at the bottom of the letter, check to be certain that the enclosure was included. Should it be missing, indicate this on the notation by writing the word "no" and circling it.	10			

Comments:

Total Points Earned _____ Divided by _____ Total Possible Points = _____ % Score

Instructor's Signature _____

Student Name _____ Date _____ Score _____

Procedure 13-5 Respond to and Initiate Written Communications: Address an Envelope According to Postal Service Optical Character Reader Guidelines

Task: To correctly address business correspondence so that the mail arrives and is processed by the U.S. Post Office as efficiently as possible.

Equipment and Supplies:
- Envelopes
- Computer or typewriter
- Correspondence

Standards: Complete the procedure and all critical steps in _____ minutes with a minimum score of _____% within three attempts.

Scoring: Divide points earned by total possible points. Failure to perform a critical step that is indicated with an asterisk (*) will result in an unsatisfactory overall score.

Time began _____ **Time ended** _____

Steps	Possible Points	First Attempt	Second Attempt	Third Attempt
1. Place the envelope into the printer or typewriter.	10	_____	_____	_____
2. Enter the word processing program, such as Microsoft Word, and check the "Tools" section for envelopes. If this is not available in the word processing program, or if a typewriter is being used, judge the area on the envelope that can be read by the optical character reader (OCR). The address block should start no higher than 2¾ inches from the bottom. Leave a bottom margin of at least ⅝ inch and left and right margins of at least 1 inch. Nothing should be written or printed below the address block or to the right of it.	20	_____	_____	_____
3. Use dark type on a light background, no script or italics, and capitalize everything in the address.	10	_____	_____	_____
4. Type the address in block format, using only approved abbreviations and eliminating all punctuation.*	20	_____	_____	_____
5. Type the city, state, and ZIP code on the last line of the address.	10	_____	_____	_____
6. No line should have more than 27 total characters, including spaces.	10	_____	_____	_____

Steps	Possible Points	First Attempt	Second Attempt	Third Attempt
7. Leave a ⅝-inch by 4¾-inch blank space in the bottom right corner of the envelope.	10			
8. Mail addressed to other countries includes the city and postal code on the third line and the name of the country on a fourth line.	10			

Comments:

Total Points Earned _____ Divided by _____ Total Possible Points = _____ % Score

Instructor's Signature _____

Student Name _____ Date _____ Score _____

Procedure 14-1 Establish the Medical Record

Task: To initiate a medical file for a new patient that will contain all the personal data necessary for a complete record and any other information required by the facility.

Equipment and Supplies:
- Computer or typewriter
- Clerical supplies
- Information on filing system
- Registration form
- File folder
- Label
- ID card for numeric system
- Cross-reference card
- Financial card
- Routing slip or encounter form
- Private conference area

Standards: Complete the procedure and all critical steps in _____ minutes with a minimum score of _____% within three attempts.

Scoring: Divide points earned by total possible points. Failure to perform a critical step that is indicated with an asterisk (*) will result in an unsatisfactory overall score.

Time began _____ Time ended _____

Steps	Possible Points	First Attempt	Second Attempt	Third Attempt
1. Determine that the patient is new to the office.	10	_____	_____	_____
2. Obtain and record the required personal data.	10	_____	_____	_____
3. Type the information onto the patient history form.	10	_____	_____	_____
4. Review entire form.	10	_____	_____	_____
5. Select the label and file folder for the record.	10	_____	_____	_____
6. Type the caption on the label, and apply to the folder	10	_____	_____	_____
7. For numeric filing, prepare a cross-reference.	10	_____	_____	_____
8. Prepare the financial card, or enter into a computerized ledger.	10	_____	_____	_____

Steps	Possible Points	First Attempt	Second Attempt	Third Attempt
9. Place the patient's history and other required forms in the folder.	**10**			
10. Clip an encounter form or routing slip on the outside of the folder	**10**			

Comments:

Total Points Earned _____ Divided by _____ Total Possible Points = _____ % Score

Instructor's Signature _____

Procedure 14-2 Establish and Maintain the Medical Record: Prepare an Informed Consent for Treatment Form

Task: To adequately and completely inform the patient regarding the treatment or procedure that he or she is to receive, and to provide legal protection for the facility and the provider.

Equipment and Supplies:
- Pen
- Consent form

Standards: Complete the procedure and all critical steps in _____ minutes with a minimum score of _____% within three attempts.

Scoring: Divide points earned by total possible points. Failure to perform a critical step that is indicated with an asterisk (*) will result in an unsatisfactory overall score.

Time began _____ **Time ended** _____

Steps	Possible Points	First Attempt	Second Attempt	Third Attempt
1. After the physician provides the details of the procedure to be done, prepare the consent form. Be sure that the form addresses the following: • The nature of the procedure or treatment • The risks and/or benefits of the procedure or treatment • Any reasonable alternatives to the procedure or treatment • The risks and/or benefits of each alternative • The risks and/or benefits of not performing the procedure or treatment	20	_____	_____	_____
2. Personalize the form with the patient's name and any other demographic information that the form lists.	10	_____	_____	_____
3. Deliver the form to the physician for use as the patient is counseled about the procedure.	10	_____	_____	_____
4. Witness the signature of the patient on the form, if necessary. The physician will usually sign the form as well.	10	_____	_____	_____
5. Provide a copy of the consent form to the patient.	10	_____	_____	_____
6. Place the consent form in the patient's chart. The facility where the procedure is to be performed may require a copy.	10	_____	_____	_____

Steps	Possible Points	First Attempt	Second Attempt	Third Attempt
7. Ask the patient if he or she has any questions about the procedure. Refer questions that the medical assistant cannot or should not answer to the physician. Be sure that all of the questions expressed by the patient are answered.	20	_____	_____	_____
8. Provide information regarding the date and time of the procedure to the patient.	10	_____	_____	_____

Comments:

Total Points Earned _____ Divided by _____ Total Possible Points = _____ % Score

Instructor's Signature _____

Procedure 14-3 Establish and Maintain the Medical Record: Add Supplementary Items to Established Patient Records

Task: To add supplementary documents and progress notes to patient histories, observing standard steps in filing, while creating an orderly file that will facilitate ready reference to any item of information.

Equipment and Supplies:
- Computer or typewriter
- Clerical supplies, sorter, stapler
- Information on filing system
- Mending tape
- Patient file folders
- Assorted correspondence and reports
- File stamp and a pen

Standards: Complete the procedure and all critical steps in _____ minutes with a minimum score of _____% within three attempts.

Scoring: Divide points earned by total possible points. Failure to perform a critical step that is indicated with an asterisk (*) will result in an unsatisfactory overall score.

Time began _____ **Time ended** _____

Steps	Possible Points	First Attempt	Second Attempt	Third Attempt
1. Group all papers according to patients' name.*	20			
2. Remove any staples or paper clips.	10			
3. Mend any damaged or torn records.	10			
4. Attach any small items to standard-size paper.	10			
5. Group any related papers together.	10			
6. Place your initials or FILE stamp in the upper left corner.	10			
7. Code the document by underlining or writing the patient's name in the upper right corner.	10			
8. Continue steps 2-7 until all documents have been conditioned, released, indexed, and coded.	10			
9. Place all documents in the sorter in filing sequence.	10			

Comments:

Total Points Earned _____ Divided by _____ Total Possible Points = _____ % Score

Instructor's Signature _____

Student Name _____ Date _____ Score _____

Procedure 14-4 Maintain the Medical Record

Task: To make certain that the medical record is usable by all parties involved in patient care.

Equipment and Supplies:
- Patient medical record
- Various forms used inside the medical record
- Results and reports, if applicable
- Clerical supplies

Standards: Complete the procedure and all critical steps in _____ minutes with a minimum score of _____% within three attempts.

Scoring: Divide points earned by total possible points. Failure to perform a critical step that is indicated with an asterisk (*) will result in an unsatisfactory overall score.

Time began _____ Time ended _____

Steps	Possible Points	First Attempt	Second Attempt	Third Attempt
1. Verify that the correct medical record has been pulled.*	20	_____	_____	_____
2. Inspect the medical record to determine which forms need to be added.	5	_____	_____	_____
3. Add all necessary forms to the record that will enable the physician to document the office visit properly.*	20	_____	_____	_____
4. Attach the forms to the record permanently or according to office policy.	10	_____	_____	_____
5. Make certain that all laboratory results and reports are available in the medical record for the physician.*	10	_____	_____	_____
6. Permanently attach laboratory results and/or reports in the record with the most recent on top.*	20	_____	_____	_____
7. Place the record in the designated place to await arrival of the patient.	5	_____	_____	_____
8. If other documents are to be added to the record, condition each document.	n/a	_____	_____	_____
9. Release each document to be added to the record.	n/a	_____	_____	_____

Steps	Possible Points	First Attempt	Second Attempt	Third Attempt
10. Index all documents to be added to the medical record.	5	_____	_____	_____
11. Code all documents to be added to the medical record.	5	_____	_____	_____

Instructor Note:

Points may be redistributed depending on the availability of materials to perform this procedure in the individual training facility.

Comments:

Total Points Earned _____ Divided by _____ Total Possible Points = _____ % Score

Instructor's Signature _____

Procedure 14-5 Establish and Maintain the Medical Record: Prepare a Record Release Form

Task: To provide a legal document to another provider or healthcare facility that indicates the patient's consent to the release of his or her medical records.

Equipment and Supplies:
- Medical record release form
- Pen
- Envelope

Standards: Complete the procedure and all critical steps in _____ minutes with a minimum score of _____% within three attempts.

Scoring: Divide points earned by total possible points. Failure to perform a critical step that is indicated with an asterisk (*) will result in an unsatisfactory overall score.

Time began _____ **Time ended** _____

Steps	Possible Points	First Attempt	Second Attempt	Third Attempt
1. Explain to the patient that a medical record release form will be necessary to obtain records from another provider. If the patient is having records sent to another provider, a release will also be required.	20	_____	_____	_____
2. Review the record release form with the patient, and ask if the form is understood or if there are any questions about the form.	20	_____	_____	_____
3. Have the patient sign the form in the space indicated. If other demographic information is required, such as a social security number or other names used, complete that information as well.	20	_____	_____	_____
4. Make a copy of the form for the file, then mail the form to the appropriate facility. Note the date that the form was sent. Provide a copy to the patient if requested.	20	_____	_____	_____
5. Follow up to ensure that the requested records actually arrive.	20	_____	_____	_____

Comments:

Total Points Earned _____ Divided by _____ Total Possible Points = _____ % Score

Instructor's Signature _____

Student Name _____ Date _____ Score _____

Procedure 14-6 Transcribe a Machine-Dictated Letter Using a Computer or Word Processor

Task: To transcribe a machine-dictated letter into a mailable document without error or corrections, using a computer or word processor.

Equipment and Supplies:
• Word processor, computer, or typewriter
• Transcribing machine
• Stationery
• Reference manual

Standards: Complete the procedure and all critical steps in _____ minutes with a minimum score of _____% within three attempts.

Scoring: Divide points earned by total possible points. Failure to perform a critical step that is indicated with an asterisk (*) will result in an unsatisfactory overall score.

Time began _____ Time ended _____

Steps	Possible Points	First Attempt	Second Attempt	Third Attempt
1. Assemble supplies.	10	_____	_____	_____
2. Set up the format for selected letter style.	20	_____	_____	_____
3. Keyboard the text while listening to the dictation.	20	_____	_____	_____
4. Edit the letter on the monitor.	20	_____	_____	_____
5. Execute a spell check.	20	_____	_____	_____
6. Direct the document to a printer.	10	_____	_____	_____

Comments:

Total Points Earned _____ Divided by _____ Total Possible Points = _____ % Score

Instructor's Signature _____

Student Name _____ Date _____ Score _____

Procedure 14-7 File Medical Records and Documents Using the Alphabetic System

Task: To file records efficiently using an alphabetic system and ensure that the records can be easily and quickly retrieved.

Equipment and Supplies:
- Medical records
- Physical filing equipment
- Cart to carry records, if needed
- Alphabetic file guide
- Staple remover
- Stapler
- Paper clips

Standards: Complete the procedure and all critical steps in _____ minutes with a minimum score of _____% within three attempts.

Scoring: Divide points earned by total possible points. Failure to perform a critical step that is indicated with an asterisk (*) will result in an unsatisfactory overall score.

Time began _____ **Time ended** _____

Steps	Possible Points	First Attempt	Second Attempt	Third Attempt
1. Using alphabetic guidelines, place the records to be filed in alphabetic order. If a stack of documents is to be filed, place them in alphabetic order inside an alphabetic file guide or sorter. Use rules for filing documents alphabetically.	20	_____	_____	_____
2. Go to the filing storage equipment (shelves, cabinets, or drawers) and locate the spot in the alphabet for the first file.	20	_____	_____	_____
3. Place the file in the cabinet or drawer in correct alphabetic order.	20	_____	_____	_____
4. If adding a document to a file, place it on top, so that the most recent information is seen first. This puts the information in the file in reverse chronologic order.	20	_____	_____	_____
5. Securely fasten documents to the chart. Do not just drop the documents inside the chart. Refile the chart in its proper place.	20	_____	_____	_____

Comments:

Total Points Earned _____ Divided by _____ Total Possible Points = _____ % Score

Instructor's Signature _____

Procedure 14-8 File Medical Records and Documents Using the Numeric System

Task: To file records efficiently using a numeric system and ensure that the records can be easily and quickly retrieved.

Equipment and Supplies:
- Medical records
- Physical filing equipment
- Cart to carry records, if needed
- Numeric file guide
- Staple remover
- Stapler
- Paper clips

Standards: Complete the procedure and all critical steps in _____ minutes with a minimum score of _____% within three attempts.

Scoring: Divide points earned by total possible points. Failure to perform a critical step that is indicated with an asterisk (*) will result in an unsatisfactory overall score.

Time began _____ **Time ended** _____

Steps	Possible Points	First Attempt	Second Attempt	Third Attempt
1. Using numeric guidelines, place the records to be filed in numeric order. If a stack of documents is to be filed, write the chart number on the document. Use rules for filing documents alphabetically.	**20**	_____	_____	_____
2. Go to the filing storage equipment (shelves, cabinets, or drawers) and locate the numericspot for the first file.	**20**	_____	_____	_____
3. Place the file in the cabinet or drawer in correct numeric order.	**20**	_____	_____	_____
4. If adding a document to a file, place it on top so that the most recent information is seen first. This puts the information in the file in reverse chronologic order.	**20**	_____	_____	_____
5. Securely fasten documents to the chart. Do not just drop the documents inside the chart.	**20**	_____	_____	_____

Comments:

Total Points Earned _____ Divided by _____ Total Possible Points = _____ % Score

Instructor's Signature _____

Procedure 14-9 Establish and Maintain the Medical Record: Color-Code Medical Records

Task: To color-code patient records using the agency's established coding system to effectively facilitate filing and finding.

Equipment and Supplies:
- 20 patient medical records
- Information on agency's coding system
- Full range of color tabs

Standards: Complete the procedure and all critical steps in _____ minutes with a minimum score of _____% within three attempts.

Scoring: Divide points earned by total possible points. Failure to perform a critical step that is indicated with an asterisk (*) will result in an unsatisfactory overall score.

Time began _____ **Time ended** _____

Steps	Possible Points	First Attempt	Second Attempt	Third Attempt
1. Assemble patient records.	10	_____	_____	_____
2. Arrange records in indexing order.	15	_____	_____	_____
3. Pick up the first chart, and note the second letter of the surname.	15	_____	_____	_____
4. Choose tab of the appropriate color.	15	_____	_____	_____
5. Type the patient's name on label in indexing order, and apply tab to folder tab.	15	_____	_____	_____
6. Repeat steps 4 and 5 until all records have been coded.	15	_____	_____	_____
7. Check all groups for any isolated color.	15	_____	_____	_____

Comments:

Total Points Earned _____ Divided by _____ Total Possible Points = _____ % Score

Instructor's Signature _____

Student Name _____ Date _____ Score _____

Procedure 14-10 Document Appropriately and Accurately

Task: To document appropriately and accurately on all patient medical records and other office paperwork that concerns the patient.

Equipment and Supplies:
- Any medical document
- Clerical supplies
- Computer or word processor
- Office policy and procedure Manual

Standards: Complete the procedure and all critical steps in _____ minutes with a minimum score of _____% within three attempts.

Scoring: Divide points earned by total possible points. Failure to perform a critical step that is indicated with an asterisk (*), will result in an unsatisfactory overall score.

Time began _____ **Time ended** _____

Steps	Possible Points	First Attempt	Second Attempt	Third Attempt
1. Determine the entry to be made into the document.	5	_____	_____	_____
2. Make the entry in legible handwriting.	20	_____	_____	_____
3. Check the entry for accuracy.	5	_____	_____	_____
4. Authenticate the entry.	20	_____	_____	_____
5. Make a correction to the same entry.	20	_____	_____	_____
6. Authenticate the corrected entry.	20	_____	_____	_____
7. Check the entry for accuracy.	5	_____	_____	_____
8. Place the document in the appropriate record or file	5	_____	_____	_____

Comments:

Total Points Earned _____ Divided by _____ Total Possible Points = _____ % Score

Instructor's Signature _____

Student Name _____ Date _____ Score _____

Procedure 16-1 Identify and Respond to Issues of Confidentiality

Task: To become proficient at identifying issues that involve confidentiality and respond to them in the manner prescribed by office policy.

Equipment and Supplies:
- Office policy manual
- Office procedure manual, if separate
- Release of information forms
- Notice of privacy practices
- Clerical supplies
- Patient medical records

Standards: Complete the procedure and all critical steps in _____ minutes with a minimum score of _____% within three attempts.

Scoring: Divide points earned by total possible points. Failure to perform a critical step that is indicated with an asterisk (*) will result in an unsatisfactory overall score.

Time began _____ **Time ended** _____

Steps	Possible Points	First Attempt	Second Attempt	Third Attempt
1. Review office policy regarding release of patient information and confidentiality in the facility.	10	_____	_____	_____
2. Review the notice of privacy practices for the facility.	10	_____	_____	_____
3. Review the facility authorization to release medical records form.	10	_____	_____	_____
4. Thoroughly read the request for information that is presented to the facility.*	10	_____	_____	_____
5. Determine if the document is valid.*	10	_____	_____	_____
6. Determine the exact information that is being requested.*	10	_____	_____	_____
7. Make certain that the release of information form either is one designed by the facility or contains all of the same information.*	10	_____	_____	_____
8. Make the requestor complete one of the facility's request forms, if necessary.	10	_____	_____	_____

Steps	Possible Points	First Attempt	Second Attempt	Third Attempt
9. Forward only the information requested to the person or representative of the organization who presented the authorization for release of information.	__10__	_____	_____	_____
10. Release the information by mail or to the agent of the requestor.	__10__	_____	_____	_____

Comments:

Total Points Earned _____ Divided by _____ Total Possible Points = _____ % Score

Instructor's Signature _____

Student Name _____ Date _____ Score _____

Procedure 17-1 Perform ICD-9 Coding

Task: To perform accurate diagnosis coding using the ICD-9-CM manual.

Equipment and Supplies:
- ICD-9-CM manual, Volumes 1 and 2, current year
- Encounter form or charge ticket
- Medical record
- Clerical supplies

Standards: Complete the procedure and all critical steps in _____ minutes with a minimum score of _____% within three attempts.

Scoring: Divide points earned by total possible points. Failure to perform a critical step that is indicated with an asterisk (*) will result in an unsatisfactory overall score.

Time began _____ **Time ended** _____

Steps	Possible Points	First Attempt	Second Attempt	Third Attempt
1. Abstract the medical record and encounter form.*	10			
2. Determine the main terms in the diagnostic statement.*	10			
3. Determine the modifying terms in the main term on the diagnostic statement.	10			
4. Locate the main terms in the Alphabetic Index.	10			
5. Locate the modifying words listed under the main term in the ICD-9-CM manual.	10			
6. Review notes and cross references.	10			
7. Choose a tentative code or codes and write them on a sheet of paper.	10			
8. Verify the tentative code's accuracy in the tabular index.*	10			
9. Carry the codes to the highest level of specificity.*	10			
10. Assign the code.*	10			

Comments:

Total Points Earned _____ Divided by _____ Total Possible Points = _____ % Score

Instructor's Signature _____

Student Name _____ Date _____ Score _____

Procedure 18-1 Perform Procedural Coding: Perform CPT-4 Coding

Task: To use the steps for procedure and service coding to obtain the most accurate and specific procedure code.

Equipment and Supplies:
- CPT-4 Coding Manual, current year
- Encounter form
- Medical record
- Clerical supplies
- Medical dictionary or medical terminology reference book

Standards: Complete the procedure and all critical steps in _____ minutes with a minimum score of _____% within three attempts.

Scoring: Divide points earned by total possible points. Failure to perform a critical step that is indicated with an asterisk (*) will result in an unsatisfactory overall score.

Time began _____ **Time ended** _____

Steps	Possible Points	First Attempt	Second Attempt	Third Attempt
1. Read medical documentation to determine what services were provided.*	10	_____	_____	_____
2. Select main term classification to begin search.*	10	_____	_____	_____
3. Select modifying terms, if needed.	10	_____	_____	_____
4. Find code or code ranges that include all or most of the medical record procedure or service description.*	10	_____	_____	_____
5. Disregard any code containing descriptions or wording not included in the medical record.	5	_____	_____	_____
6. Write down the tentative code.	5	_____	_____	_____
7. Check the code in the main index.*	10	_____	_____	_____
8. Compare the code to the medical description.	10	_____	_____	_____
9. Read the guidelines to make certain that there are no contraindications to use of the code.	5	_____	_____	_____
10. Evaluate the conventions.	5	_____	_____	_____

Steps	Possible Points	First Attempt	Second Attempt	Third Attempt
11. Determine if there are special circum-stances that require a modifier.	10			
12. Assign the code.*	10			

Comments:

Total Points Earned _____ Divided by _____ Total Possible Points = _____ % Score

Instructor's Signature _____

Student Name _____ Date _____ Score _____

Procedure 18-2 Perform Procedural Coding: Perform Evaluation and Management Coding

Task: Use the steps for evaluation and management coding to find the most accurate and specific E&M code.

Equipment and Supplies:
• CPT-4 Coding Manual, current year
• Encounter form
• Medical record
• Clerical supplies
• Medical dictionary or medical terminology reference book

Standards: Complete the procedure and all critical steps in _____ minutes with a minimum score of _____% within three attempts.

Scoring: Divide points earned by total possible points. Failure to perform a critical step that is indicated with an asterisk (*) will result in an unsatisfactory overall score.

Time began _____ **Time ended** _____

Steps	Possible Points	First Attempt	Second Attempt	Third Attempt
1. Identify the place of service.	10	_____	_____	_____
2. Identify the patient status.	10	_____	_____	_____
3. Identify the subsection, category, or subcategory of service in the E&M section.*	10	_____	_____	_____
4. Review guidelines for the selected subsection, category, or subcategory.	10	_____	_____	_____
5. Review the level of E&M service descriptions for each code in the subsection, category, or subcategory chosen.*	10	_____	_____	_____
6. Compare medical documentation to examples in Appendix C, if necessary.	10	_____	_____	_____
7. Determine the extent of the history obtained.*	10	_____	_____	_____
8. Determine the extent of the examination performed.*	10	_____	_____	_____
9. Determine the complexity of the medical decision making.*	10	_____	_____	_____

Steps	Possible Points	First Attempt	Second Attempt	Third Attempt
10. Select the appropriate level of E&M code, and document it on the medical record or the encounter form.*	__10__	_____	_____	_____

Comments:

Total Points Earned _____ Divided by _____ Total Possible Points = _____ % Score

Instructor's Signature _____

Procedure 18-3 Perform Procedural Coding: Perform Anesthesia Coding

Task: To select the most accurate and specific anesthesia code and perform the anesthesia formula calculation to determine the charge for the service.

Equipment and Supplies:
- CPT-4 Coding Manual, current year
- Encounter form
- Medical record
- Conversion factor list
- Clerical supplies
- Calculator

Standards: Complete the procedure and all critical steps in _____ minutes with a minimum score of _____% within three attempts.

Scoring: Divide points earned by total possible points. Failure to perform a critical step that is indicated with an asterisk (*) will result in an unsatisfactory overall score.

Time began _____ Time ended _____

Steps	Possible Points	First Attempt	Second Attempt	Third Attempt
1. Read medical documentation.*	10	_____	_____	_____
2. Determine anatomic site.*	10	_____	_____	_____
3. Find the anesthesia code that includes all or most of the medical record procedure or service.	5	_____	_____	_____
4. Write down the code that best matches the medical documentation.	5	_____	_____	_____
5. Find the code in the main text.*	10	_____	_____	_____
6. Read the guidelines and notes for the section, subsection, category, and subcategory.	5	_____	_____	_____
7. Evaluate conventions.	5	_____	_____	_____
8. Document the code selected.*	5	_____	_____	_____
9. Determine the Basic Unit Value from the Relative Value Guide.	5	_____	_____	_____
10. Determine the patient's physical status and document the appropriate modifier.	5	_____	_____	_____

Steps	Possible Points	First Attempt	Second Attempt	Third Attempt
11. Determine if a qualifying circumstance modifier should be used.	5			
12. Determine the total anesthesia time, divide by 15 minutes, and document the time.*	10			
13. Select the appropriate geographic conversion factor.	5			
14. Calculate the charge for the anesthesia service using the anesthesia formula.*	10			
15. Document the charge and the code in the medical record and on the encounter form.*	5			

Comments:

Total Points Earned _____ Divided by _____ Total Possible Points = _____ % Score

Instructor's Signature _____

Student Name _____ Date _____ Score _____

Procedure 18-4 Perform Procedural Coding: Perform HCPCS Coding

Task: To find the most accurate and specific HCPCS code.

Equipment and Supplies:
- HCPCS Coding Manual, current year
- Medical record
- Encounter form
- Clerical supplies

Standards: Complete the procedure and all critical steps in _____ minutes with a minimum score of _____% within three attempts.

Scoring: Divide points earned by total possible points. Failure to perform a critical step that is indicated with an asterisk (*) will result in an unsatisfactory overall score.

Time began _____ **Time ended** _____

Steps	Possible Points	First Attempt	Second Attempt	Third Attempt
1. Read medical documentation.*	10			
2. Select main term classification to begin search.*	10			
3. Select modifying terms, if needed.	5			
4. If no modifying term produces an appropriate code, repeat steps 2 and 3 until an appropriate code is found.	5			
5. Find code or code ranges that include all or most of the medical record procedure or service description.*	10			
6. Disregard any code or code range containing information not found in the medical record.	10			
7. Write down the code that best matches the description in the medical record.*	5			
8. Turn to the main text and find the code or code range.	5			
9. Compare the description of the code with the medical documentation.*	10			

Steps	Possible Points	First Attempt	Second Attempt	Third Attempt
10. Read the guidelines for the section, and make certain that there are no contraindications to using the code.*	10			
11. Evaluate the HCPCS Manual conventions.	5			
12. Determine if there are special circumstances that require a modifier.	5			
13. Record the HCPCS code selected.*	10			

Comments:

Total Points Earned _____ Divided by _____ Total Possible Points = _____ % Score

Instructor's Signature _____

Student Name _____ Date _____ Score _____

Procedure 19-1 Apply Managed Care Policies and Procedures

Task: To act within the guidelines of the managed care contracts that the physician and/or medical facility has partnered.

Equipment and Supplies:
- Managed care contracts
- Managed care handbooks
- Clerical supplies
- Forms from managed care organizations

Standards: Complete the procedure and all critical steps in _____ minutes with a minimum score of _____% within three attempts.

Scoring: Divide points earned by total possible points. Failure to perform a critical step that is indicated with an asterisk (*) will result in an unsatisfactory overall score.

Time began _____ **Time ended** _____

Steps	Possible Points	First Attempt	Second Attempt	Third Attempt
1. Determine which managed care organization the patient subscribes to.	15			
2. Read the guidelines for the policy.*	15			
3. Gather forms necessary to process the claim.	15			
4. Determine the contact person at the managed care organization who can answer questions, if necessary.*	15			
5. Attend seminars and workshops to learn more about the managed care organization.	15			
6. Use the information gained to file complete, accurate claims for reimbursement.*	25			

Comments:

Total Points Earned _____ Divided by _____ Total Possible Points = _____ % Score

Instructor's Signature _____

Student Name _____ Date _____ Score _____

Procedure 19-2 Apply Managed Care Policies and Procedures: Perform Verification of Eligibility and Benefits

Task: To confirm the patient's insurance is in effect, and what procedures and services are covered and excluded.

Equipment and Supplies:
- Managed care contracts
- Managed care handbooks
- Clerical supplies
- Forms from managed care organizations

Standards: Complete the procedure and all critical steps in _____ minutes with a minimum score of _____% within three attempts.

Scoring: Divide points earned by total possible points. Failure to perform a critical step that is indicated with an asterisk (*) will result in an unsatisfactory overall score.

Time began _____ **Time ended** _____

Steps	Possible Points	First Attempt	Second Attempt	Third Attempt
1. Determine the patient's insurance company when he or she makes the initial call for an appointment.*	15			
2. Make a copy of the patient's insurance card, front and back.*	15			
3. Complete the patient portion of the Verification and Benefit form, using one form per insurance company.	15			
4. Contact the insurance carrier by phone or fax to verify eligibility and benefits.*	15			
5. Not the name and title of the person who verified the benefits.	20			
6. Document all verification information in the patient's medical record.*	20			

Comments:

Total Points Earned _____ Divided by _____ Total Possible Points = _____ % Score

Instructor's Signature _____

Student Name _____ Date _____ Score _____

Procedure 19-3 Apply Managed Care Policies and Procedures: Perform Preauthorization (Precertification) and/or Referral

Task: To obtain authorization for patient services and referrals.

Equipment and Supplies:
- Patient medical record
- Precertification form
- Patient's insurance information
- Telephone and fax machine
- Clerical supplies

Standards: Complete the procedure and all critical steps in _____ minutes with a minimum score of _____% within three attempts.

Scoring: Divide points earned by total possible points. Failure to perform a critical step that is indicated with an asterisk (*) will result in an unsatisfactory overall score.

Time began _____ **Time ended** _____

Steps	Possible Points	First Attempt	Second Attempt	Third Attempt
1. Gather documents and forms needed.	15	_____	_____	_____
2. Examine the patient record to determine the action that needs to be taken.	15	_____	_____	_____
3. Complete the referral form.	25	_____	_____	_____
4. Proofread the completed form.	15	_____	_____	_____
5. Fax the completed form to the patient's insurance carrier.	15	_____	_____	_____
6. Place a copy of the returned approval form in the patient's medical record.	15	_____	_____	_____

Comments:

Total Points Earned _____ Divided by _____ Total Possible Points = _____ % Score

Instructor's Signature _____

Student Name _____ Date _____ Score _____

Procedure 19-4 Apply Third-Party Guidelines

Task: To ensure that claims are processed quickly and result in the highest allowable reimbursement.

Equipment and Supplies:
- Managed care contracts
- Managed care handbooks
- Clerical supplies
- Forms from managed care organizations
- Claim forms

Standards: Complete the procedure and all critical steps in _____ minutes with a minimum score of _____% within three attempts.

Scoring: Divide points earned by total possible points. Failure to perform a critical step that is indicated with an asterisk (*) will result in an unsatisfactory overall score.

Time began _____ **Time ended** _____

Steps	Possible Points	First Attempt	Second Attempt	Third Attempt
1. Determine the patient's health plan.*	10			
2. Review the rules and regulations that apply to that managed care organization.	10			
3. Make certain that there is a signature on file for the patient.*	10			
4. Determine the procedures and/or services that are to be billed.*	10			
5. Determine of all of the procedures and/or services to be billed are actually covered by the health plan.*	10			
6. Make the patient aware of any procedures and/or services that will not be covered.*	10			
7. Determine if any information needs to be added to the blocks designated "for local use."	10			
8. Make certain that all of the procedures and/or services being billed relate to at least one diagnosis.*	10			
9. Proofread the claim for accuracy.*	10			
10. Submit the claim.	10			

Comments:

Total Points Earned _____ Divided by _____ Total Possible Points = _____ % Score

Instructor's Signature _____

Student Name _____ Date _____ Score _____

Procedure 19-5 Apply Managed Care Policies and Procedures: Perform Deductible, Co-Insurance, and Allowable Amount Calculations

Task: To calculate the patient's out-of-pocket expenses or amount to be billed to a secondary insurance carrier, and to determine what amounts, if any, are to be written off or passed on to the patient for payment.

Equipment and Supplies:
- Explanation of benefits (EOB) form, explanation of medicare benefits (EOMB) form, remittance advice (RA), or Verification of Eligibility and Benefits form
- Patient accounts receivable ledger
- Calculator
- Clerical supplies

Standards: Complete the procedure and all critical steps in _____ minutes with a minimum score of _____% within three attempts.

Scoring: Divide points earned by total possible points. Failure to perform a critical step that is indicated with an asterisk (*) will result in an unsatisfactory overall score.

Time began _____ **Time ended** _____

Steps	Possible Points	First Attempt	Second Attempt	Third Attempt
1. Assemble the required materials and equipment.	15			
2. Using the EOB, EOMB, or RA: • Enter the total charge from the EOB, EOMB, or RA • Subtract the deductible amount from the total charge.*	25			
3. If the patient has met the deductible, determine the co-insurance payment due.*	15			
4. Record the deductible, and, if applicable, co-insurance amounts on separate lines on the patient ledger.*	15			
5. Subtract the allowable amount of each charge from the actual billed charge.	15			
6. Record the difference in either the adjustments or the balance due column.*	15			

Comments:

Total Points Earned _____ Divided by _____ Total Possible Points = _____ % Score

Instructor's Signature _____

Student Name _____ Date _____ Score _____

Procedure 20-1 Complete an Insurance Claim Form

Task: To accurately complete a CMS-1500 claim form.

Equipment and Supplies:
- Patient registration form
- Photocopy of patient's insurance card, front and back
- Encounter form
- CPT-4 Coding Manual
- ICD-9-CM Coding Manual
- Patient medical record
- Patient ledger
- CMS-1500 form
- Computer or typewriter
- Printer

Standards: Complete the procedure and all critical steps in _____ minutes with a minimum score of _____% within three attempts.

Scoring: Divide points earned by total possible points. Failure to perform a critical step that is indicated with an asterisk (*) will result in an unsatisfactory overall score.

Time began _____ Time ended _____

Steps	Possible Points	First Attempt	Second Attempt	Third Attempt
1. Determine the carrier to which the insurance claim will be bill in the carrier block section at the top of the form.*	10	_____	_____	_____
2. Enter the required information in the Patient/Insured section (demographic information) of the CMS-1500 form, Blocks 1-8.*	10	_____	_____	_____
3. Complete the information required in the Patient/Insured information section (insurance information) in Blocks 9-11.*	10	_____	_____	_____
4. Have th patient sign the form in Block 12 and 13, or indicate that the signature is on file by using the abbreviation SOF.*	10	_____	_____	_____
5. Complete the Physician/Supplier section, Blocks 14-23, as required by the carrier.*	10	_____	_____	_____
6. Make certain that the correct diagnosis codes are used in Block 21.*	10	_____	_____	_____

Steps	Possible Points	First Attempt	Second Attempt	Third Attempt
7. Complete the Physician/Supplier section, Blocks 24-30, including the correct procedure codes in Block 24d.*	10	_____	_____	_____
8. Obtain the signature required for Block 31 or indicate that the signature is on file by using the abbreviation SOF.*	10	_____	_____	_____
9. Complete the information required in Blocks 32 and 33.*	10	_____	_____	_____
10. Mail the insurance claim to the carrier with any attachments, if indicated.*	10	_____	_____	_____

Comments:

Total Points Earned _____ Divided by _____ Total Possible Points = _____ % Score

Instructor's Signature _____

Procedure 21-1 Explain General Office Policies:
Explain Professional Fees

Task: To explain the physician's fees so that the patient understands his or her obligations and rights for privacy.

Equipment and Supplies:
- Patient's statement
- Copy of physician's fee schedule
- Quiet, private area where the patient feels free to ask questions

Standards: Complete the procedure and all critical steps in _____ minutes with a minimum score of _____% within three attempts.

Scoring: Divide points earned by total possible points. Failure to perform a critical step that is indicated with an asterisk (*) will result in an unsatisfactory overall score.

Time began _____ **Time ended** _____

Steps	Possible Points	First Attempt	Second Attempt	Third Attempt
1. Determine that th patient has the correct bill.	10			
2. Examine the bill for possible errors.	15			
3. Refer to the fee schedule for services rendered.	15			
4. Explain itemized billing: • Date of service • Type of service rendered • Fee	15			
5. Display a professional attitude toward the patient.	15			
6. Determine whether the patient has specific concerns that my hinder payment.	15			
7. Make appropriate arrangements for a discussion between the physician and patient if further explanation is necessary for resolution of the problem.	15			

Comments:

Total Points Earned _____ Divided by _____ Total Possible Points = _____ % Score

Instructor's Signature _____

Student Name _____ Date _____ Score _____

Procedure 21-2 Post Entries on a Daysheet

Task: To post 1 day's charges and payments and compute the daily bookkeeping cycle using a pegboard.

Equipment and Supplies:
- Patient's statement
- Calculator
- Pen
- Daysheet
- Receipts
- Ledger cards
- Balances from previous day

Standards: Complete the procedure and all critical steps in _____ minutes with a minimum score of _____% within three attempts.

Scoring: Divide points earned by total possible points. Failure to perform a critical step that is indicated with an asterisk (*) will result in an unsatisfactory overall score.

Time began _____ **Time ended** _____

Steps	Possible Points	First Attempt	Second Attempt	Third Attempt
1. Prepare the board: • Place a new daysheet on the board • Place bank of receipts over the pegs, aligning the top receipt with the first open writing line on the daysheet	5	_____	_____	_____
2. Carry forward balances from the previous day.	5	_____	_____	_____
3. Pull ledger card for patient being seen that day.	5	_____	_____	_____
4. Insert the ledger card under the first receipt, aligning the first available writing line with the carbonized strip on the receipt.	5	_____	_____	_____
5. Enter the patient's name, the date, receipt numbers, and any existing balance from the ledger card.	5	_____	_____	_____
6. Detach the charge slip from the receipt and clip it to the patient's record.	5	_____	_____	_____
7. Accept the returned charge slip at the end of the visit.	5	_____	_____	_____
8. Enter the appropriate fee from the fee schedule.	5	_____	_____	_____

Steps	Possible Points	First Attempt	Second Attempt	Third Attempt
9. Locate the receipt on the board with a number matching the charge slip.	5			
10. Reinsert the patient's ledger card under the receipt.	5			
11. Write the service code number and fee on the receipt.	5			
12. Accept the patient's payment and record the amount of payment and the new balance.	5			
13. Give the completed receipt to the patient.	5			
14. Follow your agency's procedure for refiling the ledger card.	5			
15. Repeat steps 4-14 for each service of the day.	10			
16. Total all columns of the daysheet at the end of the day.	5			
17. Write preliminary totals in pencil.	5			
18. Complete proof of totals and enter totals in ink.	5			
19. Enter figures for accounts receivable control.	5			

Comments:

Total Points Earned _____ Divided by _____ Total Possible Points = _____ % Score

Instructor's Signature _____

Procedure 21-3 Post Adjustments

Task: To accurately process adjustments to patient accounts.

Equipment and Supplies:
- Patient ledgers
- Office policy manual
- Explanation of benefits (EOB)/remittance advice (RA)
- Bookkeeping system
- Clerical supplies
- Payments
- Calculator

Standards: Complete the procedure and all critical steps in _____ minutes with a minimum score of _____% within three attempts.

Scoring: Divide points earned by total possible points. Failure to perform a critical step that is indicated with an asterisk (*) will result in an unsatisfactory overall score.

Time began _____ **Time ended** _____

Steps	Possible Points	First Attempt	Second Attempt	Third Attempt
1. Open mail and set payments aside with their corresponding EOB/RA.	10			
2. Paper clip the EOB/RA to the check that arrived with it as payment.*	10			
3. Post the payment to the patient's account.*	10			
4. Determine if an adjustment is necessary on the account.	10			
5. Review the current procedure to follow in adjusting the account.	10			
6. Make sure that the ledger card is aligned properly with the day sheet, if a manual system is being used.*	10			
7. Post the adjustment in the adjustment column or other specified place on the day sheet or in the computer software.*	20			
8. Check the math calculations to make certain that the adjustment was figured correctly.*	10			
9. Determine the current balance on the patient's account.	10			

Comments:

Total Points Earned _____ Divided by _____ Total Possible Points = _____ % Score

Instructor's Signature _____

Student Name _____ Date _____ Score _____

Procedure 21-4 Process a Credit Balance

Task: To return overpayments to patients in a timely manner.

Equipment and Supplies:
- Patient ledgers
- Office policy manual
- Explanation of benefits (EOB)/remittance advice (RA)
- Bookkeeping system
- Clerical supplies
- Payments
- Calculator

Standards: Complete the procedure and all critical steps in _____ minutes with a minimum score of _____% within three attempts.

Scoring: Divide points earned by total possible points. Failure to perform a critical step that is indicated with an asterisk (*) will result in an unsatisfactory overall score.

Time began _____ **Time ended** _____

Steps	Possible Points	First Attempt	Second Attempt	Third Attempt
1. Review the office policy manual to determine the correct procedure for refunding a credit balance.	10	_____	_____	_____
2. Evaluate the payment received and the EOB.*	20	_____	_____	_____
3. Post the payment to the patient's account.	20	_____	_____	_____
4. Determine if an overpayment has been made.*	10	_____	_____	_____
5. Review the account to determine if more insurance payments are expected on the account.*	20	_____	_____	_____
6. Adjust the credit balance off of the patient's account.	20	_____	_____	_____

Comments:

Total Points Earned _____ Divided by _____ Total Possible Points = _____ % Score

Instructor's Signature _____

Student Name _____ Date _____ Score _____

Procedure 21-5 Process Refunds

Task: To return patient refunds in a timely manner.

Equipment and Supplies:
- Patient ledgers
- Office policy manual
- Explanation of benefits (EOB)/remittance advice (RA)
- Bookkeeping system
- Clerical supplies
- Payments
- Calculator

Standards: Complete the procedure and all critical steps in _____ minutes with a minimum score of _____% within three attempts.

Scoring: Divide points earned by total possible points. Failure to perform a critical step that is indicated with an asterisk (*) will result in an unsatisfactory overall score.

Time began _____ **Time ended** _____

Steps	Possible Points	First Attempt	Second Attempt	Third Attempt
1. Determine the amount of the refund to be processed.*	20	_____	_____	_____
2. Write a check for the amount of the refund.	20	_____	_____	_____
3. Present the check to the physician for a signature.	10	_____	_____	_____
4. Determine the patient's correct mailing address.	20	_____	_____	_____
5. Make a copy of the refund check and place it in the patient's medical record.*	20	_____	_____	_____
6. Mail the refund to the patient.*	10	_____	_____	_____

Comments:

Total Points Earned _____ Divided by _____ Total Possible Points = _____ % Score

Instructor's Signature _____

Student Name _____ Date _____ Score _____

Procedure 21-6 Post Nonsufficient Fund Checks

Task: To correctly note that a check was returned on a patient account as being nonsufficient.

Equipment and Supplies:
- Patient ledgers
- Office policy manual
- Bookkeeping system
- Clerical supplies
- Calculator

Standards: Complete the procedure and all critical steps in _____ minutes with a minimum score of _____% within three attempts.

Scoring: Divide points earned by total possible points. Failure to perform a critical step that is indicated with an asterisk (*) will result in an unsatisfactory overall score.

Time began _____ **Time ended** _____

Steps	Possible Points	First Attempt	Second Attempt	Third Attempt
1. Pull the ledger card that corresponds with the patient who wrote the check.	10	_____	_____	_____
2. Determine the amount to be added back to the ledger card as a result of the returned check.*	20	_____	_____	_____
3. Post that amount to the patient's ledger card.*	20	_____	_____	_____
4. Send a certified letter to the patient demanding the timely payment of the check and any fees that are assessed to the patient's account for processing.*	20	_____	_____	_____
5. Note this collection activity on the patient's medical record.*	20	_____	_____	_____
6. When the patient pays the check and fees, process it as a regular payment and return the check to the patient.	10	_____	_____	_____

Comments:

Total Points Earned _____ Divided by _____ Total Possible Points = _____ % Score

Instructor's Signature _____

Student Name _____ Date _____ Score _____

Procedure 21-7 Explain General Office Policies: Make Credit Arrangements with a Patient

Task: To assist the patient in paying for services by making mutually beneficial credit arrangements according to established office policy.

Equipment and Supplies:
- Patient ledger
- Calendar
- Truth in lending form
- Assignment of benefits form
- Patient's insurance form
- Private area for an interview

Standards: Complete the procedure and all critical steps in _____ minutes with a minimum score of _____% within three attempts.

Scoring: Divide points earned by total possible points. Failure to perform a critical step that is indicated with an asterisk (*) will result in an unsatisfactory overall score.

Time began _____ **Time ended** _____

Steps	Possible Points	First Attempt	Second Attempt	Third Attempt
1. Answer all questions about credit thoroughly and kindly.	10			
2. Inform the patient of the office policy regarding credit: • Payment at the time of first visit • Payment by bank card • Credit application	20			
3. Have the patient complete the credit application.	10			
4. Check the completed credit application.	10			
5. Discuss with the patient the possible arrangements and ask the patient to decide which of the arrangements is most suitable.	10			
6. Prepare the truth in lending form and have the patient sign it if the agreement requires more than four installments.	10			
7. Have the patient execute an assignment of insurance benefits.	10			

Steps	Possible Points	First Attempt	Second Attempt	Third Attempt
8. Make a copy of the patient's insurance ID and have the patient sign a consent for the release of the information to the insurance company.	10			
9. Keep credit information confidential.	10			

Comments:

Total Points Earned _____ Divided by _____ Total Possible Points = _____ % Score

Instructor's Signature _____

Student Name _____ Date _____ Score _____

Procedure 21-8 Perform Accounts Receivable Procedures

Task: To collect amounts due to the physician and/or medical facility.

Equipment and Supplies:
- Patient ledgers
- Office policy manual
- Telephone
- Letterhead and envelopes
- Clerical supplies

Standards: Complete the procedure and all critical steps in _____ minutes with a minimum score of _____% within three attempts.

Scoring: Divide points earned by total possible points. Failure to perform a critical step that is indicated with an asterisk (*) will result in an unsatisfactory overall score.

Time began _____ **Time ended** _____

Steps	Possible Points	First Attempt	Second Attempt	Third Attempt
1. Review office policy with regard to accounts receivable procedures.*	10	_____	_____	_____
2. Determine the billing cycle for the office.	10	_____	_____	_____
3. Determine the amounts owed to the physician and who owes the amounts.*	20	_____	_____	_____
4. Group accounts together according to office policy.*	20	_____	_____	_____
5. Print bills or copy bills from ledger cards.*	20	_____	_____	_____
6. Mail bills to patients.	10	_____	_____	_____
7. Post payments to the patients' accounts as they arrive at the office.*	10	_____	_____	_____

Comments:

Total Points Earned _____ Divided by _____ Total Possible Points = _____ % Score

Instructor's Signature _____

Procedure 21-9 Perform Billing Procedures

Task: To bill insurance companies for patient procedures and services and obtain the maximum legal reimbursement.

Equipment and Supplies:
- Patient ledgers
- Accounting system
- Calculator
- Claim forms
- Encounter forms
- Clerical supplies

Standards: Complete the procedure and all critical steps in _____ minutes with a minimum score of _____% within three attempts.

Scoring: Divide points earned by total possible points. Failure to perform a critical step that is indicated with an asterisk (*) will result in an unsatisfactory overall score.

Time began _____ **Time ended** _____

Steps	Possible Points	First Attempt	Second Attempt	Third Attempt
1. Determine the procedures and/or services that are to be billed by reading the patient's medical record.*	20			
2. Determine the diagnosis codes(s) applicable to the claim.*	10			
3. Determine the procedure code(s) applicable to the claim.*	10			
4. Complete the CMS 1500 claim form, following the directions provided for each block.*	20			
5. Insert the correct amount of money to bill in the appropriate block on the claim form.	10			
6. Address the claim to the carrier's correct address for claim submissions.	10			
7. Mail the claim form.	10			
8. Follow up on the claim to ensure timely payment.	10			

Comments:

Total Points Earned _____ Divided by _____ Total Possible Points = _____ % Score

Instructor's Signature _____

Student Name _____ Date _____ Score _____

Procedure 21-10 Perform Collection Procedures

Task: To collect the maximum amount of funds on each account.

Equipment and Supplies:
- Patient ledger
- Office policy manual
- Clerical supplies
- Scripts for telephone collections
- Letters for collection efforts
- Telephone
- Letterhead and envelopes
- Copies of claim forms previously filed

Standards: Complete the procedure and all critical steps in _____ minutes with a minimum score of _____% within three attempts.

Scoring: Divide points earned by total possible points. Failure to perform a critical step that is indicated with an asterisk (*) will result in an unsatisfactory overall score.

Time began _____ **Time ended** _____

Steps	Possible Points	First Attempt	Second Attempt	Third Attempt
1. Review office policy as it relates to collection procedures.	10			
2. Evaluate the patient ledger to determine whether it needs collection activity.*	10			
3. Determine the appropriate collection activity for the account.*	10			
4. Telephone the patient or guarantor to initiate a payment on the account.*	10			
5. If the patient or guarantor cannot be reached by phone, send a postcard or collection letter.	10			
6. Send a more demanding collection letter if past efforts by phone or letter have not produced results.*	10			
7. Once all collection efforts have failed, present the account to the physician for further disposition.	10			
8. If approved by the physician, send the account to a collection agency.	10			

Steps	Possible Points	First Attempt	Second Attempt	Third Attempt
9. If further payments arrive on the account, send them directly to the collection agency.	**10**			
10. Document the final collection activity in the patient's medical record.	**10**			

Comments:

Total Points Earned _____ Divided by _____ Total Possible Points = _____ % Score

Instructor's Signature _____

Student Name _____ Date _____ Score _____

Procedure 21-11 Perform Accounts Receivable Procedures: Age Accounts Receivables

Task: To determine the age of accounts and decide what collection activity is needed.

Equipment and Supplies:
• Patient ledger cards with a balance due
• Pen
• Computer
• Calculator

Standards: Complete the procedure and all critical steps in _____ minutes with a minimum score of _____% within three attempts.

Scoring: Divide points earned by total possible points. Failure to perform a critical step that is indicated with an asterisk (*) will result in an unsatisfactory overall score.

Time began _____ Time ended _____

Steps	Possible Points	First Attempt	Second Attempt	Third Attempt
1. Prompt the computer to compile a report on the age of accounts receivable. Many programs will have this report option that can be easily accessed.	10	_____	_____	_____
2. Divide the accounts into categories as listed below: • 0 to 30 days old • 30 to 60 days old • 60 to 90 days old • 90 to 120 days old • over 120 days old	20	_____	_____	_____
3. If the computer program does not perform this function, manually pull all ledger cards that have a balance due and divide them into the categories as listed above.	10	_____	_____	_____
4. Examine the accounts to see which are awaiting an insurance payment. Action need not be taken if an insurance payment is expected and is not long overdue. Return those ledgers to the ledger tray.	10	_____	_____	_____
5. Follow the office procedure for collections on the accounts left. Collection reminder stickers may be placed on the statements sent to the patient, or a collection letter may be sent. Be sure that the stickers are inside the envelope, not on the outside.	10	_____	_____	_____

Steps	Possible Points	First Attempt	Second Attempt	Third Attempt
6. Call patients whose accounts are over 90 days old. Attempt to make payment arrangements with the patient.	10			
7. Send a collection letter to patients whose accounts are over 120 days old, if indicated, to encourage the patient to pay the account. If it is the office policy, mention that the account is in danger of being sent to a collection agency.	10			
8. Add the total accounts receivable for each category and arrive at a figure outstanding for each. The physician may wish to have a report weekly or monthly on these figures.	10			
9. Note any arrangements made with patients regarding payment of the accounts in the chart and/or on the ledger. Send a follow-up letter to remind the patients of their payment agreements.	10			

Comments:

Total Points Earned _____ Divided by _____ Total Possible Points = _____ % Score

Instructor's Signature _____

Procedure 21-12 Post Collection Agency Payments

Task: To post payments received on an account after it has been turned over to a collection agency.

Equipment and Supplies:
- Patient ledger
- Office policy manual
- Bookkeeping system
- Clerical supplies
- Calculator

Standards: Complete the procedure and all critical steps in _____ minutes with a minimum score of _____% within three attempts.

Scoring: Divide points earned by total possible points. Failure to perform a critical step that is indicated with an asterisk (*) will result in an unsatisfactory overall score.

Time began _____ **Time ended** _____

Steps	Possible Points	First Attempt	Second Attempt	Third Attempt
1. Determine that a payment received is for an account that is currently being serviced by a collection agency.	25	_____	_____	_____
2. Notify the collection agency that a payment has been made on the account.*	25	_____	_____	_____
3. Notify the patient that the payment has been forwarded to a collection agency.*	25	_____	_____	_____
4. Instruct the patient to send any future payments to the agency.*	25	_____	_____	_____

Comments:

Total Points Earned _____ Divided by _____ Total Possible Points = _____ % Score

Instructor's Signature _____

Student Name _____ Date _____ Score _____

Procedure 22-1 Write Checks in Payment of Bills

Task: To correctly write checks for payment of bills.

Equipment and Supplies:
• Checkbook
• Bills to be paid

Standards: Complete the procédure and all critical steps in _____ minutes with a minimum score of _____% within three attempts.

Scoring: Divide points earned by total possible points. Failure to perform a critical step that is indicated with an asterisk (*) will result in an unsatisfactory overall score.

Time began _____ **Time ended** _____

Steps	Possible Points	First Attempt	Second Attempt	Third Attempt
1. Locate bill to be paid. Fill out stub first.	10			
2. Complete check and stub with pen or type-writer.	10			
3. Date the check.	10			
4. Write the payee's name on the appropriate line.	10			
5. Leave no space before the name, and follow with three dashes. Omit personal titles.	10			
6. Enter amount correctly and in a manner that prevents alteration.*	20			
7. Verify amount with check stub.	20			
8. Make a notation on the bill that is being paid. Include date and check number. File.	10			

Comments:

Total Points Earned _____ Divided by _____ Total Possible Points = _____ % Score

Instructor's Signature _____

Procedure 22-2 Prepare a Bank Deposit

Task: To prepare a bank deposit for the day's receipts and complete appropriate office records related to the deposit.

Equipment and Supplies:
- Currency
- Six checks for deposit
- Deposit slip
- Endorsement stamp (optional)
- Typewriter
- Envelope

Standards: Complete the procedure and all critical steps in _____ minutes with a minimum score of _____% within three attempts.

Scoring: Divide points earned by total possible points. Failure to perform a critical step that is indicated with an asterisk (*) will result in an unsatisfactory overall score.

Time began _____ **Time ended** _____

Steps	Possible Points	First Attempt	Second Attempt	Third Attempt
1. Organize currency.	10	_____	_____	_____
2. Total the currency, and record the amount on the deposit slip.	10	_____	_____	_____
3. Place restrictive endorsement on checks.*	20	_____	_____	_____
4. List each check separately on the deposit slip by ABA number or patient last name.	20	_____	_____	_____
5. Total the amount of currency and checks, and enter the total on the deposit slip.	10	_____	_____	_____
6. Enter the amount of the deposit in the checkbook.	10	_____	_____	_____
7. Keep a copy of the deposit slip for office records.	10	_____	_____	_____
8. Place currency, checks, and deposit slip in envelope for transport to bank.	10	_____	_____	_____

Comments:

Total Points Earned _____ Divided by _____ Total Possible Points = _____ % Score

Instructor's Signature _____

Student Name _____ Date _____ Score _____

Procedure 22-3 Reconcile a Bank Statement

Task: To reconcile a bank statement with checking account.

Equipment and Supplies:
- Ending balance of previous statement
- Current bank statement
- Cancelled checks for current month
- Checkbook stubs
- Calculator
- Pen

Standards: Complete the procedure and all critical steps in _____ minutes with a minimum score of _____% within three attempts.

Scoring: Divide points earned by total possible points. Failure to perform a critical step that is indicated with an asterisk (*) will result in an unsatisfactory overall score.

Time began _____ **Time ended** _____

Steps	Possible Points	First Attempt	Second Attempt	Third Attempt
1. Compare opening balance of the new statement with the closing balance of previous statement.	10	_____	_____	_____
2. Compare canceled checks with items on statement.	10	_____	_____	_____
3. Arrange checks in numeric order and, compare with stubs.	10	_____	_____	_____
4. Place a checkmark on the matching stub.	10	_____	_____	_____
5. List and total outstanding checks.	10	_____	_____	_____
6. Verify that all previous outstanding checks have cleared.	10	_____	_____	_____
7. Subtract the total of outstanding checks from the statement balance.	10	_____	_____	_____
8. Add to the total in step 7 any deposits made but not included in statement balance.	10	_____	_____	_____
9. Total any bank charges that appear on the bank statement, and subtract them from the checkbook balance.	10	_____	_____	_____
10. If the checkbook and statement do not agree, match bank statement entries with the checkbook entries.	10	_____	_____	_____

Comments:

Total Points Earned _____ Divided by _____ Total Possible Points = _____ % Score

Instructor's Signature _____

Student Name _____ Date _____ Score _____

Procedure 23-1 Account for Petty Cash

Task: To establish a petty cash fund, maintain an accurate record of expenditures for 1 month, and replenish the fund as necessary.

Equipment and Supplies:
- Form for petty cash fund
- Pad of vouchers
- Disbursement journal
- Two checks
- List of petty cash expenditures

Standards: Complete the procedure and all critical steps in _____ minutes with a minimum score of _____% within three attempts.

Scoring: Divide points earned by total possible points. Failure to perform a critical step that is indicated with an asterisk (*) will result in an unsatisfactory overall score.

Time began _____ Time ended _____

Steps	Possible Points	First Attempt	Second Attempt	Third Attempt
1. Determine the amount needed in the petty cash fund.	10			
2. Write a check in the determined amount.	10			
3. Record the beginning balance in the petty cash fund.	10			
4. Post the amount to miscellaneous on the disbursement record.	10			
5. Prepare a petty cash voucher for each amount withdrawn from the fund.	10			
6. Record each voucher in the petty cash record, and enter the new balance.	10			
7. Write a check to replenish the fund as necessary. *Note:* The total of the vouchers plus the fund balance must equal the beginning amount.	10			
8. Total the expense columns, and post to the appropriate accounts in the disbursement record.	10			
9. Record the amount added to the fund.	10			
10. Record the new balance in the petty cash fund.	10			

Comments:

Total Points Earned _____ Divided by _____ Total Possible Points = _____ % Score

Instructor's Signature _____

Student Name _____ Date _____ Score _____

Procedure 23-2 Process an Employee Payroll

Task: To process payroll and compensate employees, making deductions accurately.

Equipment and Supplies:
- Checkbook
- Computer and payroll software, if applicable
- Pen
- Tax withholding tables
- Federal employers tax guide

Standards: Complete the procedure and all critical steps in _____ minutes with a minimum score of _____% within three attempts.

Scoring: Divide points earned by total possible points. Failure to perform a critical step that is indicated with an asterisk (*) will result in an unsatisfactory overall score.

Time began _____ **Time ended** _____

Steps	Possible Points	First Attempt	Second Attempt	Third Attempt
1. Be sure that all information has been collected on the employees, including a copy of the social security card, a W-4 form, and an I-9 form.	20	___	___	___
2. Review the time cards for all employees. Determine if any employees need counseling because of late arrivals or habitual absences.	20	___	___	___
3. Figure the salary or hourly wages that are due the employee for the period worked.	20	___	___	___
4. Figure the deductions that must be taken from the paycheck. These usually include, but are not limited to, the following: • Federal, state, and local taxes • Social Security withholdings • Medicare withholdings • Other deductions, such as insurance, savings, etc. • Donations to organizations, such as the United Way	20	___	___	___
5. Write the check for the balance due the employee. Most software can print the checks and explanations of deductions.	20	___	___	___

Comments:

Total Points Earned _____ Divided by _____ Total Possible Points = _____ % Score

Instructor's Signature _____

Procedure 24-1 Interview a Job Candidate

Task: To evaluate job candidates fairly and choose the best person to fill an available position in the medical facility.

Equipment and Supplies:
- Candidate's completed job application
- Candidate's resume
- Private area in the medical office
- Clerical supplies

Standards: Complete the procedure and all critical steps in _____ minutes with a minimum score of _____% within three attempts.

Scoring: Divide points earned by total possible points. Failure to perform a critical step that is indicated with an asterisk (*) will result in an unsatisfactory overall score.

Time began _____ **Time ended** _____

Steps	Possible Points	First Attempt	Second Attempt	Third Attempt
1. Review the job requirements that the candidate will be required to perform.	5			
2. Match each job application with the corresponding resume	5			
3. Separate strong candidates from moderate candidates and weak candidates.*	5			
3. Review each resume and job application again and determine which candidates should be brought to the office for an interview.*	5			
4. Call each candidate, and schedule an appointment for an interview.	2			
5. Evaluate the applicant's speaking voice while making the appointment for the interview.*	5			
6. Select several interview questions in advance to ask all of the applicants.	2			
7. Note whether the applicant arrives on time for the interview.*	5			
8. Introduce yourself to the applicant, and proceed to a private area to conduct the interview.	5			

Steps	Possible Points	First Attempt	Second Attempt	Third Attempt
9. Make the applicant feel as much at ease as possible.*	5			
10. Ask the applicant the chosen questions.	2			
11. Evaluate the answers, and make notations about the candidate that are not demeaning or unprofessional.	5			
12. Ask the candidate if he or she has any questions.	5			
13. Offer strong candidates a brief tour of the facility.	2			
14. Provide a date by which a hiring decision will be made, and suggest that the candidate call the facility that day, if desired.	2			
15. Evaluate all applicants fairly according to their experience and training.	5			
16. Select the best three candidates, and call them for a second interview, if desired.*	5			
17. Discuss the final hiring decisions with the physician or others with influence.	5			
18. Make the final hiring decision.	5			
19. Call the candidate to ask him or her to come to the office to discuss the position.	5			
20. Negotiate salary and benefits.*	5			
21. Offer the position.	5			
22. If the offer is declined, call the next candidate to the office to discuss the position; repeat until a satisfactory candidate accepts and agrees to a start date.	5			

Comments:

Total Points Earned _____ Divided by _____ Total Possible Points = _____ % Score

Instructor's Signature _____

Procedure 24-2 Conduct a Performance Review

Task: To evaluate job performance fairly and determine the strengths and weaknesses of employees.

Equipment and Supplies:
- Employee's file
- Past evaluations of employee
- Notes and/or reports regarding employee behavior
- Private area in the medical office
- Clerical supplies

Standards: Complete the procedure and all critical steps in _____ minutes with a minimum score of _____% within three attempts.

Scoring: Divide points earned by total possible points. Failure to perform a critical step that is indicated with an asterisk (*) will result in an unsatisfactory overall score.

Time began _____ **Time ended** _____

Steps	Possible Points	First Attempt	Second Attempt	Third Attempt
1. Set an appointment with the employee to conduct the review.	10	_____	_____	_____
2. Allow the employee to complete a self-evaluation of his or her own work.	10	_____	_____	_____
3. Review the self-evaluation, then document additional information about the employee and his or her performance.*	15	_____	_____	_____
4. Share the information with any other supervisor or the physician, if dictated by office policy or if needed for additional input.	10	_____	_____	_____
5. Complete the final written review and proofread it for accuracy and completeness.*	10	_____	_____	_____
6. Discuss the review with the employee during the evaluation appointment.	10	_____	_____	_____
7. Progress through the interview, and explain the results of the evaluation to the employee.*	10	_____	_____	_____
8. Allow the employee to respond to any of the points raised during the evaluation, but do not allow an argumentative attitude.	5	_____	_____	_____
9. Allow the employee to respond in writing to the evaluation for a limited time, such as 5 days.	5	_____	_____	_____

Steps	Possible Points	First Attempt	Second Attempt	Third Attempt
10. Ask the employee to sign the evaluation to document that it was reviewed with him or her. (The employee does not have to agree with the evaluation to sign it.)	5			
11. Give a copy of the evaluation to the employee.	5			
12. File the evaluation in the employee's file.	5			

Comments:

Total Points Earned _____ Divided by _____ Total Possible Points = _____ % Score

Instructor's Signature _____

Student Name _____ Date _____ Score _____

Procedure 24-3 Arrange a Group Meeting

Task: To plan and execute a productive meeting that will result in achieved goals.

Equipment and Supplies:
• Meeting room
• Agenda
• Visual aids and equipment
• Handouts
• Stopwatch or clock
• Computer or word processor
• Paper
• List of items for the agenda

Standards: Complete the procedure and all critical steps in _____ minutes with a minimum score of _____% within three attempts.

Scoring: Divide points earned by total possible points. Failure to perform a critical step that is indicated with an asterisk (*) will result in an unsatisfactory overall score.

Time began _____ Time ended _____

Steps	Possible Points	First Attempt	Second Attempt	Third Attempt
1. Determine the purpose of the meeting, and draft a list of the items to be discussed. Include the desired results of the meeting.	10	_____	_____	_____
2. Determine where the meeting will be held, the time and date of the meeting, and the individuals who should attend.	10	_____	_____	_____
3. Send a memo, email, or letter to the individuals who should attend the meeting at least 10 days in advance, if possible. Send a copy to any supervisors who should be kept informed about the issues to be raised in the meeting.	10	_____	_____	_____
4. Be sure that the notice includes the following information: • Date • Time • Place • Directions, if not in a common meeting room or if away from the office • Speakers and/or meeting topics • Cost and registration information, if applicable • List of items individuals should bring to the meeting	10	_____	_____	_____

Steps	Possible Points	First Attempt	Second Attempt	Third Attempt
5. Finalize the list of items to discuss, and place them in priority order.	10			
6. Delegate any tasks that others can accomplish, and follow up to be sure that they fulfill their duties before the meeting.	10			
7. Assign a staff member the task of taking notes and keeping time during the meeting.	10			
8. Make a list of all items that need to be taken to the meeting, including equipment such as microphones, projectors, screens, computers, disks containing presentations, etc.	10			
9. Compile the final agenda for the meeting.	10			
10. On the meeting day, transport all items needed to the meeting room. Begin and end the meeting on time. Stay on track, and follow the agenda.	10			

Comments:

Total Points Earned _____ Divided by _____ Total Possible Points = _____ % Score

Instructor's Signature _____

Student Name _____ Date _____ Score _____

Procedure 25-1 Design a Presentation

Task: To gain skill in designing presentations that can be used for a variety of projects in the medical facility.

Equipment and Supplies:
- Information about presentation subject
- Software, such as PowerPoint, if needed
- Computer access
- Peripheral computer equipment, if needed

Standards: Complete the procedure and all critical steps in _____ minutes with a minimum score of _____% within three attempts.

Scoring: Divide points earned by total possible points. Failure to perform a critical step that is indicated with an asterisk (*) will result in an unsatisfactory overall score.

Time began _____ **Time ended** _____

Steps	Possible Points	First Attempt	Second Attempt	Third Attempt
1. Determine the goals of the presentation.*	10	_____	_____	_____
2. Write an outline of the entire presentation.	10	_____	_____	_____
3. Build the presentation using software, such as PowerPoint, highlighting the major points of the presentation.	5	_____	_____	_____
4. Evaluate the audience and adjust the presentation to appeal to that audience.*	10	_____	_____	_____
5. Rehearse the presentation several times in front of a mirror.	10	_____	_____	_____
6. Make a list of all equipment and materials to take to the presentation.	5	_____	_____	_____
7. Arrive for the presentation 15 to 30 minutes early, depending on the preparation and setup required.*	10	_____	_____	_____
8. Deliver the presentation within the prescribed time period.	10	_____	_____	_____
9. Ask the audience if they have any questions about the information in the presentation.	10	_____	_____	_____
10. Thank the audience, and remove all equipment and supplies when appropriate.	10	_____	_____	_____

Steps	Possible Points	First Attempt	Second Attempt	Third Attempt
11. Send a thank-you to the organization for allowing the presentation, if appropriate.	**10**			

Comments:

Total Points Earned _____ Divided by _____ Total Possible Points = _____ % Score

Instructor's Signature _____

Student Name _____ Date _____ Score _____

Procedure 25-2 Prepare a Presentation Using PowerPoint

Task: To enhance presentations using PowerPoint as a visual aid.

Equipment and Supplies:
- Information about presentation subject
- Software, such as PowerPoint, if needed
- Computer access
- Peripheral computer equipment, if needed

Standards: Complete the procedure and all critical steps in _____ minutes with a minimum score of _____% within three attempts.

Scoring: Divide points earned by total possible points. Failure to perform a critical step that is indicated with an asterisk (*) will result in an unsatisfactory overall score.

Time began _____ Time ended _____

Steps	Possible Points	First Attempt	Second Attempt	Third Attempt
1. Open the PowerPoint program.	5			
2. Have the outline of the presentation available.	5			
3. Click on the "new slide" icon on the program menu.	5			
4. Create the title slide using the slide layout section on the right side of the screen.	5			
5. Create additional slides using the slide layout section, or design the slides manually.	5			
6. Limit the number of words on the slides so that a concise message results.*	5			
7. Make certain that the font is as large as possible on the slide, beginning with a size 18 font and increasing from there.	5			
8. Do not use more than three fonts per slide.*	5			
9. Avoid using more than three text-only slides in a row.*	5			
10. Insert photos or clip art into the presentation by clicking on "Insert," then on "Picture," then choosing "Clip art" or "From file."	5			

749

Steps	Possible Points	First Attempt	Second Attempt	Third Attempt
11. Format the background of each slide, or of all slides, by clicking on "Format", then "Background," then choosing a color or fill effect.	5			
12. Click on "Slide show" and adjust the slide transitions so that the slides appear and disappear as desired and are timed correctly.	5			
13. Click on "Custom animation" to change the entrance and exit of the slides to the effect that is desired.	5			
14. Save the presentation frequently while working on it.*	5			
15. Click on "View" in the task bar, then on "Slide sorter," which will allow moving the slides around in the presentation.	5			
16. To run the show continuously, click on "Slide show", then on "Set up show", and then click in the box labeled "Loop continuously until escape" in the show options box.	5			
17. Make certain the presentation has been saved.	5			
18. Practice giving the presentation several times to smooth all transitions and to be familiar with the content.*	5			
19. Anticipate questions that the audience may ask, and have answers prepared.*	5			
20. Offer other visual aids, such as handouts, if appropriate, when giving the presentation.	5			

Comments:

Total Points Earned _____ Divided by _____ Total Possible Points = _____ % Score

Instructor's Signature _____

Student Name _____ Date _____ Score _____

Procedure 26-1 Use Standard Precautions for Removing Contaminated Gloves and Disposal of Biohazardous Material

Task: To minimize pathogen exposure by aseptically removing and discarding contaminated gloves.

Equipment and Supplies:
- Latex examination gloves
- Biohazard waste container with labeled red biohazard bag

Standards: Complete the procedure and all critical steps in _____ minutes with a minimum score of _____% within three attempts.

Scoring: Divide points earned by total possible points. Failure to perform a critical step that is indicated with an asterisk (*) will result in an unsatisfactory overall score.

Time began _____ **Time ended** _____

Steps	Possible Points	First Attempt	Second Attempt	Third Attempt
1. With the dominant hand, grasp the glove of the opposite hand near the palm and begin removing the first glove. Arms should be extended from the body, with hands pointed down.	10	_____	_____	_____
2. Pull the glove inside out until you reach the fingers, holding the contaminated glove in the dominant gloved hand.	10	_____	_____	_____
3. Insert the thumb of the nongloved hand inside the cuff of the remaining contaminated glove. Pull the glove down the hand inside out over the contaminated glove being held, leaving the contaminated side of both gloves on the inside.	10	_____	_____	_____
4. Properly dispose of the inside-out contaminated gloves in a biohazard waste container.	10	_____	_____	_____
5. Perform a medical aseptic hand wash as described in Procedure 26-2.	10	_____	_____	_____

Comments:

Total Points Earned _____ Divided by _____ Total Possible Points = _____ % Score

Instructor's Signature _____

Procedure 26-2 Perform Medical Aseptic Hand Washing

Task: To minimize the number of pathogens on your hands, thus reducing the risk of pathogenic transmission.

Equipment and Supplies:
- Sink with running water
- Antimicrobial liquid soap in a dispenser (bar soap is not acceptable)
- Nail brush or orange stick
- Paper towels in a dispenser
- Water-based antimicrobial lotion
- Biohazard waste container with labeled red biohazard bag

Standards: Complete the procedure and all critical steps in _____ minutes with a minimum score of _____% within three attempts.

Scoring: Divide points earned by total possible points. Failure to perform a critical step that is indicated with an asterisk (*) will result in an unsatisfactory overall score.

Time began _____ **Time ended** _____

Steps	Possible Points	First Attempt	Second Attempt	Third Attempt
1. Remove all jewelry except your wristwatch, which should be pulled up above your wrist or removed, and a plain gold wedding ring.	10	_____	_____	_____
2. Turn on the faucet with a paper towel and regulate the water temperature to lukewarm.	10	_____	_____	_____
3. Allow your hands to become wet, apply soap, and lather using a circular motion with friction while holding your fingertips downward. Rub well between your fingers.	10	_____	_____	_____
If this is the first hand washing of the day, use a nail brush or an orange stick and thoroughly inspect and clean under every fingernail during step 3.	10	_____	_____	_____
4. Rinse well, holding your hands so that the water flows from your wrists downward to your fingertips.	10	_____	_____	_____
5. Wet your hands again and repeat the scrubbing procedure using a vigorous, circular motion over wrists and hands for at least 1 to 2 minutes.	10	_____	_____	_____

Steps	Possible Points	First Attempt	Second Attempt	Third Attempt
6. Rinse your hands a second time, keeping fingers lower than your wrists.	10	_____	_____	_____
7. Dry your hands with paper towels. Do not touch the paper towel dispenser as you are obtaining towels.	10	_____	_____	_____
8. If faucets are not foot operated, turn off the water faucet with the paper towel.*	10	_____	_____	_____
9. After completion of drying your hands and turning off faucets, place used towels into a biohazard waste container.	10	_____	_____	_____
10. Apply a water-based antibacterial hand lotion to prevent chapped or dry skin.	10	_____	_____	_____

Comments:

Total Points Earned _____ Divided by _____ Total Possible Points = _____ % Score

Instructor's Signature _____

Student Name _____ Date _____ Score _____

Procedure 26-3 Use Standard Precautions for Sanitizing Instruments and Disposal of Biohazardous Material

Task: Following standard precautions, remove all contaminated matter from instruments in preparation for disinfection or sterilization.

Equipment and Supplies:
- Sink with hot running water
- Sanitizing agent or low-sudsing soap with enzymatic action
- Utility gloves that are decontaminated and show no signs of deterioration
- Chin-length face shield or goggles and face mask if contamination with droplets of bloodborne pathogens is possible
- Disposable brush
- Disposable paper towels
- Disposable gloves
- Disinfectant cleaner
- Biohazard waste container with labeled red biohazard bag

Standards: Complete the procedure and all critical steps in _____ minutes with a minimum score of _____% within three attempts.

Scoring: Divide points earned by total possible points. Failure to perform a critical step that is indicated with an asterisk (*) will result in an unsatisfactory overall score.

Time began _____ **Time ended** _____

Steps	Possible Points	First Attempt	Second Attempt	Third Attempt
1. Put on utility gloves.	5			
2. Put on face shield or goggles and mask if potential for splashing of infectious material exists.	10			
3. Separate sharp instruments from other instruments to be sanitized.	10			
4. Rinse the instruments under cold running water.	10			
5. Open hinged instruments and scrub all grooves, crevices, and serrations with a disposable brush.	10			
6. Rinse well with hot water.	10			

Steps	Possible Points	First Attempt	Second Attempt	Third Attempt
7. Towel dry all instruments thoroughly, and dispose of contaminated towels and disposable brush in a biohazard waste container. Do not touch the paper towel dispenser as you are obtaining towels.	10			
8. Remove utility gloves and wash hands according to Procedure 26-2.	10			
9. Towel dry your hands, and apply disposable gloves. Decontaminate utility gloves and work surfaces using disinfectant cleaner. Dispose of contaminated towels in a biohazard waste container.	10			
10. Remove disposable gloves according to Procedure 26-1. Dispose of gloves in a biohazard waste container. Wash hands according to Procedure 26-2.	10			
11. Towel dry your hands and place sanitized instruments in designated area for disinfection or sterilization.	10			

Comments:

Total Points Earned _____ Divided by _____ Total Possible Points = _____ % Score

Instructor's Signature _____

Student Name _____ Date _____ Score _____

Procedure 27-1 Obtain and Record a Patient History

Complete this procedure with another student role-playing the patient. To make the experience more realistic, choose a student about whom you know very little. To maintain the privacy of your student partner, he or she does not have to share any confidential information while participating in the role-play.

Task: To obtain an acceptable written background from the patient to help the physician determine the cause and effects of the present illness. This includes the chief complaint (CC), present illness (PI), past history (PH), family history (FH), and social history (SH).

Equipment and Supplies:
- History form
- Two pens—a red pen for recording patient allergies and a black pen to meet legal documentation guidelines
- A quiet, private area

Standards: Complete the procedure and all critical steps in _____ minutes with a minimum score of _____% within three attempts.

Scoring: Divide points earned by total possible points. Failure to perform a critical step that is indicated with an asterisk (*) will result in an unsatisfactory overall score.

Time began _____ Time ended _____

Steps	Possible Points	First Attempt	Second Attempt	Third Attempt
1. Greet and identify the patient in a pleasant manner. Introduce yourself and explain your role.	10	_____	_____	_____
2. Take the patient to a quiet, private area for the interview, and explain to the patient why the information is needed.	10	_____	_____	_____
3. Complete the history form by using therapeutic communication techniques. Make sure that all medical terminology is adequately explained. A self-history may have been mailed to the patient before the visit. If so, review the self-history for completeness.	10	_____	_____	_____
4. Speak in a pleasant, distinct manner, remembering to maintain eye contact with your patient.	10	_____	_____	_____

Steps	Possible Points	First Attempt	Second Attempt	Third Attempt
Attempt				

5. Record the following statistical information on the patient information form: **10**
   - Patient's full name, including middle initial
   - Address, including apartment number and ZIP code
   - Marital status
   - Sex (gender)
   - Age and date of birth
   - Telephone number for home and work
   - Insurance information if not already available
   - Employer's name, address, telephone number

6. Record the following medical history on the patient history (PH) form: **10**

   Chief complaint (CC)   Family history

   Present illness   Social history

   Past history

7. Ask about allergies to drugs and any other substances, and record any allergies in red ink on every page of the history form, on the front of the chart, and on each progress note page. Some practices apply allergy alert labels to the front of each chart.   **10**

8. Record all information legibly and neatly, and spell words correctly. Print rather than writing in longhand. Do not erase, scribble, or use whiteout. If you make an error, draw a single line through the error, write "error" above it, add the correction, and initial and date the entry.   **10**

9. Thank the patient for cooperating, and direct him or her back to the reception area.   **10**

10. Review the record for errors before you pass it to the physician. Use the information on the record to complete the patient's chart. Keep the information confidential.   **10**

Documentation

Your patient's CC is dizziness for 2 weeks. He denies having headaches and has no previous Hx of ear infections or hypertension. He doesn't take any prescribed medications but uses Tylenol as needed for a headache. T 97.6, P 88, R 22, BP 172/94. Document pertinent patient findings using the SOAPE method.

S: _____

O: _____

Comments:

Total Points Earned _____ Divided by _____ Total Possible Points = _____ % Score

Instructor's Signature _____

Student Name _____ Date _____ Score _____

Procedure 29-1 Provide Instruction for Health Maintenance and Disease Prevention: Teach the Patient to Read Food Labels

Task: To accurately explain the nutritional labeling of food products to the patient.

Equipment and Supplies:
- One each of three bars: Snickers candy bar, granola bar, fat-free fruit bar
- Pencil and paper

Standards: Complete the procedure and all critical steps in _____ minutes with a minimum score of _____% within three attempts.

Scoring: Divide points earned by total possible points. Failure to perform a critical step that is indicated with an asterisk (*) will result in an unsatisfactory overall score.

Time began _____ Time ended _____

Steps	Possible Points	First Attempt	Second Attempt	Third Attempt
1. Explain to the patient that you are going to teach him or her how to read a food label. Be sure to include reasons why food labels are a valuable source of nutritional information in diet planning.	10			
2. Using the labels on each bar, point out the nutritional information according to the guidelines in the text.	10			
3. Give the patient the pencil and paper to write down the serving size of each type of bar.	10			
4. Compare similarities and differences.	10			
5. Have the patient write down the total caloric amount for each product serving.	10			
6. Compare similarities and differences.	10			
7. Write down the percentage of total, saturated, trans, and unsaturated fats.	10			
8. Compare similarities and differences.	10			
9. Together, analyze the nutritional level of each.	10			

Steps	Possible Points	First Attempt	Second Attempt	Third Attempt
10. Discuss any new information that was learned.	5			
11. Ask the patient if he or she will use this information when shopping and how it will be implemented in nutritional planning.	5			

Comments:

Total Points Earned _____ Divided by _____ Total Possible Points = _____ % Score

Instructor's Signature _____

Student Name _____ Date _____ Score _____

Procedure 30-1 Obtain Vital Signs: Obtain an Oral Temperature Using a Digital Thermometer

Task: To accurately determine and record a patient's temperature using a digital thermometer.

Equipment and Supplies:
- Digital thermometer
- Probe covers
- Biohazard waste container
- Disposable gloves as appropriate

Standards: Complete the procedure and all critical steps in _____ minutes with a minimum score of _____% within three attempts.

Scoring: Divide points earned by total possible points. Failure to perform a critical step that is indicated with an asterisk (*) will result in an unsatisfactory overall score.

Time began _____ **Time ended** _____

Steps	Possible Points	First Attempt	Second Attempt	Third Attempt
1. Wash your hands and assemble equipment and supplies.	10			
2. Identify your patient and explain the procedure. Be sure that the patient has not eaten, consumed any hot or cold fluids, smoked, or exercised during the 30 minutes before the temperature is measured.*	20			
3. Prepare the probe for use as described in package directions. Make certain probe covers are always used.	10			
4. Place the probe under the patient's tongue, and instruct the patient to close the mouth tightly. Assist the patient by holding the probe end.	10			
5. When the "beep" is heard, remove the probe from the patient's mouth and immediately eject the probe cover into the appropriate waste container.*	10			
6. Note the reading in the LED window of the processing unit you are holding.	10			
7. Record the reading on the patient's medical record (e.g., T = 97.7°).*	20			
8. Wash your hands, and disinfect the equipment as indicated.	10			

Documentation in the Medical Record

A 55-year-old patient arrives today complaining of cough and congestion for 5 days. She states that she has had a fever of 100.7° F for 2 days at home. She is not taking any medication currently and is allergic to Amoxil. Obtain an oral temperature and document the case below using SOAPE format.

S: _____

O: _____

Comments:

Total Points Earned _____ Divided by _____ Total Possible Points = _____ % Score

Instructor's Signature _____

Student Name _____ Date _____ Score _____

Procedure 30-2 Obtain Vital Signs: Obtain an Aural Temperature Using the Tympanic Thermometer

Task: To accurately determine and record a patient's temperature using a tympanic thermometer.

Equipment and Supplies:
- Tympanic thermometer
- Disposable probe covers
- Biohazard waste container
- Disposable gloves as appropriate

Standards: Complete the procedure and all critical steps in _____ minutes with a minimum score of _____% within three attempts.

Scoring: Divide points earned by total possible points. Failure to perform a critical step that is indicated with an asterisk (*) will result in an unsatisfactory overall score.

Time began _____ **Time ended** _____

Steps	Possible Points	First Attempt	Second Attempt	Third Attempt
1. Wash your hands.	10	_____	_____	_____
2. Gather the necessary equipment and supplies.	10	_____	_____	_____
3. Identify your patient and explain the procedure.	20	_____	_____	_____
4. Place a disposable cover on the probe.	10	_____	_____	_____
5. Follow the package directions to start the thermometer.	10	_____	_____	_____
6. Insert the probe into the ear canal far enough to seal the opening. Do not apply pressure. For children under the age of 3, gently pull the ear lobe down and back; for patients over the age of 3, gently pull the top of the ear up and back.	10	_____	_____	_____
7. Press the button on the probe as directed. The temperature will be on the display screen in 1 to 2 seconds. Remove the probe, note the reading, and discard the probe cover without touching it.	10	_____	_____	_____
8. Wash your hands and disinfect the equipment if indicated.	10	_____	_____	_____
9. Record the temperature results (e.g., T = 98.6°[T]) on the patient's medical record.*	10	_____	_____	_____

Documentation in the Medical Record

A 3-year-old patient complains of a rash on the left forearm for 3 days. The patient is not allergic to any medication and does not take any medications daily. Obtain an aural temperature and document the case using SOAPE format.

S: _____

O: _____

Comments:

Total Points Earned _____ Divided by _____ Total Possible Points = _____ % Score

Instructor's Signature _____

Student Name _____ Date _____ Score _____

Procedure 30-3 Obtain Vital Signs: Obtain an Axillary Temperature

Task: To accurately determine and record a patient's temperature using the axillary method.

Equipment and Supplies:
- Digital unit
- Thermometer sheath or probe cover
- Supply of tissues
- Biohazard waste container
- Disposable gloves as appropriate

Standards: Complete the procedure and all critical steps in _____ minutes with a minimum score of _____% within three attempts.

Scoring: Divide points earned by total possible points. Failure to perform a critical step that is indicated with an asterisk (*) will result in an unsatisfactory overall score.

Time began _____ **Time ended** _____

Steps	Possible Points	First Attempt	Second Attempt	Third Attempt
1. Wash your hands.	10			
2. Gather equipment and supplies.	10			
3. Introduce yourself, identify your patient, and explain the procedure.*	20			
4. Prepare the thermometer or digital unit in same manner as for oral use.	10			
5. Remove the patient's clothing, and gown the patient as needed to access the axillary region. Pat the patient's axillary area dry if needed.	10			
6. Cover the thermometer or probe, and place the tip into the center of the armpit, pointing the stem toward the upper chest, making sure the thermometer is touching only skin, not clothing.*	10			
7. Instruct the patient to hold the arm snugly across the chest or abdomen until the thermometer beeps.	10			
8. Remove the thermometer, note the digital reading, and dispose of the cover in the biohazard waste container.	10			

Steps	Possible Points	First Attempt	Second Attempt	Third Attempt
9. Disinfect the thermometer if indicated.	10			
10. Wash your hands.	10			
11. Record the axillary temperature on the patient's medical record (e.g., T = 97.6° [A]).*	10			

Documentation in the Medical Record

A 7-month-old patient is brought to the office today. The child's mother states the baby has been "pulling" at the left ear for 2 days. Mother relays a lack of appetite for the patient. The mother also states that she does not have a thermometer at home, so she is unsure if the child has had a fever. Obtain an axillary temperature and document your finding using SOAPE format.

S: _____

O: _____

Comments:

Total Points Earned _____ Divided by _____ Total Possible Points = _____ % Score

Instructor's Signature _____

Student Name _____ Date _____ Score _____

Procedure 30-4 Obtain Vital Signs: Obtain an Apical Pulse

Task: To assess the patient's apical heart rate.

Equipment and Supplies:
• Watch with a second hand
• Stethoscope
• Alcohol wipes
• Patient gown

Standards: Complete the procedure and all critical steps in _____ minutes with a minimum score of _____% within three attempts.

Scoring: Divide points earned by total possible points. Failure to perform a critical step that is indicated with an asterisk (*) will result in an unsatisfactory overall score.

Time began _____ Time ended _____

Steps	Possible Points	First Attempt	Second Attempt	Third Attempt
1. Wash your hands, and clean the stethoscope earpieces and diaphragm with alcohol swabs.	10			
2. Introduce yourself, identify your patient, and explain the procedure.*	20			
3. If necessary, assist the patient in disrobing from the waist up and provide the patient with a gown, open in the front.	10			
4. Assist the patient to the sitting or supine position.	10			
5. Hold the stethoscope diaphragm against the palm of your hand for a few seconds.	10			
6. Place the stethoscope just below the left nipple in the intercostal space between the fifth and sixth ribs over the apex of the heart.	10			
7. Listen carefully for the heartbeat. Count the pulse for 1 full minute. Note any irregularities in rhythm and volume.*	10			
8. Assist the patient to sit up and dress.	5			
9. Wash your hands.	10			
10. Record the pulse in the patient chart as AP (e.g., AP = 96), and record any arrhythmias.*	10			

Documentation in the Medical Record

A patient comes to the office today complaining of left lower quadrant abdominal pain for 3 weeks. The patient also complains of nausea after eating. The patient denies any constipation or diarrhea. Obtain an apical pulse and document the case using SOAPE format.

S: _____

O: _____

Comments:

Total Points Earned _____ Divided by _____ Total Possible Points = _____ % Score

Instructor's Signature _____

Procedure 30-5 Obtain Vital Signs: Assess the Patient's Radial Pulse

Task: To determine and record a patient's pulse rate, rhythm, volume, and vessel elasticity.

Equipment and Supplies:
• Watch with a second hand

Standards: Complete the procedure and all critical steps in _____ minutes with a minimum score of _____% within three attempts.

Scoring: Divide points earned by total possible points. Failure to perform a critical step that is indicated with an asterisk (*) will result in an unsatisfactory overall score.

Time began _____ **Time ended** _____

Steps	Possible Points	First Attempt	Second Attempt	Third Attempt
1. Wash your hands.	10	_____	_____	_____
2. Introduce yourself, identify your patient, and explain the procedure.*	10	_____	_____	_____
3. Place the patient's arm in a relaxed position, palm downward.	10	_____	_____	_____
4. Gently grasp the palm side of the patient's wrist with your first three fingertips approximately 1 inch below the base of the thumb.	20	_____	_____	_____
5. Count the beats for 1 full minute, using a watch with a second hand.*	20	_____	_____	_____
6. Wash your hands.	10	_____	_____	_____
7. Record the count and any irregularities on the patient's medical record (e.g., P = 72).	20	_____	_____	_____

Documentation in the Medical Record

A 32-year-old patient arrives today to follow up on her diabetes medication. She has no other complaints. Obtain a pulse, and document the finding using SOAPE format.

S: _____

O: _____

Comments:

Total Points Earned _____ Divided by _____ Total Possible Points = _____ % Score

Instructor's Signature _____

Procedure 30-6 Obtain Vital Signs: Determine Respirations

Task: To determine and record a patient's respirations. Remember that the respiration count may be altered if the patient is aware that you are counting his or her breaths. Respirations are typically counted immediately after taking the pulse while fingers are still at the radial site.

Equipment and Supplies:
• Watch with a second hand

Standards: Complete the procedure and all critical steps in _____ minutes with a minimum score of _____% within three attempts.

Scoring: Divide points earned by total possible points. Failure to perform a critical step that is indicated with an asterisk (*) will result in an unsatisfactory overall score.

Time began _____ **Time ended** _____

Steps	Possible Points	First Attempt	Second Attempt	Third Attempt
1. Wash your hands.	10	_____	_____	_____
2. Identify your patient.	5	_____	_____	_____
3. The patient's arm will be in the same position as when counting the pulse. If having difficulty noticing breathing, place the arm across the chest to pick up movement.	10	_____	_____	_____
4. Note the rise and fall of the patient's chest.*	20	_____	_____	_____
5. Count the respirations for 30 seconds, using a watch with a second hand, and multiply by 2.	10	_____	_____	_____
6. Release the patient's wrist.	5	_____	_____	_____
7. Wash your hands.	10	_____	_____	_____
8. Record the respirations on the patient's medical record after the pulse recording (e.g., R = 18).*	10	_____	_____	_____

Documentation in the Medical Record

A 32-year-old patient arrives today to follow up on her blood pressure medication. She has no other complaints. Obtain respirations, and document the finding using SOAPE format.

S: _____

O: _____

Comments:

Total Points Earned _____ Divided by _____ Total Possible Points = _____ % Score

Instructor's Signature _____

Student Name _____ Date _____ Score _____

Procedure 30-7 Obtain Vital Signs: Determine a Patient's Blood Pressure

Task: To perform a blood pressure measurement that is correct in technique, accurate, and comfortable for the patient.

Equipment and Supplies:
- Sphygmomanometer
- Stethoscope
- Antiseptic wipes

Standards: Complete the procedure and all critical steps in _____ minutes with a minimum score of _____ % within three attempts.

Scoring: Divide points earned by total possible points. Failure to perform a critical step that is indicated with an asterisk (∗) will result in an unsatisfactory overall score.

Time began _____ Time ended _____

Steps	Possible Points	First Attempt	Second Attempt	Third Attempt
1. Wash your hands.	10			
2. Assemble the equipment and supplies needed. Clean the earpieces and diaphragm of the stethoscope with alcohol swabs.	10			
3. Introduce yourself, identify the patient, and explain the procedure.∗	20			
4. Select the appropriate arm for application of the cuff (no mastectomy on that side, without injury or disease).	10			
5. Seat the patient in a comfortable position with legs uncrossed and the arm resting at heart level on the lap or a table with the palm upward.	10			
6. Roll up the sleeve to about 5 inches above the elbow, or have the patient remove his or her arm from the sleeve.	10			
7. Determine the correct cuff size.∗	10			
8. Palpate the brachial artery at the antecubital space in both arms. If one arm has a stronger pulse, use that arm. If the pulses are equal, select the right arm.	10			

Steps	Possible Points	First Attempt	Second Attempt	Third Attempt
9. Center the cuff bladder over the brachial artery, with the connecting tube away from the patient's body and the tube to the bulb close to the body.	10			
10. Place the lower edge of the cuff about 1 inch above the palpable brachial pulse, normally located in the natural crease of the inner elbow, and wrap it snugly and smoothly.*	10			
11. Position the gauge of the sphygmo-manometer so that it is easily seen.	10			
12. Palpate the brachial pulse, tighten the screw valve on the air pump, and inflate the cuff until the pulse can no longer be felt. Make a note at the point on the gauge where the pulse could no longer be felt. Mentally add 30 mm Hg to the reading. Deflate the cuff, and wait for 15 seconds.	10			
13. Insert the earpieces of the stethoscope turned forward into the ear canals.	10			
14. Place the stethoscope bell or diaphragm over the palpated brachial artery firmly enough to obtain a seal, but not so tightly that you constrict the artery.	10			
15. Close the valve, and squeeze the bulb to inflate the cuff at a rapid but smooth rate to 30 mm above the palpated pulse level, which was previously determined.	10			
16. Open the valve slightly, and deflate the cuff at the constant rate of 2 to 3 mm Hg per heartbeat.*	10			
17. Listen throughout the entire deflation; note the point on the gauge at which you hear the first sound (systolic) and the last sound (diastolic) until the sounds have stopped for at least 10 mm Hg. Read the pressure to the closest even number. Do not reinflate the cuff once the air has been released. Wait 30 to 60 seconds to repeat the procedure if needed.	10			
18. Remove the stethoscope from your ears, and record the systolic and diastolic readings as BP systolic/diastolic (e.g., BP 120/80).	10			

Steps	Possible Points	First Attempt	Second Attempt	Third Attempt
19. Remove the cuff from the patient's arm and return it to its proper storage area. Clean the earpieces of the stethoscope with alcohol and return it to storage.	10	_____	_____	_____
20. Wash your hands.	10	_____	_____	_____

Documentation in the Medical Record

A 32-year-old patient arrives today to follow up on her blood pressure medication. She has no other complaints. She states she has stopped taking her Diovan 80 mg because of lack of prescription coverage. Obtain the blood pressure, and document the finding using SOAPE format.

S: _____

O: _____

Comments:

Total Points Earned _____ Divided by _____ Total Possible Points = _____ % Score

Instructor's Signature _____

Procedure 30-8 Obtain Vital Signs: Measure a Patient's Weight and Height

Task: To accurately weigh and measure a patient as part of the physical assessment procedure.

Note: Be sure the scale is located in an area away from traffic to maintain patient privacy.

Equipment and Supplies:
• Balance scale with a measuring bar

Standards: Complete the procedure and all critical steps in _____ minutes with a minimum score of _____% within three attempts.

Scoring: Divide points earned by total possible points. Failure to perform a critical step that is indicated with an asterisk (*) will result in an unsatisfactory overall score.

Time began _____ **Time ended** _____

Steps	Possible Points	First Attempt	Second Attempt	Third Attempt
1. Wash your hands.	10	_____	_____	_____
2. Identify your patient, and explain the procedure.*	20	_____	_____	_____
3. If the patient is to remove his or her shoes for weighing, place a paper towel on the scale platform. The patient may be given disposable slippers to wear. Check to see that the balance bar pointer floats in the middle of the balance frame when all weights are at zero.	10	_____	_____	_____
4. Help the patient onto the scale. Make certain that the female patient is not holding a purse and that the male or female patient has removed any heavy objects from pockets.	10	_____	_____	_____
5. Move the large weight into the groove closest to the estimated weight of the patient. While the patient is standing still, slide the small upper weight to the right along the pound markers until the pointer balances in the middle of the balance frame.*	10	_____	_____	_____
6. Leave the weights in place.	10	_____	_____	_____
7. Ask the patient to stand up straight and to look straight ahead. On some scales the patient may need to turn with the back to the scale.	10	_____	_____	_____

Steps	Possible Points	First Attempt	Second Attempt	Third Attempt
8. Adjust the height bar so that it just touches the top of the patient's head. Leave the elevation bar set but fold down the horizontal bar.*	10			
9. Assist the patient off the scale. Make certain that all items removed for weighing are given back to the patient.	10			
10. Read the weight scale. Add the numbers at the markers of the large and the small weights and record the total to the nearest ¼ lb on the patient's medical record (e.g., Wt: 136½).	10			
11. Record the height. Read the marker at the movable point of the ruler, and record the measurement to the nearest quarter inch on the patient's medical record (e.g., Ht: 64¼).	10			
12. Use the patient's weight and height to record the BMI level if part of office procedure.	10			
13. Return the weights and the measuring bar to zero.	5			
14. Wash your hands.	10			
15. Record the results on the patient's medical record.*	10			

Documentation on the Medical Record

A patient arrives today for a general physical. Obtain and record the weight and height of the patient below using SOAPE format.

S: _____

O: _____

Comments:

Total Points Earned _____ Divided by _____ Total Possible Points = _____ % Score

Instructor's Signature

Procedure 31-1 Prepare and Maintain Examination and Treatment Areas

Task: Prepare an examination room for a patient procedure, maintain equipment and supplies needed for the physical examination, and demonstrate maintenance of the room after a patient visit.

Equipment and Supplies:
- Disfectant
- Table paper
- Patient gowns
- Sheets
- Disposable gloves,
- Sink with antibacterial hand-washing agent,
- Paper towels,
- Biohazard waste containers
- Sharps containers
- Impervious gowns
- Face guards

Standards: Complete the procedure and all critical steps in _____ minutes with a minimum score of _____% within three attempts.

Scoring: Divide points earned by total possible points. Failure to perform a critical step that is indicated with an asterisk (*) will result in an unsatisfactory overall score.

Time began _____ **Time ended** _____

Steps	Possible Points	First Attempt	Second Attempt	Third Attempt
1. Check the area at the beginning of each day and between patients to make sure that it is completely stocked with equipment and supplies and that equipment is functioning properly.	10	_____	_____	_____
2. Check the expiration date of all packages and supplies.	5	_____	_____	_____
3. Discard any expired supplies*	2	_____	_____	_____
4. Check to be sure the room is well lit and a comfortable temperature for the patient.	5	_____	_____	_____
5. Clean and disinfect the area daily, and between patients*	5	_____	_____	_____
6. Restock supplies and clean all potentially contaminated surfaces, including the examination table, between patients with an appropriate disinfectant. After cleaning the table, change the examination paper by unrolling a new piece.	10	_____	_____	_____

Steps	Possible Points	First Attempt	Second Attempt	Third Attempt
7. Arrange drapes, gowns, and any other patient supplies before the patient enters the room so they are ready for use.	5			
8. Prepare instruments and equipment needed for the examination and arrange these items for easy access.	5			
9. Be sure the examination room contains all required materials for standard precautions. Replace biohazard containers when they are two-thirds full.	5			
10. Wash your hands before the patient is escorted to the room.*	5			

Comments:

Total Points Earned _____ Divided by _____ Total Possible Points = _____ % Score

Instructor's Signature _____

Student Name _____ Date _____ Score _____

Procedure 31-2 Prepare Patient for and Assist with Routine and Specialty Examinations: Fowler's and Semi-Fowler's Positions

Task: To position and drape the patient for examinations of the head, neck, and chest or for patients who have difficulty breathing when lying flat.

Equipment and Supplies:
- Examination table
- Table paper
- Patient gown
- Drape

Standards: Complete the procedure and all critical steps in _____ minutes with a minimum score of _____% within three attempts.

Scoring: Divide points earned by total possible points. Failure to perform a critical step that is indicated with an asterisk (*) will result in an unsatisfactory overall score.

Time began _____ Time ended _____

Steps	Possible Points	First Attempt	Second Attempt	Third Attempt
1. Prepare the examination room according to acceptable medical aseptic rules.	__10__	_____	_____	_____
2. Wash your hands.	__10__	_____	_____	_____
3. Greet and identify the patient, and determine whether the patient understands the procedure. If the patient does not understand, explain what to expect.	__10__	_____	_____	_____
4. Give the patient a gown, and explain the clothing that must be removed for the particular examination being done and whether the gown should be open in the front or the back. Provide assistance as needed. Give the patient privacy while changing. Knock on the examination room door before reentering to make sure the patient has completed undressing and gowning.*	__10__	_____	_____	_____
5. Either elevate the head of the bed 90 degrees or instruct the patient to sit at the end of the table. Extend the footrest for patient comfort. The patient may be more comfortable in a semi-Fowler's position. This modification of Fowler's position has the head of the table elevated 45 degrees and may be used for postsurgical follow-up or for patients with fevers, head injuries, or pain. It is also a comfortable, supported position for patients with breathing disorders.	__10__	_____	_____	_____

Steps	Possible Points	First Attempt	Second Attempt	Third Attempt
6. Drape the patient according to the type of examination and the needed patient exposure.	10			
7. After the examination is completed, assist the patient as needed to get off of the table and get dressed.	5			
8. Clean and disinfect the examination room according to standard precautions. Roll clean paper over the table.	10			
9. Wash your hands.	10			

Comments:

Total Points Earned _____ Divided by _____ Total Possible Points = _____ % Score

Instructor's Signature _____

Student Name _____ Date _____ Score _____

Procedure 31-3 Prepare Patient for and Assist with Routine and Specialty Examinations: Horizontal Recumbent and Dorsal Recumbent Positions

Task: To position and drape the patient for examinations of the abdomen, heart, and breasts in the horizontal recumbent (supine) position and the rectal, vaginal, and perineal areas in the dorsal recumbent position.

Equipment and Supplies:
- Examination table
- Table paper
- Patient gown
- Drape

Standards: Complete the procedure and all critical steps in _____ minutes with a minimum score of _____% within three attempts.

Scoring: Divide points earned by total possible points. Failure to perform a critical step that is indicated with an asterisk (*) will result in an unsatisfactory overall score.

Time began _____ **Time ended** _____

Steps	Possible Points	First Attempt	Second Attempt	Third Attempt
1. Prepare the examination room according to acceptable medical aseptic rules.	10	_____	_____	_____
2. Wash your hands.	10	_____	_____	_____
3. Greet and identify the patient, and determine whether the patient understands the procedure.	10	_____	_____	_____
4. Give the patient a gown, and explain the clothing that must be removed for the particular examination being done and whether the gown should be open in the front or the back. Provide assistance as needed. For the horizontal recumbent position, the gown should be open in the front. Give the patient privacy while changing. Knock on the examination room door before reentering to make sure the patient has completed undressing and gowning.*	10	_____	_____	_____
5. Do not place the patient in these positions until the physician is ready for that part of the examination.	5	_____	_____	_____

Steps	Possible Points	First Attempt	Second Attempt	Third Attempt
6. Pull out the table extension that supports the patient's legs. For the horizontal recumbent (supine) position, help the patient lie flat on the table with the face upward. For the dorsal recumbent position, have the patient lie flat on the back and flex the knees so the feet are flat on the table. If needed, help the patient move down toward the foot of the table for the examination.	10			
7. Drape the patient from nipple line to feet in the supine position, and diagonally with the point of the drape between the feet for the dorsal recumbent position.	10			
8. After the examination is completed, assist the patient as needed to get off of the table and get dressed.	5			
9. Clean and disinfect the examination room according to standard precautions. Roll clean paper over the table.	10			
10. Wash hands.	10			

Comments:

Total Points Earned _____ Divided by _____ Total Possible Points = _____ % Score

Instructor's Signature _____

Student Name _____ Date _____ Score _____

Procedure 31-4 Prepare Patient for and Assist with Routine and Specialty Examinations: Lithotomy Position

Task: To position and drape the patient primarily for vaginal and pelvic examinations and Pap smears.

Equipment and Supplies:
- Examination table
- Table paper
- Patient gown
- Drape

Standards: Complete the procedure and all critical steps in _____ minutes with a minimum score of _____% within three attempts.

Scoring: Divide points earned by total possible points. Failure to perform a critical step that is indicated with an asterisk (*) will result in an unsatisfactory overall score.

Time began _____ **Time ended** _____

Steps	Possible Points	First Attempt	Second Attempt	Third Attempt
1. Prepare the examination room according to acceptable medical aseptic rules.	10			
2. Wash your hands.	10			
3. Greet and identify the patient, and determine whether the patient understands the procedure.	10			
4. Give the patient a gown, and instruct the patient to undress from the waist down with the gown open in the back. If the physician will also be doing a breast examination the gown should be open in the front. Provide assistance as needed. Give the patient privacy while changing. Knock on the examination room door before reentering to make sure the patient has completed undressing and gowning. Do not place the patient in this position until the physician is ready for that part of the examination.*	10			

Steps	Possible Points	First Attempt	Second Attempt	Third Attempt
5. Pull out the table extension that supports the patient's legs, and help the patient lay face upward on the table. Pull out the stirrups, adjusting their extension length for patient comfort, and lock them in place. Reinsert the table extension and have the patient move toward the foot of the table with her buttocks on the bottom table edge. Gently place the patient's legs in the stirrups, checking for comfort. Some offices may stock cloth or paper stirrup covers to protect the patient and make the position more comfortable. The patient's arms can be placed alongside the body or across the chest.	10			
6. Drape the patient diagonally with the point of the drape between the feet. The drape should be large enough to cover the patient from the nipple line to the ankles and wide enough so the patient's thighs are not exposed.	10			
7. After the examination is completed, assist the patient as needed to get off of the table and get dressed.	10			
8. Clean and disinfect the examination room according to standard precautions. Roll clean paper over the table.	10			
9. Wash hands.	10			

Comments:

Total Points Earned _____ Divided by _____ Total Possible Points = _____ % Score

Instructor's Signature _____

Student Name _____ Date _____ Score _____

Procedure 31-5 Prepare Patient for and Assist with Routine and Specialty Examinations: Sims' Position

Task: To position and drape the patient for examinations of the rectum, rectal thermometer readings, instillation of rectal medications, perineal examinations, and some pelvic examinations.

Equipment and Supplies:
- Examination table
- Table paper
- Patient gown
- Drape

Standards: Complete the procedure and all critical steps in _____ minutes with a minimum score of _____% within three attempts.

Scoring: Divide points earned by total possible points. Failure to perform a critical step that is indicated with an asterisk (*) will result in an unsatisfactory overall score.

Time began _____ **Time ended** _____

Steps	Possible Points	First Attempt	Second Attempt	Third Attempt
1. Prepare the examination room according to acceptable medical aseptic rules.	10			
2. Wash your hands.	10			
3. Greet and identify the patient, and determine whether the patient understands the procedure. If the patient does not understand, explain what to expect.	10			
4. Give the patient a gown and explain the clothing that must be removed for the particular examination being done. Tell the patient to open the gown in the back. Provide assistance as needed. Give the patient privacy while changing. Knock on the examination room door before reentering to make sure the patient has completed undressing and gowning. Do not place the patient in this position until the physician is ready for that part of the examination.*	10			
5. Help the patient turn onto the left side; the left arm and shoulder should be drawn back behind the body so that the patient is tilted onto the chest. Flex the right arm upward for support, slightly flex the left leg, and sharply flex the right leg upward. Help the patient move the buttocks to the side edge of the table.	10			

Steps	Possible Points	First Attempt	Second Attempt	Third Attempt
6. Drape the patient diagonally in a diamond shape, with the point of the diamond dropping below the buttocks. Make sure that the drape is large enough so that the patient is not exposed.	10			
7. After the examination is completed, assist the patient as needed to get off of the table and get dressed.	5			
8. Clean and disinfect the examination room according to standard precautions. Roll clean paper over the table.	10			
9. Wash hands.	10			

Comments:

Total Points Earned _____ Divided by _____ Total Possible Points = _____ % Score

Instructor's Signature _____

Student Name _____ Date _____ Score _____

Procedure 31-6 Prepare Patient for and Assist with Routine and Specialty Examinations: Prone Position

Task: To position and drape the patient for examinations of the back and certain surgical procedures.

Equipment and Supplies:
- Examination table
- Table paper
- Patient gown
- Drape

Standards: Complete the procedure and all critical steps in _____ minutes with a minimum score of _____% within three attempts.

Scoring: Divide points earned by total possible points. Failure to perform a critical step that is indicated with an asterisk (*) will result in an unsatisfactory overall score.

Time began _____ **Time ended** _____

Steps	Possible Points	First Attempt	Second Attempt	Third Attempt
1. Prepare the examination room according to acceptable medical aseptic rules.	10	_____	_____	_____
2. Wash your hands.	10	_____	_____	_____
3. Greet and identify the patient, and determine whether the patient understands the procedure.	10	_____	_____	_____
4. Give the patient a gown, and explain the clothing that must be removed for the particular examination being done. Tell the patient to open the gown in the back. Provide assistance as needed. Give the patient privacy while changing. Knock on the examination room door before reentering to make sure the patient has completed undressing and gowning. Do not place the patient in this position until the physician is ready for that part of the examination.*	10	_____	_____	_____
5. Pull out the table extension if necessary, and help the patient lie down on his or her back.	5	_____	_____	_____

Steps	Possible Points	First Attempt	Second Attempt	Third Attempt
6. Drape the patient over any exposed area that is not included in the examination. For female patients the drape should be large enough to cover from the breasts to the feet so if the patient is asked to roll over she is not exposed accidentally.	10			
7. After the examination is completed, assist the patient as needed to get off of the table and get dressed.	5			
8. Clean and disinfect the examination room according to standard precautions. Roll clean paper over the table.	10			
9. Wash hands.	10			

Comments:

Total Points Earned _____ Divided by _____ Total Possible Points = _____ % Score

Instructor's Signature _____

Student Name _____ Date _____ Score _____

Procedure 31-7 Prepare Patient for and Assist with Routine and Specialty Examinations: Knee-Chest Position

Task: To position and drape the patient for examinations of the back and certain surgical procedures.

Equipment and Supplies:
- Examination table
- Table paper
- Patient gown
- Drape

Standards: Complete the procedure and all critical steps in _____ minutes with a minimum score of _____% within three attempts.

Scoring: Divide points earned by total possible points. Failure to perform a critical step that is indicated with an asterisk (*) will result in an unsatisfactory overall score.

Time began _____ **Time ended** _____

Steps	Possible Points	First Attempt	Second Attempt	Third Attempt
1. Prepare the examination room according to acceptable medical aseptic rules.	10	_____	_____	_____
2. Wash your hands.	10	_____	_____	_____
3. Greet and identify the patient, and determine whether the patient understands the procedure. If the patient does not understand, explain what to expect.	10	_____	_____	_____
4. Give the patient a gown and explain the clothing that must be removed for the particular examination being done. Tell the patient to open the gown in the back. Provide assistance as needed. Give the patient privacy while changing. Knock on the examination room door before reentering to make sure the patient has completed undressing and gowning. Do not place the patient in this position until the physician is ready for that part of the examination.*	10	_____	_____	_____

Steps	Possible Points	First Attempt	Second Attempt	Third Attempt
5. Pull out the table extension if necessary, and help the patient lie down on his or her back then turn over to the prone position. Ask the patient to move up onto the knees, spread the knees apart, and lean forward onto the head so that the buttocks are raised. Tell the patient to keep the back straight and turn the face to either side. The patient should rest his or her weight on the chest and shoulders. If the patient has difficulty maintaining this position, an alternative is to place weight on bent elbows with head off of the table.	10			
6. Drape the patient diagonally so that the point of the drape is on the table between the legs.	10			
7. After the examination is completed, assist the patient as needed to get off of the table and get dressed.	10			
8. Clean and disinfect the examination room according to standard precautions. Roll clean paper over the table.	10			
9. Wash your hands.	10			

Comments:

Total Points Earned _____ Divided by _____ Total Possible Points = _____ % Score

Instructor's Signature _____

Student Name _____ Date _____ Score _____

Procedure 31-8 Prepare Patient for and Assist with Routine and Specialty Examinations: Prepare for and Assist with the Physical Examination

Task: To help the physician examine patients by preparing the patient and the necessary equipment and ensuring patient safety and comfort during the examination.

Equipment and Supplies:
- Stethoscope
- Ophthalmoscope
- Scale with height measurement bar
- Tongue depressor
- Cotton balls
- Examination light
- Percussion hammer
- Lubricating gel
- Examination gloves
- Sphygmomanometer
- Otoscope with disposable speculum
- Tape measure
- Gauze sponges
- Pen light
- Nasal speculum
- Tuning fork
- Biohazard container
- Laboratory request forms
- Specimen bottles and laboratory requisitions
- Patient gown
- Drapes
- Thermometer
- Cotton-tipped applicators
- Hemoccult supplies

Standards: Complete the procedure and all critical steps in _____ minutes with a minimum score of _____% within three attempts.

Scoring: Divide points earned by total possible points. Failure to perform a critical step that is indicated with an asterisk (*) will result in an unsatisfactory overall score.

Time began _____ **Time ended** _____

Steps	Possible Points	First Attempt	Second Attempt	Third Attempt
1. Prepare the examining room according to acceptable medical aseptic rules.	10	_____	_____	_____
2. Wash your hands.	10	_____	_____	_____
3. Locate the instruments for the procedure. Set them out in order of use within reach of the physician and cover them until the physician enters the examination room.	10	_____	_____	_____

Steps	Possible Points	First Attempt	Second Attempt	Third Attempt
4. Identify the patient, and determine whether the patient understands the procedure. If the patient does not understand, explain what to expect.	10			
5. Review the medical history with the patient, and investigate the purpose of the visit. Record interview results.*	20			
6. Measure and record the patient's vital signs, height, weight, and BMI.	10			
7. Instruct the patient on how to collect a urine specimen if ordered, and hand the patient the properly labeled specimen container. Obtain blood samples for any tests that are ordered. Obtain resting ECG if ordered.	10			
8. Hand the patient a gown and drape. Instruct the patient regarding what clothes should be removed for the examination and whether the gown should be open in the front or back. Help the patient with undressing as needed; however, most patients prefer to undress in privacy. Knock on the door before reentry to protect patient privacy.*	10			
9. Assist the patient in sitting at the foot examination table; place the drape over the patient's lap and legs. If the patient is elderly, confused, or feeling faint or dizzy, do not leave him or her alone.	10			
10. Place the patient chart in the chart holder on the door, or inform the physician that the patient is ready. Be careful to place patient identity information out of sight to protect patient privacy.*	5			
11. Assist during the examination by handing the physician each instrument as it is needed and by positioning and draping the patient.	10			
12. When the physician has completed the examination, allow the patient to rest for a moment, then help the patient from the table. Assist with dressing, if necessary. Use proper body mechanics if assistance in transfer is needed.	10			

Steps	Possible Points	First Attempt	Second Attempt	Third Attempt
13. Return to the patient and ask if he or she has any questions. Give the patient any final instructions, and schedule tests as ordered by the physician and/or the next appointment.	10	_____	_____	_____
14. Put on gloves and dispose of used supplies and linens in designated biohazard waste containers. Clean surfaces with disinfectant. Disinfect all equipment.	10	_____	_____	_____
15. Remove gloves, discard them in the biohazard waste container, and wash hands.	10	_____	_____	_____

Documentation in the Medical Record

A 31-year-old woman arrives in the office for an annual physical and Pap smear. Her only complaint is the presence of some abnormal moles on the right side of her neck. She takes a multivitamin daily and has no allergies to medication. Document the case using SOAPE format.

S: _____

O: _____

Comments:

Total Points Earned _____ Divided by _____ Total Possible Points = _____ % Score

Instructor's Signature _____

Procedure 32-1 Maintain Medication and Immunization Records: Prepare a Prescription for the Physician's Signature

Task: To accurately prepare a prescription for the physician's signature using appropriate abbreviations and prescription format.

Equipment and Supplies:
- Prescription pad
- Drug reference materials if needed
- Black pen
- Patient chart

Standards: Complete the procedure and all critical steps in _____ minutes with a minimum score of _____% within three attempts.

Scoring: Divide points earned by total possible points. Failure to perform a critical step that is indicated with an asterisk (*) will result in an unsatisfactory overall score.

Time began _____ **Time ended** _____

Steps	Possible Points	First Attempt	Second Attempt	Third Attempt
1. Refer to the physician's written order for the prescription. If the physician gives a verbal order to write a prescription, write down the order and review it with the physician for accuracy.	10	_____	_____	_____
2. If unfamiliar with the medication, look up the drug in a drug reference book (such as the PDR).*	10	_____	_____	_____
3. Ask the patient about drug allergies.*	10	_____	_____	_____
4. Using a prescription pad that has the physician's name, address, telephone number, and DEA registration number preprinted on the slip, begin to transcribe the physician order.	10	_____	_____	_____
5. Record the patient's name and address and the date on which the prescription is being written.	10	_____	_____	_____
6. Next to the Rx, write in legible handwriting the name of the drug (correctly spelled), the dosage form (such as tablet, capsule, and so forth, using correct abbreviations), and the strength ordered.	10	_____	_____	_____

Steps	Possible Points	First Attempt	Second Attempt	Third Attempt
7. On the next line write Disp. This is the subscription, which includes directions to the pharmacist on the amount to be dispensed and the form of the drug.	10			
8. Next comes the signature. This includes directions for the patient, such as how and when to take the medicine, and is usually preceded by the symbol Sig.	10			
9. The physician tells you the patient can get three refills of the prescription, so this information should be added at the bottom of the prescription on the designated line.	10			
10. The physician must review and sign the prescription before it is given to the patient.	5			
11. Document on the patient's chart the medication order and any pertinent details, including patient education and refill information.	10			

Prepare a prescription for Lipitor 20 mg, taken once daily with food at bedtime. Provide the patient with a 1-month supply, and allow for three refills.

_____

_____

_____

Comments:

Total Points Earned _____ Divided by _____ Total Possible Points = _____ % Score

Instructor's Signature _____

Procedure 33-1 Apply Pharmacology Principles to Prepare and Administer Oral and Parenteral (Excluding IV) Medications: Calculate the Correct Dosage for Administration

Task: To calculate the correct dose amount and choose the correct equipment when the physician orders 2.4 million IU of penicillin G benzathine (Bicillin).

Equipment and Supplies:
- Premixed syringes of Bicillin in the following two strengths are available:
- 0.6 million IU/syringe
- 1.2 million IU/syringe

Standards: Complete the procedure and all critical steps in _____ minutes with a minimum score of _____% within three attempts.

Scoring: Divide points earned by total possible points. Failure to perform a critical step that is indicated with an asterisk (*) will result in an unsatisfactory overall score.

Time began _____ **Time ended** _____

Steps	Possible Points	First Attempt	Second Attempt	Third Attempt
1. Read the order in quiet surroundings to make sure that you fully understand it.	15	_____	_____	_____
2. Write out the order.	15	_____	_____	_____
3. Examine the drug labels to see what strengths and amounts are available.	15	_____	_____	_____
4. Write down the standard formula. $$\frac{\text{Available strength}}{\text{Ordered strength}} = \frac{\text{Available amount}}{\text{Amount to give}}$$	15	_____	_____	_____
5. Rewrite the formula, replacing the unknown values with the known quantities. The unknown x will be the amount of the drug to give.	10	_____	_____	_____
6. Work the proportion problem by cross-multiplying to solve for x.	10	_____	_____	_____
7. State your answer by filling in the blanks, as follows: To administer 2.4 million IU of Bicillin, I would select _____ of the premixed syringes labeled _____.	10	_____	_____	_____

Comments:

Total Points Earned _____ Divided by _____ Total Possible Points = _____ % Score

Instructor's Signature _____

Procedure 33-2 Apply Pharmacology Principles to Prepare and Administer Oral and Parenteral (Excluding IV) Medications: Calculate the Correct Dosage for Administration Using Two Systems of Measurement

Task: To choose the correct system of measurement and calculate the correct dose amount when the physician orders 120 mg of a drug to be administered to a patient. (tablet label reads 1 gr each.)

Equipment and Supplies:
- Tablets labeled 1 gr (grain) each
- Standard mathematical formula:

$$\frac{\text{Available strength}}{\text{Ordered strength}} = \frac{\text{Available amount}}{\text{Amount to give}}$$

- Conversion equivalent: 1 gr = 60 mg

Standards: Complete the procedure and all critical steps in _____ minutes with a minimum score of _____% within three attempts.

Scoring: Divide points earned by total possible points. Failure to perform a critical step that is indicated with an asterisk (*) will result in an unsatisfactory overall score.

Time began _____ **Time ended** _____

Steps	Possible Points	First Attempt	Second Attempt	Third Attempt
1. Read the order in quiet surroundings to make sure that you fully understand it.	5	_____	_____	_____
2. Write out the order.	5	_____	_____	_____
3. Examine the drug labels to see what strengths and amounts are available.*	10	_____	_____	_____
4. Convert the ordered system of measurement to the system of measurement on the label.	20	_____	_____	_____
5. Place the amount ordered on the left side of the equation and the conversion factor on the right side so that similar units can be cancelled when cross-multiplied.	10	_____	_____	_____
6. Write down the standard formula.	10	_____	_____	_____

Steps	Possible Points	First Attempt	Second Attempt	Third Attempt
7. Rewrite the formula, replacing the unknown values with the known quantities and using the system of measurement on the label. The unknown *x* will be the amount of the drug to give (amount to give).	10			
8. Work the proportion problem by cross-multiplying to solve for *x*.	10			
9. State your answer by filling in the blank, as follows: To administer 120 mg of a drug from tablets labeled *1 gr* (grain) *each*, give _____ tablet(s).	10			

Comments:

Total Points Earned _____ Divided by _____ Total Possible Points = _____ % Score

Instructor's Signature _____

Student Name _____ Date _____ Score _____

Procedure 33-3 Apply Pharmacology Principles to Prepare and Administer Oral and Parenteral (Excluding IV) Medications: Calculate the Correct Pediatric Dosage Using the Body Surface Area Method

Task: To calculate the correct dose amount using the body surface area (BSA) method for a 90-pound child who is 48 inches tall when the adult dose is 250 mg.

Equipment and Supplies:
- Balance scale with length measurement
- Conversion data

Adult dosage 250 mg/mL

$$\text{Pediatric dose} = \frac{\text{(BSA) of child in m}^2}{1.7 \text{ m2 (average adult BSA)}} \times \text{Adult dose}$$

Standards: Complete the procedure and all critical steps in _____ minutes with a minimum score of _____% within three attempts.

Scoring: Divide points earned by total possible points. Failure to perform a critical step that is indicated with an asterisk (*) will result in an unsatisfactory overall score.

Time began _____ **Time ended** _____

Steps	Possible Points	First Attempt	Second Attempt	Third Attempt
1. Read the order in quiet surroundings to make sure that you fully understand it.	5			
2. Write out the order.	10			
3. Examine the drug labels to see what strengths and amounts are available.*	10			
4. Write down the BSA formula.	10			
5. Using the BSA method, determine the BSA in m^2 by intersecting the child's weight and height on the right column (child is overweight).	10			
6. Divide the child's BSA by 1.7 m^2 (the average adult BSA)	10			
7. Multiply this calculation by the adult dose (250 mg)	10			
8. State your answer by filling in the blank, as follows: To administer an adult medication labeled 250 mg/mL to a 90-pound child, give _____ mg.	10			

Comments:

Total Points Earned _____ Divided by _____ Total Possible Points = _____ % Score

Instructor's Signature _____

Procedure 33-4 Apply Pharmacology Principles to Prepare and Administer Oral and Parenteral (Excluding IV) Medications: Calculate the Correct Pediatric Dosage for Administration Using Body Weight

Task: To calculate correct dosage by using body weight method.

Ordered: Zithromax suspension, 5 mg/kg bid times 5 days for a patient who has a diagnosis of otitis media. The patient weighs 22 pounds. The suspension is labeled 100 mg/5 mL.

Weight conversion: 2.2 lb = 1 kg

Equipment and Supplies:
- Suspension labeled 100 mg/5 mL
- Balance scale
- Formula for conversion of pounds to kilograms
- Standard math formula:

$$\frac{\text{Available strength}}{\text{Ordered strength}} = \frac{\text{Available amount}}{\text{Amount to give}}$$

- Paper and pencil

Standards: Complete the procedure and all critical steps in _____ minutes with a minimum score of _____% within three attempts.

Scoring: Divide points earned by total possible points. Failure to perform a critical step that is indicated with an asterisk (*) will result in an unsatisfactory overall score.

Time began _____ **Time ended** _____

Steps	Possible Points	First Attempt	Second Attempt	Third Attempt
1. Read the order in quiet surroundings to make sure that you fully understand it.	5	_____	_____	_____
2. Write out the order.	10	_____	_____	_____
3. Examine the drug label to check the strength and amount.*	10	_____	_____	_____
4. Convert the patient's weight from pounds to kilograms.	10	_____	_____	_____
5. Calculate the total daily amount of medication by multiplying the weight in kilograms by the mg/kg factor.	10	_____	_____	_____

Steps	Possible Points	First Attempt	Second Attempt	Third Attempt
6. Calculate the individual dose of Zithromax; divide the daily dose by 2 (bid is twice a day).	10			
7. Compare the ordered daily dose with the dose information on the medication label (100 mg = 5 mL).	10			
8. Write down the standard formula.	10			
9. Rewrite the formula, replacing the unknown values with the known quantities. The unknown x will be the amount of the drug to give.	10			
10. Work the problem by cross-multiplying to solve for x. State your answer by filling in the blank: To administer 5 mg/kg of body weight of Zithromax from capsules labeled 100 mg/5 mL, I would give _____ mL.	10			

Comments:

Total Points Earned _____ Divided by _____ Total Possible Points = _____ % Score

Instructor's Signature _____

Procedure 34-1 Apply Pharmacology Principles to Prepare and Administer Oral and Parenteral (Excluding IV) Medications: Safety Measures in Preparing, Administering, and Documenting Medication

Task: To safely prepare, administer, and document completion of a medication order.

Equipment and Supplies:
- Written physician order, including the drug name, strength, dose, and route
- PDR reference
- Container of ordered medication
- Correct equipment for dispensing the drug

Dr. Thau writes the following order: Administer Recombivax 10 mcg IM to Chris MacCarthy.

Standards: Complete the procedure and all critical steps in _____ minutes with a minimum score of _____% within three attempts.

Scoring: Divide points earned by total possible points. Failure to perform a critical step that is indicated with an asterisk (*) will result in an unsatisfactory overall score.

Time began _____ **Time ended** _____

Steps	Possible Points	First Attempt	Second Attempt	Third Attempt
1. Read the order and clarify any questions with the physician.	10	_____	_____	_____
2. If you are unfamiliar with the drug, refer to the PDR or the package insert to determine the purpose of the drug, common side effects, typical dose, and any pertinent precautions or contraindications. Recombivax is a hepatitis B immunization. Use the "seven rights" to prevent errors.	10	_____	_____	_____
3. Take the written order with you to the medication room, and compare the Recombivax label with the physician's order. Based on the information printed on the medication label, perform calculations needed to match the physician's order. Confirm the answer with the physician if you have any questions.	10	_____	_____	_____
4. Dispense medication in a well-lit, quiet area.	10	_____	_____	_____
5. Wash your hands.	10	_____	_____	_____

Steps	Possible Points	First Attempt	Second Attempt	Third Attempt
6. Compare the written order with the label on the multidose vial when you remove it from storage. Check the expiration date on the container and dispose of the medication if it has expired.	10			
7. Compare the order with the label on the multidose vial just before drawing it up into the appropriate syringe unit. Make certain that the strength on the label matches the order or that you dispense the correctly calculated dose.	10			
8. Compare the label and the physician order before returning the vial to storage.	10			
9. Greet and identify Chris by name and inform him you are going to administer a hepatitis B immunization.	10			
10. Mention the name of the drug and why it is being given, and ask the patient if he has any allergies to the medication.	10			
11. If necessary, help the patient into a sitting position.	5			
12. Administer the medication into the left deltoid muscle using correct administration techniques and Occupational Safety and Health Administration (OSHA) precautions.	20			
13. Conduct patient education on the purpose of the drug, typical side effects, and dosage and storage recommendations. Refer to the physician to clarify information if needed.	10			
14. The patient must remain in the office for 20 to 30 minutes after drug administration as a precaution against untoward effects.	10			
15. If the patient experiences any discomfort after taking a medication, the physician should be notified immediately and the incident documented completely and accurately.	10			
16. Wash your hands.	10			
17. Document the administration of the drug, including the date and time; the drug name, dose, strength, and route of administration; any patient side effects; and patient education conducted about the drug.	10			

Documentation in the Medical Record

_____

_____

_____

Comments:

Total Points Earned _____ Divided by _____ Total Possible Points = _____ % Score

Instructor's Signature _____

Procedure 34-2 Apply Pharmacology Principles to Prepare and Administer Oral and Parenteral (Excluding IV) Medications: Maintain Medication Records

Task: To document completion of medication orders.

Equipment and Supplies:
- Written physician order, including the name, strength, dose, and route of administration of the medication ordered
- PDR reference
- Patient chart

Dr. Thau writes the following orders for control of Mrs. Lange's hypertension:
Lasix 20 mg PO qd
Potassium Chloride 20 mEq PO qd to Alice Lange

You reviewed the orders for clarification, completed the three label checks, confirmed the identity of the patient, asked the patient about drug allergies, administered the medications as ordered, and answered patient questions about the continuation of drug therapy at home. You must now document this process in the patient chart.

Standards: Complete the procedure and all critical steps in _____ minutes with a minimum score of _____% within three attempts.

Scoring: Divide points earned by total possible points. Failure to perform a critical step that is indicated with an asterisk (*) will result in an unsatisfactory overall score.

Time began _____ Time ended _____

Steps	Possible Points	First Attempt	Second Attempt	Third Attempt
1. Greet and identify Alice by name and inform her you are going to administer a diuretic and potassium supplement.	10	_____	_____	_____
2. Mention the names of the drugs and why they are being given, and ask Alice if she has any allergies to the medication.*	10	_____	_____	_____
3. Administer the medications orally as ordered, making sure Alice swallows the pills without difficulty.	5	_____	_____	_____
4. Conduct patient education about the purpose of the drugs, typical side effects, and dosage and storage recommendations. Refer to the physician to clarify information if needed.	10	_____	_____	_____
5. The patient must remain in the office for 20 to 30 minutes after drug administration as a precaution against untoward effects.	10	_____	_____	_____

Steps	Possible Points	First Attempt	Second Attempt	Third Attempt
6. If the patient experiences any discomfort after taking a medication, the physician should be notified immediately and the incident documented completely and accurately.	10			
7. Wash your hands.	10			
8. Document the administration of the medications, including the date and time; the drug names, dose, strength, and route of administration; any patient side effects; and patient education conducted about the drug.*	10			

Practice documenting the following orders:

1. Tylenol elixir 120 mg PO to Anthony Baker, 8 years old, for a fever

_____

_____

_____

_____

2. Gantrisin Pediatric 500 mg PO to Samantha Carpassi, 3 years old, for a urinary tract infection

_____

_____

_____

_____

3. Dilaudid cough syrup 2 mg PO to Roberto Alphonse, 43 years old, for bronchitis

_____

_____

_____

_____

4. Diflucan 400 mg PO loading dose to Anastasia Smith, 19 years old, for a vaginal yeast infection.

_____

_____

_____

_____

Comments:

Total Points Earned _____ Divided by _____ Total Possible Points = _____ % Score

Instructor's Signature _____

Student Name _____ Date _____ Score _____

Procedure 34-3 Apply Pharmacology Principles to Prepare and Administer Oral and Parenteral (Excluding IV) Medications: Dispense, Administer, and Document Oral Medications

Task: To safely dispense, administer to a patient, and document the administration of an oral medication.

Equipment and Supplies:
- Container of ordered medication
- Calibrated medication cup
- Written physician order, including the drug name, strength, dose, and route
- Water if appropriate
- Patient medical record

Order: Administer hydrochlorothiazide (HydroDIURIL) 100 mg PO tab stat for hypertension

Standards: Complete the procedure and all critical steps in _____ minutes with a minimum score of _____% within three attempts.

Scoring: Divide points earned by total possible points. Failure to perform a critical step that is indicated with an asterisk (*) will result in an unsatisfactory overall score.

Time began _____ **Time ended** _____

Steps	Possible Points	First Attempt	Second Attempt	Third Attempt
1. Read the order and clarify any questions with the physician.	10	_____	_____	_____
2. If you are unfamiliar with HydroDIURIL, refer to the PDR or the package insert to determine the purpose of the drug, common side effects, typical dose, and any pertinent precautions or contraindications. Be prepared to answer patient questions about the medication. Use the "seven rights" to prevent errors.	10	_____	_____	_____
3. Perform calculations needed to match the physician's order. Confirm the answer with the physician if you have any questions.	10	_____	_____	_____
4. Dispense medication in a well-lit, quiet area.	10	_____	_____	_____
5. Wash your hands.	10	_____	_____	_____
6. Compare the order with the label on the container of medicine when you remove it from storage. Check the expiration date on the container and dispose of the medication if it has expired.	10	_____	_____	_____

Steps	Possible Points	First Attempt	Second Attempt	Third Attempt
7. Compare the order with the label on the container of medicine just before dispensing the ordered dose. Make certain that the strength on the label matches the order or that you dispense the correctly calculated dose.	10			

To Dispense Solid Oral Medications (Hydro-DIURIL Tablet)

8. Gently tap the prescribed dose into the lid of the medication container. Avoid touching the inside of the lid as well as the medication.	10			
9. Empty the medication in the container lid into a medicine cup.	10			

To Dispense Liquid Oral Preparations (Hydro-DIURIL Solution)

10. Shake medication well if required.	5			
11. When liquid medications are poured, the label should be held in the palm of the hand.*	10			
12. Place the medicine cup on a flat surface and, at eye level, pour the medication to the prescribed dose mark on the medicine cup.	20			

For Both Solid and Liquid Oral Medications

13. Recap the container and compare the label and the physician order before replacing the container in storage.	10			
14. Transport the medication to the patient.	10			
15. Greet and identify the patient by name.	10			
16. Mention the name of the drug and why it is being given, and ask the patient if she or he has any allergies to the medication.*	10			
17. If necessary, help the patient into a sitting position.	5			
18. Administer tablets, capsules, or caplets with water. If the patient is receiving liquid medication, offer water after the medication is taken if appropriate. Make sure the patient swallows the entire dose.	10			

Steps	Possible Points	First Attempt	Second Attempt	Third Attempt
19. Conduct patient education regarding the purpose of the drug, typical side effects, and dosage and storage recommendations. Refer to the physician to clarify information if needed.*	10			
20. The patient must remain in the office for 20 to 30 minutes after drug administration as a precaution against untoward effects.	5			
21. If the patient experiences any discomfort after taking a medication, the physician should be notified immediately and the incident documented completely and accurately.	10			
22. Wash your hands.	10			
23. Document the administration of the drug, including the date and time; the drug name, dose, strength, and route of administration; any patient side effects; and patient education conducted about the drug.	10			

Documentation in the Medical Record

_____

_____

_____

Comments:

Total Points Earned _____ Divided by _____ Total Possible Points = _____ % Score

Instructor's Signature _____

Procedure 34-4 Apply Pharmacology Principles to Prepare and Administer Oral and Parenteral (Excluding IV) Medications: Fill a Syringe Using an Ampule

Task: To correctly and safely remove medication for administration from a glass ampule.

Equipment and Supplies:
- Syringe/needle unit
- Filter needle
- Sterile gauze squares
- Sharps container
- Biohazard waste container
- Medication ampule
- Physician order
- Alcohol squares
- Disposable gloves

Standards: Complete the procedure and all critical steps in _____ minutes with a minimum score of _____% within three attempts.

Scoring: Divide points earned by total possible points. Failure to perform a critical step that is indicated with an asterisk (*) will result in an unsatisfactory overall score.

Time began _____ **Time ended** _____

Steps	Possible Points	First Attempt	Second Attempt	Third Attempt
1. Review physician's medication order for clarity. If unfamiliar with the drug, look it up in a reference book.	10			
2. Wash hands and assemble equipment.	10			
3. Perform medication label and physician order check when removing the ampule from storage. Check the expiration date on the ampule.	10			
4. Gently tap the top of the ampule with your fingers to settle all the medication to the bottom portion of the flask.	5			
5. Thoroughly disinfect the neck of the ampule with alcohol squares. Check the label against the order a second time.	10			
6. Wrap the top of the ampule with a gauze square to protect yourself from the glass. Hold the covered ampule between your thumb and finger, in front of you and above waist level.	10			

Steps	Possible Points	First Attempt	Second Attempt	Third Attempt
7. Push the top of the ampule away from your body to break the neck. You will hear a pop because the ampule is vacuum sealed. The glass is designed not to shatter, and the medication will not spill out. Dispose of the gauze square and glass top in the sharps container.	10			
8. Open the sterile syringe and needle unit. Touching the needle covers only, unscrew the needle from the syringe, place it on the counter, and attach the sterile filter needle.*	10			
9. Without touching the sides of the opened ampule, insert the syringe unit with the filter needle attached into the ampule and withdraw the ordered dose. Then recover the needle.	10			
10. Before discarding the ampule in the sharps container, check the physician order against the label one more time to complete the three label checks. If you are drawing the medication up for the physician to administer, take the ampule and the syringe unit to the physician for the final safety check.	10			
11. Change the filter needle, safeguarding the sterility of the injection unit, for an appropriate length and gauge needle based on the physician-ordered route of administration and patient characteristics. Discard the used filter needle into the sharps container.	10			
12. Dispose of used alcohol and gauze squares.	10			
13. Transport ordered medication in the injection unit to the patient. Identify the patient. Apply gloves and administer the medication as ordered. Discard the used syringe unit into a sharps container in the patient room. Remove gloves and discard in biohazard waste container and wash hands.	10			
14. Answer patient questions and document the procedure on the patient chart.	10			

Comments:

Total Points Earned _____ Divided by _____ Total Possible Points = _____ % Score

Instructor's Signature _____

Procedure 34-5 Apply Pharmacology Principles to Prepare and Administer Oral and Parenteral (Excluding IV) Medications: Fill a Syringe Using a Vial

Task: To fill a syringe from a multidose vial, using sterile technique.

Equipment and Supplies:
- Multidose vial containing the medication ordered
- Alcohol wipes
- Sterile needle and syringe unit
- Written order, including the drug name, strength, and route of administration

Standards: Complete the procedure and all critical steps in _____ minutes with a minimum score of _____% within three attempts.

Scoring: Divide points earned by total possible points. Failure to perform a critical step that is indicated with an asterisk (*) will result in an unsatisfactory overall score.

Time began _____ **Time ended** _____

Steps	Possible Points	First Attempt	Second Attempt	Third Attempt
1. Wash your hands.	10	_____	_____	_____
2. Read the order, and choose the correct vial of medication.	10	_____	_____	_____
3. Choose the correct syringe and needle size, depending on the site and the quantity of medication to be injected.	10	_____	_____	_____
4. Compare the order with both the name of the drug on the vial of medication and the amount to be withdrawn in the syringe.	10	_____	_____	_____
5. Gently agitate the medication by rolling the vial between your palms.	10	_____	_____	_____
6. Check the quality of the medication and the expiration date.	10	_____	_____	_____
7. Cleanse the rubber stopper of the vial with the alcohol wipe, using a circular motion. Place the vial on a secure flat surface, leaving the alcohol swab over the rubber stopper.	10	_____	_____	_____
8. With the needle cover in place, grasp the syringe plunger and draw up an amount of air equal to the amount of medication ordered.	10	_____	_____	_____

Steps	Possible Points	First Attempt	Second Attempt	Third Attempt
9. Remove the needle cover and insert the needle into the center of the rubber stopper. Hold the vial firmly against a flat surface, and watch carefully that the needle touches only the cleaned rubber area.	20			
10. Inject the aspirated air in the syringe into the vial.	10			
11. Keeping the syringe unit in the vial, pick up and invert them. Slowly pull back on the plunger with the unit at eye level until the proper amount of medication is withdrawn.	20			
12. While the needle is still in the vial, check that no air bubbles are in the syringe.	10			
13. If air bubbles are present, slip the fingers holding the vial down to grasp the vial and syringe as a single unit.	5			
14. With your free hand, tap the syringe until the air bubbles dislodge and float into the tip of the syringe.	5			
15. Gently expel these tiny air bubbles through the needle, then continue withdrawing until the accurate amount of medication has been withdrawn.	5			
16. Withdraw the needle from the vial, and carefully replace the needle cover without letting the needle touch the outside of the cover.	10			
17. Return the medication to the shelf or the refrigerator, checking that you have the correct drug and dosage.	10			

Comments:

Total Points Earned _____ Divided by _____ Total Possible Points = _____ % Score

Instructor's Signature _____

Procedure 34-6 Apply Pharmacology Principles to Prepare and Administer Oral and Parenteral (Excluding IV) Medications: Reconstitute a Powdered Drug for Administration

Task: To reconstitute a powdered drug for intramuscular injection as ordered by the physician.

Equipment and Supplies:
- Vial containing the ordered powdered medication
- Diluent: Sterile saline
- Alcohol wipes
- Cotton ball
- Two sterile needle and syringe units
- Disposable gloves
- Sharps container
- Written order, including the patient's name, when to give the drug, the route of administration, and the name and strength of the drug

Standards: Complete the procedure and all critical steps in _____ minutes with a minimum score of _____% within three attempts.

Scoring: Divide points earned by total possible points. Failure to perform a critical step that is indicated with an asterisk (*) will result in an unsatisfactory overall score.

Time began _____ **Time ended** _____

Steps	Possible Points	First Attempt	Second Attempt	Third Attempt
1. Wash your hands. Follow standard precautions.	10	_____	_____	_____
2. Select the correct vial of powdered medication from the shelf and the recommended diluent for reconstitution. Perform the three drug label and physician order checks during preparation, and verify the seven rights throughout the procedure.*	20	_____	_____	_____
3. Read the label to determine the correct amount of diluent to add to create the dose ordered by the physician. Calculate the correct dose, if necessary, and continue with the three label checks.	20	_____	_____	_____
4. Remove the tops from each vial, and clean each with an alcohol wipe. Leave the wipes in place on top of each vial.	5	_____	_____	_____

Steps	Possible Points	First Attempt	Second Attempt	Third Attempt
5. Using one of the syringe units with the needle cover in place, grasp the syringe plunger and draw up the amount of air equal to the amount of diluent needed to reconstitute the drug.	10			
6. Remove the needle cover, and insert the needle into the center of the rubber stopper of the diluent. Hold the vial firmly against a flat surface and watch carefully that the needle touches only the cleaned rubber area.	10			
7. Inject the aspirated air in the syringe into the diluent vial.	10			
8. Invert the diluent vial, and aspirate the calculated or recommended amount of diluent.*	10			
9. Remove the needle from the diluent vial, and inject the diluent into the drug vial. Remove the needle, and discard the syringe unit into the sharps container.	10			
10. Roll the vial with the drug and diluent mixture between the palms of your hands to mix it thoroughly. Do not shake the vial unless directed to do so on the drug label. When the medication is completely mixed there is no residue or crystals on the bottom of the vial.	10			
11. Aspirate air into the second syringe unit that is equal to the calculated amount of medication to be administered.	10			
12. Inject the air into the mixed drug vial, invert the vial, and withdraw the ordered amount of medication.	10			

Comments:

Total Points Earned _____ Divided by _____ Total Possible Points = _____ % Score

Instructor's Signature _____

Procedure 34-7 Apply Pharmacology Principles to Prepare and Administer Oral and Parenteral (Excluding IV) Medications: Give an Intradermal Injection

Task: To inject 0.1 mL of purified protein derivative (PPD) to perform a Mantoux test as ordered by the physician.

Equipment and Supplies:
- Vial of tuberculin PPD
- Alcohol wipes
- 27-gauge, ⅜-inch sterile needle and syringe unit with safety needle cover device
- Physician order, including the patient's name, when to give the drug, the route of administration, and the name and strength of the drug
- Disposable gloves
- Gauze squares
- Sharps container
- Patient medical record
- Written patient instructions for follow-up

Standards: Complete the procedure and all critical steps in _____ minutes with a minimum score of _____% within three attempts.

Scoring: Divide points earned by total possible points. Failure to perform a critical step that is indicated with an asterisk (*) will result in an unsatisfactory overall score.

Time began _____ **Time ended** _____

Steps	Possible Points	First Attempt	Second Attempt	Third Attempt
1. Wash your hands. Follow standard precautions.	10	_____	_____	_____
2. Select the correct medication from the shelf or the refrigerator.	10	_____	_____	_____
3. Read the label to be sure that you have the right drug (PPD) and the right strength. Perform the three label and order checks as the medication is dispensed.*	10	_____	_____	_____
4. Warm refrigerated medications by gently rolling the container between your palms.	5	_____	_____	_____
5. Prepare the syringe as described in Procedure 34-5, withdrawing the correct dose of 0.1 mL.	20	_____	_____	_____
6. Transport the medication to the patient.	10	_____	_____	_____
7. Greet and identify the patient by name.	10	_____	_____	_____

Steps	Possible Points	First Attempt	Second Attempt	Third Attempt
8. Ask the patient if he or she has ever had a positive reaction to a PPD (TB test) injection before. If yes, then report this information to the physician before administering the test. An individual who has a history of a positive PPD test result will always have a positive result because of antibody action.*	10			
9. Apply gloves, and position the patient comfortably.	10			
10. Locate the antecubital space, then find a site several fingerwidths down the midanterior aspect of the forearm. Avoid any scarred, discolored, or pigmented areas.	20			
11. Cleanse the patient's skin with an alcohol wipe using a circular motion, moving from the center outward.	10			
12. Allow the antiseptic to dry.	5			
13. Remove the cap from the needle.	5			
14. With the thumb and first two fingers of your nondominant hand, stretch the skin of the forearm apart and taut at the location of the injection.	10			
15. Grasp the syringe between the thumb and first two fingers of your dominant hand, palm down, with the needle bevel upward. Hold the syringe close to the plunger end.	10			
16. At a 15-degree angle, with the syringe unit parallel to the surface of the skin, carefully insert the needle just until the bevel point is under the skin surface	20			
17. Slowly and steadily inject the medication by depressing the plunger with your little finger. Do not aspirate. A wheal should appear.*	20			
18. After administering all of the medication (0.1 mL), withdraw the needle.	10			
19. Immediately cover the contaminated needle with the safety device and dispose of the syringe unit in a sharps container.	10			
20. Do not massage, but you may blot the area with a cotton ball or gauze square. Do not cover the site with a bandage.	5			
21. Make sure that your patient is comfortable and safe.	5			

Steps	Possible Points	First Attempt	Second Attempt	Third Attempt
22. Observe the patient for any adverse reaction.	10	_____	_____	_____
23. Dispose of the gloves in the biohazard container, and wash your hands.	10	_____	_____	_____
24. Record the procedure and any reactions that occurred at the site of the injection on the patient's medical record. Include the exact site of the injection.	10	_____	_____	_____
25. Tell the patient when to return to the office for any reaction to be read, or give the patient a postcard to be completed and returned.*	10	_____	_____	_____

Reading the Mantoux Test Results

26. Apply latex gloves; using good lighting and with the patient's arm slightly flexed, measure the induration at the site of the injection. Measure only the raised area; do not include any areas of inflammation.*	10	_____	_____	_____
27. Discard the gloves in the biohazard waste container and wash your hands.	5	_____	_____	_____
28. Document the results of the Mantoux test in the patient chart, including a complete description of the size of the induration, if any, and the appearance of the test site. Notify the physician.	10	_____	_____	_____

Documentation in the Medical Record

_____

_____

_____

Comments:

Total Points Earned _____ Divided by _____ Total Possible Points = _____ % Score

Instructor's Signature _____

Student Name _____ Date _____ Score _____

Procedure 34-8 Apply Pharmacology Principles to Prepare and Administer Oral and Parenteral (Excluding IV) Medications: Give a Subcutaneous Injection

Task: To inject 0.5 mL of medication into the subcutaneous tissue using a 25-gauge, ⅝-inch needle and syringe of correct size and type, as directed by the physician.

Equipment and Supplies:
- A vial of ordered medication
- Alcohol wipes
- Gauze squares or cotton balls
- A sterile needle and syringe unit with safety cover device
- Disposable gloves
- Sharps container
- A written order, including the patient's name, when to give the drug, the route of administration, and the name and strength of the drug
- Patient's medical record

Order: Administer 0.5 mL Varicella vaccine SC stat to Mandy Leno, age 11.

Standards: Complete the procedure and all critical steps in _____ minutes with a minimum score of _____% within three attempts.

Scoring: Divide points earned by total possible points. Failure to perform a critical step that is indicated with an asterisk (*) will result in an unsatisfactory overall score.

Time began _____ Time ended _____

Steps	Possible Points	First Attempt	Second Attempt	Third Attempt
1. Wash your hands. Follow standard precautions.	10	_____	_____	_____
2. Select the correct medication from the shelf or the refrigerator.	10	_____	_____	_____
3. Read the label to be sure that you have the right drug and the right strength. Perform the three label and order checks while dispensing the medication, and verify the seven rights. Perform any necessary dose calculations.*	20	_____	_____	_____
4. Warm refrigerated medications by gently rolling the container between your palms.	5	_____	_____	_____
5. Prepare the syringe, withdrawing the correct dose.	10	_____	_____	_____
6. Transport the medication to the patient.	5	_____	_____	_____

Steps	Possible Points	First Attempt	Second Attempt	Third Attempt
7. Greet and identify the patient by name. Explain the purpose of the immunization.*	10			
8. Ask the patient to sit upright, and help position her comfortably if necessary.	5			
9. Expose the upper posterior arm.	5			
10. Apply gloves, and with the thumb and fingers of your nondominant hand, grasp the tissue of the posterior upper arm. Cleanse the patient's skin with the antiseptic sponge, using a circular motion, moving outward from the center.	10			
11. Remove the cap from the needle.	5			
12. Hold the syringe between the thumb and the first two fingers of your dominant hand, and with one swift movement, insert the entire needle up to the hub at a 45-degree angle.	20			
13. Aspirate (except when administering heparin or insulin) by withdrawing the plunger slightly to be sure that no blood enters the syringe.	10			
14. If blood appears, immediately withdraw the unit without injecting the medication and dispose of it in the sharps container. Compress the injection site with an alcohol swab or gauze bandage.	10			
15. Begin again with step 1.	10			
16. If no blood appears in the syringe, push in the plunger slowly and steadily until all medication has been administered.	10			
17. Place the gauze square next to the needle, and withdraw it at the same angle of insertion. Immediately place the safety device over the contaminated needle.	10			
18. Gently massage the site with the gauze square (do not massage insulin or heparin injections).	5			
19. Discard the needle and syringe into the sharps container.	10			
20. Make sure that your patient is comfortable and safe.	5			
21. Dispose of the gloves in the biohazard waste, and wash your hands.	10			

Steps	Possible Points	First Attempt	Second Attempt	Third Attempt
22. Observe the patient for any adverse reaction. You may need to keep the patient under observation for 20 to 30 minutes.	5	_____	_____	_____
23. Record the drug administration on the patient's medical record, including the exact injection site, and on the immunization record.	10	_____	_____	_____

Documentation in the Medical Record

_____

_____

_____

Comments:

Total Points Earned _____ Divided by _____ Total Possible Points = _____ % Score

Instructor's Signature _____

Student Name _____ Date _____ Score _____

Procedure 34-9 Apply Pharmacology Principles to Prepare and Administer Oral and Parenteral (Excluding IV) Medications: Give an Intramuscular Injection into the Deltoid

Task: To inject ordered medication into the muscle, using a 22-gauge, 11/2-inch needle and 3-mL syringe, as directed by the physician.

Equipment and Supplies:
- A vial containing ordered medication
- Alcohol wipes
- Cotton ball
- Sterile needle and syringe unit with safety needle cover
- Disposable gloves
- Sharps container
- Written order, including the patient's name, when to give the drug, the route of administration, and the name and strength of the drug
- Patient medical record

Order: Administer 300,000 U Penicillin G IM stat to Ramon Diez, age 23.

Standards: Complete the procedure and all critical steps in _____ minutes with a minimum score of _____% within three attempts.

Scoring: Divide points earned by total possible points. Failure to perform a critical step that is indicated with an asterisk (*) will result in an unsatisfactory overall score.

Time began _____ **Time ended** _____

Steps	Possible Points	First Attempt	Second Attempt	Third Attempt
1. Wash your hands. Follow standard precautions.	10	_____	_____	_____
2. Select the correct medication from storage.	10	_____	_____	_____
3. Read the label to be sure that you have the right drug and the right strength.*	10	_____	_____	_____
4. Warm refrigerated medications by gently rolling between your palms.	5	_____	_____	_____
5. Calculate the correct dose if necessary, and continue with the three label checks while drawing the medication into the syringe.	10	_____	_____	_____
6. Transport the medication to the patient.	5	_____	_____	_____
7. Greet and identify the patient by name.	5	_____	_____	_____
8. Ask patient if he is allergic to penicillin or any other antibiotics.*	10	_____	_____	_____

Steps	Possible Points	First Attempt	Second Attempt	Third Attempt
9. Help the patient into an upright sitting position.	5			
10. Apply gloves, and expose the deltoid site. The mid-deltoid site is located approximately two to three fingerwidths below the acromial process.	10			
11. Cleanse the patient's skin with the alcohol wipe using a circular motion, moving outward from the center.	10			
12. Remove the needle cover. Place your non-dominant hand on the patient's shoulder, and with the thumb and first two fingers spread the skin tightly.	10			
13. Grasp the syringe as you would a dart, and with one swift movement, insert the entire needle up to the hub, at a 90-degree angle, into the muscle.	10			
14. Aspirate: Withdraw the plunger slightly to be sure that no blood enters the syringe.*	10			
15. If blood appears, immediately withdraw the syringe, discard it in the sharps container, and compress the injection site with the cotton ball.	10			
16. Begin again with step 1.	5			
17. If no blood appears in the syringe, push in the plunger slowly and steadily until all medication has been administered.	10			
18. Place the cotton ball next to the needle and apply counterpressure to the area while you withdraw the needle at the same angle of insertion. Immediately place the safety cover over the contaminated needle and discard the syringe unit into the sharps container.	10			
19. Gently massage the site with the cotton ball.	10			
20. Make sure that your patient is comfortable and safe.	5			
21. Observe the patient for any adverse reaction. You may need to keep the patient under observation for 20 to 30 minutes.	5			
22. Dispose of the gloves in the biohazard waste and wash your hands.	10			

Steps	Possible Points	First Attempt	Second Attempt	Third Attempt
23. Record the drug administration on the patient's medical record, and on the required DEA record if the medication is a controlled substance.	__10__	_____	_____	_____

Documentation in the Medical Record

_____

_____

_____

Comments:

Total Points Earned _____ Divided by _____ Total Possible Points = _____ % Score

Instructor's Signature _____

Procedure 34-10 Apply Pharmacology Principles to Prepare and Administer Oral and Parenteral (Excluding IV) Medications: Administer a Pediatric Intramuscular Vastus Lateralis Injection

Task: To inject 0.5 mL of vaccine into the vastus lateralis muscle, using a 22-gauge, ⅝-inch needle.

Equipment and Supplies:
- A vial containing Hib vaccine
- Alcohol wipes
- Cotton ball or 2 × 2 gauze square
- Sterile needle and syringe unit with safety device
- Disposable gloves
- Sharps container
- Written order, including the patient's name, when to give the drug, the route of administration, and the name and strength of the drug
- Patient's medical record

Order: Administer 0.5 mL of *Haemophilus Influenzae* (Hib) vaccine IM to Lizzy Dearborne, age 4 months, stat.

Standards: Complete the procedure and all critical steps in _____ minutes with a minimum score of _____% within three attempts.

Scoring: Divide points earned by total possible points. Failure to perform a critical step that is indicated with an asterisk (*) will result in an unsatisfactory overall score.

Time began _____ **Time ended** _____

Steps	Possible Points	First Attempt	Second Attempt	Third Attempt
1. Check the patient's medical record for a previous allergic reaction to Hib vaccine; check the baby's temperature and ask caregiver about recent illnesses, because those with moderate to severe illness should not receive the vaccination.	10	_____	_____	_____
2. Wash your hands. Follow standard precautions.	10	_____	_____	_____
3. Select the correct medication from storage.	10	_____	_____	_____
4. Read the label to be sure that you have the right drug and the right strength, and check the expiration date.*	10	_____	_____	_____
5. Warm refrigerated medications by gently rolling between your palms.	5	_____	_____	_____

Steps	Possible Points	First Attempt	Second Attempt	Third Attempt
6. Calculate the correct dose if needed, and continue with the three label checks while drawing the medication into the syringe. Follow the steps explained in Procedure 34-5 to correctly draw up the vaccination.	10			
7. Complete the vaccination log according to office procedure.	5			
8. Transport the medication to the patient.	5			
9. Greet and identify the patient's caregiver and child by name.	10			
10. Explain the procedure to the child's caregiver.*	10			
11. Position the infant on her back. Ask the caregiver to remove any clothing necessary to expose the infant's thighs. Choose either the right or the left thigh for the injection.	10			
12. Apply gloves, and cleanse the patient's skin with the alcohol wipe using a circular motion, moving outward from the center.	10			
13. Ask for caregiver assistance in holding the child still if necessary.	5			
14. Remove the needle cover, and with the thumb and first two fingers of your non-dominant hand, spread the skin at the site tightly.	10			
15. Grasp the syringe as you would a dart, and with one swift movement insert the needle at a 45-degree angle into the muscle, with the needle pointing toward the feet.	10			
16. Aspirate: Withdraw the plunger slightly to be sure that no blood enters the syringe.*	10			
17. If blood appears, immediately withdraw the syringe, discard it in the sharps container, and compress the injection site with the cotton ball. Begin again with step 2.	10			
18. If no blood appears in the syringe, push in the plunger slowly and steadily until all medication has been administered.	10			

Steps	Possible Points	First Attempt	Second Attempt	Third Attempt
19. Place the cotton ball next to the needle, and apply counterpressure to the area while you withdraw the needle at the same angle of insertion. Immediately place the safety cover over the contaminated needle and discard the syringe unit into the sharps container.	10			
20. Gently massage the site with the cotton ball.	5			
21. Make sure that the infant is safely held by the caregiver.	5			
22. Dispose of gloves in the biohazard waste, and wash your hands.	10			
23. Record drug administration in the patient's medical record and on the vaccination log.*	10			
24. Observe the patient for 20 to 30 minutes for any adverse reaction.	10			

Documentation in the Medical Record

_____

_____

_____

Comments:

Total Points Earned _____ Divided by _____ Total Possible Points = _____ % Score

Instructor's Signature _____

Procedure 34-11 Apply Pharmacology Principles to Prepare and Administer Oral and Parenteral (Excluding IV) Medications: Give a Z-Track Intramuscular Injection into the Dorsogluteal Site

Task: To inject 1 mL of medication into the muscle using a 23-gauge, 2-inch needle and 3-mL syringe and the Z-track method, as directed by the physician.

Equipment and Supplies:
- Vial containing the ordered medication
- Alcohol wipes
- Cotton ball
- Disposable gloves
- Sharps container
- Sterile needle and syringe unit with safety needle cover
- Additional sterile needle
- Written order, including the patient's name, when to give the drug, the route of administration, and the name and strength of the drug

Standards: Complete the procedure and all critical steps in _____ minutes with a minimum score of _____% within three attempts.

Scoring: Divide points earned by total possible points. Failure to perform a critical step that is indicated with an asterisk (*) will result in an unsatisfactory overall score.

Time began _____ **Time ended** _____

Steps	Possible Points	First Attempt	Second Attempt	Third Attempt
1. Wash your hands. Follow standard precautions.	10	____	____	____
2. Select the correct medication from the shelf or the refrigerator.	10	____	____	____
3. Perform the three order and label checks as well as verifying the seven rights.*	10	____	____	____
4. Warm refrigerated medications by gently rolling the container between your palms.	5	____	____	____
5. Draw up the ordered amount of medication into the syringe unit.	10	____	____	____
6. Replace the needle cover, and give a slight turn to loosen the needle. Secure a new needle, still in its sheath, to the tip of the syringe, being careful not to contaminate the needle or hub of the syringe. Discard the contaminated needle.	10	____	____	____
7. Transport the medication to the patient.	5	____	____	____

Steps	Possible Points	First Attempt	Second Attempt	Third Attempt
8. Greet and identify the patient by name.	5			
9. Position the patient comfortably in Sims' position.	5			
10. Expose the site and apply gloves. The dorsogluteal site is found by placing the palm of the nondominant hand on the greater trochanter of the femur, pointing your fingers toward the posterior iliac spine and index finger toward the anterior iliac spine. The injection site is in the upper outer area of the gluteus medius. This area needs to be seen for Z-track injection.*	20			
11. Cleanse the patient's skin with the alcohol wipe, using a circular motion, moving outward from the center. Make sure to clean the actual area of injection.	10			
12. Remove the needle cover.	5			
13. Push the skin to one side, and hold it firmly in place. If the skin is slippery, use a dry gauze sponge to hold the skin in place.	10			
14. Grasp the syringe as you would a dart, and with one swift movement insert the entire needle up to the hub at a 90-degree angle into the upper outer area of the gluteus medius muscle.	10			
15. Aspirate: Withdraw the plunger slightly to be sure that no blood enters the syringe.*	10			
16. If blood appears, immediately withdraw the syringe, dispose of the syringe unit in the sharps container, and compress the injection site with a gauze square or cotton ball.	10			
17. Begin again with step 1.	5			
18. If no blood appears in the syringe, push in the plunger slowly and steadily until all medication has been administered.	10			
19. Wait 10 seconds for medication to be dispersed, then withdraw the needle at the same angle of insertion. As the needle is withdrawn, release the displaced skin to prevent the tracking of medication to the surface.*	10			

Steps	Possible Points	First Attempt	Second Attempt	Third Attempt
20. If the manufacturer recommends it, gently massage the site with the gauze square or cotton ball. Many medications requiring Z-track administration should not be massaged.	10			
21. Immediately place the safety needle cover over the contaminated needle and dispose of the needle and syringe unit into a sharps container.	10			
22. Make sure your patient is comfortable and safe.	5			
23. Dispose of gloves in the biohazard waste, and wash your hands.	10			
24. Observe the patient for any adverse reaction. You may need to keep the patient under observation for 20 to 30 minutes.	5			
25. Record the drug administration on the patient's medical record, including the exact site of injection.	10			

Documentation in the Medical Record

_____

_____

_____

Comments:

Total Points Earned _____ Divided by _____ Total Possible Points = _____ % Score

Instructor's Signature _____

Student Name _____ Date _____ Score _____

Procedure 35-1 Use an Automated External Defibrillator (AED)

Task: To defibrillate adult victims with cardiac arrest.

Equipment and Supplies:
- Practice automated external defibrillator (AED)
- Approved mannequin

Standards: Complete the procedure and all critical steps in _____ minutes with a minimum score of _____% within three attempts.

Scoring: Divide points earned by total possible points. Failure to perform a critical step that is indicated with an asterisk (*) will result in an unsatisfactory overall score.

Time began _____ **Time ended** _____

Steps	Possible Points	First Attempt	Second Attempt	Third Attempt
1. Place the AED near the victim's left ear. Turn the AED on.	20	_____	_____	_____
2. Attach electrode pads as pictured on the AED. Place electrodes at the sternum and apex of the heart. Make sure pads have complete contact with the victim's chest and they do not overlap.	20	_____	_____	_____
3. All rescuers must clear away from the victim. Press the ANALYZE button. The AED will analyze the victim's coronary status, will announce if the victim is going to be shocked, and automatically charges the electrodes.	20	_____	_____	_____
4. All rescuers must clear away from the victim. Press the SHOCK button if the machine is not automated. May repeat three analyze-shock cycles.*	20	_____	_____	_____
5. After three shocks are delivered, reassess the patient's status. If there is no pulse, perform CPR for 1 minute. Then repeat.	10	_____	_____	_____
6. If the machine gives the "no shock indicated" signal, assess the victim. Check the carotid pulse and breathing status and keep the AED attached until emergency medical services arrive.	20	_____	_____	_____
7. Keep AED pads in place to quickly diagnose ventricular fibrillation if it occurs.	10	_____	_____	_____

Documentation in the Medical Record

_____

_____

_____

_____

Comments:

Total Points Earned _____ Divided by _____ Total Possible Points = _____ % Score

Instructor's Signature _____

Student Name _____ Date _____ Score _____

Procedure 35-2 Perform Telephone Screening and Appropriate Documentation

Task: To asses the direction of emergency care and document information appropriately in the patient record.

Equipment and Supplies:
- Note pad with pen or pencil
- Patient record
- Facility's emergency procedures manual
- Appointment book or program
- Area emergency numbers

Practice Scenario: Cheryl is working with the phone triage staff, when they receive a call from the mother of a 5-year-old patient; the mother reports that her son fell and cut his arm. What type of information should Cheryl gather about the injury? What action should be taken? How should the incident be documented?

Standards: Complete the procedure and all critical steps in _____ minutes with a minimum score of _____% within three attempts.

Scoring: Divide points earned by total possible points. Failure to perform a critical step that is indicated with an asterisk (*) will result in an unsatisfactory overall score.

Time began _____ Time ended _____

Steps	Possible Points	First Attempt	Second Attempt	Third Attempt
1. Stay calm and reassure the caller.	5	_____	_____	_____
2. Verify the identity of the caller and the injured patient.	5	_____	_____	_____
3. Immediately record the name of the caller and the patient, location, and phone number.*	10	_____	_____	_____
4. Determine if the patient's condition is life-threatening. Quantify the amount of blood loss, if the patient is alert and responsive, if breathing is normal. Notify EMS if necessary*.	10	_____	_____	_____
5. If EMS is notified, stay on the line with the caller until EMS personnel arrive at the scene.	10	_____	_____	_____

Steps	Possible Points	First Attempt	Second Attempt	Third Attempt
6. If emergency services are not needed, gather details about the injury to determine if the patient can be seen in the office or should be referred to an emergency room (ER). Consider the following questions: • Is there a suspected head or neck injury? Has the patient been moved? • Is there a possible fracture? If so, where? • Are there any other symptoms? • Is there anything pertinent in the patient's health history that would complicate the situation? • Has the caller administered any first aid? What?	10			
7. Based on information gathered, determine when the patient should be seen in the office if he or she has not been referred to an ER.	10			
8. At any point in this process, do not hesitate to consult the physician or experienced staff or refer to the facility's emergency procedures manual to determine how to manage the patient's problem.	10			
9. Always allow the caller to hang up first, just in case more information or assistance is needed.	5			
10. Document information gathered, actions taken or recommended, any home care recommendations, and whether the physician was notified.*	10			

Documentation in the Medical Record

_____

_____

_____

_____

Comments:

Total Points Earned _____ Divided by _____ Total Possible Points = _____ % Score

Instructor's Signature _____

Student Name _____ Date _____ Score _____

Procedure 35-3 Perform Adult Rescue Breathing and One-Rescuer CPR

Task: To restore a victim's breathing and blood circulation when respiration and/or pulse stop.

Equipment and Supplies:
- Disposable gloves
- CPR ventilator mask
- Approved mannequin

Standards: Complete the procedure and all critical steps in _____ minutes with a minimum score of _____% within three attempts.

Scoring: Divide points earned by total possible points. Failure to perform a critical step that is indicated with an asterisk (*) will result in an unsatisfactory overall score.

Time began _____ **Time ended** _____

Steps	Possible Points	First Attempt	Second Attempt	Third Attempt
1. Establish unresponsiveness. Tap the victim and ask, "Are you OK?" Wait for victim to respond.	10	_____	_____	_____
2. Activate the emergency response system. Put on gloves and get ventilator mask.	5	_____	_____	_____
3. Tilt the victim's head by placing one hand on the forehead and applying enough pressure to push the head back and with the fingers of the other hand under the chin, lift up and pull the jaw forward. Look, listen, and feel for signs of breathing. Place your ear over the mouth and listen for breathing. Watch the rising and falling of the chest for evidence of breathing. If breathing is absent or inadequate, open the airway and place the ventilator mask over the victim's nose and mouth.	10	_____	_____	_____
4. Give two slow breaths (1½ to 2 seconds per breath for an adult and 1 to 2 seconds per breath for an infant or child), holding the ventilator mask tightly against the face while tilting the victim's chin back to keep the airway open. Remove your mouth from the mouthpiece between breaths to allow time for patient exhalation between breaths.	10	_____	_____	_____

853

Steps	Possible Points	First Attempt	Second Attempt	Third Attempt
5. Check the patient's pulse (at the carotid for an adult or older child or brachial artery for an infant). If a pulse is present, continue rescue breathing (one breath every 4 to 5 seconds, about 10 to 12 breaths per minute for an adult, or one breath every 3 seconds for an infant or child). If no signs of circulation are present, begin cycles of 15 chest compressions (at a rate of about 100 compressions per minute for an adult) followed by two slow breaths.*	10	_____	_____	_____
6. To deliver chest compressions, kneel at the victim's side a couple of inches away from the chest. Move your fingers up the ribs to the point where the sternum and the ribs join in the center of the lower part of the sternum but above the xiphoid process.	10	_____	_____	_____
7. Place the heel of your hand on the chest over the lower part of the sternum.*	5	_____	_____	_____
8. Place your other hand on top of the first and either interlace or lift your fingers upward off of the chest.*	5	_____	_____	_____
9. Bring your shoulders directly over the victim's sternum as you compress downward, and keep your elbows locked.	5	_____	_____	_____
10. Depress the sternum 1½ to 2 inches in an adult victim. Relax the pressure on the sternum after each compression, but do not remove your hands from the victim's sternum.	10	_____	_____	_____
11. After performing 15 compressions (at a rate of about 100 compressions per minute), open the airway and give two slow rescue breaths.	5	_____	_____	_____
12. After four cycles of compressions and breaths (15:2 ratio, about 1 minute) recheck breathing and carotid pulse. If there is a pulse but no breathing, continue rescue breathing (one breath every 5 seconds, about 10 to 12 breaths per minute) and reevaluate the victim's breathing and pulse every few minutes. If no signs of circulation are present, continue 15:2 cycles of compressions and ventilations, starting with chest compressions. Continue giving CPR until EMS relieves you.	5	_____	_____	_____
13. Remove gloves and the ventilator mask valve and dispose in the biohazard container. Disinfect the ventilator mask per manufacturer recommendations. Wash hands.	5	_____	_____	_____

Steps	Possible Points	First Attempt	Second Attempt	Third Attempt
14. Document the procedure and patient condition.	5			

Documentation in the Medical Record

_____

_____

_____

_____

Comments:

Total Points Earned _____ Divided by _____ Total Possible Points = _____ % Score

Instructor's Signature _____

Student Name _____ Date _____ Score _____

Procedure 35-4 Administer Oxygen

Task: To provide oxygen for a patient in respiratory distress.

Equipment and Supplies:
- Portable oxygen tank
- Pressure regulator
- Flow meter
- Nasal cannula with connecting tubing

Standards: Complete the procedure and all critical steps in _____ minutes with a minimum score of _____% within three attempts.

Scoring: Divide points earned by total possible points. Failure to perform a critical step that is indicated with an asterisk (*) will result in an unsatisfactory overall score.

Time began _____ **Time ended** _____

Steps	Possible Points	First Attempt	Second Attempt	Third Attempt
1. Gather equipment and wash hands.	10	_____	_____	_____
2. Identify the patient and explain the procedure.	10	_____	_____	_____
3. Check the pressure gauge on the tank to determine the amount of oxygen in the tank.	10	_____	_____	_____
4. If necessary, open the cylinder on the tank one full counterclockwise turn, then attach the cannula tubing to the flow meter.	20	_____	_____	_____
5. Adjust the administration of the oxygen according to the physician's order. Usually the flow meter is set at 12 to 15 liters per minute (LPM). Check to make sure oxygen is flowing through the cannula.*	10	_____	_____	_____
6. Insert cannula tips into the nostrils and adjust the tubing around the back of the patient's ears.	10	_____	_____	_____
7. Make sure the patient is comfortable and answer any questions.	10	_____	_____	_____
8. Wash hands.	10	_____	_____	_____
9. Document the procedure, including the number of liters of oxygen being adminis-tered and the patient's condition. Continue to monitor the patient throughout the procedure, and document any changes in condition.	10	_____	_____	_____

Documentation in the Medical Record

_____

_____

_____

_____

Comments:

Total Points Earned _____ Divided by _____ Total Possible Points = _____ % Score

Instructor's Signature _____

Student Name _____ Date _____ Score _____

Procedure 35-5 Respond to an Adult with an Obstructed Airway

Task: To remove an airway obstruction and restore ventilation.

Equipment and Supplies:
- Disposable gloves
- Ventilation mask (for unconscious victim)
- Approved mannequin to practice unconscious foreign body airway obstruction (FBAO)

Standards: Complete the procedure and all critical steps in _____ minutes with a minimum score of _____% within three attempts.

Scoring: Divide points earned by total possible points. Failure to perform a critical step that is indicated with an asterisk (*) will result in an unsatisfactory overall score.

Time began _____ **Time ended** _____

Steps	Possible Points	First Attempt	Second Attempt	Third Attempt
1. Ask "Are you choking?" If victim indicates yes, ask "Can you speak?" If the victim is unable to speak, tell the victim you are going to help.	10	_____	_____	_____
2. Stand behind the victim with feet slightly apart.	5	_____	_____	_____
3. Reach around the victim's abdomen and place an index finger into the victim's navel or at the level of the belt buckle. Make a fist of the opposite hand (do not tuck the thumb into the fist) and place the thumb side of the fist against the victim's abdomen above the navel. If the victim is pregnant, place the fist above the enlarged uterus. If the victim is obese, it may be necessary to place the fist higher in the abdomen. It may be necessary to perform chest thrusts on a victim who is pregnant or obese.	5	_____	_____	_____
4. Place the opposite hand over the fist and give abdominal thrusts in a quick inward and upward movement.*	5	_____	_____	_____
5. Repeat the abdominal thrusts until the object is expelled or the victim becomes unresponsive.	5	_____	_____	_____

Steps	Possible Points	First Attempt	Second Attempt	Third Attempt
Unresponsive Victim				
6. Activate the emergency response system.	10			
7. Put on disposable gloves and get ventilation mask. Open the victim's mouth with a tongue-jaw lift (hold the tongue down with the thumb and lift the jaw) and perform a finger sweep to determine if the foreign object is in the mouth; attempt to remove it if possible.*	5			
8. If the obstruction is still lodged, open the airway with a head-tilt, jaw-thrust maneuver and attempt to ventilate using the barrier device with two slow breaths. If breaths do not go in (chest does not rise), retilt the head and try to ventilate again.	5			
9. If ventilation is unsuccessful, move to the victim's feet and kneel astride the victim's thighs. Place the heel of one hand above the navel but below the xiphoid process of the sternum. Place the other hand on top of the first, with the fingers elevated off of the abdomen. Administer five quick abdominal thrusts, pushing in and up.*	5			
10. Move back beside the head of the victim and repeat the finger sweep. If the obstruction is not found, continue cycles of two rescue breaths, five abdominal thrusts, and finger sweep until either the obstruction is removed or EMS arrives.	5			
11. If the obstruction is removed, assess the victim for breathing and circulation. If a pulse is present, but the patient is not breathing, begin rescue breathing. If no pulse is present, begin CPR.	5			
12. Once either the patient is stabilized or EMS has taken over care, remove gloves and the ventilator mask valve and dispose in the biohazard container. Disinfect the ventilator mask per manufacturer recommendations. Wash hands.	5			
13. Document the procedure and patient condition.	5			

Documentation in the Medical Record

_____

_____

_____

_____

Comments:

Total Points Earned _____ Divided by _____ Total Possible Points = _____ % Score

Instructor's Signature _____

Student Name _____ Date _____ Score _____

Procedure 35-6 Care for a Patient Who Has Fainted

Task: To provide emergency care for and assessment of a patient who has fainted.

Equipment and Supplies:
- Sphygmomanometer
- Stethoscope
- Watch with second hand
- Blanket
- Foot stool or box
- Oxygen equipment, if ordered by physician
  - Portable oxygen tank
  - Pressure regulator
  - Flow meter
  - Nasal cannula with connecting tubing

Standards: Complete the procedure and all critical steps in _____ minutes with a minimum score of _____% within three attempts.

Scoring: Divide points earned by total possible points. Failure to perform a critical step that is indicated with an asterisk (*) will result in an unsatisfactory overall score.

Time began _____ **Time ended** _____

Steps	Possible Points	First Attempt	Second Attempt	Third Attempt
1. If warning is given that the patient feels faint, have the patient lower the head to the knees to increase the blood supply to the brain.* If this does not stop the episode, either have the patient lie down on the examination table or lower the patient to the floor. If the patient collapses to the floor when fainting, treat with caution because of possible head or neck injuries.	10	_____	_____	_____
2. Immediately notify the physician of the patient's condition, and assess the patient for life-threatening emergencies such as respiratory or cardiac arrest. If the patient is breathing and has a pulse, monitor the patient's vital signs.	10	_____	_____	_____
3. Loosen any tight clothing and keep the patient warm, applying a blanket if needed.	20	_____	_____	_____
4. If there is no concern about a head or neck injury, elevate the patient's legs above the level of the heart.*	10	_____	_____	_____

Steps	Possible Points	First Attempt	Second Attempt	Third Attempt
5. Continue to monitor vital signs, and apply oxygen via nasal cannula if ordered by the physician.	10			
6. If vital signs are unstable or the patient does not respond quickly, activate emergency medical services.	10			
7. If the patient vomits, roll the patient on his or her side to avoid aspiration of vomitus into the lungs.	10			
8. Once the patient has completely recovered, assist the patient into a sitting position. Do not leave the patient unattended on the examination table.	10			
9. Document the incident, including a description of the episode, patient symptoms, vital signs, length of time, and any complaints. If oxygen was administered, document the number of liters and length of administration.	10			

Documentation in the Medical Record

_____

_____

_____

_____

Comments:

Total Points Earned _____ Divided by _____ Total Possible Points = _____ % Score

Instructor's Signature _____

Student Name _____ Date _____ Score _____

Procedure 35-7 Control Bleeding

Task: To stop hemorrhaging from an open wound.

Equipment and Supplies:
- Gloves, sterile if available
- Appropriate personal protective equipment (PPE) according to OSHA guidelines including:
  - Impermeable gown
  - Goggles or face shield
  - Impermeable mask
- Sterile dressings
- Bandaging material
- Biohazard waste container

Standards: Complete the procedure and all critical steps in _____ minutes with a minimum score of _____% within three attempts.

Scoring: Divide points earned by total possible points. Failure to perform a critical step that is indicated with an asterisk (*) will result in an unsatisfactory overall score.

Time began _____ Time ended _____

Steps	Possible Points	First Attempt	Second Attempt	Third Attempt
1. Wash hands, and apply appropriate personal protective equipment.	10	_____	_____	_____
2. Assemble equipment and supplies.	10	_____	_____	_____
3. Apply several layers of sterile dressing material directly to the wound, and exert pressure.	10	_____	_____	_____
4. Wrap the wound with bandage material. Add more dressing and bandaging material if bleeding continues.	10	_____	_____	_____
5. If bleeding persists and the wound is located on an extremity, elevate the extremity above the level of the heart. Notify the physician immediately if bleeding cannot be controlled.	10	_____	_____	_____

Steps	Possible Points	First Attempt	Second Attempt	Third Attempt
6. If bleeding still continues, maintain direct pressure and elevation; also apply pressure to the appropriate artery. If bleeding is in the arm, apply pressure to the brachial artery by squeezing the inner aspect of the upper mid-arm. If bleeding is in the leg, apply pressure to the femoral artery on the affected side by pushing with the heel of the hand into the femoral crease at the groin. If bleeding cannot be controlled, it may be necessary to activate the emergency medical system.	10			
7. Once the bleeding is controlled and the patient is stabilized, dispose of contaminated materials into the biohazard waste container.	10			
8. Disinfect the area, remove gloves, and dispose into biohazard waste.	10			
9. Wash hands.	10			
10. Document the incident, including the details of the wound, when and how it occurred, patient symptoms, vital signs, physician treatment, and the patient's current condition.	10			

Documentation in the Medical Record

_____

_____

_____

_____

Comments:

Total Points Earned _____ Divided by _____ Total Possible Points = _____ % Score

Instructor's Signature _____

Procedure 36-1 Prepare Patient for and Assist with Routine and Specialty Examinations: Measure Distance Visual Acuity Using the Snellen Chart

Task: To determine the patient's degree of visual clarity at a measured distance of 20 feet using the Snellen chart.

Equipment and Supplies:
- Snellen eye chart
- Eye occluder
- Pen or pencil and paper
- Patient record

Standards: Complete the procedure and all critical steps in _____ minutes with a minimum score of _____% within three attempts.

Scoring: Divide points earned by total possible points. Failure to perform a critical step that is indicated with an asterisk (*) will result in an unsatisfactory overall score.

Time began _____ **Time ended** _____

Steps	Possible Points	First Attempt	Second Attempt	Third Attempt
1. Wash your hands.	10	_____	_____	_____
2. Prepare the examination room. Make sure that (a) the room is well lit, (b) a distance marker is 20 feet from the chart, and (c) the chart is placed at the eye level of the patient.	10	_____	_____	_____
3. Identify the patient and explain the procedure. Instruct the patient not to squint during the test, because this temporarily improves vision. The patient should not have an opportunity to study the chart before the test is given. If the patient wears corrective lenses, they should be worn during the test.	10	_____	_____	_____
4. Position the patient in a standing or sitting position at the 20-foot marker.*	10	_____	_____	_____
5. Position the Snellen chart at eye level to the patient.	5	_____	_____	_____
6. Instruct the patient to cover the left eye with the occluder and to keep both eyes open throughout the test to prevent squinting.*	10	_____	_____	_____

Steps	Possible Points	First Attempt	Second Attempt	Third Attempt
7. Stand beside the chart and point to each row as the patient orally reads down the chart, starting with the 20/70 row.*	10			
8. Proceed down the rows of the chart until the smallest row the patient can read with a maximum of two errors is reached. If one or two letters are missed, the outcome is recorded with a minus sign and the number of errors. If more than two errors are made, the previous line should be documented.	10			
9. Record any patient reactions in reading the chart.	5			
10. Repeat the procedure with the left eye.	10			
11. Document the date and time, the procedure, visual acuity results, and any patient reactions on the patient's record. Also record whether corrective lenses were worn.	10			

Documentation in the Medical Record

_____

_____

_____

Comments:

Total Points Earned _____ Divided by _____ Total Possible Points = _____ % Score

Instructor's Signature _____

Procedure 36-2 Prepare Patient for and Assist with Routine and Specialty Examinations: Assess Color Acuity Using the Ishihara Test

Task: To correctly assess a patient's color acuity and record the results.

Equipment and Supplies:
- Room area with natural light
- Ishihara color plate book
- Pen, pencil, and paper
- Watch with a second hand
- Patient record

Standards: Complete the procedure and all critical steps in _____ minutes with a minimum score of _____% within three attempts.

Scoring: Divide points earned by total possible points. Failure to perform a critical step that is indicated with an asterisk (*) will result in an unsatisfactory overall score.

1. Assemble the necessary equipment and prepare the room for testing. The room should be quiet and illuminated with natural light.   __10__   _____   _____   _____

2. Identify the patient, and explain the procedure. Use a practice card during the explanation, and be sure that the patient understands that he or she has 3 seconds to identify each plate.   __10__   _____   _____   _____

3. Hold up the first plate at a right angle to the patient's line of vision and 30 inches from the patient. Be sure both of the patient's eyes are kept open during the test.*   __20__   _____   _____   _____

4. Ask the patient to tell you what number is on the plate, and record the plate number and the patient's answer.*   __10__   _____   _____   _____

5. Continue this sequence until all 11 plates have been read. If the patient cannot identify the number on the plate, place an X in the record for that plate number.   __10__   _____   _____   _____

6. Include any unusual signs in your record, such as eye rubbing, squinting, or excessive blinking.   __10__   _____   _____   _____

7. Place the book back into its cardboard sleeve, and return the book to its storage space.   __10__   _____   _____   _____

Steps	Possible Points	First Attempt	Second Attempt	Third Attempt
8. Record the procedure, including the date and time, the testing results, and any patient signs exhibited during the test in the patient's record.*	20			

Documentation in the Medical Record

_____

_____

_____

Comments:

Total Points Earned _____ Divided by _____ Total Possible Points = _____ % Score

Instructor's Signature _____

Procedure 36-3 Prepare Patient for and Assist with Procedures, Treatments, and Minor Office Surgeries: Irrigate a Patient's Eyes

Task: To cleanse the eye (or eyes), as ordered by the physician.

Equipment and Supplies:
- Prescribed sterile irrigation solution
- Sterile irrigating bulb syringe and sterile basin or prepackaged solution with dispenser
- Basin for drainage
- Sterile gauze squares
- Disposable drape
- Towel
- Nonsterile disposable gloves
- Biohazard waste container
- Patient record

Standards: Complete the procedure and all critical steps in _____ minutes with a minimum score of _____% within three attempts.

Scoring: Divide points earned by total possible points. Failure to perform a critical step that is indicated with an asterisk (*) will result in an unsatisfactory overall score.

Time began _____ **Time ended** _____

Steps	Possible Points	First Attempt	Second Attempt	Third Attempt
1. Wash your hands.	10	_____	_____	_____
2. Check the physician's orders to determine which eye requires irrigation (or whether both eyes require it) and the type of solution to be used.	10	_____	_____	_____
3. Assemble the materials needed.	10	_____	_____	_____
4. Check the expiration date of the solution, and read the label three times.*	10	_____	_____	_____
5. Identify the patient, and explain the procedure.*	10	_____	_____	_____
6. Assist the patient into a sitting or supine position, making certain that the head is turned toward the side of the affected eye. Place the disposable drape over the patient's neck and shoulder.	10	_____	_____	_____
7. Put on gloves, and rinse your gloved hands under warm water to remove all powder from the gloves.	10	_____	_____	_____

Steps	Possible Points	First Attempt	Second Attempt	Third Attempt
8. Place or have the patient hold a drainage basin next to the affected eye to receive the solution from the eye. Place a polylined drape under the basin to avoid getting the solution on the patient.	10			
9. Moisten a gauze square with solution, and cleanse the eyelid and lashes. Start at the inner canthus (near nose) to the outer canthus (farthest from nose) and dispose of the gauze square in the biohazard container after each wipe.*	10			
10. If using a bulb syringe, pour the required volume of body-temperature irrigating solution into the basin and withdraw solution into the bulb syringe. If using an irrigating solution in a prepackaged dispenser, remove the lid.	10			
11. Separate and hold the eyelids with the index finger and thumb of one hand. With the other hand, place the syringe or dispenser on the bridge of the nose parallel to the eye.	10			
12. Squeeze the bulb or dispenser, directing the solution toward the lower conjunctiva of the inner canthus, allowing the solution to flow steadily and slowly from the inner to outer canthus. Do not touch the eye or eyelids with the applicator.	10			
13. Refill the syringe or continue to gently squeeze the prepackaged bottle, and continue the procedure until the amount of solution ordered by the physician has been administered or until drainage from the eye is clear.	10			
14. Dry the eyelid from the inner to outer canthus with sterile gauze. Do not use cotton balls because fibers might remain in the eye.	5			
15. Dispose of the irrigation results, and clean the work area.	5			
16. Remove gloves and wash your hands.	10			
17. Document the procedure in the patient's record using appropriate abbreviations; including the date and time; the type and amount of solution used; which eye was irrigated; any significant patient reactions; and the results.*	20			

Documentation in the Medical Record

_____

_____

_____

Comments:

Total Points Earned _____ Divided by _____ Total Possible Points = _____ % Score

Instructor's Signature _____

Procedure 36-4 Prepare Patient for and Assist with Procedures, Treatments, and Minor Office Surgeries: Instill Eye Medication

Task: To apply medication to the eye(s), as ordered by the physician.

Equipment and Supplies:
- Sterile medication with sterile eye dropper or ophthalmic ointment
- Disposable drape
- Sterile gauze squares
- Disposable nonsterile gloves
- Patient record

Standards: Complete the procedure and all critical steps in _____ minutes with a minimum score of _____% within three attempts.

Scoring: Divide points earned by total possible points. Failure to perform a critical step that is indicated with an asterisk (*) will result in an unsatisfactory overall score.

Time began _____ **Time ended** _____

Steps	Possible Points	First Attempt	Second Attempt	Third Attempt
1. Wash your hands.	10	_____	_____	_____
2. Check the physician's order to determine which eye requires medication (or whether medication is ordered for both eyes) and the name and strength of the medication you will be using.	10	_____	_____	_____
3. Assemble equipment and supplies.	10	_____	_____	_____
4. Read the label of the medication three times.	10	_____	_____	_____
5. Identify the patient, and explain the procedure.*	10	_____	_____	_____
6. Put on nonsterile gloves, and rinse your gloved hands under warm water to remove all powder from the gloves.	5	_____	_____	_____
7. Assist the patient into a sitting or supine position. Ask the patient to tilt the head backward and look up.	5	_____	_____	_____
8. Pull the lower conjunctival sac downward.*	5	_____	_____	_____

Steps	Possible Points	First Attempt	Second Attempt	Third Attempt
9. Insert the prescribed number of drops or amount of ointment into the eye. For eye-drops, place drops in the center of the lower conjunctival sac, with the tip of the dropper held parallel to the eye and ½ inch above the eye sac. For eye ointment (ung), squeeze a thin ribbon along the lower conjunctival sac from inner to outer canthus, making sure not to touch the eye with the applicator.	20			
10. Instruct the patient to gently close the eye and rotate the eyeball.	10			
11. Dry any excess drainage from inner to outer canthus, and explain that the medication may temporarily blur vision.	10			
12. Discard the unused medication, and clean the procedure area.	5			
13. Remove gloves, and wash hands.	10			
14. Record the procedure on the patient's chart, including the date and time; the name and strength of the medication; the amount of the dose administered; which eye was treated; teaching instructions given if the treatment is to continue at home; and any observations.*	20			

Documentation in the Medical Record

_____

_____

_____

Comments:

Total Points Earned _____ Divided by _____ Total Possible Points = _____ % Score

Instructor's Signature _____

Procedure 36-5 Prepare Patient for and Assist with Routine and Specialty Examinations: Measure Hearing Acuity Using an Audiometer

Task: To perform audiometric testing of hearing acuity.

Equipment and Supplies:
- Audiometer with adjustable headphones
- Quiet area
- Patient record

Standards: Complete the procedure and all critical steps in _____ minutes with a minimum score of _____% within three attempts.

Scoring: Divide points earned by total possible points. Failure to perform a critical step that is indicated with an asterisk (*) will result in an unsatisfactory overall score.

Time began _____ **Time ended** _____

Steps	Possible Points	First Attempt	Second Attempt	Third Attempt
1. Wash hands, assemble the equipment, and conduct the patient into a quiet area.	10	_____	_____	_____
2. Explain that the audiometer will measure whether the patient can hear various sound wave frequencies through the headphones. Each ear will be tested separately. When the patient hears a frequency, he or she should raise a hand to signal the medical assistant.*	10	_____	_____	_____
3. Place the headphones over the patient's ears, making sure the headphones are adjusted for comfort.	10	_____	_____	_____
4. The audiometer tests each ear separately, starting at a low frequency. If the results are not automatically recorded by the machine, the medical assistant documents the patient response to the frequencies on a graph or audiogram.	20	_____	_____	_____
5. Frequencies are gradually increased to test patient ability to hear. The medical assistant continues to document each response by the patient.	10	_____	_____	_____

Steps	Possible Points	First Attempt	Second Attempt	Third Attempt
6. The other ear is then tested, and the results are documented.	10			
7. Patient results are given to the physician for interpretation.	10			
8. Disinfect the equipment according to the manufacturer's guidelines.	10			
9. Wash hands.	10			

Documentation in the Medical Record

_____

_____

_____

Comments:

Total Points Earned _____ Divided by _____ Total Possible Points = _____ % Score

Instructor's Signature _____

Student Name _____ Date _____ Score _____

Procedure 36-6 Prepare Patient for and Assist with Procedures, Treatments, and Minor Office Surgeries: Irrigate a Patient's Ear

Task: To remove excessive or impacted cerumen from a patient's ear (or ears).

Equipment and Supplies:
- Irrigating solution
- Basin for irrigating solution
- Bulb syringe or an approved otic irrigation device
- Gauze squares
- Otoscope
- Drainage basin
- Disposable drape with polylined barrier
- Cotton-tipped applicators
- Disposable gloves
- Patient record

Standards: Complete the procedure and all critical steps in _____ minutes with a minimum score of _____% within three attempts.

Scoring: Divide points earned by total possible points. Failure to perform a critical step that is indicated with an asterisk (*) will result in an unsatisfactory overall score.

Time began _____ **Time ended** _____

Steps	Possible Points	First Attempt	Second Attempt	Third Attempt
1. Wash your hands.	5	_____	_____	_____
2. Check the physician's order and assemble the materials needed.	5	_____	_____	_____
3. Check the label of the solution three times: (a) when you remove it from the shelf, (b) when you pour it, and (c) when you return it to the shelf.	5	_____	_____	_____
4. Prepare the solution as ordered. The solution should be at body temperature to help loosen the cerumen.	10	_____	_____	_____
5. Identify the patient, and explain the procedure.*	5	_____	_____	_____
6. View the affected ear with an otoscope to locate cerumen impaction.	5	_____	_____	_____

Steps	Possible Points	First Attempt	Second Attempt	Third Attempt
7. Place the patient in a sitting position with the head tilted toward the affected ear. A water-absorbent towel is placed over a polylined barrier on the patient's shoulder, and the collecting basin is placed on the towel at the base of the ear. The patient can assist you by holding the collecting basin in place.*	5			
8. Apply gloves, and wipe any particles from the outside of the ear with gauze squares.	5			
9. Test to be certain that the solution is warm, fill the syringe, and expel air.	5			
10. Straighten the external ear canal. For adults and children over the age of 3, gently pull the pinna of the ear up and back; for children younger than 3, pull the ear lobe down and back.	10			
11. Place the tip of the syringe into the meatus of the ear.	5			
12. Gently direct the flow of the solution toward the roof of the canal.	5			
13. Refill the syringe with warm solution, and continue until the material has been removed. Note the particles in the collecting basin to evaluate when the material has been successfully removed.	5			
14. Dry the patient's external ear with gauze squares and the visible ear canal gently with cotton-tipped applicators.	5			
15. Inspect the ear with an otoscope to determine the results.	5			
16. Place a clean, absorbent towel on the examination table, and allow the patient to rest quietly with the head turned to the irrigated side while you wait for the physician to return to check the affected ear.	5			
17. Clean the work area, and return all equipment after it has been properly disinfected. Wash your hands.	5			

Steps	Possible Points	First Attempt	Second Attempt	Third Attempt
18. Record the procedure, including the date and time; which ear was irrigated, using the appropriate abbreviations—AU (both ears), AD (right ear), AS (left ear); the type and amount of irrigating solution used; the characteristics of the material returned from the irrigation; the visibility of the tympanic membrane after irrigation; and any patient reactions.	5			

You are ordered to perform an irrigation of both ears on Mrs. Ophelia Black because of impacted cerumen. Otoscopic examination before the irrigation revealed a large amount of dark brown ear wax in both ears. After irrigation both tympanic membranes were visible and Mrs. Black had no complaints of discomfort.

Documentation in the Medical Record

_____

_____

_____

Comments:

Total Points Earned _____ Divided by _____ Total Possible Points = _____ % Score

Instructor's Signature _____

Procedure 36-7 Prepare Patient for and Assist with Procedures, Treatments, and Minor Office Surgeries: Instill Medicated Ear Drops

Task: To instill the correct medication in the accurate dose directly into the external auditory canal.

Equipment and Supplies:
- Prescribed otic drops in dispenser bottle
- Cotton balls
- Disposable gloves
- Patient record

Standards: Complete the procedure and all critical steps in _____ minutes with a minimum score of _____% within three attempts.

Scoring: Divide points earned by total possible points. Failure to perform a critical step that is indicated with an asterisk (*) will result in an unsatisfactory overall score.

Time began _____ **Time ended** _____

Steps	Possible Points	First Attempt	Second Attempt	Third Attempt
1. Wash hands, and gather the needed equipment and supplies.	10			
2. Check the medication label three times: (a) when you remove it from the shelf, (b) when you prepare it, and (c) when you return it to the shelf.	10			
3. Identify your patient, and explain the procedure.*	10			
4. Have the patient sit up and tilt head away from the affected ear or lie down on the side with the affected ear upward.	10			
5. Check the temperature of the medication bottle. If it feels cold, gently roll the bottle back and forth between your hands to warm the drops.	10			
6. Hold the dropper firmly in your dominant hand. With the other hand, gently pull the pinna up and back if the patient is an adult or the ear lobe down and back if the patient is younger than 3 years old.	10			
7. Place the tip of the dropper in the ear canal meatus, and instill the medication drops along the side of the canal.*	10			

Steps	Possible Points	First Attempt	Second Attempt	Third Attempt
8. Instruct the patient to rest on the opposite side of the affected ear and to remain in this position for approximately 3 minutes.	5			
9. If instructed by the physician, place a moistened cotton ball into the ear canal.	5			
10. Clean the work area, and wash your hands.	10			
11. Record the procedure using the appropriate abbreviations, including the date and time; name, dose, and strength of the medication; which ear was treated; and patient reactions on the chart.*	10			

Documentation in the Medical Record

_____

_____

_____

Comments:

Total Points Earned _____ Divided by _____ Total Possible Points = _____ % Score

Instructor's Signature _____

Procedure 36-8 Prepare Patient for and Assist with Procedures, Treatments, and Minor Office Surgeries: Collect a Specimen for a Throat Culture

Task: To collect a throat culture, using sterile technique, for either immediate testing or transportation to the laboratory.

Equipment and Supplies:
- Nonsterile gloves
- Face protection barrier if the patient is coughing or if there is danger of splattering of body fluids
- Sterile swab
- Sterile tongue depressor
- Transport medium
- Biohazard waste container
- Laboratory requisition if sample is being sent out for examination
- Patient record

Standards: Complete the procedure and all critical steps in _____ minutes with a minimum score of _____% within three attempts.

Scoring: Divide points earned by total possible points. Failure to perform a critical step that is indicated with an asterisk (*) will result in an unsatisfactory overall score.

Time began _____ **Time ended** _____

Steps	Possible Points	First Attempt	Second Attempt	Third Attempt
1. Wash and dry your hands.	5	_____	_____	_____
2. Gather the materials needed.	5	_____	_____	_____
3. Don gloves and face protection if needed.	10	_____	_____	_____
4. Position the patient so that the light shines into the mouth.	10	_____	_____	_____
5. Remove the sterile swab from the sterile wrap with your dominant hand, and grasp the sterile tongue depressor with your non-dominant hand.	10	_____	_____	_____
6. Instruct the patient to open the mouth and say "ah." Depress the tongue with the depressor.	10	_____	_____	_____
7. Swab the back of the throat between the tonsillar pillars and especially any reddened, patchy areas of the throat, white pus pockets, purulent areas, and the tonsils.*	10	_____	_____	_____

Steps	Possible Points	First Attempt	Second Attempt	Third Attempt
8. Place the swab into the transport medium, label it, and send it to the laboratory. If direct slide testing is requested, return the labeled swab to the laboratory.	10			
9. Dispose of contaminated supplies in bio-hazard waste container.	5			
10. Disinfect the work area.	5			
11. Remove gloves; place in a biohazard waste container.	5			
12. Wash your hands.	5			
13. Record procedure in the patient's record.*	10			

Documentation in the Medical Record

_____

_____

_____

Comments:

Total Points Earned _____ Divided by _____ Total Possible Points = _____ % Score

Instructor's Signature _____

Procedure 37-1 Obtain Specimens for Microbiologic Testing: Collect a Wound Specimen for Testing and/or Culture

Task: To obtain an adequate sample for culture without contaminating the specimen.

Equipment and Supplies:
- Sterile culture kit containing tube, swabs, and transport media (for swabbing)
- Sterile culture kit containing syringe and transport media (for aspirating)
- Laboratory requisition
- Sterile gauze squares
- Recommended wound-cleansing solution
- Sterile dressing
- Gloves
- Biohazard container
- Face guard
- Patient record

Standards: Complete the procedure and all critical steps in _____ minutes with a minimum score of _____% within three attempts.

Scoring: Divide points earned by total possible points. Failure to perform a critical step that is indicated with an asterisk (*) will result in an unsatisfactory overall score.

Time began _____ **Time ended** _____

Steps	Possible Points	First Attempt	Second Attempt	Third Attempt
1. Wash your hands, gather supplies, and don gloves and face protection.	10	_____	_____	_____
2. Remove dressing from the wound, and dispose of it in a biohazard waste container.	10	_____	_____	_____
3. Observe the wound, and make note of the color, odor, and amount of exudate present.	10	_____	_____	_____
4. Swabbing. Remove the swab from the culture kit, insert the swab into the wound, and saturate it with the exudate. If necessary, use more than one swab, properly labeling each container, to obtain exudates from the entire wound. If preparing an anaerobic culture, place the specimen in the culture tube as quickly as possible to avoid oxygen exposure and possible destruction of microbes.*	10	_____	_____	_____
5. Aspirating. Remove the syringe from the kit, insert the tip into the wound exudate, and draw back the plunger, drawing the exudate up into the syringe.	10	_____	_____	_____

Steps	Possible Points	First Attempt	Second Attempt	Third Attempt
6. Place the swab into the culture tube, and crush the transport media ampule, which is in the transport tube, by squeezing the walls of the transport tube slightly, or place the exudate-filled syringe directly into the transport tube.	10			
7. Label the culture tube accurately. Include on the laboratory slip the patient's recent antibiotic therapy, the wound site, and the suspected organism.	10			
8. Clean the wound as ordered by the physician, and apply a sterile dressing to the area.	10			
9. Clean the area, disposing of all waste materials in a biohazard waste container. Remove gloves and wash your hands.	10			
10. Place culture tube in the laboratory collection area. Chart the procedure and all wound data on the patient's record.	10			

Documentation in the Medical Record

_____

_____

_____

Comments:

Total Points Earned _____ Divided by _____ Total Possible Points = _____ % Score

Instructor's Signature _____

Student Name _____ Date _____ Score _____

Procedure 38-1 Perform Telephone Screening of a GI Patient Complaint

Task: To answer the telephone professionally and manage patient phone calls according to physician guidelines.

Scenario: A 22-year-old woman reports acute abdominal pain.

Equipment and Supplies:
- Telephone
- Message pad
- Pen
- Access to appointment schedule
- Access to patient records
- Physician policy manual for managing patient phone calls

Standards: Complete the procedure and all critical steps in _____ minutes with a minimum score of _____% within three attempts.

Scoring: Divide points earned by total possible points. Failure to perform a critical step that is indicated with an asterisk (*) will result in an unsatisfactory overall score.

Time began _____ **Time ended** _____

Steps	Possible Points	First Attempt	Second Attempt	Third Attempt
1. Answer the telephone by the third ring, speaking directly into the mouthpiece.	5	_____	_____	_____
2. Speak distinctly with a pleasant tone and expression, at a moderate rate, and with sufficient volume.	5	_____	_____	_____
3. Identify the office and/or physician as well as yourself.	5	_____	_____	_____
4. Verify the identity of the caller, and access the patient's record.*	10	_____	_____	_____
5. Determine the needs of the caller.	10	_____	_____	_____

Steps	Possible Points	First Attempt	Second Attempt	Third Attempt
6. Considering the patient's complaint, formulate questions that are designed to gather the information required to make a decision about when the patient should be seen and the physician notified. Given the patient's sex, age, and complaint of acute abdominal pain, consider the following questions: • What are the onset, frequency, and duration of the abdominal pain? • What is the exact anatomic location of the discomfort? • What is the quality of the pain? Is it sharp, dull, stabbing, etc.? • On a scale of 1 to 10, what is the patient's level of pain? • Does the patient have a history of this occurrence? Does she have a history of gynecologic or pelvic disorders? • Has she taken any medication for the discomfort, and has it been effective?	10			
7. Refer to the physician's policies regarding patient phone calls as needed.	10			
8. Depending on the patient's answers to your questions and the physician's policies regarding the management of abdominal discomfort, refer to the appointment schedule and make her an appointment or take a message for the physician to return her call.	10			
9. Document the details of the interaction and the results in the patient's chart.*	10			

Documentation in the Medical Record

_____

_____

_____

_____

Comments:

Total Points Earned _____ Divided by _____ Total Possible Points = _____ % Score

Instructor's Signature _____

Procedure 38-2 Instruct Patients in the Collection of Fecal Specimens: Assist with Hemoccult Screening

Task: To assist the physician with collection of a fecal sample and process the sample for hemoccult screening; to instruct the patient on hemoccult screening at home.

Equipment and Supplies:
- Hemoccult slides
- Hemoccult developer
- Applicator sticks
- Patient record

Standards: Complete the procedure and all critical steps in _____ minutes with a minimum score of _____ % within three attempts.

Scoring: Divide points earned by total possible points. Failure to perform a critical step that is indicated with an asterisk (*) will result in an unsatisfactory overall score.

Time began _____ **Time ended** _____

Steps	Possible Points	First Attempt	Second Attempt	Third Attempt
1. Wash your hands, and assemble all needed equipment and supplies.	10	_____	_____	_____
2. Identify the patient, and explain the procedure.*	10	_____	_____	_____
3. Give the patient an examination gown, and instruct him or her to remove all clothing below the waist and put on the gown with the opening to the back. Provide a drape for additional privacy.	5	_____	_____	_____
4. Assist the patient onto the table. When the physician is ready, place the patient in the appropriate position for the type of examination ordered.	5	_____	_____	_____
5. Drape the patient so that only the anus is exposed. A fenestrated drape (drape with a circular opening placed over the anus) may be used in place of the rectangular drape.	5	_____	_____	_____

Steps	Possible Points	First Attempt	Second Attempt	Third Attempt
6. Don gloves, and assist the physician as requested during the examination. This includes the following: • Handing the needed supplies to the physician. • Collecting specimens by holding the container to accept the sample. • Placing a thin smear of fecal material inside Box A. • Applying a second sample from a different part of the stool inside Box B. • Closing the cover and disposing of contaminated supplies as you are given them by the physician	10			
7. On completion of the examination, remove gloves, wash hands, and assist the patient into a sitting position.	5			
8. Wait 3 to 5 minutes before developing the sample.	5			
9. Don gloves, and open the flap in the back of the slides. Apply 2 drops of Hemoccult Developer directly over the smear.*	10			
10. Interpret the results in 60 seconds.	10			
11. The hemoccult test is negative if there is no detectable trace of color on or at the edge of the smear, and it is positive if there is any trace of blue on or at the edge of the smear.	5			
12. Apply gloves and clean the work area and all equipment used. Dispose of gloves in biohazard waste container and wash your hands.	5			
13. Record the procedure and any pertinent information on the patient's record.*	10			
14. Give the patient a kit for collecting stool samples as ordered by the physician. Typically the physician will order a sample from three different bowel movements. The patient must follow the recommended medication restrictions and dietary guidelines throughout the testing period. • No aspirin or NSAIDs for 7 days before the test • No more than 250 mg of vitamin C per day; avoid eating red meats including processed meats or cold cuts; and avoid raw fruits and vegetables, especially melons, radishes, turnips, and horseradish, for 72 hours before the stool collections.	10			

Steps	Possible Points	First Attempt	Second Attempt	Third Attempt
15. Store the kit in the bathroom at home or carry it with you while you are away from home until the three different stool samples are collected.	10	_____	_____	_____
16. Write your name and other required information on the front of the collection slides.	5	_____	_____	_____
17. Flush the toilet twice before your bowel movement or cover the toilet with plastic wrap to collect the stool specimen.	5	_____	_____	_____
18. Use one of the applicator sticks to collect a small fecal sample. Place a smear of stool on the designated area in the first slide.	5	_____	_____	_____
19. Close the slide and store it away from heat, light, and strong chemicals such as bleach. Do not place it in a plastic bag.	5	_____	_____	_____
20. Repeat this procedure for 2 more days or two more bowel movements as ordered by the physician, using a different card for each sample.	5	_____	_____	_____
21. After collecting all samples as ordered, seal the test envelope and return the kit to the physician's office. Do not send stool samples in the mail unless you have a special envelope from the physician.	5	_____	_____	_____

Documentation in the Medical Record

_____

_____

_____

Comments:

Total Points Earned _____ Divided by _____ Total Possible Points = _____ % Score

Instructor's Signature _____

Procedure 38-3 Prepare Patient for and Assist with Routine and Specialty Examinations: Assist with a Colon Endoscopic Examination

Task: To assist the physician with the examination, to prepare collected specimens as requested, and to promote patient comfort and safety.

Equipment and Supplies:
- Nonsterile gloves (for medical assistant and physician)
- Appropriate instrument: sigmoidoscope or proctoscope
- Water-soluble lubricant
- Drape and patient gown
- Long cotton-tipped swabs
- Suction source
- Sterile biopsy forceps
- Rectal speculum
- Specimen containers with appropriate preservative added
- Laboratory requisition forms
- Tissue wipes
- Biohazard container
- Patient record

Standards: Complete the procedure and all critical steps in _____ minutes with a minimum score of _____ % within three attempts.

Scoring: Divide points earned by total possible points. Failure to perform a critical step that is indicated with an asterisk (*) will result in an unsatisfactory overall score.

Time began _____ **Time ended** _____

Steps	Possible Points	First Attempt	Second Attempt	Third Attempt
1. Wash your hands, and assemble all needed equipment and supplies.	5	_____	_____	_____
2. Identify the patient and explain the procedure. Be sure the patient has completed the proper preparation procedures.*	5	_____	_____	_____
3. Ask the patient to empty his or her bladder.	5	_____	_____	_____
4. Give the patient an examination gown, and instruct him or her to remove all clothing below the waist and put on the gown with the opening to the back. Provide a drape for additional privacy.	5	_____	_____	_____
5. Obtain and record the patient's vital signs.	10	_____	_____	_____

Steps	Possible Points	First Attempt	Second Attempt	Third Attempt
6. Assist the patient onto the table. When the physician is ready, place the patient in the appropriate position for the type of examination ordered.	5			
7. Drape the patient so that only the anus is exposed. A fenestrated drape (drape with a circular opening placed over the anus) may be used in place of the rectangular drape.	10			
8. Don gloves, and assist the physician as requested during the examination. This includes the following: • Lubricating the physician's gloved index finger for the digital examination • Lubricating the obturator tip of the instrument before insertion • Plugging in the scope's light source when the physician is ready • Handing the needed supplies to the physician • Collecting specimens by holding the container to accept the sample • Labeling specimens immediately because several specimens may be taken from different areas • Disposing of contaminated supplies as you are given them by the physician	20			
9. Throughout the examination, observe the patient for any undue reactions. Encourage the patient to breathe slowly through pursed lips to facilitate relaxation.	10			
10. On completion of the examination, provide the patient with tissues to cleanse the anal area. Remove gloves, wash hands, and assist the patient into a resting position; allow the patient time to recover from the procedure. Monitor the patient's blood pressure if indicated.	5			
11. Once the patient's condition is stabilized, assist the patient off the table and instruct him or her to get dressed. Show the patient where the sink, towels, and tissues are, and provide assistance if needed.	5			
12. Complete all laboratory request forms and specimen-container labels, and place specimens in the appropriate location for laboratory pickup.	5			

Steps	Possible Points	First Attempt	Second Attempt	Third Attempt
13. Apply gloves, and clean the work area and all equipment used. The endoscope is first sanitized, then sterilized according to the manufacturer's recommendations. Dispose of gloves in biohazard waste container, and wash your hands.	5			
14. Record the procedure and any pertinent information on the patient's record.	5			

Documentation in the Medical Record

_____

_____

_____

Comments:

Total Points Earned _____ Divided by _____ Total Possible Points = _____ % Score

Instructor's Signature _____

Procedure 39-1 Provide Instruction for Health Maintenance and Disease Prevention: Teach Testicular Self-Examination

Task: To instruct the patient in the steps of testicular self-examination.

Equipment and Supplies:
- Self-examination pamphlet and shower card
- Demonstration model
- Nonsterile gloves
- Patient record

Standards: Complete the procedure and all critical steps in _____ minutes with a minimum score of _____% within three attempts.

Scoring: Divide points earned by total possible points. Failure to perform a critical step that is indicated with an asterisk (*) will result in an unsatisfactory overall score.

Time began _____   **Time ended** _____

Steps	Possible Points	First Attempt	Second Attempt	Third Attempt
1. Wash your hands and collect needed supplies.	10	_____	_____	_____
2. Explain to the patient what you are going to do.	10	_____	_____	_____
3. Begin by explaining to the patient that testicular cancer may produce no symptoms in the early stages, so it is important to examine the testes once a month for abnormal changes and early detection of the disease. This should begin at puberty or approximately 15 years of age. It is best to do the examination in the shower or in a warm bath. The total examination takes about 3 minutes.*	10	_____	_____	_____
4. Examination of the testes: Start by holding the scrotum in the palms of the hands. Then feel one testicle. Apply a small amount of pressure. Slowly roll it between the thumb and fingers and feel for any hard, painless lumps.	10	_____	_____	_____
5. Examination of the epididymis: This comma-shaped cord is found behind the testis. Its job is to store and transport sperm. Tender when touched, it is the location of most noncancerous problems. Check for hard spots and lumps.	10	_____	_____	_____

Steps	Possible Points	First Attempt	Second Attempt	Third Attempt
6. Examination of the vas deferens: Continue by examining the sperm-carrying tube that runs up the epididymis. Normally, the vas feels like a firm, movable, smooth tube.	10			
7. Now repeat the entire examination on the other side, beginning with the opposite testis.	10			
8. After completing the examination on the model, ask the patient to do a return-examination using the model. A male assistant can have the patient do a self-testicular examination.*	10			
9. Give the pamphlet to the patient, along with the shower card, with instructions to hang it in the shower as a monthly reminder and guide.	10			
10. Record the instructional interaction in the patient's medical record.	10			

Documentation in the Medical Record

_____

_____

_____

Comments:

Total Points Earned _____ Divided by _____ Total Possible Points = _____ % Score

Instructor's Signature _____

Student Name _____ Date _____ Score _____

Procedure 40-1 Prepare Patient for and Assist with Routine and Specialty Examinations: Assist with Examination of the Female Patient and Pap Smear

Task: To assist the physician in examination of a female patient and diagnostic Pap smear.

Equipment and Supplies:
- Patient gown
- Lubricant
- 4- × 4-inch gauze squares
- Laboratory requisition slips
- Drape sheet
- Examination light
- Cervical spatula and Cytobrush
- ThinPrep container
- Vaginal speculum
- Uterine sponge forceps
- Disposable examination gloves
- Fixative for Pap smear
- Urine specimen container if needed
- Stool for occult blood test if needed
- Biohazard waste container
- Patient record
- Appropriate patient education materials

Standards: Complete the procedure and all critical steps in _____ minutes with a minimum score of _____% within three attempts.

Scoring: Divide points earned by total possible points. Failure to perform a critical step that is indicated with an asterisk (*) will result in an unsatisfactory overall score.

Time began _____ Time ended _____

Steps	Possible Points	First Attempt	Second Attempt	Third Attempt
1. Assemble the materials needed, and prepare the room. Prepare the equipment and supplies needed for the Pap smear.	10			
2. Wash your hands. Follow standard precautions.	10			
3. Identify the patient, and briefly explain the procedure.	10			
4. Instruct the patient to empty the bladder and collect a urine specimen if needed.	5			
5. Instruct the patient to disrobe completely and to put on a gown with the opening in the front.	5			

Steps	Possible Points	First Attempt	Second Attempt	Third Attempt
6. Assist the physician with the breast examination. Patient should start by sitting at the end of the examination table. Drape the patient, and assist the physician with the examination. Provide reassurance to the patient as needed.	10			
7. When the physician is ready to examine the breasts and the abdomen with the patient in the supine position, assist the patient into the supine position and drape as needed.	10			
8. When the physician is ready to begin the vaginal examination, assist the patient into the lithotomy position. Have the patient slide down to the end of the table, placing her legs in the stirrups, the knees should be relaxed and rotated outward. Remember always to position the patient underneath the drape.	10			
9. Direct the light source onto the perineal area.*	5			
10. Don gloves. Warm the stainless steel vaginal speculum in warm water (physician may prefer disposable plastic speculum). Pass the proper instruments to the physician in proper sequence. Physician will need the Cytobrush for cervical cells and spatula for the cervical sample.	10			
11. Assist the physician with ThinPrep preparation if desired by swirling the cervical specimen in the preservative solution at least 10 times to ensure that the specimen has been mixed with the preservative solution.	10			
12. Label the specimen container, and place it in a biohazard bag.	10			
13. Apply water-soluble lubricant to the physician's fingers.	n/a			
14. Physician may prepare stool for occult blood testing after rectal examination. Have materials ready.	10			
15. Instruct the patient to breathe deeply through the mouth with hands crossed over the chest.	5			
16. Place the soiled instruments in a basin.	5			

Steps	Possible Points	First Attempt	Second Attempt	Third Attempt
17. Assist the patient off the table and with dressing if needed.	5			
18. While patient is in the dressing room, clean the room, removing used equipment.	10			
19. Sanitize and sterilize stainless steel equipment. Remove gloves and wash your hands.	10			
20. Prepare the Pap smear and other samples for transportation to the laboratory. Complete the requisitions including patient's LMP date and whether she is on hormone therapy.	10			
21. Record all procedures on the patient's medical record.	10			

Documentation in the Medical Record

_____

_____

_____

Comments:

Total Points Earned _____ Divided by _____ Total Possible Points = _____ % Score

Instructor's Signature _____

Procedure 40-2 Prepare Patient for and Assist with Procedures, Treatments, and Minor Office Surgeries: Prepare the Patient for Cryosurgery

Task: To prepare the patient and assist the physician in cryosurgery.

Equipment and Supplies:
- Cryosurgery machine equipped with liquid nitrogen canister
- Cryoprobe
- Cervical tenaculum
- Cervical ring forceps or disposable cervical swabs
- Vaginal speculum
- 44-inch gauze squares
- Disposable examination gloves
- Gowns and face protection
- Specimen containers
- Biohazard waste container
- Cytology request forms
- Patient record

Standards: Complete the procedure and all critical steps in _____ minutes with a minimum score of _____% within three attempts.

Scoring: Divide points earned by total possible points. Failure to perform a critical step that is indicated with an asterisk (*) will result in an unsatisfactory overall score.

Time began _____ **Time ended** _____

Steps	Possible Points	First Attempt	Second Attempt	Third Attempt
1. Assemble equipment.	10	_____	_____	_____
2. Wash your hands.	10	_____	_____	_____
3. Take the patient's temperature and blood pressure, and record them on the patient's record.*	10	_____	_____	_____
4. Drape and assist the patient into the lithotomy position. Don gloves.	10	_____	_____	_____
5. Assist the physician with the procedure by handing the equipment needed.	5	_____	_____	_____
6. Encourage the patient to take deep breaths to promote relaxation of the pelvic muscles during the procedure. Observe the patient for any signs of distress.	5	_____	_____	_____

Steps	Possible Points	First Attempt	Second Attempt	Third Attempt
7. When the procedure is completed, place the patient in a supine position and allow her to rest while you tidy the room and remove the used supplies. Retake temperature and blood pressure.	10			
8. Help patient sit up, and assist her in dressing if needed.	5			
9. Remove gloves and wash hands.	10			
10. Disinfect and sterilize equipment per manufacturer's directions, and return equipment to the proper storage area.	10			
11. Record procedure and final vital sign measurements on the patient's record.	10			

Documentation in the Medical Record

_____

_____

_____

Comments:

Total Points Earned _____ Divided by _____ Total Possible Points = _____ % Score

Instructor's Signature _____

Student Name _____ Date _____ Score _____

Procedure 40-3 Provide Instruction for Health Maintenance and Disease Prevention: Teach the Patient Breast Self-Examination

Task: To teach the patient how to palpate her breast for possible abnormalities.

Equipment and Supplies:
- Instruction pamphlet
- Teaching model (to use to demonstrate the technique before a return demonstration by the patient)
- Patient record

Standards: Complete the procedure and all critical steps in _____ minutes with a minimum score of _____% within three attempts.

Scoring: Divide points earned by total possible points. Failure to perform a critical step that is indicated with an asterisk (*) will result in an unsatisfactory overall score.

Time began _____ **Time ended** _____

Steps	Possible Points	First Attempt	Second Attempt	Third Attempt
1. Assemble equipment.	10	_____	_____	_____
2. Tell the patient to examine the breasts while bathing or showering in warm water. The best time to perform this examination is immediately after the menstrual period is completed because at this time there is minimal breast engorgement. Nonmenstruating women should examine breasts the first of the month.	10	_____	_____	_____
3. Have the patient raise one arm. With her fingers flat, she should press gently in small circles, starting at the outermost top edge of the breast and spiraling in toward the nipple. Touch every part of each breast, including the axillary region, gently feeling for a lump or thickening. Use the right hand to examine the left breast and the left hand for the right breast.	10	_____	_____	_____
4. After the bath or shower is completed, the patient should continue the examination in front of a mirror with arms at the sides. Then, with the arms raised above the head, look carefully for changes in the size, shape, and contour of each breast. Look for puckering, dimpling, or changes in skin texture.*	10	_____	_____	_____
5. Gently squeeze both nipples and look for discharge.	10	_____	_____	_____

Steps	Possible Points	First Attempt	Second Attempt	Third Attempt
6. Before dressing, the patient should lie on a bed. Place a towel or pillow under the right shoulder and the right hand behind the head. Examine the right breast using the left hand. Press gently in small circles, starting at the outermost top edge, including the axillary region, and spiraling in toward the nipple. Repeat with left breast.	10			
7. The patient should return the demonstration of how to do the breast examination to confirm understanding.	5			
8. Give the patient the instruction pamphlet to use at home. If you have given her the shower card to follow, show her how it will hang inside the shower on a faucet or the shower nozzle and be a quick reference for her.	5			
9 Record all procedures on the patient's medical record.	10			

Documentation in the Medical Record

_____

_____

_____

Comments:

Total Points Earned _____ Divided by _____ Total Possible Points = _____ % Score

Instructor's Signature _____

Procedure 40-4 Prepare Patient for and Assist with Routine and Specialty Examinations: Assist with the Prenatal Examination

Task: To promote a healthy pregnancy for the mother and fetus and screen for potential problems.

Equipment and Supplies:
- Scale with height measure
- Sphygmomanometer
- Stethoscope
- Tape measure
- Doppler fetoscope
- Urine specimen container
- Disposable examination gloves, vaginal speculum, and lubricant if vaginal examination conducted
- STD test setups
- Laboratory requisition slips
- Biohazard waste container
- Biohazard bags for specimen transport
- Patient education materials
- Patient chart

Standards: Complete the procedure and all critical steps in _____ minutes with a minimum score of _____% within three attempts.

Scoring: Divide points earned by total possible points. Failure to perform a critical step that is indicated with an asterisk (*) will result in an unsatisfactory overall score.

Time began _____ **Time ended** _____

Steps	Possible Points	First Attempt	Second Attempt	Third Attempt
1. Wash your hands, assemble equipment, and identify the patient.	10	_____	_____	_____
2. Measure and record the patient's weight.	10	_____	_____	_____
3. Collect a urine specimen, perform urinalysis, and record urinalysis results to determine the presence of protein, glucose, or ketones in the urine.	10	_____	_____	_____
4. Measure and record the mother's blood pressure.	10	_____	_____	_____
5. Instruct the patient to disrobe from the waist down and put on a gown open to the front so the uterine fundal height can be measured.	10	_____	_____	_____
6. Assist the patient onto the examination table if needed and provide a drape for privacy.	10	_____	_____	_____

Steps	Possible Points	First Attempt	Second Attempt	Third Attempt
7. Assist the physician as needed throughout the examination.	5			
8. After the examination is completed, assist the patient off the examination table, making sure to observe for signs of dizziness or problems with balance.	5			
9. Answer the patient's questions and provide patient education materials as needed.*	10			
10. Collect and package all specimens for transport. Complete labels as needed.	10			
11. Discard supplies and disinfect the equipment according to manufacturer's guidelines. Wear disposable examination gloves and follow OSHA guidelines if handling any contaminated items.	10			
12. Wash your hands.	10			
13. Document pertinent information in the patient chart.	10			

Documentation in the Medical Record

_____

_____

_____

Comments:

Total Points Earned _____ Divided by _____ Total Possible Points = _____ % Score

Instructor's Signature _____

Student Name _____ Date _____ Score _____

Procedure 40-5 Prepare Patient for and Assist with Procedures, Treatments, and Minor Office Surgeries: Establish the Estimated Date of Delivery Using Nägele's Rule and Lunar Method

Task: To establish the patient's due date.

Equipment and Supplies:
- Calendar for present and following year
- Paper and pencil
- Commercial EDD wheel (optional)

Standards: Complete the procedure and all critical steps in _____ minutes with a minimum score of _____% within three attempts.

Scoring: Divide points earned by total possible points. Failure to perform a critical step that is indicated with an asterisk (*) will result in an unsatisfactory overall score.

Time began _____ Time ended _____

Steps	Possible Points	First Attempt	Second Attempt	Third Attempt
1. Ask the patient for the date of the onset of the LMP. Be sure that this is the date of the onset and not the date of the termination of the menses.	10	_____	_____	_____
2. Patient informs you that her LMP was June 7, 2002.	5	_____	_____	_____
3. Calculate her EDD using Nägele's method: Begin with the date of the first day of her LMP. Count back 3 months and add 1 year plus 7 days.	10	_____	_____	_____
4. Using the same LMP, calculate her EDD using the lunar rule.	10	_____	_____	_____
5. Compare the results for accuracy. Did you obtain the same EDD using both methods?	5	_____	_____	_____
6. Record the EDD in the patient's chart.	10	_____	_____	_____

Comments:

Total Points Earned _____ Divided by _____ Total Possible Points = _____ % Score

Instructor's Signature _____

Student Name _____ Date _____ Score _____

Procedure 41-1 Maintain Medication and Immunization Records: Documentation of Immunizations.

Task: To accurately document the administration of a pediatric immunization.

Case Study: Document the administration of the second dose of the hepatitis B immunization to a 5-week-old infant, Samantha Anderson.

Equipment and Supplies:
- Vaccine immunization administration record
- Parent immunization booklet
- Patient chart
- VIS form for hepatitis B

Standards: Complete the procedure and all critical steps in _____ minutes with a minimum score of _____% within three attempts.

Scoring: Divide points earned by total possible points. Failure to perform a critical step that is indicated with an asterisk (*) will result in an unsatisfactory overall score.

Time began _____ **Time ended** _____

Steps	Possible Points	First Attempt	Second Attempt	Third Attempt
1. Gather forms.	10	_____	_____	_____
2. Make sure the physician obtained informed consent from the parent, the hepatitis B VIS form was given, and that any parental questions were answered.	10	_____	_____	_____
3. After dispensing the vaccine dose and before administration, complete the information required on the Vaccine Administration Record, including the name of the vaccine, the date given, route of administration and site, vaccine lot number and manufacturer, the date on the VIS form, the date it was given to the parent, and your signature or initials.*	10	_____	_____	_____
4. Administer the vaccine IM as taught in Chapter 34.	10	_____	_____	_____
5. Record the date of administration, the name and address of the physician practice, and the type of vaccine administered in the parent's immunization booklet.	10	_____	_____	_____

913

Steps	Possible Points	First Attempt	Second Attempt	Third Attempt
6. After administration of the hepatitis vaccine, record in the child's chart the following details:*	10			

a. Date the vaccine was administered
b. Vaccine manufacturer, batch and lot numbers, expiration date
c. Type of vaccine administered and dose
d. Route of administration and exact site if an injection is given
e. Any reported or observed side effects
f. Publication date of the VIS form given to the parent (on the bottom of the form)
g. Parent education regarding possible side effects of the vaccination
h. Name and title of the person administering the vaccine

Documentation in the Medical Record: Administered hepatitis B, second dose, IM to the right vastus lateralis site.

_____

_____

_____

Comments:

Total Points Earned _____ Divided by _____ Total Possible Points = _____ % Score

Instructor's Signature _____

Student Name _____ Date _____ Score _____

Procedure 41-2 Prepare Patient for and Assist with Routine and Specialty Examinations: Measure the Circumference of an Infant's Head

Task: To obtain an accurate measurement of the circumference of an infant's head.

Equipment and Supplies:
- Flexible disposable tape measure
- Age- and sex-specific growth chart
- Patient's chart
- Pen

Standards: Complete the procedure and all critical steps in _____ minutes with a minimum score of _____% within three attempts.

Scoring: Divide points earned by total possible points. Failure to perform a critical step that is indicated with an asterisk (*) will result in an unsatisfactory overall score.

Time began _____ **Time ended** _____

Steps	Possible Points	First Attempt	Second Attempt	Third Attempt
1. Wash your hands.	10	_____	_____	_____
2. Identify the patient and gain infant cooperation through conversation.	5	_____	_____	_____
3. Place the infant in the supine position; an older child may sit on the examination table; alternatively, the infant may be held by the parent.	5	_____	_____	_____
4. Hold the tape measure with the zero mark against the infant's forehead, slightly above the eyebrows and the top of the ears. Ask the parent for assistance if necessary.*	10	_____	_____	_____
5. Bring the tape measure around the head, just above the ears, until it meets. Read to the nearest 0.01 cm or ¼ inch.	10	_____	_____	_____
6. Record the measurement on the growth chart and the patient's chart.	10	_____	_____	_____
7. Dispose of the tape measure.	5	_____	_____	_____
8. Wash your hands.	10	_____	_____	_____

Documentation in the Medical Record

_____

_____

_____

Comments:

Total Points Earned _____ Divided by _____ Total Possible Points = _____ % Score

Instructor's Signature _____

Student Name _____ Date _____ Score _____

Procedure 41-3 Prepare Patient for and Assist with Routine and Specialty Examinations: Measure Infant Length and Weight

Task: To accurately measure infant length and weight so growth patterns can be monitored and recorded.

Equipment and Supplies:
- Infant scale with paper cover
- Flexible measuring tape
- Examination table paper
- Pen
- Sex-specific infant growth chart
- Patient's chart
- Biohazard waste container

Standards: Complete the procedure and all critical steps in _____ minutes with a minimum score of _____% within three attempts.

Scoring: Divide points earned by total possible points. Failure to perform a critical step that is indicated with an asterisk (*) will result in an unsatisfactory overall score.

Time began _____ **Time ended** _____

Steps	Possible Points	First Attempt	Second Attempt	Third Attempt
Measuring Infant Length				
1. Wash your hands, assemble equipment, and explain the procedure to the infant's caregiver.	10	_____	_____	_____
2. Undress the infant in preparation for measurement of length and weight. You may leave the diaper on while the length measurement is taken, but it must be removed before the infant is weighed.	10	_____	_____	_____
3. Ask the caregiver to place the infant on his or her back on the examination table, which is covered with paper. If it is a pediatric table with a headboard, ask the caregiver to gently hold the infant's head against the board while you straighten the infant's leg and mark on the paper the location of the heel. If there is no headboard, ask the caregiver to gently hold the infant's head still while you extend the leg for measurement.*	10	_____	_____	_____
4. Measure and record the infant's length with the tape measure.	10	_____	_____	_____

Steps	Possible Points	First Attempt	Second Attempt	Third Attempt
5. Document the results in either inches or centimeters, depending on office policy, on the infant's growth chart, in the progress notes, and in the caregiver's record if requested. Complete the growth chart graph by connecting the dot from the last visit.*	10			
Measuring Infant Weight				
6. Wash your hands, assemble equipment, and explain the procedure to the infant's caregiver.	10			
7. Prepare the scale by sliding weights to the left and covering it with disposable paper to reduce the risk of pathogen transmission.	5			
8. Completely undress the infant, including the diaper.	5			
9. Place the infant gently onto the center of the scale, keeping your hand directly above the infant's trunk for safety.	5			
10. Slide the weights across the scale until balance is achieved. Attempt to read the infant's weight while he or she is still.	10			
11. Return the weights to the far left of the scale and remove the baby. The caregiver can apply a diaper while you discard the paper covering the scale. If it has become contaminated during the procedure, follow OSHA guidelines for gloves and disposal of contaminated waste. Disinfect the equipment according to manufacturer guidelines.	10			
12. Wash your hands.	10			
13. Document the results in either pounds or kilograms, depending on office policy, on the infant's growth chart, in the progress notes, and in the caregiver's record if requested. Complete the growth chart graph by connecting the dot from the last visit.*	10			

Documentation in the Medical Record

_____

_____

_____

Comments:

Total Points Earned _____ Divided by _____ Total Possible Points = _____ % Score

Instructor's Signature _____

Procedure 41-4 Prepare Patient for and Assist with Routine and Specialty Examinations: Obtain Pediatric Vital Signs and Vision Screening

Task: To accurately obtain vital signs for and assess vision of a pediatric patient.

Equipment and Supplies:
- Digital or tympanic thermometer
- Pediatric blood pressure cuff
- Wristwatch with sweep second hand
- Weight scale with height bar
- Stethoscope
- Snellen E eye chart and oculator
- Pen
- Patient's chart

Standards: Complete the procedure and all critical steps in _____ minutes with a minimum score of _____% within three attempts.

Scoring: Divide points earned by total possible points. Failure to perform a critical step that is indicated with an asterisk (*) will result in an unsatisfactory overall score.

Time began _____ **Time ended** _____

Steps	Possible Points	First Attempt	Second Attempt	Third Attempt
1. Gather equipment.	5	_____	_____	_____
2. Wash your hands.	5	_____	_____	_____
3. Explain the procedure to the parent, and if you want the parent to help by holding the child, explain the technique you want him or her to employ.*	5	_____	_____	_____
4. Help the child stand in the center of the scale, and weigh the child. Ask the child to turn around, and obtain the child's height. Record your findings.	5	_____	_____	_____
5. Obtain tympanic or axillary temperature.	5	_____	_____	_____
6. Record the temperature. Indicate the method used: A = axillary, T = tympanic.	5	_____	_____	_____
7. Place the stethoscope on the child's chest at the midpoint between the sternum and the left nipple. Listen for the apical beat.	5	_____	_____	_____

Steps	Possible Points	First Attempt	Second Attempt	Third Attempt
8. Count the apical beat for 1 full minute.	10			
9. Record the apical pulse. Be sure to place an Ap before the rate to indicate that this is an apical pulse reading.	5			
10. Place your flat hand on the child's chest, and count the respirations for 1 full minute.	5			
11. Record the respiration rate.	5			
12. Check to be sure that you have the correct-size blood pressure cuff, then proceed with taking the blood pressure.	10			
13. Record the blood pressure.	5			
14. If vision screening is to be done, familiarize the child with the E chart by asking him to make an E point the same way as your E is pointing. Then position the child in front of the pediatric E Snellen chart and have him match the E sign (using his fingers) with the E on the chart that you are pointing to.*	5			
15. Record the vision results: OD = right eye; OS = left eye; OU = both eyes.	5			
16. Compliment the child on his or her performance, and if the parent is present, share the praise with the parent.	5			
17. Wash your hands.	5			
18. Perform appropriate disinfection, and return all equipment used to proper storage area.	5			

Documentation in the Medical Record

_____

_____

_____

Comments:

Total Points Earned _____ Divided by _____ Total Possible Points = _____ % Score

Instructor's Signature _____

Student Name _____ Date _____ Score _____

Procedure 41-5 Prepare Patient for and Assist with Procedures, Treatments, and Minor Office Surgeries: Apply a Urinary Collection Device

Task: To properly apply a pediatric urinary collection device.

Equipment and Supplies:
- Pediatric urine collection bag
- Labeled laboratory urinary container
- Laboratory test request form
- Antiseptic wipes
- Biohazard waste container
- Disposable examination gloves

Standards: Complete the procedure and all critical steps in _____ minutes with a minimum score of _____% within three attempts.

Scoring: Divide points earned by total possible points. Failure to perform a critical step that is indicated with an asterisk (*) will result in an unsatisfactory overall score.

Time began _____ **Time ended** _____

Steps	Possible Points	First Attempt	Second Attempt	Third Attempt
1. Assemble all needed supplies.	10	_____	_____	_____
2. Wash your hands, and don gloves.	10	_____	_____	_____
3. Ask the parent to remove the diaper from the child, or place the child in a supine position on the examination table and remove the diaper.	5	_____	_____	_____
4. Cleanse the genitalia with antiseptic wipes.	10	_____	_____	_____

Male: Cleanse the urinary meatus in a circular motion, starting directly on the meatus, and work in an outward pattern. Repeat with a clean wipe. If the child is not circumcised, retract the foreskin to expose the meatus, and when you have completed cleansing, return the foreskin to its natural position.

Female: Hold the labia open with your non-dominant hand and with your dominant hand, cleanse the inner labia, from the clitoris to the vaginal meatus, in a superior to inferior pattern.

5. Discard the first wipe and repeat with a clean wipe.*	5	_____	_____	_____

Steps	Possible Points	First Attempt	Second Attempt	Third Attempt
6. Make sure the area is dry. Unfold the collection device, remove the paper from the upper portion, place this portion over the mons pubis, and press it securely into place. Continue by removing the lower portion of the paper and securing this portion against the perineum. Be sure that the device is attached smoothly and that you have not taped it to part of the infant's thigh.	10	_____	_____	_____
7. Rediaper the infant, or if the parent is helping, the parent may rediaper the infant at this time. The diaper will help hold the bag in place.	5	_____	_____	_____
8. Suggest that the parent give the child liquids if allowed and check the bag for urine at frequent intervals.	5	_____	_____	_____
9. When there is a noticeable amount of urine in the bag, apply gloves, remove the device, cleanse the skin area that was attached to the device, and rediaper the child.	10	_____	_____	_____
10. Pour the urine carefully into the laboratory urine container, and handle the sample in a routine manner.	5	_____	_____	_____
11. Dispose of all used equipment in a biohazard waste container.	10	_____	_____	_____
12. Remove gloves, dispose of them in a biohazard container, and wash your hands.	10	_____	_____	_____
13. Record the procedure in the patient's record.	10	_____	_____	_____

Documentation in the Medical Record

_____

_____

_____

Comments:

Total Points Earned _____ Divided by _____ Total Possible Points = _____ % Score

Instructor's Signature _____

Student Name _____ Date _____ Score _____

Procedure 42-1 Prepare Patient for and Assist with Procedures, Treatments, and Minor Office Surgeries: Assist the Patient with Cold Application

Task: To apply a cold compress to a body area to decrease pain, prevent further swelling, and/or decrease inflammation.

Equipment and Supplies:
- Ice bag or closeable disposable plastic kitchen food bag
- Small ice cubes or ice chips
- Towel
- Patient record

Standards: Complete the procedure and all critical steps in _____ minutes with a minimum score of _____% within three attempts.

Scoring: Divide points earned by total possible points. Failure to perform a critical step that is indicated with an asterisk (*) will result in an unsatisfactory overall score.

Time began _____ **Time ended** _____

Steps	Possible Points	First Attempt	Second Attempt	Third Attempt
1. Wash your hands.	10	_____	_____	_____
2. Explain the procedure to the patient, and answer any questions.*	10	_____	_____	_____
3. Check the bag for possible leaks.	10	_____	_____	_____
4. Fill the bag with small cubes or chips of ice until it is about two thirds full.	10	_____	_____	_____
5. Push down on the top of the bag to expel excess air, and apply the cap.	10	_____	_____	_____
6. Dry the outside, and cover it with one or two towel layers.	10	_____	_____	_____
7. Help the patient position the ice bag on the injured area.	10	_____	_____	_____
8. Advise the patient to leave the ice bag in place for about 20 to 30 minutes or until the area feels numb, whichever is first.*	10	_____	_____	_____
9. Check the skin for color, feeling, and pain.	10	_____	_____	_____
10. Record the procedure in the patient's chart.	10	_____	_____	_____

Documentation in the Medical Record

_____

_____

_____

Comments:

Total Points Earned _____ Divided by _____ Total Possible Points = _____ % Score

Instructor's Signature _____

Procedure 42-2 Prepare Patient for and Assist with Procedures, Treatments, and Minor Office Surgeries: Assist with Hot Moist Heat Application in the Office

Task: To apply moist heat to a body area to increase circulation, increase metabolism, and relax muscles.

Equipment and Supplies:
• Commercial hot moist heat packs
• Towel
• Patient record

Standards: Complete the procedure and all critical steps in _____ minutes with a minimum score of _____% within three attempts.

Scoring: Divide points earned by total possible points. Failure to perform a critical step that is indicated with an asterisk (*) will result in an unsatisfactory overall score.

Time began _____ **Time ended** _____

Steps	Possible Points	First Attempt	Second Attempt	Third Attempt
1. Wash your hands.	10	_____	_____	_____
2. Explain the procedure to the patient, and answer any questions.*	10	_____	_____	_____
3. Ask the patient to remove all jewelry from the area to be treated.	10	_____	_____	_____
4. Place one or two towel layers over the area to be treated.	10	_____	_____	_____
5. Apply the commercial moist heat packs.	5	_____	_____	_____
6. Cover with the remaining portion of the towel.	10	_____	_____	_____
7. Advise the patient to leave the heat pack in place no longer than 20 to 30 minutes, off for the same amount of time, and repeat if needed.*	10	_____	_____	_____

Documentation in the Medical Record

_____

_____

_____

Comments:

Total Points Earned _____ Divided by _____ Total Possible Points = _____ % Score

Instructor's Signature _____

Student Name _____ Date _____ Score _____

Procedure 42-3 Prepare Patient for and Assist with Procedures, Treatments, and Minor Office Surgeries: Assist with Therapeutic Ultrasonography

Task: To apply ultra-high-frequency sound waves to a patient's deep tissues for therapy. The medical assistant should perform ultrasound therapy only under the supervision of the physician or a physical therapist.

Equipment and Supplies:
- Ultrasound machine
- Ultrasound gel or lotion
- Patient record

Standards: Complete the procedure and all critical steps in _____ minutes with a minimum score of _____% within three attempts.

Scoring: Divide points earned by total possible points. Failure to perform a critical step that is indicated with an asterisk (*) will result in an unsatisfactory overall score.

Time began _____ **Time ended** _____

Steps	Possible Points	First Attempt	Second Attempt	Third Attempt
1. Prepare your equipment and wash your hands.	5			
2. Confirm the patient's identity.	5			
3. Explain the procedure, and tell the patient to notify you of any discomfort during the procedure.*	5			
4. Ask the patient about the presence of any internal or external metal objects.	5			
5. Position the patient comfortably, with the area to be treated exposed.	5			
6. Apply a warmed ultrasound gel liberally over the area to be treated and to the applicator head.	5			
7. Begin the treatment with the intensity control at the lowest setting.	5			
8. Set the timer on the machine to the ordered time.	5			
9. Slowly increase the intensity control to the ordered amount.	5			

Steps	Possible Points	First Attempt	Second Attempt	Third Attempt
10. Hold the applicator with the head firmly and completely against the patient's skin over the area to be treated.	5			
11. Work the applicator over the area to be treated by moving it continuously in a circular fashion at a speed of 2 inches per second or as directed by the physician.	5			
12. Keep the applicator head in contact with the patient's skin at all times while the machine is on, and keep it moving continuously during the treatment time.	5			
13. When the timer sounds, it shuts off the machine automatically. Then you can safely lift the applicator head away from the patient.	5			
14. Return the intensity control to zero.	5			
15. Remove the ultrasound gel from the patient's skin and from the applicator head with a tissue or paper wipe. Wash your hands.	5			
16. Assist the patient to get dressed if necessary.	5			
17. Record the procedure in the patient's chart, including the date, area treated, intensity setting, duration of treatment, and any unusual reactions that may have occurred during treatment. If none occurred, indicate that also.	20			

Documentation in the Medical Record

_____

_____

_____

Comments:

Total Points Earned _____ Divided by _____ Total Possible Points = _____ % Score

Instructor's Signature _____

Student Name _____ Date _____ Score _____

Procedure 42-4 Prepare Patient for and Assist with Procedures, Treatments, and Minor Office Surgeries: Assist with Cast Application

Task: To assist the physician in applying a fiberglass cast.

Equipment and Supplies:
- Rolls of fiberglass casting material
- Stockinette
- Sheet wadding and/or spongy padding
- Tape
- Scissors
- Water
- Basin
- Bandage
- Gloves for physician and medical assistant
- Stand to support foot (lower extremity)
- Patient record

Standards: Complete the procedure and all critical steps in _____ minutes with a minimum score of _____% within three attempts.

Scoring: Divide points earned by total possible points. Failure to perform a critical step that is indicated with an asterisk (*) will result in an unsatisfactory overall score.

Time began _____ Time ended _____

Steps	Possible Points	First Attempt	Second Attempt	Third Attempt
1. Wash your hands.	10			
2. Identify the patient.	5			
3. Explain the procedure for applying a cast, and answer questions before application.*	10			
4. Assemble equipment.	10			
5. Seat the patient comfortably, as directed by the physician. If the cast is being applied to the lower extremity, the toes must be supported by a stand.	5			
6. Clean the area that the cast will cover. Note any objective signs and ask about subjective symptoms (chart them at the end of the procedure).	10			
7. Cut stockinette to fit the area the cast will cover.	10			

Steps	Possible Points	First Attempt	Second Attempt	Third Attempt
8. Apply stockinette smoothly to the area that the cast will cover. Leave 1 or 2 inches of excess stockinette above and below the cast area to finish the cast.	10			
9. Excess stockinette may be cut away where wrinkles form (e.g., at the front of the ankle).	10			
10. Sheet wadding is applied along the length of the cast using a spiral bandage turn. Extra padding may be used over bony prominences such as the bones of the elbow or ankle.	10			
11. Don gloves.	5			
12. With lukewarm water in the basin, wet the fiberglass tape as directed by the physician.	10			
13. Assist as directed as the physician applies the inner layer of fiberglass tape. A length of 1 to 2 inches of stockinette is rolled over the inner layer of the cast to form a smooth edge when the outer layer is applied.	10			
14. Assist as directed by the physician to open and apply an outer layer of fiberglass tape.	10			
15. Assist to shape the cast as directed. All contours must be smooth.	5			
16. Discard the water and excess materials. Remove gloves, and wash hands.	10			
17. Reassure the patient, review cast care verbally, and provide written instructions.*	10			
18. Document observations and procedure in patient record.	10			

Documentation in the Medical Record

_____

_____

_____

Comments:

Total Points Earned _____ Divided by _____ Total Possible Points = _____ % Score

Instructor's Signature _____

Student Name _____ Date _____ Score _____

Procedure 42-5 Prepare Patient for and Assist with Procedures, Treatments, and Minor Office Surgeries: Triangular Arm Sling Application

Task: To properly place a casted arm in a triangular sling.

Equipment and Supplies:
- Triangular-shaped arm sling
- Large safety pins
- Patient record

Standards: Complete the procedure and all critical steps in _____ minutes with a minimum score of _____% within three attempts.

Scoring: Divide points earned by total possible points. Failure to perform a critical step that is indicated with an asterisk (*) will result in an unsatisfactory overall score.

Time began _____ Time ended _____

Steps	Possible Points	First Attempt	Second Attempt	Third Attempt
1. Review the physician's order for a triangular arm sling.	10			
2. Wash your hands and obtain the desired sling.	10			
3. Explain the procedure to the patient.*	10			
4. Position the patient's injured arm across the chest so that it is parallel to the floor and the patient's waist, with the hand slightly elevated.	10			
5. Carefully slide the triangular sling between the patient's chest and the affected arm.	10			
6. Bring the lower front corner up over the shoulder of the affected side to the neck.	10			
7. Grasp the opposite corner, and tie or pin the ends together at the side of the neck.	10			
8. Fold in the tail and fasten with a safety pin to secure the elbow.	10			
9. Fold the sling edge to form a smooth edge along the wrist.	10			
10. Record the procedure in the patient's chart.	10			

Documentation in the Medical Record

_____

_____

_____

Comments:

Total Points Earned _____ Divided by _____ Total Possible Points = _____ % Score

Instructor's Signature _____

Student Name _____ Date _____ Score _____

Procedure 42-6 Prepare Patient for and Assist with Procedures, Treatments, and Minor Office Surgeries: Assist with Cast Removal

Task: To remove a cast.

Equipment and Supplies:
- Cast cutter
- Cast spreader
- Large bandage scissors
- Basin of warm water
- Mild soap
- Towel
- Skin lotion
- Patient record

Standards: Complete the procedure and all critical steps in _____ minutes with a minimum score of _____% within three attempts.

Scoring: Divide points earned by total possible points. Failure to perform a critical step that is indicated with an asterisk (*) will result in an unsatisfactory overall score.

Time began _____ Time ended _____

Steps	Possible Points	First Attempt	Second Attempt	Third Attempt
1. Explain the procedure to the patient.*	10	_____	_____	_____
2. Provide adequate support for the limb throughout the entire procedure.	10	_____	_____	_____
3. Make a cut on both the medial side and the lateral side of the long axis of the cast.	10	_____	_____	_____
4. Pry the two halves apart using the cast spreader.	10	_____	_____	_____
5. Carefully remove the two parts of the cast.	10	_____	_____	_____
6. Use the large bandage scissors to cut away the stockinette and padding remaining.	10	_____	_____	_____
7. Gently wash the area that was covered by the cast with mild soap and warm water.*	10	_____	_____	_____
8. Dry and apply a gentle skin lotion.	10	_____	_____	_____
9. Give the patient appropriate instructions about exercising and using the limb, as directed by the physician.	10	_____	_____	_____
10. Record the procedure in the patient's medical record.	10	_____	_____	_____

Documentation in the Medical Record

_____

_____

_____

Comments:

Total Points Earned _____ Divided by _____ Total Possible Points = _____ % Score

Instructor's Signature _____

Procedure 42-7 Prepare Patient for and Assist with Procedures, Treatments, and Minor Office Surgeries: Assist the Patient with Crutch Walking

Task: To properly fit crutches for your patient and teach the patient how to use the crutches properly in three-point walking.

Equipment and Supplies:
- Crutches with arm pads and foam handgrips
- Patient record

Standards: Complete the procedure and all critical steps in _____ minutes with a minimum score of _____% within three attempts.

Scoring: Divide points earned by total possible points. Failure to perform a critical step that is indicated with an asterisk (*) will result in an unsatisfactory overall score.

Time began _____ **Time ended** _____

Steps	Possible Points	First Attempt	Second Attempt	Third Attempt
1. Fit the crutches to the patient so they are 1-1½ inches below the armpits while they are standing up straight. The handgrips should be even with the top of the hip line.	10	_____	_____	_____
2. Be sure that all wingnuts are tight.	5	_____	_____	_____
3. Make sure the foam pads at the armpits and around the handgrips are comfortable.	10	_____	_____	_____
4. Instruct the patient to keep the injured leg as relaxed as possible and slightly bent at the knee. The patient's elbow should be bent from 23 to 30 degrees when holding the handgrip.	10	_____	_____	_____
5. Place the crutch tips approximately 6 inches away from and parallel to the toes.	10	_____	_____	_____
6. Ask the patient to push down on the crutches and lift the body slightly, nearly straightening the arms. The patient should hold the top of the crutches tightly to his or her sides, and use the hands to absorb the weight. Do not let the tops of the crutches press into the armpits.	10	_____	_____	_____
7. Have the patient swing the body forward about 12 inches.	10	_____	_____	_____

Steps	Possible Points	First Attempt	Second Attempt	Third Attempt
8. Instruct the patient to stand on the good leg, and then move the crutches just ahead of the good foot and repeat.	10			
9. Stairs: To walk up and down stairs with crutches, face the steps, hold the handrail with one hand and tuck both crutches under the armpit on the other side. To go up the steps, start with the uninjured side keeping the injured side raised behind. When going down, hold the injured foot up in front, and hop down each stair on the good foot. If the stairway does not have handrails, use the crutches under both arms and hop up or down each step on the uninjured leg. If necessary the patient can sit on the stairs and move up or down each step.	10			
10. Document the patient education intervention in the patient record.*	10			

Documentation in the Medical Record

_____

_____

_____

Comments:

Total Points Earned _____ Divided by _____ Total Possible Points = _____ % Score

Instructor's Signature _____

Student Name _____ Date _____ Score _____

Procedure 43-1 Prepare Patient for and Assist with Routine and Specialty Examinations: Assist with the Neurologic Examination

Task: To assist the physician in obtaining an accurate neurologic examination of the patient.

Equipment and Supplies:
- Otoscope
- Ophthalmoscope
- Percussion hammer
- Disposable pinwheel
- Penlight
- Tuning fork
- Cotton ball
- Tongue depressor
- Small vials of warm and cold liquids prepared according to the physician's instructions
- Small vials of sweet and salty liquids prepared according to the physician's instructions
- Small vials containing substances with distinct odors, such as instant coffee, cinnamon, and vanilla, prepared according to the physician's instructions
- Patient record

Standards: Complete the procedure and all critical steps in _____ minutes with a minimum score of _____% within three attempts.

Scoring: Divide points earned by total possible points. Failure to perform a critical step that is indicated with an asterisk (*) will result in an unsatisfactory overall score.

Time began _____ **Time ended** _____

Steps	Possible Points	First Attempt	Second Attempt	Third Attempt
1. Greet the patient, and help him or her onto the examination table. Explain the procedure to the patient.	20	_____	_____	_____
2. During the examination, be prepared to assist the patient in changing positions as necessary. Have the necessary examination instruments ready for the physician at the appropriate time during the examination. Record all results from the examination as indicated by the physician.	10	_____	_____	_____

Steps	Possible Points	First Attempt	Second Attempt	Third Attempt
3. The neurologic examination will generally follow the following order but can be modified according to physician preference: a. Mental status examination b. Proprioception and cerebellar function c. Cranial nerve assessment d. Sensory nerve function e. Reflexes	10			
4. Complete the documentation of the examination in the patient's medical record.*	10			

Documentation in the Medical Record

_____

_____

_____

Comments:

Total Points Earned _____ Divided by _____ Total Possible Points = _____ % Score

Instructor's Signature _____

Procedure 43-2 Prepare Patient for and Assist with Procedures, Treatments, and Minor Office Surgeries: Prepare the Patient for an EEG

Task: To prepare a patient properly both physically and psychologically to obtain an accurate and useful EEG recording.

Standards: Complete the procedure and all critical steps in _____ minutes with a minimum score of _____% within three attempts.

Scoring: Divide points earned by total possible points. Failure to perform a critical step that is indicated with an asterisk (*) will result in an unsatisfactory overall score.

Time began _____ **Time ended** _____

Steps	Possible Points	First Attempt	Second Attempt	Third Attempt
1. Greet the patient, and introduce yourself. Explain to the patient that you will go over what is going to happen step by step to ensure the best results.*	10	_____	_____	_____
2. Explain to the patient the purpose of the EEG, how the procedure will be carried out, and what will be expected of the patient during the test.	10	_____	_____	_____
3. Tell the patient that the electrodes pick up tiny electrical signals from the body and that there is no danger of electrical shock.	10	_____	_____	_____
4. Explain that the test is painless because the electrodes are attached to the scalp with paste.	10	_____	_____	_____
5. If this is a sleep EEG, suggest that the patient stay up later than usual the night before the test so that it will be easier to fall asleep.	5	_____	_____	_____
6. Go over the physical preparation, including the diet to be followed for the 48 hours before the test. This usually includes no stimulants like coffee, chocolate, or sodas, and no meal skipping.	10	_____	_____	_____
7. Tell the patient that a baseline EEG will be taken at the beginning of the test, and during this time the patient will be asked to avoid all movement, even eye and tongue movement.	5	_____	_____	_____

943

Steps	Possible Points	First Attempt	Second Attempt	Third Attempt
8. If a stimulation examination is ordered, explain that the brain will be stimulated by the patient viewing flickering lights. The EEG will be measuring the brain's response to this stimulation.	5			
9. Ask the patient whether he or she has any questions. If so, answer the questions so that the patient understands the procedure clearly.*	5			
10. Document the procedure in the patient record.	5			

Documentation in the Medical Record

_____

_____

_____

Comments:

Total Points Earned _____ Divided by _____ Total Possible Points = _____ % Score

Instructor's Signature _____

Procedure 43-3 Prepare Patient for and Assist with Procedures, Treatments, and Minor Office Surgeries: Prepare the Patient for and Assist with a Lumbar Puncture

Task: To prepare a patient properly both physically and mentally for a lumbar puncture to obtain a specimen of CSF for testing.

Equipment and Supplies:
- Local anesthetic
- Sterile, disposable lumbar puncture kit
- Mayo stand
- Sterile gloves
- Permanent marker to label tubes
- Patient record

Standards: Complete the procedure and all critical steps in _____ minutes with a minimum score of _____% within three attempts.

Scoring: Divide points earned by total possible points. Failure to perform a critical step that is indicated with an asterisk (*) will result in an unsatisfactory overall score.

Time began _____ **Time ended** _____

Steps	Possible Points	First Attempt	Second Attempt	Third Attempt
1. Greet the patient and introduce yourself. Explain to the patient that you will go over what is going to happen step by step to ensure the best results.	10	_____	_____	_____
2. Explain to the patient the purpose of the lumbar puncture, how the procedure will be carried out, and what will be expected of the patient during the test.*	20	_____	_____	_____
3. Have the patient void just before the procedure.	5	_____	_____	_____
4. Give the patient a hospital gown, and have him or her put it on with the opening down the back.	5	_____	_____	_____
5. Place the patient in a left, side-lying fetal position for the lumbar puncture.	5	_____	_____	_____
6. Support the patient's head with a pillow as necessary, and also provide a pillow for between the knees if needed.	5	_____	_____	_____

Steps	Possible Points	First Attempt	Second Attempt	Third Attempt
7. Perform a sterile skin preparation of the patient's lumbar region in the usual manner.	10			
8. Place the sterile disposable lumbar puncture kit on the Mayo stand and open it, establishing a sterile field. Put on sterile gloves, take the fenestrated drape from the kit, and drape the lumbar region of the patient, so that only the L3-L4 region of the lower spine is exposed.	10			
9. When the physician is ready to do the lumbar puncture, provide the local anesthetic by holding the vial for the physician or pouring it into the sterile medicine cup on the sterile field of the Mayo stand.	10			
10. Reassure the patient, and help him or her to hold still during the injection of the local anesthetic and the insertion of the spinal needle.*	10			
11. Be prepared to hold the top of the manometer steady if requested by the physician.	10			
12. Using the permanent marker, label the specimens #1, #2, and #3 in the order in which they were collected. This is a critically important step in this procedure.*	20			
13. Complete the laboratory requisition form, and prepare the CSF specimens for transport to the laboratory.	10			
14. Break down the Mayo stand sterile field setup by disposing of sharps, biohazard materials, and regular waste in the normal manner.	10			
15. Monitor the patient, and give liquids as directed by the physician.	10			
16. Document the procedure in the patient's chart.	10			

Documentation in the Medical Record

_____

_____

_____

Comments:

Total Points Earned _____ Divided by _____ Total Possible Points = _____ % Score

Instructor's Signature _____

Procedure 44-1 Prepare Patient for and Assist with Procedures, Treatments, and Minor Office Surgeries: Perform a Blood Glucose Accu-Chek Test

Task: To perform accurately a blood test for possible diabetes mellitus.

Equipment and Supplies:
- Accu-Chek glucose monitor or similar glucose monitoring device
- Accu-Chek glucose testing strip
- Lancet and autoloading finger-puncturing device
- Alcohol preps
- Gauze squares
- Disposable gloves
- Patient record

Standards: Complete the procedure and all critical steps in _____ minutes with a minimum score of _____% within three attempts.

Scoring: Divide points earned by total possible points. Failure to perform a critical step that is indicated with an asterisk (*) will result in an unsatisfactory overall score.

Time began _____ **Time ended** _____

Steps	Possible Points	First Attempt	Second Attempt	Third Attempt
1. Reread the physician's order, and collect the necessary equipment and supplies needed to complete the testing procedure. Perform quality-control measures according to manufacturer guidelines and office policy.	10	_____	_____	_____
2. Wash your hands, and put on gloves.	5	_____	_____	_____
3. Ask the patient to wash his or her hands in warm soapy water, then to rinse them in warm water and dry them completely.	5	_____	_____	_____
4. Check the patient's index and ring fingers, and select the site for puncture.	5	_____	_____	_____
5. Turn on the Accu-Chek monitor by pressing the ON button.	5	_____	_____	_____
6. Make sure the code number on the LED display matches the code number on the container of test strips.*	10	_____	_____	_____
7. Remove a test strip from the vial, and immediately replace the vial cover.	10	_____	_____	_____

Steps	Possible Points	First Attempt	Second Attempt	Third Attempt
8. Check the strip for discoloration by comparing the color of the round window on the back of the test strip with the designated "unused" color chart provided on the test strip vial label.	10			
9. Do not touch the yellow test pad or round window on the back of the strip when handling the strip.	10			
10. When the test strip symbol begins flashing in the lower right-hand corner of the display screen, insert the test strip into the designated testing slot until it locks into place. When the test strip is inserted correctly, the arrows on the test strip will be facing up and pointing toward the monitor.	10			
11. Cleanse the selected site on the patient's fingertip with the alcohol wipe, and allow the finger to air dry.*	10			
12. Perform the finger puncture, and wipe away the first drop of blood.	10			
13. Apply a large hanging drop of blood to the center of the yellow testing pad. a. Do not touch the pad with the patient's finger. b. Do not apply a second drop of blood. c. Do not smear the blood with your finger. d. Be certain the yellow test pad is saturated with blood.	10			
14. Give the patient a gauze square to hold securely over the puncture site.	10			
15. The monitor will automatically begin the measurement process as soon as it senses the drop of blood. Read the test result when it is displayed in the display window in milligrams per deciliter. Turn off the monitor by pressing the "O" button.	20			
16. Discard all biohazard waste into the proper waste containers.	10			
17. Clean the glucometer according to manufacturer guidelines, disinfect the work area, remove gloves and dispose of them properly, and wash your hands.	10			

Steps	Possible Points	First Attempt	Second Attempt	Third Attempt
18. Record the testing results in the patient's medical record.	10	_____	_____	_____

Documentation in the Medical Record

_____

_____

_____

Comments:

Total Points Earned _____ Divided by _____ Total Possible Points = _____ % Score

Instructor's Signature _____

Procedure 45-1 Prepare Patient for and Assist with Procedures, Treatments, and Minor Office Surgeries: Teach a Patient How to Use a Peak Flow Meter

Task: To instruct the patient in the proper method of performing a peak flow meter test.

Equipment and Supplies:
- Peak flow meter
- Disposable mouthpiece
- Notebook with pen
- Patient record
- Biohazard waste container

Standards: Complete the procedure and all critical steps in _____ minutes with a minimum score of _____ % within three attempts.

Scoring: Divide points earned by total possible points. Failure to perform a critical step that is indicated with an asterisk (*) will result in an unsatisfactory overall score.

Time began _____ Time ended _____

Steps	Possible Points	First Attempt	Second Attempt	Third Attempt
1. Wash your hands	10			
2. Place the mouthpiece on the peak flow meter and slide the marker to the bottom of the scale.*	10			
3. Introduce yourself and confirm the identity of the patient.	10			
4. Explain the purpose of the test	10			
5. Explain the actual maneuver of forced expiration.	5			
6. Be certain the patient is comfortable and in a proper position either sitting upright or standing (standing is preferred)	5			
7. Loosen any tight clothing, such as a necktie, bra, or belt.	5			
8. Hold the meter upright, being careful not to block the opening with the fingers	5			

Steps	Possible Points	First Attempt	Second Attempt	Third Attempt
9. Instruct the patient to inhale as deeply as possible, place the mouthpiece into mouth beyond the teeth, and form a tight seal with the lips. Caution the patient not to put the tongue in the mouthpiece when exhaling.	10			
10. Instruct the patient to exhale as hard and as fast as possible into the peak flow meter.	10			
11. The forced exhalation will move the marker up the scale and stop at the point of the peak expiratory flow. Record this number and return the marker to the bottom of the scale.	10			
12. Repeat the procedure two more times, sliding the indicator to the bottom of the scale before each reading, and record each result.*	10			
13. Encourage the patient to inhale as deeply as possible and exhale as fast and as forcefully as possible with each effort	10			
14. Place the test results on the patient's chart for physician review, noting the time and date of the highest reading.	10			
15. Clean and disinfect the equipment, discarding waste in a biohazard waste container, or give the patient the meter for continued use at home with instructions to follow the manufacturer's cleaning recommendations.	10			
16. Wash your hands.	10			
17. Record testing information on the patient's chart.	10			

Comments:

Total Points Earned _____ Divided by _____ Total Possible Points = _____ % Score

Instructor's Signature _____

Procedure 45-2 Prepare Patient for and Assist with Procedures, Treatments, and Minor Office Surgeries: Perform a Nebulizer Treatment

Task: To perform a nebulizer treatment.

Equipment and Supplies:
- Nebulizer machine
- Disposable connector tubing with medication dispenser
- Disposable mouthpiece or mask as ordered
- Medication as ordered and sterile saline or water for mixing
- Patient record and pen
- Biohazard waste container

Standards: Complete the procedure and all critical steps in _____ minutes with a minimum score of _____% within three attempts.

Scoring: Divide points earned by total possible points. Failure to perform a critical step that is indicated with an asterisk (*) will result in an unsatisfactory overall score.

Time began _____   Time ended _____

Steps	Possible Points	First Attempt	Second Attempt	Third Attempt
1. Plug the nebulizer into a properly grounded electrical outlet.	5	_____	_____	_____
2. Introduce yourself and confirm the identity of the patient.*	10	_____	_____	_____
3. Explain the purpose of the treatment	10	_____	_____	_____
4. Wash your hands.	10	_____	_____	_____
5. Measure the prescribed dose of drug and diluent and place it into the nebulizer medication cup.	10	_____	_____	_____
6. Replace the top of the medication cup and connect it to the mouthpiece or face mask.	10	_____	_____	_____
7. Connect the disposable tubing to both the nebulizer and the medication cup.	10	_____	_____	_____
8. The patient should be sitting upright to allow for total lung expansion.	5	_____	_____	_____
9. Turn the nebulizer on (should see a mist coming from the back of the tube opposite the mouthpiece or into the face mask).	10	_____	_____	_____

Steps	Possible Points	First Attempt	Second Attempt	Third Attempt
10. If using a mask, position it comfortably but securely over the patient's mouth and nose.	10			
11. If using a mouthpiece, instruct the patient to hold it between the teeth with the lips pursed around the mouthpiece.	10			
12. Encourage the patient to take slow, deep breath through the mouth. Hold each breath 2-3 seconds to allow the medication to disperse through the lungs	10			
13. Continue the treatment until aerosol is no longer produced (about 10 minutes).	5			
14. Turn the nebulizer off.	5			
15. Encourage the patient to take several deep breaths and cough loosened secretions into disposable tissues.*	10			
16. Dispose of the mouthpiece or mask, tubing, and contaminated tissues in a biohazard container.	5			
17. Wash your hands.	10			
18. Record the nebulizer treatment, the patient's response, including the amount of coughing, whether coughing was productive or nonproductive, and any side effects of the medication.	10			
19. If the patient is to continue home nebulizer treatments, conduct patient education with both the patient and caregivers as appropriate. Make sure they demonstrate treatment steps to confirm understanding.	10			

Comments:

Total Points Earned _____ Divided by _____ Total Possible Points = _____ % Score

Instructor's Signature _____

Procedure 45-3 Prepare Patient for and Assist with Procedures, Treatments, and Minor Office Surgeries: Perform Volume Capacity Spirometric Testing

Task: To perform volume capacity testing.

Equipment and Supplies:
- Scale with height measuring device
- Sphygmomanometer and stethoscope
- Spirometer with recording paper in place
- External spirometric tubing
- Disposable mouthpiece
- Nasal clip if needed
- Biohazard waste container
- Patient record

Standards: Complete the procedure and all critical steps in _____ minutes with a minimum score of _____% within three attempts.

Scoring: Divide points earned by total possible points. Failure to perform a critical step that is indicated with an asterisk (*) will result in an unsatisfactory overall score.

Time began _____ **Time ended** _____

Steps	Possible Points	First Attempt	Second Attempt	Third Attempt
1. Wash your hands and assemble the spirometer.	10	_____	_____	_____
2. Introduce yourself, and confirm the identity of the patient. Determine whether any special preparation was needed by this patient and if it was followed.	10	_____	_____	_____
3. Explain the purpose of the test.	10	_____	_____	_____
4. Measure and record the patient's vital signs, height, and weight.*	10	_____	_____	_____
5. Explain the actual maneuver.	10	_____	_____	_____
6. Be certain the patient is comfortable and in proper sitting or standing position.	5	_____	_____	_____
7. Loosen any tight clothing, such as necktie, bra or belt.	5	_____	_____	_____
8. Show the patient the proper chin and neck position.	5	_____	_____	_____

Steps	Possible Points	First Attempt	Second Attempt	Third Attempt
9. Practice the maneuver with the patient before you begin.	5			
10. Place a soft nose clip on the patient's nose.*	10			
11. Place the mouthpiece in the mouth and instruct the patient to seal the lips around the piece.	10			
12. The patient should inhale according to instructions.	10			
13. Use active, forceful coaching during exhalation.*	10			
14. Give the patient feedback after the maneuver is completed.	10			
15. Carefully observe the patient for indications of vertigo or dyspnea or any other signs of difficulty. If complications occur, stop the test and inform the physician.	10			
16. Continue testing until three acceptable maneuvers have been performed.	10			
17. Place the test results on the patient's chart for physician review. Dismiss the patient only if results are satisfactory.	10			
18. Clean and disinfect the equipment. Discard waste in a biohazard waste container.	10			
19. Wash your hands.	10			
20. Record testing information on the patient's chart.	10			

Documentation in the Medical Record

_____

_____

_____

Comments:

Total Points Earned _____ Divided by _____ Total Possible Points = _____ % Score

Instructor's Signature _____

Student Name _____ Date _____ Score _____

Procedure 45-4 Prepare Patient for and Assist with Procedures, Treatments, and Minor Office Surgeries: Obtain a Sputum Sample for Culture

Task: To collect a sputum sample while observing standard precautions.

Equipment and Supplies:
- Sterile laboratory specimen cup, accurately labeled
- Biohazard laboratory specimen bag with laboratory requisition
- Disposable examination gloves
- Face shield with goggles
- Impervious gown
- Biohazard waste container
- Cup of water
- Ginger ale or juice
- Patient record

Standards: Complete the procedure and all critical steps in _____ minutes with a minimum score of _____% within three attempts.

Scoring: Divide points earned by total possible points. Failure to perform a critical step that is indicated with an asterisk (*) will result in an unsatisfactory overall score.

Time began _____ **Time ended** _____

Steps	Possible Points	First Attempt	Second Attempt	Third Attempt
1. Assemble the equipment, and label the specimen cup.	10	_____	_____	_____
2. Identify the patient, and explain the procedure.	10	_____	_____	_____
3. Wash your hands and don gloves, face shield, and lab coat.	10	_____	_____	_____
4. Have the patient rinse his or her mouth with water.	5	_____	_____	_____
5. Carefully remove the specimen cup lid, taking care not to touch the inside of the lid or the inside of the container, and place it upside down on a side table.	10	_____	_____	_____
6. Instruct the patient to take three deep breaths then cough deeply to bring up secretions from the lower respiratory tract.	10	_____	_____	_____
7. Tell the patient to spit directly into the specimen container during the procedure.	5	_____	_____	_____

Steps	Possible Points	First Attempt	Second Attempt	Third Attempt
8. Place the lid on the container securely, taking care not to touch the inside of the lid, then place the container into the plastic specimen bag.	10			
9. Offer the patient a glass of juice or ginger ale.	5			
10. If another test is ordered for the next morning, instruct the patient when to come to the office or explain how to complete the procedure at home. Remind him or her to follow the same instructions for preparation. Stress the importance of maintaining the sterility of the container and collecting the specimen first thing in the morning.	10			
11. Clean the work area, and properly dispose of all supplies.	10			
12. Wash your hands	10			
13. Process the specimen immediately to ensure optimal test results	10			
14. Record the procedure in the patient's record.	10			

Docmentation in the Medical Record

_____

_____

_____

Comments:

Total Points Earned _____ Divided by _____ Total Possible Points = _____ % Score

Instructor's Signature _____

Student Name _____ Date _____ Score _____

Procedure 47-1 Instruct Individuals According to Their Needs: Sensorimotor Changes of Aging

Task: Role-play to better understand the needs of aging persons.

Equipment and Supplies:
- Yellow glasses, ski goggles, or laboratory goggles
- Pink, white, yellow "pills" (various colors of Tic Tacs work)
- Vaseline
- Cotton balls
- Eye patches
- Tape
- Thick gloves
- Utility glove
- Tongue depressors
- Ace bandages
- Medical forms in small print
- Pennies
- Button shirts
- Walker

Standards: Complete the procedure and all critical steps in _____ minutes with a minimum score of _____% within three attempts.

Scoring: Divide points earned by total possible points. Failure to perform a critical step that is indicated with an asterisk (*) will result in an unsatisfactory overall score.

Time began _____ Time ended _____

Steps	Possible Points	First Attempt	Second Attempt	Third Attempt
1. Role-play vision and hearing loss: • Put two cotton balls in each ear and an eye patch over one eye. Follow your partner's instructions. • Partner: Stand out of the line of vision (to prevent lip-reading). Without using gestures or changing voice volume, tell your partner to cross the room and pick up a book.	10	_____	_____	_____
2. Role-play yellowing of lens: • Line up "pills" of different pastel colors. • Partner: Pick out the different colors while wearing the yellow glasses.	10	_____	_____	_____

Steps	Possible Points	First Attempt	Second Attempt	Third Attempt
3. Role-play difficulty with focusing: • Put on goggles smeared with Vaseline, and follow your partner's directions. • Partner: Stand at least 3 feet in front of your partner and motion for him or her to come to you (your partner is deaf, so talking will not help).	10			
4. Role-play loss of peripheral vision: • Put on goggles with black paper taped to sides. • Partner: Stand to the side out of the field of vision and motion for your patient to follow you.	10			
5. Role-play aphasia and partial paralysis: • You are unable to use your right arm or leg. Place tape over your mouth. Let your partner know you need to go to the bathroom. • Partner: Stand at least 3 feet away with your back to your partner and wait for instructions.	10			
6. Role-play problems with dexterity: • Put thick gloves on your hands and try to sign your name, button a shirt, tie your shoes, and pick up pennies.	10			
7. Role-play problems with mobility: • Use the walker to cross the room. • Partner: After your partner starts to use the walker, hand him or her a book to carry.	10			
8. Role-play changes in sensation: • Put a rubber utility glove on; turn on hot water; test the difference in temperature between the gloved hand and nongloved hand.	10			
9. Summarize and share with the group your impressions of the effect of age-related sensorimotor changes.*	20			

Comments:

Total Points Earned _____ Divided by _____ Total Possible Points = _____ % Score

Instructor's Signature _____

Procedure 48-1 Perform Electrocardiography: Obtain a 12-lead ECG

Task: To obtain an accurate, artifact-free recording of the electrical activity of the heart.

Equipment and Supplies:
- ECG machine with patient lead cable
- 10 disposable, self-adhesive electrodes
- Patient gown and drape
- ECG mounting card if necessary
- Patient record

Standards: Complete the procedure and all critical steps in _____ minutes with a minimum score of _____% within three attempts.

Scoring: Divide points earned by total possible points. Failure to perform a critical step that is indicated with an asterisk (*) will result in an unsatisfactory overall score.

Time began _____ **Time ended** _____

Steps	Possible Points	First Attempt	Second Attempt	Third Attempt
1. Wash your hands.	5	_____	_____	_____
2. Explain the procedure to the patient.*	5	_____	_____	_____
3. Ask the patient to disrobe to the waist (including the female patient's bra), and remove socks, stockings, or pantyhose as necessary.	5	_____	_____	_____
4. Position the patient on the examination table, and drape appropriately.	5	_____	_____	_____
5. Turn on the machine to allow the stylus to warm up (may not be necessary in newer machines).	5	_____	_____	_____
6. Label the beginning of the tracing paper with the patient's name, date, time, and current cardiovascular medications, or input information into the machine.	5	_____	_____	_____
7. At each location you are going to place an electrode, clean the skin with an alcohol wipe.	5	_____	_____	_____

Steps	Possible Points	First Attempt	Second Attempt	Third Attempt
8. Apply the self-adhesive electrodes to clean, dry, fleshy areas of the extremities. It may be necessary to shave extremely hairy areas to achieve adequate electrode attachment or to place a piece of tape over the electrode to make sure it is secure.	10			
9. Apply the self-adhesive electrodes to clean areas on the chest.*	10			
10. Carefully connect the lead wires to the correct electrode with the alligator clips on the end of each lead. Make sure the lead wires are not crossed.	10			
11. Press the AUTO button on the machine, and run the ECG tracing. The machine will automatically place the standardization at the beginning, then the 12 leads will follow in the three-channel matrix with a lead II rhythm strip across the bottom of the page.	5			
12. Watch for artifacts during the recording. If artifacts are present, make appropriate corrections, and repeat the recording to get a clean reading.	5			
13. Remove the lead wires from the electrodes, then remove the electrodes from the patient.	5			
14. Assist the patient with getting dressed as needed. Clean and return the ECG machine to its storage area.	5			
15. Mount the ECG or give the unmounted ECG recording to the physician as directed.	5			
16. Wash your hands.	5			
17. Document the procedure in the patient's chart.	5			

Documentation in the Medical Record

_____

_____

_____

Comments:

Total Points Earned _____ Divided by _____ Total Possible Points = _____ % Score

Instructor's Signature _____

Procedure 48-2 Prepare Patient for and Assist with Routine and Specialty Examinations: Apply a Holter Monitor

Task: To establish a possible correlation between coronary disorders and the patient's 24-hour daily activities.

Equipment and Supplies:
- Holter monitor with new battery and blank recording tape
- Disposable electrodes
- Razor
- Gauze pads or abrasive tool as needed
- Activity diary
- Carrying case with belt or shoulder strap
- Alcohol swabs
- Cloth tape (nonallergenic)
- Patient record

Standards: Complete the procedure and all critical steps in _____ minutes with a minimum score of _____% within three attempts.

Scoring: Divide points earned by total possible points. Failure to perform a critical step that is indicated with an asterisk (*) will result in an unsatisfactory overall score.

Time began _____ **Time ended** _____

Steps	Possible Points	First Attempt	Second Attempt	Third Attempt
1. Wash your hands.	5	_____	_____	_____
2. Assemble equipment needed.	5	_____	_____	_____
3. Install a new battery or fully charged rechargeable battery into the monitor.	5	_____	_____	_____
4. Greet the patient, and explain the procedure.*	5	_____	_____	_____
5. Ask the patient to disrobe to the waist and to sit at the end of the examination table or lie down.	5	_____	_____	_____
6. Clean each electrode application site with the alcohol swab, and allow the sites to air dry.	5	_____	_____	_____
7. If the patient has a hairy chest, dry shave the area at each of the electrode sites.	5	_____	_____	_____
8. Fold a gauze pad over your index finger and briskly rub the sites or use an abrasive tool as indicated.	5	_____	_____	_____

Steps	Possible Points	First Attempt	Second Attempt	Third Attempt
9. Apply the electrodes to the sites recommended by the manufacturer, making sure to use enough pressure that they adhere completely to the skin. Rub the edges of each electrode a second time to make certain that the electrode will stay in place.	5			
10. Attach the lead wires to the electrodes, and connect the end terminal to the patient cable.	5			
11. Place a strip of cloth tape over each electrode.	5			
12. Attach the test cable to the monitor and plug it into the electrocardiograph. Run a baseline test tracing as directed by manufacturer guidelines.	5			
13. Help the patient get dressed without disturbing the connected electrodes. Be certain that the cable extends through the buttoned front or out the bottom of the shirt or blouse.	5			
14. Place the monitor in the carrying case, and attach it to the patient's belt or place it over the shoulder. Be sure the wires are not being pulled or bent in half.	5			
15. Plug the electrode cable into the monitor.	5			
16. Record the patient's name, date of birth, and starting date and time in the patient's activity diary.	5			
17. Give the patient the activity diary, and advise him or her to begin by writing in his or her present activity. Include patient education information on the importance of continually recording activities in the diary; using the event marker on the monitor if he or she experiences any symptoms; and correlating the event with a recording in the diary including the time and details regarding the related activity before or during the event.	5			
18. Schedule the patient for a return appointment in 24 hours.	5			
19. Wash your hands.	5			
20. Record the procedure in patient's chart.	5			

Documentation in the Medical Record

_____

_____

_____

Comments:

Total Points Earned _____ Divided by _____ Total Possible Points = _____ % Score

Instructor's Signature _____

Procedure 49-1 Prepare Patient for and Assist with Routine and Specialty Examinations: General Procedure for X-Ray Examination

Task: To assist with an x-ray examination under the supervision of a physician.

Equipment and Supplies:
- Physician's order for an x-ray examination
- Patient identification card to imprint radiographs
- X-ray machine
- X-ray cassettes, loaded with film
- Appropriate accessory items for patient comfort and shielding
- X-ray darkroom with automatic processor
- Patient record

Standards: Complete the procedure and all critical steps in _____ minutes with a minimum score of _____% within three attempts.

Scoring: Divide points earned by total possible points. Failure to perform a critical step that is indicated with an asterisk (*) will result in an unsatisfactory overall score.

Time began _____ **Time ended** _____

Steps	Possible Points	First Attempt	Second Attempt	Third Attempt
1. Check order and equipment needed. Ascertain whether any special preparations are needed.	10	_____	_____	_____
2. Introduce yourself, and confirm the identity of the patient. Ascertain whether any necessary preparations were implemented.	10	_____	_____	_____
3. Explain the procedure to the patient, and respond appropriately to any questions or concerns.*	10	_____	_____	_____
4. Ask childbearing women if pregnancy is possible, and confirm that patient does not have allergies to iodine dye and/or shellfish if iodine dye will be used.*	10	_____	_____	_____
5. Place the x-ray cassette correctly.	5	_____	_____	_____
6. Check to make certain that the patient has removed all metal objects from the area to be examined.	5	_____	_____	_____
7. Position the patient properly, and immobilize the part, if necessary.	10	_____	_____	_____

Steps	Possible Points	First Attempt	Second Attempt	Third Attempt
8. Drape the patient as necessary, and shield the gonads if appropriate.	10			
9. Align the x-ray tube with the cassette at the proper distance.	10			
10. Measure the patient's thickness through the path of the central ray, and set the control panel for the correct exposure.	10			
11. Stand behind a lead shield during the exposure.*	10			
12. Ask the patient to assume a comfortable position after the examination is completed, and wait until the films are processed.	5			
13. In the darkroom, remove the film from the cassette, identify the film, and process the film in the automatic processor.	10			
14. Dismiss the patient when all films are satisfactory.	5			
15. Place the finished radiograph(s) in a properly labeled envelope, and present it to the physician for interpretation. When it has been read, file it according to the policies of the office.	10			
16. Record the x-ray examination on the patient's chart, along with the final written x-ray findings.	10			

Documentation in the Medical Record

_____

_____

_____

Comments:

Total Points Earned _____ Divided by _____ Total Possible Points = _____ % Score

Instructor's Signature _____

Procedure 50-1 Use the Microscope

Task: To focus the microscope properly, using a prepared slide, under low power, high power, and oil immersion

Equipment and Supplies:
• Microscope
• Lens cleaner
• Lens tissue
• Slide containing specimen

Standards: Complete the procedure and all critical steps in _____ minutes with a minimum score of _____ % within three attempts.

Scoring: Divide points earned by total possible points. Failure to perform a critical step that is indicated with an asterisk (*) will result in an unsatisfactory overall score.

Time began _____ **Time ended** _____

Steps	Possible Points	First Attempt	Second Attempt	Third Attempt
1. Wash your hands.	5	_____	_____	_____
2. Gather the materials needed.	5	_____	_____	_____
3. Clean the lenses with lens tissue and lens cleaner.*	10	_____	_____	_____
4. Adjust seating to a comfortable height.	5	_____	_____	_____
5. Plug the microscope into an electric outlet, and turn on the light switch.	10	_____	_____	_____
6. Place the slide specimen on the stage and secure it.	10	_____	_____	_____
7. Turn the revolving nosepiece to low power.	10	_____	_____	_____
8. Carefully raise the stage while observing with the naked eye from the side.	10	_____	_____	_____
9. Focus the specimen, using the coarse adjustment knob.	10	_____	_____	_____
10. Switch to fine adjustment, and focus the specimen in detail.	10	_____	_____	_____
11. Adjust the amount of light by closing the iris diaphragm and lowering the condenser.	10	_____	_____	_____
12. Place a small drop of oil on the slide.	10	_____	_____	_____

Steps	Possible Points	First Attempt	Second Attempt	Third Attempt
13. Carefully swing the oil immersion objective into place.	10			
14. Adjust the focus with the fine adjustment knob.	10			
15. Increase the light by opening the iris diaphragm and raising the condenser.	10			
16. Identify the specimen.	10			
17. Return to low power.	10			
18. Lower the stage.	10			
19. Center the stage.	10			
20. Remove the slide.	10			
21. Switch off the light, and unplug the microscope.	10			
22. Clean the lenses with lens tissue, and remove oil with lens cleaner.	10			
23. Wipe the microscope with a cloth.	10			
24. Cover the microscope.	5			
25. Clean the work area.	10			
26. Wash your hands.	10			

Comments:

Total Points Earned _____ Divided by _____ Total Possible Points = _____ % Score

Instructor's Signature _____

Student Name _____ Date _____ Score _____

Procedure 51-1 Instruct Individuals According to Their Needs: Instruct a Patient in the Collection of a Clean-Catch Midstream Urine Specimen

Task: To collect a contaminant-free urine sample for culture or analysis using clean-catch midstream specimen (CCMS) technique.

Equipment and Supplies:
- Sterile container with lid and label
- Antiseptic towelettes

Standards: Complete the procedure and all critical steps in _____ minutes with a minimum score of _____% within three attempts.

Scoring: Divide points earned by total possible points. Failure to perform a critical step that is indicated with an asterisk (*) will result in an unsatisfactory overall score.

Time began _____ **Time ended** _____

Steps	Possible Points	First Attempt	Second Attempt	Third Attempt
1. Label the container and give the patient the supplies.	10			
2. Explain the following instructions to adult patients or to the guardians of child patients.	10			
Obtaining a Clean-Catch Midstream Specimen (Female Patient)				
1. Wash your hands, and remove your underclothing.	5			
2. Expose the urinary meatus by spreading apart the labia with one hand	5			
3. Cleanse each side of the urinary meatus with a front-to-back motion, from the pubis to the anus. Use a separate antiseptic wipe to cleanse each side of the meatus.	5			
4. Cleanse directly across the meatus, front-to-back, using a third cotton ball or antiseptic wipe	5			
5. Hold the labia apart throughout this procedure.	5			

977

Steps	Possible Points	First Attempt	Second Attempt	Third Attempt
6. Void a small amount of urine into the toilet.	5			
7. Move the specimen container into position and void the next portion of urine into it. remember, this is a sterile container. do not put your fingers on the inside of the container.	5			
8. Remove the cup, and void the last amount of urine into the toilet. (This means that the first part and the last part of the urinary flow have been excluded from the specimen. Only the middle portion of the flow is included.)	5			
9. Wipe in your usual manner, redress, and return the sterile specimen to the place designated by the medical facility.	5			

Obtaining a Clean-Catch Midstream Specimen (Male Patient)

Steps	Possible Points	First Attempt	Second Attempt	Third Attempt
1. Wash your hands, and expose the penis.	5			
2. Retract the foreskin of the penis (if not circumcised).	5			
3. Cleanse the area around the glans penis (meatus) and the urethral opening by washing each side of the glans with a separate antiseptic wipe.	5			
4. Cleanse directly across the urethral opening using a third cotton ball or antiseptic wipe.	5			
5. Void a small amount of urine into the toilet or urinal.	5			
6. Collect the next portion of the urine in the sterile container without touching the inside of the container with hands or penis.	5			
7. Void the last amount of urine into the toilet or urinal.	5			
8. Wipe and redress.	5			
9. Return the specimen to the designated area provided.	5			

Documentation in the Medical Record

_____

_____

_____

Comments:

Total Points Earned _____ Divided by _____ Total Possible Points = _____ % Score

Instructor's Signature _____

Student Name _____ Date _____ Score _____

Procedure 51-2 Perform Urinalysis: Assess Urine for Color and Turbidity

Task: To assess and record the color of a urine specimen.

Equipment and Supplies:
- Urine specimen
- Centrifuge tube

Standards: Complete the procedure and all critical steps in _____ minutes with a minimum score of _____% within three attempts.

Scoring: Divide points earned by total possible points. Failure to perform a critical step that is indicated with an asterisk (*) will result in an unsatisfactory overall score.

Time began _____ **Time ended** _____

Steps	Possible Points	First Attempt	Second Attempt	Third Attempt
1. Wash and dry your hands and don gloves.	10	_____	_____	_____
2. Mix the urine by swirling.	10	_____	_____	_____
3. Label a centrifuge tube if a complete urinalysis is being done.	10	_____	_____	_____
4. Pour the specimen into a standard-size centrifuge tube.	10	_____	_____	_____
5. Assess and record the color • Pale straw • Yellow • Dark yellow • Amber	20	_____	_____	_____
6. Assess the clarity: • Clear—no cloudiness • Slightly turbid—can see light print through tube • Moderately turbid—can see only dark print through tube • Very turbid—cannot see through tube	20	_____	_____	_____
7. Clean the work area, remove gloves, and wash your hands.*	10	_____	_____	_____
8. Record the results in the patient's record.	10	_____	_____	_____

Documentation in the Medical Record

_____

_____

_____

Comments:

Total Points Earned _____ Divided by _____ Total Possible Points = _____ % Score

Instructor's Signature _____

Procedure 51-3 Perform Routine Maintenance of Administrative and Clinical Equipment: Measure Urine Specific Gravity with a Refractometer

Task: To calibrate a refractometer and measure the refractive index of urine. A refractometer is also known as a *total solids (TS) meter*.

Equipment and Supplies:
- Urinary refractometer
- Disposable pipet
- Distilled water
- Biohazard waste container

Standards: Complete the procedure and all critical steps in _____ minutes with a minimum score of _____% within three attempts.

Scoring: Divide points earned by total possible points. Failure to perform a critical step that is indicated with an asterisk (*) will result in an unsatisfactory overall score.

Time began _____ **Time ended** _____

Steps	Possible Points	First Attempt	Second Attempt	Third Attempt
1. Wash your hands and assemble equipment while the urine specimen reaches room temperature.	10	_____	_____	_____
2. Apply gloves and mix the urine specimen in the collection container.	10	_____	_____	_____
3. Using a disposable pipet, apply a drop of water to the prism of the refractometer by lifting the plastic cover. Close the cover and point the device toward a light source such as a window or lamp. Look into the refractometer and rotate the eyepiece so the scale can be clearly read. The scale reads from 1.000 to 1.035 in increments of 0.001.	10	_____	_____	_____
4. Calibrate the refractometer by inserting the small screwdriver provided by the manufacturer in the screw on the underside of the instrument. Turn the screw so that the line is positioned over 1.000.	10	_____	_____	_____

Steps	Possible Points	First Attempt	Second Attempt	Third Attempt
5. Wipe the prism with a soft, lint-free tissue, and apply a drop of mixed urine. Close the cover, point the device at a light source, and read the specific gravity on the scale. Discard the pipet in a biohazard waste container. The value for specific gravity shown in Figure 47-9 is 1.020. Note that specific gravity has no units following the value.	10			
6. Wipe the urine from the prism with a disposable, soft, lint-free tissue between samples. When finished, clean with tissue moistened with alcohol or with a disposable alcohol wipe. Discard these tissues in a biohazard waste container.	10			
7. Record the results, and discard the urine sample.	10			
8. Remove and discard gloves, and wash your hands.	10			

Documentation in the Medical Record

_____

_____

_____

Comments:

Total Points Earned _____ Divided by _____ Total Possible Points = _____ % Score

Instructor's Signature _____

Student Name _____ Date _____ Score _____

Procedure 51-4 Perform Urinalysis: Test Urine with Chemical Reagent Strips—the Chemical Analysis

Task: To perform chemical testing on a urine sample.

Equipment and Supplies:
- Urine specimen
- Reagent strips
- Timer

Standards: Complete the procedure and all critical steps in _____ minutes with a minimum score of _____% within three attempts.

Scoring: Divide points earned by total possible points. Failure to perform a critical step that is indicated with an asterisk (*) will result in an unsatisfactory overall score.

Time began _____ **Time ended** _____

Steps	Possible Points	First Attempt	Second Attempt	Third Attempt
1. Wash and dry your hands. Put on nonsterile gloves and eye protection.	5			
2. Check the time of collection, the container, and the mode of preservation.	5			
3. If the specimen has been refrigerated, allow it to warm to room temperature.*	5			
4. Check the reagent strip container for expiration date.	5			
5. Remove the reagent strip from the container. Hold it in your hand, or place it on a clean paper towel. Recap the container tightly.	5			
6. Compare nonreactive test pads with the negative color blocks on the color chart on the container.	10			
7. Thoroughly mix the specimen by swirling.	10			
8. Following manufacturer's directions, note the time and dip the strip into the urine, then remove.	10			
9. Quickly remove the excess urine from the strip by touching the side of the strip to a paper towel or the side of the urine container.	10			

Steps	Possible Points	First Attempt	Second Attempt	Third Attempt
10. Hold the strip horizontally. At the exact time, compare the strip with the appropriate color chart on the reagent container. Alternately, the strip can be placed on a paper towel.	10			
11. Read the concentration by comparing the strip to the color chart on the side of the bottle. *Do not touch the strip to the bottle.*	10			
12. Clean the work area, remove your gloves, and wash your hands. If a paper towel was used, dispose of it in the biohazard container.	10			
13. Record the results in the patient's record.	10			

Documentation in the Medical Record

_____

_____

_____

Comments:

Total Points Earned _____ Divided by _____ Total Possible Points = _____ % Score

Instructor's Signature _____

Student Name _____ Date _____ Score _____

Procedure 51-5 Perform Urinalysis: Prepare Urine Specimen for Microscopic Examination

Task: To perform a microscopic examination of urine to determine the presence of normal and abnormal elements.

Equipment and Supplies:
- Urine specimen
- Centrifuge tube
- Centrifuge
- Disposable pipet
- Microscope slide and coverslip
- Microscope
- Permanent marker

Standards: Complete the procedure and all critical steps in _____ minutes with a minimum score of _____% within three attempts.

Scoring: Divide points earned by total possible points. Failure to perform a critical step that is indicated with an asterisk (*) will result in an unsatisfactory overall score.

Time began _____ **Time ended** _____

Steps	Possible Points	First Attempt	Second Attempt	Third Attempt
1. Wash and dry your hands. Don nonsterile gloves and face protection.	5			
2. Gently mix the urine specimen.	5			
3. Pour 10 mL of urine into a labeled centrifuge tube, and cap the tube.	5			
4. Place the tube in the centrifuge.	5			
5. Place another tube containing 10 mL of water in the opposite cup.*	5			
6. Secure the lid, and centrifuge for 5 minutes or for the time specified for your instrument.	5			
7. Remove the tube from the centrifuge after the instrument has come to a full stop.	5			
8. Pour off the clear supernatant from the top of the specimen by inverting the centrifuge tube over the sink drain. Do not turn the tube upright until the supernatant is fully decanted.*	10			

Steps	Possible Points	First Attempt	Second Attempt	Third Attempt
9. Prevent the loss of sediment down the drain.	5			
10. Thoroughly mix the sediment by grasping the tube near the top and rapidly flicking it with the fingers of the other hand until all sediment is thoroughly resuspended.*	5			
11. Transfer one drop of sediment to a clean, labeled slide using a clean disposable transfer pipet.*	5			
12. Place a clean coverslip over the drop, and place the slide on the microscope stage. Remove face protection.	5			
13. Focus under low power, and reduce the light.	5			
14. First, scan the entire coverslip for abnormal findings.	5			
15. Examine five low-power fields. Count and classify each type of cast seen, if any, and note mucus if present.	5			
16. Switch to high-power magnification, and adjust the light.	5			
17. In five high-power fields, count the following elements: red blood cells, white blood cells, and round, transitional, and squamous epithelial cells.	5			
18. In the same five fields, report the following as few, moderate, or many: crystals (identify and report each type seen separately), bacteria (identify as rods or cocci), sperm, yeast, and parasites.	5			
19. Average the five fields, and report the results. Do not remove the slide from the microscope until the physician has verified the results.	5			
20. Clean up the work area, remove gloves, and wash your hands	5			

Documentation in the Medical Record

_____

_____

_____

Comments:

Total Points Earned _____ Divided by _____ Total Possible Points = _____ % Score

Instructor's Signature _____

Student Name _____ Date _____ Score _____

Procedure 51-6 Use Methods of Quality Control: Determine the Reliability of Chemical Reagent Strips

Task: To reconstitute a control sample and to test the reliability of the urinalysis chemical testing strip.

Equipment and Supplies:
- Chek-Stix Control Strips for Urinalysis (Bayer)
- Distilled water
- Capped tube with milliliter markings
- Test tube rack
- Forceps
- Timer
- Chemical strips for urine testing
- Color chart for chemical strips

Standards: Complete the procedure and all critical steps in _____ minutes with a minimum score of _____% within three attempts.

Scoring: Divide points earned by total possible points. Failure to perform a critical step that is indicated with an asterisk (*) will result in an unsatisfactory overall score.

Time began _____ **Time ended** _____

Steps	Possible Points	First Attempt	Second Attempt	Third Attempt
1. Assemble equipment and supplies. Record lot number and the expiration date of the Chek-Stix.	10	_____	_____	_____
2. Wash and dry your hands, and put on non-sterile gloves.	5	_____	_____	_____
3. Place a conical tube in the rack and remove the cap.	5	_____	_____	_____
4. Pour 15 mL of distilled water into the tube.	5	_____	_____	_____
5. Using forceps, remove one strip from the bottle. Inspect the strips for mottling or discoloration.	5	_____	_____	_____
6. Place the strip in the water, and tightly cap the tube.	5	_____	_____	_____
7. Invert the tube for 2 minutes.	5	_____	_____	_____
8. Allow the tube to sit in the rack for 30 minutes.	5	_____	_____	_____
9. Invert the tube one time, and remove the strip with forceps.	5	_____	_____	_____

Steps	Possible Points	First Attempt	Second Attempt	Third Attempt
10. Discard the strip in a biohazard waste container. Once reconstituted, the control solution is stable for 8 hours at room temperature.	5			
11. Perform quality control of the chemical reagent strip by dipping it into the control solution according to Procedure 51-4.	5			
12. Read and record the results.	5			
13. Compare the results to the Chek-Stix package insert or chart on the bottle provided by the manufacturer.	5			
14. Discard the chemical reagent strip and the urine control in the biohazard container.	5			
15. Clean up the work area, remove gloves, and wash your hands.	5			

Documentation in the Medical Record

_____

_____

_____

Comments:

Total Points Earned _____ Divided by _____ Total Possible Points = _____ % Score

Instructor's Signature _____

Procedure 51-7 Perform Urinalysis: Test Urine for Glucose with the Clinitest Method

Task: To perform confirmatory testing for glucose in the urine using the Clinitest procedure for reducing substances.

Equipment and Supplies:
- Urine specimen
- Clinitest tablet, tube, and dropper
- Distilled water
- Test tube rack
- Color chart
- Timer

Standards: Complete the procedure and all critical steps in _____ minutes with a minimum score of _____% within three attempts.

Scoring: Divide points earned by total possible points. Failure to perform a critical step that is indicated with an asterisk (*) will result in an unsatisfactory overall score.

Time began _____ **Time ended** _____

Steps	Possible Points	First Attempt	Second Attempt	Third Attempt
1. Wash and dry your hands, and don nonsterile gloves and eye protection.	5			
2. Holding a Clinitest dropper vertically, add 10 drops of distilled water then five drops of urine to a Clinitest tube.	10			
3. Place the prepared tube into the rack.	5			
4. With dry hands, remove a Clinitest tablet from the bottle by shaking a tablet into the bottle cap.	5			
5. Tap the tablet into the test tube, and recap the container.	5			
6. Observe the entire reaction to detect the rapid pass-through phenomenon, which means that the glucose level in the urine is very high. (See step 9.)	5			
7. When boiling ceases, time exactly 15 seconds then gently shake the tube to mix the entire contents.*	5			

Steps	Possible Points	First Attempt	Second Attempt	Third Attempt
8. Immediately compare the color of the specimen with the five-drop color chart, and record your findings.	10			
9. If an orange color briefly develops during the reaction, rapid pass-through has occurred, and the test must be repeated using the two-drop color chart.	5			

Documentation in the Medical Record

_____

_____

_____

Comments:

Total Points Earned _____ Divided by _____ Total Possible Points = _____ % Score

Instructor's Signature _____

Student Name _____ Date _____ Score _____

Procedure 51-8 Perform Urinalysis: Perform a Pregnancy Test

Task: To perform a pregnancy testing of urine using the QuickVue (Quidel) pregnancy test method.

Equipment and Supplies:
• Urine specimen
• QuickVue test kit

Standards: Complete the procedure and all critical steps in _____ minutes with a minimum score of _____% within three attempts.

Scoring: Divide points earned by total possible points. Failure to perform a critical step that is indicated with an asterisk (*) will result in an unsatisfactory overall score.

Time began _____ **Time ended** _____

Steps	Possible Points	First Attempt	Second Attempt	Third Attempt
1. Wash and dry your hands. Put on nonsterile gloves.	5	_____	_____	_____
2. Prepare the testing equipment.*	5	_____	_____	_____
3. Collect the needed specimen.	5	_____	_____	_____
4. Remove the test cassette from the foil pouch.	5	_____	_____	_____
5. Add three drops of urine using the dropper that accompanies the kit. Dispose of the dropper in a biohazard bag.*	5	_____	_____	_____
6. Wait 3 minutes and read the test results.	5	_____	_____	_____
7. Interpret the results. • *Negative:* A blue control line next to the letter C will be present. No line will be present next to the letter T. • *Positive:* A blue control line next to the letter C will appear along with a pink line next to the letter T.	10	_____	_____	_____
8. If a blue line does not appear in the C area, the test is invalid and the specimen must be retested using another kit. Check the expiration date of the kit before proceeding.	10	_____	_____	_____
9. Discard the cassette in a biohazard waste container, remove the gloves, and wash the hands.	5	_____	_____	_____

Steps	Possible Points	First Attempt	Second Attempt	Third Attempt
10. Record the results as either positive or negative.	5			

Documentation in the Medical Record

_____

_____

_____

Comments:

Total Points Earned _____ Divided by _____ Total Possible Points = _____ % Score

Instructor's Signature _____

Student Name _____ Date _____ Score _____

Procedure 51-9 Perform Urinalysis: Perform a Multidrug Screen Urine Test

Task: To screen a urine specimen for drugs or drug metabolites at their specified cutoff levels.

Equipment and Supplies:
- Instant-View Multi-Drug Screen Urine Test in a sealed pouch
- Freshly voided urine sample
- Timer
- Biohazard container

Standards: Complete the procedure and all critical steps in _____ minutes with a minimum score of _____% within three attempts.

Scoring: Divide points earned by total possible points. Failure to perform a critical step that is indicated with an asterisk (*) will result in an unsatisfactory overall score.

Time began _____ **Time ended** _____

Steps	Possible Points	First Attempt	Second Attempt	Third Attempt
1. Wash your hands, and assemble the equipment and specimen. Check the expiration date on the test kit.	10			
2. Determine urine temperature (within 4 minutes of voiding).*	10			
3. Bring specimen and the testing device to room temperature.	5			
4. Remove the device from the foil pouch, and label it with specimen identification.	5			
Dip Method				
5. Remove the cap of the specimen and dip the device into the specimen for 10 seconds. The surface of the urine must be above the sample well and below the arrowheads in the window.	5			
Alternate Method				
6. Remove the pipet from the pouch, and fill the pipet to the line on the barrel with urine. Dispense the entire volume onto the sample well on the testing device.	5			
7. Recap the urine specimen.	5			
8. Set the timer for 4 to 7 minutes. Do not read results after 7 minutes.	5			

Steps	Possible Points	First Attempt	Second Attempt	Third Attempt
9. Interpret results • Positive—If the C line appears and there is no T line, the test indicates a positive result for that drug. • Negative—If the C line and the T line both appear, the test indicates that the level for the drug or its metabolites is below the cutoff level. • Invalid—If no C line develops within 5 minutes on any test strip, the assay is invalid. Ensure that the urine has not been adulterated (Procedure 51-10) and/or repeat the assay with a new test device.	10			
10. Record the results.	5			
11. Color photocopying will provide a permanent record of results, but the copy must be made within 7 minutes of adding the urine. Ensure that the photocopier does not become contaminated; wipe the glass with alcohol or another manufacturer-approved disinfectant after making the copy.	5			
12. Discard urine and device in biohazard container.	5			
13. Remove gloves and wash hands.	5			

Documentation in the Medical Record

_____

_____

_____

Comments:

Total Points Earned _____ Divided by _____ Total Possible Points = _____ % Score

Instructor's Signature _____

Procedure 51-10 Perform Urinalysis: Assess a Urine Specimen for Adulteration Before Drug Testing

Task: To assess a urine specimen for additive adulteration.

Equipment and Supplies:
- Quik Test Adulterant Strips (Quik Test USA, Boca Raton, Fla.)
- Urine sample (freshly voided; urine should be stored at room temperature for no longer than 2 hours or at refrigerator temperature for longer than 4 hours before testing)
- Paper towels
- Timer
- Biohazard waste container

Standards: Complete the procedure and all critical steps in _____ minutes with a minimum score of _____% within three attempts.

Scoring: Divide points earned by total possible points. Failure to perform a critical step that is indicated with an asterisk (*) will result in an unsatisfactory overall score.

Time began _____ **Time ended** _____

Steps	Possible Points	First Attempt	Second Attempt	Third Attempt
1. Wash your hands, assemble equipment and specimen. Check the expiration date on the test kit.	10			
2. Remove one strip from the container, and recap tightly.	10			
3. Dip test strip briefly into the urine, and remove.	5			
4. Blot the strip by touching the side of the strip to paper toweling.	5			
5. Read results within 1 minute by comparing each pad to the color strips on the canister.	5			
6. Dispose of paper towels and strip in the biohazard container.	5			
7. Remove gloves and wash hands.	5			
8. Record results.*	5			

Documentation in the Medical Record

_____

_____

_____

Comments:

Total Points Earned _____ Divided by _____ Total Possible Points = _____ % Score

Instructor's Signature _____

Procedure 52-1   Perform Venipuncture: Collect a Venous Blood Sample Using the Syringe Method

Task: To collect a venous blood specimen.

Equipment and Supplies:
- Needle, syringe with 21- or 22-gauge safety needle
- Vacutainer tubes appropriate for tests ordered
- 70% isopropyl alcohol
- Sterile gauze pads
- Tourniquet
- Syringe adapter for transfer to Vacutainer tubes
- Nonallergenic tape or bandage
- Permanent marking pen

Standards: Complete the procedure and all critical steps in _____ minutes with a minimum score of _____ % within three attempts.

Scoring: Divide points earned by total possible points. Failure to perform a critical step that is indicated with an asterisk (*) will result in an unsatisfactory overall score.

Time began _____   **Time ended** _____

Steps	Possible Points	First Attempt	Second Attempt	Third Attempt
1. Check the requisition form to determine the tests ordered. Gather the correct tubes and supplies you will need.	10	_____	_____	_____
2. Wash and dry your hands, and put on non-sterile gloves.	5	_____	_____	_____
3. Identify the patient, explain the procedure, and obtain permission to perform the venipuncture.*	10	_____	_____	_____
4. Assist the patient to sit with the arm well supported in a slightly downward position.	5	_____	_____	_____
5. Assemble equipment. Choice of syringe barrel size and needle size depends on your inspection of the patient's veins and the amount of blood required for the ordered tests. Attach the needle to the syringe. Pull and depress the plunger several times to loosen it in the barrel. Keep the cover on the needle.	10	_____	_____	_____

Steps	Possible Points	First Attempt	Second Attempt	Third Attempt
6. Apply the tourniquet around the patient's arm 3 to 4 inches above the elbow. The tourniquet should never be tied so tightly that it restricts blood flow in the artery.* The tourniquet should remain in place no longer than 1 minute.	10			
7. Ask the patient to make a fist.	5			
8. Select the venipuncture site by palpating the antecubital space, and use your index finger to trace the path of the vein and to judge its depth. The vein most often used is the median cephalic, which lies in the middle of the elbow.*	10			
9. Cleanse the site, starting in the center of the area and working outward in a circular pattern with the alcohol pad. Allow the area to dry before proceeding.	10			
10. Hold the syringe in your dominant hand. Your thumb should be on top and your fingers underneath. Remove the needle sheath.	10			
11. Grasp the patient's arm with the nondominant hand while using your thumb and forefinger to draw the skin taut over the site to anchor the vein.	10			
12. Insert the needle through the skin and into the vein with the bevel of the needle up, aligned parallel to the vein, at a 15-degree angle, rapidly, and smoothly. Observe for a "flash" of blood in the hub of the syringe. Request that the patient release his or her fist.	10			
13. Slowly pull back the plunger of the syringe with the nondominant hand. Do not allow more than 1 mL of headspace between the blood and the top of the plunger. Make sure that you do not move the needle after entering the vein. Fill the barrel to the needed volume.	10			
14. Release the tourniquet when venipuncture is complete. It must be released before the needle is removed from the arm*.	10			
15. Place sterile gauze over the puncture site at the time of needle withdrawal. Immediately activate the needle safety device.	10			

Steps	Possible Points	First Attempt	Second Attempt	Third Attempt
16. Instruct the patient to apply direct pressure on the puncture site with sterile gauze. The patient may elevate the arm, but it should not be bent.	10	_____	_____	_____
17. Transfer the blood immediately to the required tube or tubes using a syringe adapter. Do not push on the plunger during transfer. Discard the entire unit when transfer is complete. Invert tubes after addition of blood, and label with the necessary patient information.	10	_____	_____	_____
18. Inspect the puncture site for bleeding or hematoma.	5	_____	_____	_____
19. Apply a hypoallergenic bandage.*	5	_____	_____	_____
20. Clean the work area, remove gloves, and wash your hands.	10	_____	_____	_____
21. Complete the laboratory requisition form, and route the specimen to the proper place. Record the procedure in the patient's record.	10	_____	_____	_____

Documentation in the Medical Record

_____

_____

_____

Comments:

Total Points Earned _____ Divided by _____ Total Possible Points = _____ % Score

Instructor's Signature _____

Procedure 52-2 Perform Venipuncture: Collect a Venous Blood Sample Using the Evacuated Tube Method

Task: To collect a venous blood specimen.

Equipment and Supplies:
- Vacutainer needle, needle holder, and proper tubes for requested tests
- 70% isopropyl alcohol
- Gauze pads
- Tourniquet
- Nonallergenic tape or bandage
- Permanent marking pen

Standards: Complete the procedure and all critical steps in _____ minutes with a minimum score of _____% within three attempts.

Scoring: Divide points earned by total possible points. Failure to perform a critical step that is indicated with an asterisk (*) will result in an unsatisfactory overall score.

Time began _____ **Time ended** _____

Steps	Possible Points	First Attempt	Second Attempt	Third Attempt
1. Check the requisition form to determine the tests ordered. Gather the correct tubes and supplies that you will need.	10	_____	_____	_____
2. Wash and dry your hands, and put on non-sterile gloves.	5	_____	_____	_____
3. Identify the patient, explain the procedure, and obtain permission for the venipuncture.	10	_____	_____	_____
4. Assist the patient to sit with the arm well supported in a slightly downward position.	5	_____	_____	_____
5. Assemble equipment. Choice of needle size depends on your inspection of the patient's veins. Attach the needle firmly to the Vacutainer holder. Keep the cover on the needle.	10	_____	_____	_____
6. Apply the tourniquet around the patient's arm 3 to 4 inches above the elbow. The tourniquet should never be tied so tightly that it restricts blood flow in the artery. Tourniquets should remain in place no longer than 60 seconds.	10 5	_____	_____	_____
7. Ask the patient to make a fist.				

Steps	Possible Points	First Attempt	Second Attempt	Third Attempt
8. Select the venipuncture site by palpating the antecubital space, and use your index finger to trace the path of the vein and to judge its depth. The vein most often used is the median cephalic, which lies in the middle of the elbow.	10			
9. Cleanse the site, starting in the center of the area and working outward in a circular pattern with the alcohol pad.*	10			
10. Dry the site with a gauze pad.	5			
11. Hold the Vacutainer assembly in your dominant hand. Your thumb should be on top and your fingers underneath. You may wish to position the first tube to be drawn in the needle holder, but do not push it onto the double pointed needle past the marking on the holder. Remove the needle sheath.	10			
12. Grasp the patient's arm with the nondominant hand while using your thumb and forefinger to draw the skin taut over the site, to anchor the vein.	10			
13. Insert the needle through the skin and into the vein with the bevel of the needle up, aligned parallel to the vein, at a 15-degree angle, rapidly, and smoothly.	10			
14. Place two fingers on the flanges of the needle holder and, with the thumb, push the tube onto the double-pointed needle. Make sure that you do not change the needle's position in the vein. When blood begins to flow into the tube, ask the patient to release the fist.	10			
15. Allow the tube to fill to maximum capacity. Remove the tube by curling the fingers underneath and pushing on the needle holder with the thumb. Take care not to move the needle when removing the tube.	10			
16. Insert the second tube into the needle holder, following the instructions in the previous steps. Continue filling tubes until the order on the requisition is filled. Gently invert each tube immediately after removing from the needle holder to mix anticoagulants and blood. As the last tube is filling, release the tourniquet.	10			

Steps	Possible Points	First Attempt	Second Attempt	Third Attempt
17. Remove the last tube from the holder. Place gauze over the puncture site, and quickly remove the needle, engaging the safety device. Dispose of the entire unit in the sharps container.	10			
18. Apply pressure to the gauze, or instruct the patient to do so. The patient may elevate the arm but should not bend it.	10			
19. Label tubes with the patient's name, the date, and the time.	10			
20. Check the puncture site for bleeding and hematoma formation.	5			
21. Apply a hypoallergenic bandage.	5			
22. Clean the work area, remove gloves, and wash your hands.	10			
23. Complete the laboratory requisition, and route to the proper place. Record the procedure in the patient's record.	10			

Documentation in the Medical Record

_____

_____

_____

Comments:

Total Points Earned _____ Divided by _____ Total Possible Points = _____ % Score

Instructor's Signature _____

Student Name _____ Date _____ Score _____

Procedure 52-3 Perform Venipuncture: Perform Venipuncture with a Winged Infusion Set (Butterfly Needle)

Task: To obtain the venous sample accurately from a hand vein using a winged infusion set.

Equipment and Supplies:
- Tourniquet
- Alcohol pads or other antiseptic preps
- Gauze pads
- Winged infusion ("butterfly") needle set
- Appropriate tubes with a needle and needle adapter
- Syringe with needle
- Sharps disposal container
- Nonallergenic bandage
- Permanent marking pen

Standards: Complete the procedure and all critical steps in _____ minutes with a minimum score of _____% within three attempts.

Scoring: Divide points earned by total possible points. Failure to perform a critical step that is indicated with an asterisk (*) will result in an unsatisfactory overall score.

Time began _____ Time ended _____

Steps	Possible Points	First Attempt	Second Attempt	Third Attempt
1. Check the requisition, and gather the appropriate tubes for the needed tests. Assemble the balance of your supplies.	10	_____	_____	_____
2. Wash your hands, and put on gloves.	5	_____	_____	_____
3. Identify the patient, and explain the procedure.*	10	_____	_____	_____
4. Remove the butterfly device from the package, and stretch the tubing slightly. Take care not to accidentally activate the needle-retracting safety device.	5	_____	_____	_____
5. Attach the butterfly device to the syringe or needle holder.	5	_____	_____	_____
6. Seat the first tube into the evacuated tube holder, and place the unit carefully in a place where it will not roll away.	5	_____	_____	_____
7. Apply a tourniquet to the patient's wrist, just proximal to the wrist bone. Do not apply the tourniquet so tightly that blood flow in the arteries is impeded.	10	_____	_____	_____

Steps	Possible Points	First Attempt	Second Attempt	Third Attempt
8. Hold the patient's hand in your nondominant hand, with the fingers lower than the wrist	10			
9. Select a vein, and cleanse the site at the bifurcation (forking) of the veins.	5			
10. Using your thumb, pull the patient's skin taut over the knuckles.	5			
11. With the needle at a 10- to 15-degree angle, bevel up, align it with the vein.	5			
12. Insert the needle by holding the wings or the rear of the set. After insertion the wings are never to be touched again. Ensure that the safety device is not activated.	10			
13. Push the blood-collecting tube onto the end of the holder or draw blood into the syringe. Note the position of the hands while drawing the blood. When drawing blood into the syringe, ensure that the vacuum you create is slow and steady and that no more than 1 mL of head space between the blood and the plunger is seen.	10			
14. Release the tourniquet when the blood appears in the tube or a "flash" of blood is seen in the hub of the syringe.	10			
15. Always keep the tube and the holder in a downward position so that the tube will fill from the bottom up.	10			
16. Place a gauze pad over the puncture site, and gently remove the needle.	10			

Documentation in the Medical Record

_____

_____

_____

Comments:

Total Points Earned _____ Divided by _____ Total Possible Points = _____ % Score

Instructor's Signature _____

Student Name _____ Date _____ Score _____

Procedure 52-4 Perform Capillary Puncture

Task: To collect a capillary blood specimen suitable for testing, using fingertip puncture technique.

Equipment and Supplies:
- Sterile disposable safety lancet
- 70% alcohol prep pads
- Sterile gauze pads
- Nonallergenic tape
- Appropriate collection containers such as capillary tubes or Microtainer devices
- Sealing clay or caps for capillary tubes
- Permanent marking pen

Standards: Complete the procedure and all critical steps in _____ minutes with a minimum score of _____% within three attempts.

Scoring: Divide points earned by total possible points. Failure to perform a critical step that is indicated with an asterisk (*) will result in an unsatisfactory overall score.

Time began _____ Time ended _____

Steps	Possible Points	First Attempt	Second Attempt	Third Attempt
1. Read requisition, and gather all needed supplies.	10			
2. Wash and dry your hands. Put on nonsterile gloves.	10			
3. Identify the patient, and explain the procedure.*	10			
4. Assemble the needed materials based on the physician's requisition.	10			
5. Select a puncture site depending on the age of the patient and the sample to be obtained (side of middle finger of nondominant hand, medial or lateral curved surface of the heel, or the great toe for an infant).	10			
6. Gently rub the finger along the sides.	5			
7. Clean the site with alcohol, and dry it with sterile gauze.	5			
8. Grasp the patient's finger on the sides near the puncture site with your nondominant forefinger and thumb.	5			

Steps	Possible Points	First Attempt	Second Attempt	Third Attempt
9. Hold the lancet at a right angle to the patient's finger, and make a rapid, deep puncture on the patient's fingertip.	10	____	____	____
10. Wipe away the first drop of blood with clean gauze. Dispose of the lancet in the sharps container.*	10	____	____	____
11. Apply gentle pressure to cause the blood to flow freely.	10	____	____	____
12. Collect blood samples.	10	____	____	____
a. Express a large drop of blood, touch the end of the tube to the drop of blood (not the finger), fill capillary tubes, place the finger over the blood-free end of the tube, and seal the other end of the tube by inserting it into the sealing clay. The tube should be approximately three quarters full before it is sealed.				
b. Wipe the finger with a clean sterile gauze pad, express another large drop of blood, and fill a Microtainer. Do not touch the container to the finger. If more blood is needed, wipe the puncture with clean gauze and gently squeeze another drop. Cap the tube when the collection is complete.				
13. Apply pressure to the site with clean sterile gauze when collection is complete. The patient may be able to assist with this step.	10	____	____	____
14. Select an appropriate means for labeling the containers. Capillary tubes can be placed in a red-topped tube, which is subsequently labeled. Microtainers can be placed in zipper-lock bags that are subsequently labeled.	10	____	____	____
15. Check the patient for bleeding, clean the site if traces of blood are visible, and apply a nonallergenic bandage if indicated.	5	____	____	____
16. Dispose of used materials in proper containers.	10	____	____	____
17. Clean the work area. Remove gloves. Wash your hands.	10	____	____	____
18. Record the procedure in the patient's record.	10	____	____	____

Documentation in the Medical Record

_____

_____

_____

Comments:

Total Points Earned _____ Divided by _____ Total Possible Points = _____ % Score

Instructor's Signature _____

Student Name _____ Date _____ Score _____

Procedure 53-1 Perform Hematology Testing:
Perform a Microhematocrit

Task: To perform a microhematocrit accurately.

Equipment and Supplies:
- EDTA-anticoagulant blood
- Capillary tubes
- Sealing clay
- Centrifuge

Standards: Complete the procedure and all critical steps in _____ minutes with a minimum score of _____% within three attempts.

Scoring: Divide points earned by total possible points. Failure to perform a critical step that is indicated with an asterisk (*) will result in an unsatisfactory overall score.

Time began _____ **Time ended** _____

Steps	Possible Points	First Attempt	Second Attempt	Third Attempt
1. Wash and dry your hands. Put on nonsterile gloves.	10	_____	_____	_____
2. Assemble the materials needed.	10	_____	_____	_____
3. Fill two plain (blue-tipped) capillary tubes two thirds to three fourths full with well-mixed EDTA-anticoagulant blood by tipping the blood tube slightly and touching the capillary tube end opposite the blue band to the blood. If the capillary tube and the blood tube are held almost parallel to the table, the capillary tube will fill easily by capillary action.	10	_____	_____	_____
4. Wipe the outside of a tube with clean gauze without touching the wet open end of the tube.	10	_____	_____	_____
5. Tip the tube until the blood runs toward the end with the colored band.	10	_____	_____	_____
6. Seal the end with the blue band with sealing clay by holding the tube horizontally and inserting the tube. Insert the tube as many times as needed to achieve a plug up to the blue band.	10	_____	_____	_____
7. Place the tubes opposite each other in the centrifuge, with sealed ends securely against the gasket.	10	_____	_____	_____

Steps	Possible Points	First Attempt	Second Attempt	Third Attempt
8. Note the numbers on the centrifuge slots, and record them.	5			
9. Secure the locking top, fasten the lid down, and lock.*	10			
10. Set the timer, and adjust the speed as needed.	10			
11. Allow the centrifuge to come to a complete stop. Unlock the lids.*	10			
12. Remove the tubes immediately, and read the results. If this is not possible, store the tubes in an upright position	10			
13. Determine the microhematocrit values using one of the following methods: a. Centrifuge with built-in reader using calibrated capillary tubes. • Position the tubes as directed by manufacturer's instructions. • Read both tubes. • The average of the two results is reported. • The two values should not vary by more than 2%. b. Centrifuge without built-in reader. • Carefully remove the tubes from the centrifuge. • Place a tube on the microhematocrit reader. • Align the clay-RBC junction with the zero line on the reader. Align the plasma meniscus with the 100% line. The value is read at the junction of the red cell layer and the buffy coat. The buffy coat is not included in the reading. • Read both tubes. • The average of the two results is reported. • The two values should not vary by more than 2%.	10			
14. Dispose of the capillary tubes in a sharps container.	10			
15. Clean the work area, and properly dispose of all biohazard materials. Remove gloves, and wash your hands.	10			
16. Record the results in the patient's medical record.	10			

Documentation in the Medical Record

_____
_____
_____

Comments:

Total Points Earned _____ Divided by _____ Total Possible Points = _____ % Score

Instructor's Signature _____

Procedure 53-2 Perform Routine Maintenance of Clinical Equipment: Preventative Maintenance for the Microhematocrit Centrifuge

Task: To perform daily, monthly, and quarterly quality control on a microhematocrit centrifuge

Equipment and Supplies:
- Microhematocrit centrifuge
- Quality-control logbook
- High-, normal-, and low-quality control samples

Standards: Complete the procedure and all critical steps in _____ minutes with a minimum score of _____% within three attempts.

Scoring: Divide points earned by total possible points. Failure to perform a critical step that is indicated with an asterisk (*) will result in an unsatisfactory overall score.

Time began _____ Time ended _____

Steps	Possible Points	First Attempt	Second Attempt	Third Attempt
Note: These are generic recommendations. Always check manufacturer's guidelines for specific instructions. Always unplug the power cord before cleaning or servicing the centrifuge. Wear protective gloves and clothing.				
Daily Maintenance				
1. Clean the inside of the centrifuge and the gasket with a disinfectant recommended by the manufacturer. Plastic and nonmetal parts may be cleaned with a fresh solution of 5% sodium hypochlorite (bleach) mixed 1:10 with water (one part bleach plus nine parts water).	10	_____	_____	_____
Monthly Maintenance				
1. Check the reading device. Misuse and zeroing of the reading devices can promote considerable error. Always use a second, simple reading device as a cross-check. Use a ruler or a flat plastic card. These cards are used by laying the spun hematocrit tube on the card and aligning the red cells with a line on the card to obtain the reading.	10	_____	_____	_____
2. Check the rotor for cracks or corrosion, and check the interior for signs of white powder.	10	_____	_____	_____

Steps	Possible Points	First Attempt	Second Attempt	Third Attempt
3. Record all preventative maintenance in the laboratory logbook.	10			
Semiannual Maintenance				
1. Check the gasket for cuts and breaks.	10			
2. Check the timer with a stopwatch.	10			
3. Perform a maximum cell pack to verify the time required for complete packing by reading a sample after centrifugation then recentrifuging for 1 minute. The results should be the same. If they are not, perform preventive maintenance and/or call the service technician.	10			
4. Record all preventative measures in the laboratory logbook.	10			
Annual Maintenance or Maintenance Performed as Needed				
1. The centrifuge functions and maintenance verification should be performed by qualified personnel. This would include checking the centrifuge mechanism, rotors, timer, speed, and electrical leaks.	10			
2. Record all professional service calls in the laboratory logbook.	10			

Comments:

Total Points Earned _____ Divided by _____ Total Possible Points = _____ % Score

Instructor's Signature _____

Procedure 53-3 Perform Hematology Testing:
Perform a Hemoglobin Test

Task: To determine accurately the level of hemoglobin present in a blood sample using the HemoCue B-Hemoglobin System.

Equipment and Supplies:
- Hemo-Cue (Hemo-Cue, Lake Forest, Calif.)
- Hemo-Cue cuvette
- Autolet or blood lancet
- Alcohol preps
- Gauze squares

Standards: Complete the procedure and all critical steps in _____ minutes with a minimum score of _____% within three attempts.

Scoring: Divide points earned by total possible points. Failure to perform a critical step that is indicated with an asterisk (*) will result in an unsatisfactory overall score.

Time began _____ **Time ended** _____

Steps	Possible Points	First Attempt	Second Attempt	Third Attempt
1. Perform instrument quality control by inserting the control cuvette into the instrument. Ensure that the reading is within acceptable limits before proceeding.*	10	_____	_____	_____
2. Wash and dry hands.	10	_____	_____	_____
3. Collect and assemble all equipment and supplies needed.	10	_____	_____	_____
4. Explain the procedure to the patient.*	10	_____	_____	_____
5. Put on gloves.	10	_____	_____	_____
6. Examine the fingers, and choose the site to be used to obtain the blood sample.	10	_____	_____	_____
7. Clean the site with alcohol or other recommended antiseptic preparation.	10	_____	_____	_____
8. Perform a capillary puncture, and obtain the blood sample.	10	_____	_____	_____
9. Wipe away the first drop of blood.*	10	_____	_____	_____

Steps	Possible Points	First Attempt	Second Attempt	Third Attempt
10. Touch the microcuvette to the drop of blood. Do not touch the finger. The correct volume will be drawn into the cuvette by capillary action. Wipe off any excess blood from the sides of the cuvette.	10			
11. Place the cuvette in the cuvette holder, and insert it into the instrument.	10			
12. Read the result, and record it on the patient's medical record.	10			
13. Dispose of the biohazard waste in correct containers, and properly clean the work area. Turn the instrument off, and return it to the proper storage location.	10			
14. Remove gloves and wash hands.	10			

Student Name _____ Date _____ Score _____

Procedure 53-4 Prepare a Blood Smear Stained with Wright's Stain

Task: To prepare and stain a slide that meets the criteria for the performance of a differential examination.

Equipment and Supplies:
- Clean glass slides
- Transfer pipette or capillary tube
- Wright's stain materials
- EDTA-anticoagulated blood specimen
- Diff-Safe blood dispenser (Alpha Scientific, Malvern, Pa.)

Standards: Complete the procedure and all critical steps in _____ minutes with a minimum score of _____% within three attempts.

Scoring: Divide points earned by total possible points. Failure to perform a critical step that is indicated with an asterisk (*) will result in an unsatisfactory overall score.

Time began _____ **Time ended** _____

Steps	Possible Points	First Attempt	Second Attempt	Third Attempt
1. Wash and dry your hands. Put on nonsterile gloves.	10			
2. Assemble the materials needed.	10			
3. Mix the blood specimen.	10			
4. Insert a Diff-Safe blood dispenser (Alpha Scientific, Malvern, Pa.) into the top of the vacuum tube. Invert the tube, and dispense a drop of blood onto a slide about ½ to ¾ inch from the right end by pressing on the tube.	10			
5. Hold one side of this slide with your non-dominant hand.	5			
6. Place the spreader slide in front of the drop of blood at an angle of 30 to 35 degrees. Use your dominant hand.	10			
7. Pull back the spreader slide into the drop of blood, and allow the blood to spread to the edges of the slide.	10			
8. Push the spreader slide forward with a quick smooth motion, maintaining the same angle throughout.	10			
9. Rapidly but gently wave the slide to accelerate the drying process.	10			

Steps	Possible Points	First Attempt	Second Attempt	Third Attempt
10. Stand the slide with the thick end down, and allow the slide to complete drying.	10			
11. Label the slide when it is dry. Use a pencil, and write the name in the thick end of the smear or on the frosted area.	10			

12. Stain according to method used.
• Two-step method:
  a. Place the smear on a staining rack, with the blood side up.
  b. Flood the smear with Wright's stain.
  c. Wait for 1 to 3 minutes.
  d. Add an equal amount of buffer, drop by drop, on top of the Wright stain.
  e. Blow gently, and mix the two solutions until a green metallic sheen appears. This should appear within 2 to 4 minutes.
  f. Rinse thoroughly with distilled water.
  g. Drain water from the slide.
  h. Wipe the back of the smear with gauze.
  i. Stand the smear to dry.
 	
• Quick stain:
  a. Place the smear into solutions according to the manufacturer's instructions.
  b. Proceed with steps f through i as listed for the two-step method.
	10			

13. Clean the work area. Properly dispose of all biohazard materials. Remove gloves, and wash your hands.	10			

Comments:

Total Points Earned _____ Divided by _____ Total Possible Points = _____ % Score

Instructor's Signature _____

Student Name _____ Date _____ Score _____

Procedure 53-5 Perform a Differential Examination of a Smear Stained with Wright's Stain

Task: To perform a differential cell count, evaluate RBC morphology, and estimate the number of platelets.

Equipment and Supplies:
- Microscope
- Immersion oil
- Lens tissue
- Lens cleaner

Standards: Complete the procedure and all critical steps in _____ minutes with a minimum score of _____% within three attempts.

Scoring: Divide points earned by total possible points. Failure to perform a critical step that is indicated with an asterisk (*) will result in an unsatisfactory overall score.

Time began _____ **Time ended** _____

Steps	Possible Points	First Attempt	Second Attempt	Third Attempt
1. Wash and dry your hands.	5			
2. Assemble the materials needed.	5			
3. Clean the microscope with lens tissue and lens cleaner.	5			
4. Place the slide on the stage, with the smear facing up. Position the feathered edge of the smear over the stage aperture.	5			
5. Locate an area of the smear where the RBCs barely touch one another or slightly overlap, using the low-power objective.	5			
6. Rotate the objective to high power and refocus. Apply a drop of immersion oil to the slide, and rotate the oil immersion lens into place. Increase the light as needed using the iris diaphragm.	5			
7. Count 100 consecutive WBCs in as many viewing fields as necessary using a winding pattern, identifying each cell encountered.*	10			
8. Record each white cell on the differential cell counter by depressing the appropriate key for each cell.	15			

Steps	Possible Points	First Attempt	Second Attempt	Third Attempt
9. Evaluate the RBCs observed in 10 fields. Record any variations in the following: • Size—microcytosis, macrocytosis, aniso-cytosis • Shape—poikilocytosis, ovalocytosis, target cells, sickle cells, and so forth • Content—normochromic or hypochromic	20			
10. Count the platelets in 10 fields, calculate an average, and multiply that average by 15,000 to give an estimate of the platelet count. The normal platelet count is 150,000 to 400,000/mm^3. Report the count as normal, decreased, or increased.	10			
11. Clean the microscope with lens tissue and lens cleaner, paying special attention to removing the oil from the 100× objective.*	5			
12. Clean the work area and properly dispose of all materials.	5			
13. Record the testing results in the patient's record.	5			

Documentation in the Medical Record

_____

_____

_____

Comments:

Total Points Earned _____ Divided by _____ Total Possible Points = _____ % Score

Instructor's Signature _____

Procedure 53-6 Perform Hematology Testing: Perform an Erythrocyte Sedimentation Rate Using a Modified Westergren Method

Task: To fill a Westergren tube properly and to observe and record an erythrocyte sedimentation rate (ESR) obtained by using the Westergren method.

Equipment and Supplies:
- EDTA-anticoagulated blood specimen
- Safety tube decapper
- Sediplast ESR system
- Sediplast rack
- Timer

Standards: Complete the procedure and all critical steps in _____ minutes with a minimum score of _____% within three attempts.

Scoring: Divide points earned by total possible points. Failure to perform a critical step that is indicated with an asterisk (*) will result in an unsatisfactory overall score.

Time began _____ **Time ended** _____

Steps	Possible Points	First Attempt	Second Attempt	Third Attempt
1. Wash and dry your hands. Put on face protection and nonsterile gloves.	10	_____	_____	_____
2. Assemble the materials needed.	10	_____	_____	_____
3. Check the leveling bubble of the Sediplast rack.	10	_____	_____	_____
4. Bring the blood sample to room temperature if it has been refrigerated, and mix the sample well by inverting the tube gently several times.*	10	_____	_____	_____
5. Remove the stopper on the blood sample using a tube decapper and on the prefilled Sediplast vial.	10	_____	_____	_____
6. Fill the vial to the indicated line, replace the stopper on the prefilled vial, and invert several times to mix. Recap the blood collection tube.	10	_____	_____	_____
7. Insert the Sediplast pipette through the pierceable stopper on the vial, and push down until the pipette touches the bottom of the vial. The pipette will automatically draw the blood up to the zero mark.	10	_____	_____	_____

Steps	Possible Points	First Attempt	Second Attempt	Third Attempt
8. Insert the pipette and the vial into the rack, ensuring that it is vertical.	10			
9. Allow the tube to stand undisturbed for 60 minutes.	10			
10. Measure the distance the erythrocytes have fallen. The scale reads in millimeters, and each line is 1 mm.	10			
11. Clean the work area, and properly dispose of all biohazard materials. Remove face protection and gloves, and wash your hands. Dispose of the pipette in a biohazard container.	10			
12. Record the findings in the patient's medical record.	10			

Documentation in the Medical Record

_____

_____

_____

Comments:

Total Points Earned _____ Divided by _____ Total Possible Points = _____ % Score

Instructor's Signature _____

Procedure 53-7 Determine ABO Group Using a Slide Test

Student Name _____ **Date** _____ **Score** _____

Task: To determine a patient's ABO group accurately using the slide test technique.

Equipment and Supplies:
- Glass slides with frosted ends
- Anti-A and anti-B serum
- Applicator sticks
- Lancet and automatic finger puncture device
- Alcohol preps
- Sterile gauze squares
- Laboratory marking pen or pencil

Standards: Complete the procedure and all critical steps in _____ minutes with a minimum score of _____% within three attempts.

Scoring: Divide points earned by total possible points. Failure to perform a critical step that is indicated with an asterisk (*) will result in an unsatisfactory overall score.

Time began _____ **Time ended** _____

Steps	Possible Points	First Attempt	Second Attempt	Third Attempt
1. Assemble all of the supplies and equipment needed to complete the testing procedure.	10			
2. Wash your hands, and put on face protection and gloves.	10			
3. Explain the procedure to the patient.*	10			
4. Label the slides in the frosted area with the patient's name.	10			
5. Place one drop of anti-A serum on slide 1, one drop of anti-B serum on slide 2, and one drop of anti-A and anti-B on slide 3.	10			
6. Select the puncture site, and perform a finger puncture procedure.	10			
7. Wipe away the first drop of blood.*	10			
8. Place one large drop of blood on each of the three prepared slides, close to but not touching the drop of antiserum	10			
9. Cover the puncture site with a sterile gauze square and instruct the patient to apply gentle pressure to the site.	10			

Steps	Possible Points	First Attempt	Second Attempt	Third Attempt
10. Mix the antiserum and blood thoroughly, using a clean applicator stick for each slide. The mixture should be spread over an area measuring approximately 20 × 40 mm	10			
11. Read and interpret the results of the reaction for all slides.	10			
12. Ensure the patient has stopped bleeding, and apply a bandage to the puncture site if necessary.	10			
13. Discard all biohazard testing waste in the appropriate container.	10			
14. Clean the testing area.	10			
15. Record the testing results.	10			

Note: Because of the serious implications of incorrect blood typing, ABO and Rh typing are not routinely performed in a physician's office laboratory. Instead, these tests are performed in a hospital or blood banking facility.

Documentation in the Medical Record

_____

_____

_____

Comments:

Total Points Earned _____ Divided by _____ Total Possible Points = _____ % Score

Instructor's Signature _____

Student Name _____ Date _____ Score _____

Procedure 53-8 Determine Rh Factor Using the Slide Method

Task: To determine accurately the presence or absence of anti-D agglutinations.

Equipment and Supplies:
- Two glass slides with frosted ends
- Anti-D serum
- Applicator sticks
- Lancet and automatic finger puncture device
- Alcohol preps
- Sterile gauze squares
- Laboratory marker or pencil

Standards: Complete the procedure and all critical steps in _____ minutes with a minimum score of _____% within three attempts.

Scoring: Divide points earned by total possible points. Failure to perform a critical step that is indicated with an asterisk (*) will result in an unsatisfactory overall score.

Time began _____ Time ended _____

Steps	Possible Points	First Attempt	Second Attempt	Third Attempt
1. Assemble all the equipment and supplies needed to complete the testing procedure.	10			
2. Wash your hands, and put on face protection and gloves.	10			
3. Label one slide "D" and one slide "C."	10			
4. Place one drop of anti-D serum on the D slide.	10			
5. Place one drop of the appropriate control reagent on the C slide.	10			
6. Perform a capillary puncture to secure a blood specimen.	10			
7. To each slide, add one large drop of the patient's blood, close to but not touching the antiserum.	10			
8. Thoroughly mix the blood with the anti-D serum and the control, using a clean applicator stick for each slide, and spread the reaction mixture over an area measuring approximately 20 × 40 mm on each slide.	10			
9. Place the slide on an Rh viewbox.	10			

Steps	Possible Points	First Attempt	Second Attempt	Third Attempt
10. Read the results immediately.	10			
11. Discard all disposable equipment in the proper biohazardous waste containers.	10			
12. Clean area. Remove gloves and face protection, and wash your hands.	10			
13. Record the testing results.	10			

Documentation in the Medical Record

_____

_____

_____

Comments:

Total Points Earned _____ Divided by _____ Total Possible Points = _____ % Score

Instructor's Signature _____

Procedure 53-9 Perform Chemistry Testing: Perform a Blood Glucose Accu-Chek Test

Task: To accurately perform a blood test for possible diabetes mellitus.

Equipment and Supplies:
- Accu-Chek glucose monitor or similar glucose monitoring device
- Accu-Chek glucose testing strip
- Lancet and autoloading finger-puncturing device
- Alcohol preps
- Gauze squares
- Disposable gloves
- Patient record

Standards: Complete the procedure and all critical steps in _____ minutes with a minimum score of _____% within three attempts.

Scoring: Divide points earned by total possible points. Failure to perform a critical step that is indicated with an asterisk (*) will result in an unsatisfactory overall score.

Time began _____ **Time ended** _____

Steps	Possible Points	First Attempt	Second Attempt	Third Attempt
1. Reread the physician's order, and collect the necessary equipment and supplies needed to complete the testing procedure. Perform quality-control measures according to manufacturer guidelines and office policy.	10			
2. Wash your hands, and put on gloves.	5			
3. Ask the patient to wash his or her hands in warm soapy water, then to rinse them in warm water and dry them completely.	5			
4. Check the patient's index and ring fingers, and select the site for puncture.	5			
5. Turn on the Accu-Chek monitor by pressing the ON button.	5			
6. Make sure the code number on the LED display matches the code number on the container of test strips.*	10			
7. Remove a test strip from the vial, and immediately replace the vial cover.	10			

Steps	Possible Points	First Attempt	Second Attempt	Third Attempt
8. Check the strip for discoloration by comparing the color of the round window on the back of the test strip with the designated "unused" color chart provided on the test strip vial label.	10			
9. Do not touch the yellow test pad or round window on the back of the strip when handling the strip.	10			
10. When the test strip symbol begins flashing in the lower right-hand corner of the display screen, insert the test strip into the designated testing slot until it locks into place. When the test strip is inserted correctly, the arrows on the test strip will be facing up and pointing toward the monitor.	10			
11. Cleanse the selected site on the patient's fingertip with the alcohol wipe, and allow the finger to air dry.*	10			
12. Perform the finger puncture, and wipe away the first drop of blood.	10			
13. Apply a large hanging drop of blood to the center of the yellow testing pad. a. Do not touch the pad with the patient's finger. b. Do not apply a second drop of blood. c. Do not smear the blood with your finger. d. Be certain the yellow test pad is saturated with blood.	10			
14. Give the patient a gauze square to hold securely over the puncture site.	10			
15. The monitor will automatically begin the measurement process as soon as it senses the drop of blood. Read the test result when it is displayed in the display window in milligrams per deciliter. Turn off the monitor by pressing the "O" button.	20			
16. Discard all biohazard waste into the proper waste containers.	10			
17. Clean the glucometer according to manufacturer guidelines, disinfect the work area, remove gloves and dispose of them properly, and wash your hands.	10			
18. Record the testing results in the patient's medical record.	10			

Documentation in the Medical Record

_____

_____

_____

Comments:

Total Points Earned _____ Divided by _____ Total Possible Points = _____ % Score

Instructor's Signature _____

Student Name _____ Date _____ Score _____

Procedure 53-10 Perform Chemistry Testing: Determine Cholesterol Level Using a ProAct Testing Device

Task: To perform and report accurately a ProAct test for cholesterol level.

Equipment and Supplies:
- ProAct testing device
- Lithium heparin capillary tube and capillary pipette
- Lancets and lancet device
- Sterile gauze
- Alcohol preps
- Biohazard waste container
- Biohazard sharps container

Standards: Complete the procedure and all critical steps in _____ minutes with a minimum score of _____% within three attempts.

Scoring: Divide points earned by total possible points. Failure to perform a critical step that is indicated with an asterisk (*) will result in an unsatisfactory overall score.

Time began _____ Time ended _____

Steps	Possible Points	First Attempt	Second Attempt	Third Attempt
1. Reread the physician's order, and assemble all the supplies and equipment needed to complete the test.	10			
2. Wash your hands, and put on gloves.	10			
3. Explain the procedure to the patient.*	10			
4. Load the lancet device with a sterile lancet.	10			
5. Examine the patient's index and ring fingers, and pick a puncture site.	10			
6. Cleanse the chosen puncture site with alcohol, and allow the site to air dry.	10			
7. Puncture the site, and wipe away the first drop of blood with a sterile gauze square.	10			
8. Hold the capillary tube horizontally by the colored end of the tube, and allow the tube to fill. Do not allow air bubbles to enter the tube; if this occurs, discard the capillary tube and continue drawing the sample with a new tube.	10			

Steps	Possible Points	First Attempt	Second Attempt	Third Attempt
9. Give the patient a clean gauze square, and ask the patient to apply pressure to the puncture site.	10			
10. Remove a cholesterol testing strip from the container, and close the container immediately.	10			
11. Remove the foil protecting the test area of the strip, and place the strip on a dry, hard, flat surface.	10			
12. Attach the capillary tube filled with blood to the pipette.	10			
13. Squeeze the plunger of the pipette completely to allow a drop of blood to form at the end of the capillary tube.	10			
14. Allow the drop of blood to fall onto the center of the red mesh application zone. Make sure that the tip of the capillary tube does not touch the test strip and that all blood is dispensed.	10			
15. Allow the sample to soak into the red mesh for 3 to 15 seconds.	10			
16. Insert the cholesterol strip into the test port. The ProAct device will count down approximately 160 seconds.	10			
17. Remove the capillary tube from the pipette, and discard it in a biohazard container.	10			
18. When the measurement time is completed, REMOVE STRIP will appear in the LED display window. Remove the used test strip, and the test result will appear on the display.	10			
19. Examine the test area of the used testing strip for uneven color development before discarding it into the biohazard waste container.	10			
20. Discard all biohazard testing waste in appropriate containers, clean the testing area, remove gloves, and wash your hands.	10			
21. Record the test results in the patient's medical record.	10			

Documentation in the Medical Record

_____

_____

_____

Comments:

Total Points Earned _____ Divided by _____ Total Possible Points = _____ % Score

Instructor's Signature _____

Procedure 54-1 Instruct Patients in the Collection of Fecal Specimens for Ova and Parasites

Task: To instruct a patient in the proper collection of stool for an ova and parasite microscopic examination.

Equipment and Supplies:
- Clean, dry container for stool collection
- Parasitology collection vials
- Plastic zipper-lock bag

Standards: Complete the procedure and all critical steps in _____ minutes with a minimum score of _____% within three attempts.

Scoring: Divide points earned by total possible points. Failure to perform a critical step that is indicated with an asterisk (*) will result in an unsatisfactory overall score.

Time began _____ **Time ended** _____

Steps	Possible Points	First Attempt	Second Attempt	Third Attempt
1. Ensure the patient has not taken any antacids, laxatives, or stool softeners before collection.	10	_____	_____	_____
2. Instruct the patient to urinate before collecting the specimen.*	10	_____	_____	_____
3. Collect the specimen. a. From adults: Instruct the patient to defecate into the container. Stool cannot be retrieved from the toilet bowl. b. From children: Loosely drape the toilet rim with plastic wrap and lower the seat. Instruct the child to defecate into the toilet, onto the wrap. Remove the stool using a disposable plastic spoon. c. From infants: Fasten a "diaper" made of plastic wrap over the child using tape or diaper pins. Remove the plastic wrap immediately after defecation, and remove the stool using a plastic spoon. *Never leave the child unattended with the plastic wrap in place as it could cause suffocation should it be removed.*	10	_____	_____	_____

Steps	Possible Points	First Attempt	Second Attempt	Third Attempt

4. Instruct the patient to add stool to the collection container.
   a. If the stool is formed, use the scoop on the lid of the container to add large jelly-bean sized piece of stool to the liquid in the containers.
   b. If the stool is liquid, pour it into the container until the preservative in the vial reaches the indicated level in the containers.
	10			

5. Instruct the patient to tighten the caps completely and wipe the outside of the vials with rubbing alcohol or wash carefully with soap and water.	10			
6. The vials should be labeled and transported to the laboratory immediately if possible. Do not refrigerate the vials.	10			
7. Instruct the patient to wash his or her hands after the procedure.	10			

Comments:

Total Points Earned _____ Divided by _____ Total Possible Points = _____ % Score

Instructor's Signature _____

Student Name _____ Date _____ Score _____

Procedure 54-2 Inoculate a Blood Agar Plate for Culture of *Streptococcus pyogenes*

Task: To inoculate a blood agar plate for the detection of the etiologic agent of "strep throat."

Equipment and Supplies:
- Blood agar plate
- Bacitracin disk or strep A disk
- Incinerator
- Inoculating loop
- Permanent marker
- Swab from patient's throat (see Procedure 36-8)
- Forceps

Standards: Complete the procedure and all critical steps in _____ minutes with a minimum score of _____% within three attempts.

Scoring: Divide points earned by total possible points. Failure to perform a critical step that is indicated with an asterisk (*) will result in an unsatisfactory overall score.

Time began _____ Time ended _____

Steps	Possible Points	First Attempt	Second Attempt	Third Attempt
1. Wash and dry your hands and put on gloves.	10	_____	_____	_____
2. Remove the swab from the transport device. Grasp the plate by the bottom (media side), and lift the cover, or lift the cover while the plate is on the table.	10	_____	_____	_____
3. Roll the swab down the middle of the top half of the plate, then use the swab to streak back and forth on the same half of the plate. Dispose of the swab properly.	10	_____	_____	_____
4. Sterilize a loop in the Bacti-Cinerator, and allow it to cool.	10	_____	_____	_____
5. Pull the loop over the surface of the agar, pulling some of the inoculum into the uninoculated portion of the plate, and spread it around. Flame the loop again, and pull some of the inoculum from the second area into the third area.	10	_____	_____	_____
6. Use the loop to make three slices approximately 1 cm long in the agar in the swabbed area. Sterilize the loop.*	10	_____	_____	_____

Steps	Possible Points	First Attempt	Second Attempt	Third Attempt
7. Sterilize the forceps, and remove one disk from the vial. Place a bacitracin differentiation disk on the agar in the first quadrant. Sterilize the forceps.	10			
8. With permanent marker, label the agar side of the plate with the patient's name and identification number and the date.	10			
9. Place the plate in the incubator, with the agar side of the plate on the top.	10			
10. Incubate for 24 hours, then examine.	10			
11. Incubate negative cultures for an additional 24 hours.	10			
12. Clean the work area, and properly dispose of all biohazard waste.	10			
13. Remove your gloves, and wash your hands.	10			

Comments:

Total Points Earned _____ Divided by _____ Total Possible Points = _____ % Score

Instructor's Signature _____

Student Name _____ Date _____ Score _____

Procedure 54-3 Perform a Urine Culture

Task: To inoculate three plates with 1 µl of urine in order to quantitate the number of bacteria and aid in the diagnosis of a urinary tract infection.

Equipment and Supplies:
- Urine specimen, collected CCMS in a sterile container
- Bacti-Cinerator
- 1-µL calibrated inoculating loop
- Blood agar plate, MacConkey agar plate, and Columbia nutrient agar plate (or an appropriate selection of all-purpose, differential, and selective media)

Standards: Complete the procedure and all critical steps in _____ minutes with a minimum score of _____% within three attempts.

Scoring: Divide points earned by total possible points. Failure to perform a critical step that is indicated with an asterisk (*) will result in an unsatisfactory overall score.

Time began _____ Time ended _____

Steps	Possible Points	First Attempt	Second Attempt	Third Attempt
1. Wash and dry your hands, and put on gloves.	10			
2. With the screw-cap lid in place, mix the urine specimen thoroughly by swirling.	10			
3. Sterilize the calibrated loop, cool, and dip the tip into the specimen.	10			
4. Spread the urine on the plate by "painting" the specimen down the center of the plate then streaking thoroughly at right angles to the inoculum.	10			
5. Inoculate the second and third plates in the same manner.	10			
6. Label the bottom of the plates with the patient's name and identification number and the date.	10			
7. Record all information in the patient's medical record.	10			
8. Place the plates in the incubator, with the agar sides of the plates facing up.	10			
9. Incubate for 24 hours, then count the colonies on the all-purpose medium.	10			

Steps	Possible Points	First Attempt	Second Attempt	Third Attempt
10. The results will be interpreted by a physician or medical technologist as follows: • >100 colonies = >100,000 colony-forming units (cfu)/mL of urine indicates a urinary tract infection • 10 to 100 colonies = 10,000 to 100,000 cfu/mL of urine indicates suspicion. The urine may have been allowed to stand at room temperature, which facilitated overgrowth of bacteria, or the patient may have a subclinical infection. Recollection of the specimen is recommended. • <10 colonies = 10,000 cfu/mL of urine; indicates normal urethral microbiota	__10__	_____	_____	_____
11. Clean the work area, dispose of all biohazard waste, remove gloves, and wash your hands.	__10__	_____	_____	_____

Documentation in the Medical Record

_____

_____

_____

Comments:

Total Points Earned _____ Divided by _____ Total Possible Points = _____ % Score

Instructor's Signature _____

Procedure 54-4 Perform Microbiology Testing: Perform a Screening Urine Culture Test

Task: To assess the level of bacteriuria using a dip and count method in order to aid in diagnosis of urinary tract infections.

Equipment and Supplies:
- Clean-catch midstream urine specimen
- Uricult test kit
- Incubator
- Biohazard waste container

Standards: Complete the procedure and all critical steps in _____ minutes with a minimum score of _____% within three attempts.

Scoring: Divide points earned by total possible points. Failure to perform a critical step that is indicated with an asterisk (*) will result in an unsatisfactory overall score.

Time began _____ **Time ended** _____

Steps	Possible Points	First Attempt	Second Attempt	Third Attempt
1. Wash your hands, assemble equipment and specimen, and put on gloves. Check the expiration date on the test kit. Label the vial with the patient information.	10	_____	_____	_____
2. Remove the slide from the test kit. Do not touch the slide or lay it down.	10	_____	_____	_____
3. Dip the slide into the urine specimen, tipping the cup carefully if necessary. Alternately, the urine may be poured over the slide, catching it in another container.	10	_____	_____	_____
4. Allow excess urine to drain, then replace the slide in the protective vial. Screw the cap on loosely.	10	_____	_____	_____
5. Incubate the vial upright in a 35° to 37° C (90° to 98.6° F) incubator for 18 to 24 hours.	10	_____	_____	_____
6. After incubation, the test results will be interpreted by removing the slide from its protective vial, assessing bacterial colony density, and comparing the density on the slide with the density chart provided. No actual colony counting is necessary.*	10	_____	_____	_____

Steps	Possible Points	First Attempt	Second Attempt	Third Attempt
7. The results are interpreted as follows. • Normal: Less than 10,000 colony-forming units (cfu)/mL of urine; no UTI is present. • Borderline: 10,000 to 100,000 cfu/mL of urine; a chronic or relapsing infection may be present, and the test should be repeated. • Positive: More than 100,000 cfu/mL of urine; a UTI is likely.	10			
8. Return the vial to the protective case and replace the cap.	10			
9. Dispose of the test in a biohazard waste container.*	10			
10. Remove gloves, and wash your hands.	10			
11. Record the results.	10			

Documentation in the Medical Record

_____

_____

_____

Comments:

Total Points Earned _____ Divided by _____ Total Possible Points = _____ % Score

Instructor's Signature _____

Student Name _____ Date _____ Score _____

Procedure 54-5 Prepare a Direct Smear or Culture Smear for Staining

Task: To prepare a smear for staining from a clinical specimen or from a culture medium.

Equipment and Supplies:
- Clean glass slides
- Permanent marker
- Incinerator
- Normal saline solution
- Specimen collected on a smear
- 24-hour culture on agar

Standards: Complete the procedure and all critical steps in _____ minutes with a minimum score of _____% within three attempts.

Scoring: Divide points earned by total possible points. Failure to perform a critical step that is indicated with an asterisk (*) will result in an unsatisfactory overall score.

Time began _____ **Time ended** _____

Steps	Possible Points	First Attempt	Second Attempt	Third Attempt
Direct Smear				
1. Wash and dry your hands. Put on face protection and gloves.	10	_____	_____	_____
2. Label the slide with a permanent marking pen.	10	_____	_____	_____
3. Prepare a thin smear by rolling the swab on the slide. Make certain that all areas of the swab touch the slide.	10	_____	_____	_____
4. Allow the smear to air dry. Do not wave it or heat dry it.*	10	_____	_____	_____
5. Hold the slide with the smear up. Heat-fix the slide using an incinerator. Check the heating process by touching the slide to the back of the hand The slide should feel warm, not hot. Check it often by touching the back of the slide to the back of the hand. Cool the slide.	10	_____	_____	_____

Steps	Possible Points	First Attempt	Second Attempt	Third Attempt
Culture Smear				
1. Wash and dry your hands. Don face protection and gloves.	10			
2. Identify the colonies to be stained by circling them on the back of the plate and numbering them with a permanent marker. Label the slide accordingly.	10			
3. Apply a small drop of saline solution to the slide, using a loop.	10			
4. Touch, with a sterile loop, only the top of the colony chosen. Transfer the material picked up to the appropriate area of the slide, and spread it in a circular motion to the size of a dime. Repeat for each colony chosen using a separate slide.	10			
5. Allow the smear to air dry.	10			
6. Heat fix the smear as described for a direct smear.	10			
7. Properly dispose of all biohazard materials, and clean the work area.	10			
8. Remove gloves, and wash your hands.	10			

Comments:

Total Points Earned _____ Divided by _____ Total Possible Points = _____ % Score

Instructor's Signature _____

Procedure 54-6 Stain a Smear with Gram Stain

Task: To stain a slide, using the Gram stain, so that the organisms present are colored appropriately.

Equipment and Supplies:
• Gram stain reagents
• Staining rack
• Forceps
• Wash bottle of water
• Prepared smear for staining
• Absorbent paper

Standards: Complete the procedure and all critical steps in _____ minutes with a minimum score of _____% within three attempts.

Scoring: Divide points earned by total possible points. Failure to perform a critical step that is indicated with an asterisk (*) will result in an unsatisfactory overall score.

Time began _____ Time ended _____

Steps	Possible Points	First Attempt	Second Attempt	Third Attempt
1. Wash and dry your hands.	__10__	_____	_____	_____
2. Place the slide face up on a level staining rack.	__10__	_____	_____	_____
3. Flood the slide with crystal violet. Time for 30 seconds.	__10__	_____	_____	_____
4. Flood the stain off with a sharp stream of water from the wash bottle. With forceps, tip the slide to remove the water.*	__10__	_____	_____	_____
5. Flood the slide with Gram iodine (mordant). Time for 30 seconds.	__10__	_____	_____	_____
6. Flood the iodine off with water. Grasp the slide with forceps, and hold it nearly vertical.*	__10__	_____	_____	_____
7. Decolorize by running the decolorizer (alcohol) down the slide until the smear stops, giving off purple stain in all but the thickest portions (about 10 seconds).	__10__	_____	_____	_____
8. Rinse the slide with water, and return it to the staining rack.	__10__	_____	_____	_____
9. Flood the slide with safranin, and time for 30 seconds.	__10__	_____	_____	_____

Steps	Possible Points	First Attempt	Second Attempt	Third Attempt
10. Rinse the slide well with water.*	10			
11. Wipe off the back of the slide with an alcohol tissue.	10			
12. Blot the slide dry between sheets of absorbent paper.	10			
13. Clean the work area. Remove gloves, and wash your hands.	10			
14. Record the procedure in the patient's record.	10			

Documentation in the Medical Record

_____

_____

_____

Comments:

Total Points Earned _____ Divided by _____ Total Possible Points = _____ % Score

Instructor's Signature _____

Procedure 54-7 Screen and Follow up Test Results: Perform a Rapid Strep Test

Task: To perform a rapid strep screening test to assist in the diagnosis of strep throat and to follow up negative results by performing a throat culture collection.

Equipment and Supplies:
- Directigen Strep A test kit
- Timer or wristwatch with sweep second hand
- Throat swab specimen (see Procedure 36-8)

Standards: Complete the procedure and all critical steps in _____ minutes with a minimum score of _____% within three attempts.

Scoring: Divide points earned by total possible points. Failure to perform a critical step that is indicated with an asterisk (*) will result in an unsatisfactory overall score.

Time began _____ Time ended _____

Steps	Possible Points	First Attempt	Second Attempt	Third Attempt
1. Collect all supplies and equipment needed to perform the test. Bring all reagents and reaction disks to room temperature (minimum of 30 minutes).	10	_____	_____	_____
2. Wash and dry your hands. Put on gloves and face protection.	10	_____	_____	_____
3. Position all bottles vertically, and dispense reagents slowly as free-falling drops. Avoid reagent contact with your eyes because the reagent is an irritant.	10	_____	_____	_____
4. Add three drops of reagent 1 to an extraction tube. This solution is pink.	10	_____	_____	_____
5. Add three drops of reagent 2 to the same tube. The solution should turn yellow.	10	_____	_____	_____
6. Place the specimen swab in the tube, twirling the swab in the mix.	10	_____	_____	_____
7. Let stand for exactly 1 minute.	10	_____	_____	_____
8. Add three drops of reagent 3 to the same tube, again twirling the swab in the tube to mix. This solution should be pink.	10	_____	_____	_____

Steps	Possible Points	First Attempt	Second Attempt	Third Attempt
9. Express the liquid from the swab by squeezing the tube with the thumb and forefinger and rotating the swab as it is withdrawn. The liquid must be thoroughly removed from the swab. Best results are achieved when the liquid reaches or exceeds the line on the tube.	10			
10. Discard the swab in a biohazard waste container.	10			
11. Remove the reaction disk from the pouch, and place it on a dry, flat surface.	10			
12. Pour the entire contents of the tube into the reaction disk.	10			
13. Read the test results when the entire end of assay window turns red (5 to 10 minutes).	10			
14. Properly dispose of all contaminated waste.	10			
15. Clean work area, remove gloves, and wash your hands.	10			
16. Record the test results in the patient's medical record.	10			
17. If the test results are negative, a second throat swab should be obtained and a throat culture should be performed. Often two swabs are used simultaneously when the sample is collected from the throat so as to avoid recollecting a specimen.	10			

Documentation in the Medical Record

_____

_____

_____

Comments:

Total Points Earned _____ Divided by _____ Total Possible Points = _____ % Score

Instructor's Signature _____

Procedure 54-8 Obtain a Specimen for Microbiologic Testing: Perform a Cellulose Tape Collection for Pinworms

Task: To obtain a rectal sample using cellulose tape for the purpose of testing for pinworm eggs.

Equipment and Supplies:
- Glass slide
- Clear cellulose tape
- Wooden tongue depressor
- Toluene
- Microscope
- Gauze or cotton balls

Standards: Complete the procedure and all critical steps in _____ minutes with a minimum score of _____% within three attempts.

Scoring: Divide points earned by total possible points. Failure to perform a critical step that is indicated with an asterisk (*) will result in an unsatisfactory overall score.

Time began _____ **Time ended** _____

Steps	Possible Points	First Attempt	Second Attempt	Third Attempt
1. Gather and prepare supplies and equipment needed for obtaining the specimen.	_10_	_____	_____	_____
2. Place a strip of cellulose tape on a glass slide, starting ½ inch from one end and running toward the same end. Continue around this end lengthwise. Tear off the strip so that it is even with the other end*. Note: Do not use Magic transparent tape; use regular clear cellulose tape.	_10_	_____	_____	_____
3. Place a strip of paper measuring ½ × 1 inch between the slide and the tape at the end where the tape is torn flush. This will be the specimen-labeling area. As soon as the child arrives, place the child with the attending parent in the prepared examination room.	_10_	_____	_____	_____
4. Wash hands, put on gloves, and apply face protection.	_10_	_____	_____	_____
5. Remove the clothing and diaper from the child and lay the child in a prone position, over the parent's lap, with the buttocks in a superior plane.	_10_	_____	_____	_____

Steps	Possible Points	First Attempt	Second Attempt	Third Attempt
6. To obtain the perianal sample, first peel back the tape on the slide by gripping the label. With the tape looped (adhesive side outward) over a wooden tongue depressor that is held against the slide and extended about 1 inch beyond it, press the tape firmly against the right and left anal folds.	10			
7. Spread the tape back on the slide, adhesive side down.	10			
8. Smooth the tape using a cotton ball or gauze square.	10			
9. Write the patient's name and date on the slide label.	10			
10. Advise the parent that the child can be dressed, or assist with dressing the child if needed.	10			
Testing the Sample				
11. Lift one side of the tape, and apply one drop of toluene before pressing the tape back down on the glass slide.	10			
12. Place the prepared slide under the microscope's low-power objective for examination by a physician or medical technologist under low illumination.	10			
13. Dispose of all biohazard waste, clean the work area, remove gloves, and wash your hands.	10			

Comments:

Total Points Earned _____ Divided by _____ Total Possible Points = _____ % Score

Instructor's Signature _____

Student Name _____ Date _____ Score _____

Procedure 54-9 Perform Immunology Testing: Perform the Mono-Test for Infectious Mononucleosis

Task: To perform and interpret a slide test for infectious mononucleosis.

Equipment and Supplies:
- Mono-Test kit
- Serum or plasma from a blood specimen

Standards: Complete the procedure and all critical steps in _____ minutes with a minimum score of _____% within three attempts.

Scoring: Divide points earned by total possible points. Failure to perform a critical step that is indicated with an asterisk (*) will result in an unsatisfactory overall score.

Time began _____ **Time ended** _____

Steps	Possible Points	First Attempt	Second Attempt	Third Attempt
1. Remove the test kit from the refrigerator, and allow the reagents to warm to room temperature. Check the expiration date of the kit.	10	_____	_____	_____
2. Wash and dry your hands. Put on gloves.	10	_____	_____	_____
3. Fill a disposable capillary tube to the calibration mark with serum or plasma. Using the rubber bulb included in the kit, deposit the specimen in the first circle of the clean glass slide also provided in the kit.	10	_____	_____	_____
4. Place one drop of negative control in the second circle and one drop of positive control in the third circle.	10	_____	_____	_____
5. Thoroughly mix the Mono-Test reagent by rolling the bottle gently between the palms of the hands. Squeeze the enclosed dropper to mix all the contents of the bottle.	10	_____	_____	_____
6. Hold the dropper in a vertical position, and add one drop of Mono-Test reagent to each area of the slide. Do not touch the dropper to the slide.	10	_____	_____	_____
7. Using separate stirrers, quickly and thoroughly mix each area, spreading each area out to 1 inch in diameter.	10	_____	_____	_____

Steps	Possible Points	First Attempt	Second Attempt	Third Attempt
8. Rock the slide gently for exactly 2 minutes; observe immediately for agglutination. A dark background is best for viewing.	10			
9. Interpret the test results, and record them. Agglutination is positive, and no agglutination is negative.	10			
10. Clean the work area. Remove gloves, and wash your hands.	10			
11. Record the test results in the patient's medical record.	10			

Documentation in the Medical Record

_____

_____

_____

Comments:

Total Points Earned _____ Divided by _____ Total Possible Points = _____ % Score

Instructor's Signature _____

Student Name _____ Date _____ Score _____

Procedure 55-1 Identify Surgical Instruments

Task: To identify, correctly spell the names of, and determine the use(s) of standard office instruments or those selected by your instructor.

Equipment and Supplies:
- Curved hemostat
- Straight hemostat
- Dressing (thumb) forceps
- Paper and pen
- Disposable scalpel and blade
- Dissecting scissors
- Towel clamp
- Vaginal speculum
- Bandage scissors
- Allis tissue forceps

Standards: Complete the procedure and all critical steps in _____ minutes with a minimum score of _____% within three attempts.

Scoring: Divide points earned by total possible points. Failure to perform a critical step that is indicated with an asterisk (*) will result in an unsatisfactory overall score.

Time began _____ **Time ended** _____

Steps	Possible Points	First Attempt	Second Attempt	Third Attempt
1. Look for the following parts that determine usage: box-lock, serrations, finger rings, cutting edge, noncutting edge, thumb type, teeth ratchets, and electric attachments.	10	_____	_____	_____
2. Consider the general classification of the instrument: cutting and dissection, grasping and clamping, retracting, or probing and dilating.	10	_____	_____	_____
3. Carefully examine the teeth and serrations.	10	_____	_____	_____
4. Look at the length of the instrument to determine the area of the body for which it is used.*	10	_____	_____	_____
5. Try to remember whether the instrument was named for a famous physician, university, or clinic.	10	_____	_____	_____
6. If the instrument is a pair of scissors, look at the points and determine whether the tips are sharp-sharp, sharp-blunt, or blunt-blunt.	10	_____	_____	_____

Steps	Possible Points	First Attempt	Second Attempt	Third Attempt
7. Carefully compare the instrument with similar instruments that you know to determine whether it is in the same category or has the same name.	10			
8. Write, with correct spelling, the complete name of each instrument, including its category and use.	30			

Comments:

Total Points Earned _____ Divided by _____ Total Possible Points = _____ % Score

Instructor's Signature _____

Procedure 56-1 Wrap Items for Autoclaving: Wrap Instruments and Supplies for Sterilization in an Autoclave

Task: To place dry, checked, sanitized, and disinfected supplies and instruments inside appropriate wrapping materials for sterilization and storage without contamination.

Equipment and Supplies:
- Dry, checked, sanitized, and disinfected items
- Autoclave paper or cloth wrapping material
- Autoclave tape
- Indicator tape
- A waterproof felt-tipped pen

Standards: Complete the procedure and all critical steps in _____ minutes with a minimum score of _____% within three attempts.

Scoring: Divide points earned by total possible points. Failure to perform a critical step that is indicated with an asterisk (*) will result in an unsatisfactory overall score.

Time began _____ Time ended _____

Steps	Possible Points	First Attempt	Second Attempt	Third Attempt
1. Collect and assemble already sanitized and disinfected items to be wrapped. Gloves may be worn.	5	_____	_____	_____
2. Place the wrapping material on a clean flat surface.	5	_____	_____	_____
3. Place the item (or items) diagonally at the approximate center of the wrapping material. Make sure the size of the square is large enough for the items.	10	_____	_____	_____
4. With the squares that are cloth fabric, use two pieces if the cloth is single layered, or follow the manufacturer's recommendation when using commercial autoclave wrapping paper.	10	_____	_____	_____
5. Open any hinged instruments. If the instrument is sharp, its teeth or tip should be shielded with cotton or gauze.	10	_____	_____	_____
6. If the package is to contain several items, place a commercial sterilization indicator inside the package at the approximate center.	10	_____	_____	_____
7. Bring up the bottom corner of the wrap, and fold back a portion of it.	10	_____	_____	_____

Steps	Possible Points	First Attempt	Second Attempt	Third Attempt
8. Repeat the above step with each corner, making sure to turn back a portion each time.	10	_____	_____	_____
9. Fold the last flap over.	10	_____	_____	_____
10. Secure with autoclave tape.	10	_____	_____	_____
11. Secure with autoclave tape and label package with the date including year, contents, and your initials.	10	_____	_____	_____

Comments:

Total Points Earned _____ Divided by _____ Total Possible Points = _____ % Score

Instructor's Signature _____

Student Name _____ Date _____ Score _____

Procedure 56-2 Perform Sterilization Techniques: Operate the Autoclave

Task: To sterilize properly prepared supplies and instruments using the autoclave.

Equipment and Supplies:
- An autoclave
- Wrapped items ready to be sterilized

Standards: Complete the procedure and all critical steps in _____ minutes with a minimum score of _____% within three attempts.

Scoring: Divide points earned by total possible points. Failure to perform a critical step that is indicated with an asterisk (*) will result in an unsatisfactory overall score.

Time began _____ **Time ended** _____

Steps	Possible Points	First Attempt	Second Attempt	Third Attempt
The specific instructions for operating an autoclave may vary based on the model number and manufacturer. Refer to instructions that accompany the autoclave to be sure that the appropriate steps are followed.				
1. Check the water level in the reservoir, and add distilled water as necessary.	5	_____	_____	_____
2. Turn the control to "fill" to allow water to flow into the chamber. The water will flow until you turn the control to its next position. Do not let the water overflow.	5	_____	_____	_____
3. Load the chamber with wrapped items, then space them for maximum circulation and penetration.	5	_____	_____	_____
4. Close and seal the door.	5	_____	_____	_____
5. Turn the control setting to "on" or "autoclave" to start the cycle.	5	_____	_____	_____
6. Watch the gauges until the temperature gauge reaches at least 121° C (250° F) and the pressure gauge reaches 15 lb of pressure.	10	_____	_____	_____
7. Set the timer for the desired time.	10	_____	_____	_____
8. At the end of the timed cycle, turn the control setting to "vent."	10	_____	_____	_____

Steps	Possible Points	First Attempt	Second Attempt	Third Attempt
9. Wait for the pressure gauge to reach zero.	10			
10. Carefully open the chamber door ¼ inch.	10			
11. Leave the autoclave control at "vent" to continue producing heat.	10			
12. Allow complete drying of all articles.	10			
13. Using heat-resistant gloves or pads, remove the items from the chamber and place the sterilized packages on dry, covered shelves or open autoclave door and allow items to cool.	5			
14. Turn the control knob to "off," and keep the door slightly ajar.	5			

Comments:

Total Points Earned _____ Divided by _____ Total Possible Points = _____ % Score

Instructor's Signature _____

Procedure 56-3 Prepare Patients for and Assist with Procedures, Treatments, and Minor Office Surgeries: Perform Skin Prep for Surgery

Task: To prepare the patient's skin and remove hair from the surgical site to reduce the risk of wound contamination.

Equipment and Supplies:
- A disposal skin prep kit containing the following:
  - Gauze sponges
  - Cotton-tipped applicators
  - Antiseptic soap
  - Disposable gloves
  - Two small bowls
  - Antiseptic
  - Optional: cotton balls, nail pick, scrub brush
- Sterile drape
- Biohazard sharps container and waste receptacle

Standards: Complete the procedure and all critical steps in _____ minutes with a minimum score of _____% within three attempts.

Scoring: Divide points earned by total possible points. Failure to perform a critical step that is indicated with an asterisk (*) will result in an unsatisfactory overall score.

Time began _____ **Time ended** _____

Steps	Possible Points	First Attempt	Second Attempt	Third Attempt
1. Wash your hands, and dry them carefully.	10			
2. Instruct the patient on the skin preparation procedure.*	5			
3. Ask the patient to remove any clothing that might interfere with exposure of the site, and provide a gown if needed.	5			
4. Assist the patient into the proper position for site exposure. Provide a drape if necessary to protect patient privacy.*	10			
5. Expose the site. Use a light if necessary.	10			
6. Apply gloves, and open the skin prep pack.	10			
7. Add the surgical soap and antiseptic solutions to the two bowls.	10			

Steps	Possible Points	First Attempt	Second Attempt	Third Attempt
8. Start at the incision site and begin washing with the antiseptic soap on a gauze sponge in a circular motion, moving from the center to the edges of the area to be scrubbed.	10			
9. After one complete wipe, discard the sponge, and begin again with a new sponge soaked in the antiseptic solution.	10			
10. When you return to the incision site for the next circular sweep, you must use clean material.	10			
11. Repeat the process, using sufficient friction for 5 minutes (or follow office policy for the length of time required for a particular prep).	10			
12. If there is hair growth, the area may need to be shaved. Hold skin taut, and shave in the direction of growth. Use caution to avoid injury to yourself or your patient. Immediately after completion, dispose of the razor in the sharps container.	10			
13. After shaving, scrub the skin a second time.	10			
14. Rinse the area with a sterile solution.	10			
15. Dry the area, using the same circular technique with dry sponges. The area may be dried by blotting with a third sterile towel.	10			
16. Paint on the antiseptic with the cotton-tipped applicators or gauze sponges, using the same circular technique and never returning to an area that has already been painted.	10			
17. Place a sterile drape and/or towel over the area.	10			
18. Answer all patient questions to relieve anxiety about the upcoming surgical procedure.	10			
19. Document completion of the skin prep in the patient's chart.	10			

Documentation in the Medical Record

_____

_____

_____

Comments:

Total Points Earned _____ Divided by _____ Total Possible Points = _____ % Score

Instructor's Signature _____

Procedure 56-4 Perform Hand Washing: Perform a Surgical Hand Scrub

Task: To scrub your hands with surgical soap, using friction, running water, and a sterile brush to sanitize your skin before assisting with any procedure that requires surgical asepsis.

Equipment and Supplies:
- Sink with foot or arm control for running water
- Surgical soap in a dispenser
- Towels
- Nail file or orange stick
- Sterile brush

Standards: Complete the procedure and all critical steps in _____ minutes with a minimum score of _____% within three attempts.

Scoring: Divide points earned by total possible points. Failure to perform a critical step that is indicated with an asterisk (*) will result in an unsatisfactory overall score.

Time began _____ **Time ended** _____

Steps	Possible Points	First Attempt	Second Attempt	Third Attempt
1. Remove all jewelry.	5	_____	_____	_____
2. Roll long sleeves above the elbows.	5	_____	_____	_____
3. Inspect your fingernails for length and your hands for skin breaks.	5	_____	_____	_____
4. Turn on the faucet and regulate the water to a comfortable temperature, being careful to stand away from the sink to prevent contamination of clothing.	5	_____	_____	_____
5. Keep your hands upright and held at or above waist level.*	10	_____	_____	_____
6. Clean your fingernails with a file, discard it (in most situations you will drop the file into the sink and discard it later to prevent contamination by lowering your hands and/or touching a waste receptacle), and rinse your hands under the faucet without touching the faucet or the inside of the sink basin.	10	_____	_____	_____
7. Allow the water to run over your hands from the fingertips to the elbows without moving the arm back and forth under the water.	10	_____	_____	_____

Steps	Possible Points	First Attempt	Second Attempt	Third Attempt
8. Apply surgical soap from the dispenser to the sterile brush (or use a preprepared disposable brush), and start the scrub by scrubbing the palm of the hand in a circular fashion.	10			
9. Continue from the palm to the base of the thumb, then move on to the other fingers, scrubbing from the base, along each side, and across the nail, holding fingertips upward, remembering to rub between the fingers. After fingers are completely scrubbed, clean the posterior surface of the hand in a circular fashion, then proceed to the wrist. The scrub process should take at least 5 minutes for each hand and arm.	10			
10. Do not return to a clean area after you have moved to the next part of the hand.*	10			
11. Wash wrists and forearms in a circular fashion around the arm while holding your hands above waist level.	10			
12. Rinse arms and forearms from the fingertips upward, holding the fingers up, without touching the faucet or the inside of the sink basin.	10			
13. Apply more solution without touching any dirty surface, and repeat the scrub on the other side, remembering to wash and use friction between each finger with a firm, circular motion.	10			
14. Scrub all surfaces with a brush, being careful not to abrade your skin. The second hand and arm should take at least 5 minutes.	10			
15. Rinse thoroughly, keeping your hands up and above waist level. Discard scrub brush without lowering arms below the waist.	10			
16. Turn off the faucet with the foot or forearm lever, if available.	10			
17. Dry your hands with a sterile towel, being careful to keep fingers pointing upward and hands above the waist. Do not rub back and forth, dragging contaminants from the dirtier area of the upper arm down toward the hands. Use the opposite end of the towel for the other hand.	10			

Steps	Possible Points	First Attempt	Second Attempt	Third Attempt
18. Using a patting motion, continue to dry the forearms. Discard the towel and keep your hands up and above waist level.	__10__	_____	_____	_____

Comments:

Total Points Earned _____ Divided by _____ Total Possible Points = _____ % Score

Instructor's Signature _____

Student Name _____ Date _____ Score _____

Procedure 56-5 Prepare Patients for and Assist with Procedures, Treatments, and Minor Office Surgeries: Open a Sterile Pack and Create a Sterile Field

Task: To open a sterile pack that contains a table drape using correct aseptic technique.

Equipment and Supplies:
- A sterile pack (autoclaved linen or disposable) that will serve as a sterile table drape or field
- Mayo stand or countertop
- Disinfectant and gauze sponges

Standards: Complete the procedure and all critical steps in _____ minutes with a minimum score of _____% within three attempts.

Scoring: Divide points earned by total possible points. Failure to perform a critical step that is indicated with an asterisk (*) will result in an unsatisfactory overall score.

Time began _____ **Time ended** _____

Steps	Possible Points	First Attempt	Second Attempt	Third Attempt
1. Check that the Mayo stand or countertop is dust free and clean. If it is not, clean with 70% alcohol or another disinfectant, and dry carefully.	5	_____	_____	_____
2. Wash your hands, and dry them carefully. If you will be assisting with a surgical procedure immediately after opening the sterile pack, perform the surgical hand scrub as explained in Procedure 56-4.	10	_____	_____	_____
3. Place the sterile pack on the Mayo stand or countertop, and read the label.	5	_____	_____	_____
4. Check the expiration date. If using an autoclaved pack, check the indicator tape for color change.*	10	_____	_____	_____
5. Open outside cover. Position the package so that the outer envelope flap is at the top and facing you.	10	_____	_____	_____
6. Open the outermost flap. Next open the first flap away from you. Do not cross over the pack.	10	_____	_____	_____
7. Open the second corner, pulling to side.	10	_____	_____	_____

Steps	Possible Points	First Attempt	Second Attempt	Third Attempt
8. While holding the two corners of the sterile pack, position it in the center of the Mayo tray. Do not drop the wrapper below the surface of the tray until the pack is positioned.	**10**	_____	_____	_____
9. Be careful to lift the flap by touching only the small folded-back tab and without touching or crossing over the inner surface of the pack or its contents.	**10**	_____	_____	_____
10. Open the remaining two corners of the pack. You now have a sterile drape as a sterile field to work from and for the distribution of additional sterile supplies and instruments.	**10**	_____	_____	_____

Comments:

Total Points Earned _____ Divided by _____ Total Possible Points = _____ % Score

Instructor's Signature _____

Student Name _____ Date _____ Score _____

Procedure 56-6 Prepare Patients for and Assist with Procedures, Treatments, and Minor Office Surgeries: Use Transfer Forceps

Task: To move sterile items on a sterile field or transfer sterile items to a gloved team member.

Equipment and Supplies:
- Sterile item to move or transfer
- Sterile wrapped transfer forceps
- Mayo stand setup with a sterile field and sterile instruments

Standards: Complete the procedure and all critical steps in _____ minutes with a minimum score of _____% within three attempts.

Scoring: Divide points earned by total possible points. Failure to perform a critical step that is indicated with an asterisk (*) will result in an unsatisfactory overall score.

Time began _____ **Time ended** _____

Steps	Possible Points	First Attempt	Second Attempt	Third Attempt
1. Wash your hands, and dry them carefully. If you will be assisting with a surgical procedure immediately after this procedure, perform the surgical hand scrub as explained in Procedure 56-4.	10	_____	_____	_____
2. Open a package containing a sterile transfer forceps.	10	_____	_____	_____
3. Using aseptic technique, handle sterile forceps by ring handle only. Always point forceps tips down.	20	_____	_____	_____
4. Grasp an item on the sterile field with sterile forceps, points down, and move it to its proper position for the procedure, making sure not to cross the sterile field with the hand or contaminated end of the forceps.	20	_____	_____	_____
5. Or, transfer an instrument from the autoclave to the sterile field.	20	_____	_____	_____
6. Remove the transfer forceps after one-time use.	20	_____	_____	_____

Comments:

Total Points Earned _____ Divided by _____ Total Possible Points = _____ % Score

Instructor's Signature _____

Student Name _____ Date _____ Score _____

Procedure 56-7 Prepare Patients for and Assist with Procedures, Treatments, and Minor Office Surgeries: Pour Sterile Solution onto a Sterile Field(s)

Task: Pour a sterile solution into a sterile stainless-steel bowl or container that is sitting at the edge of a sterile field.

Equipment and Supplies:
- A bottle of sterile solution
- A sterile bowl or container
- A sterile field
- A sink or waste receptacle

Note: The sterile bowl should be placed near one edge of the field and the perimeter of the 1-inch barrier.

Standards: Complete the procedure and all critical steps in _____ minutes with a minimum score of _____% within three attempts.

Scoring: Divide points earned by total possible points. Failure to perform a critical step that is indicated with an asterisk (*) will result in an unsatisfactory overall score.

Time began _____ **Time ended** _____

Steps	Possible Points	First Attempt	Second Attempt	Third Attempt
1. Wash your hands, and dry them carefully. If you will be assisting with a surgical procedure immediately after this procedure, perform the surgical hand scrub as explained in Procedure 56-4.	_10_	_____	_____	_____
2. Read the label of the ordered solution.*	_10_	_____	_____	_____
3. Place your hand over the label and lift the bottle. *Note:* If the container has a double cap, set the outer cap on the counter inside up, then proceed.	_10_	_____	_____	_____
4. Lift the lid of the bottle straight up, then slightly to one side, and hold the lid in your nondominant hand facing downward.	_10_	_____	_____	_____
5. Pour away from the label.	_10_	_____	_____	_____
6. If the container does not have a double cap, before pouring the solution into the sterile container pour off a small amount of the solution into a waste receptacle.	_10_	_____	_____	_____

Steps	Possible Points	First Attempt	Second Attempt	Third Attempt
7. Pour away from the label, into the bowl, without allowing any part of the bottle to touch the bowl and without crossing over the sterile field.	10			
8. Tilt the bottle up to stop the pouring while it is still over the bowl.	10			
9. Replace the cap (or caps) off to the side, away from the sterile field.	10			

Comments:

Total Points Earned _____ Divided by _____ Total Possible Points = _____ % Score

Instructor's Signature _____

Procedure 56-8 Prepare Patients for and Assist with Procedures, Treatments, and Minor Office Surgeries: Apply Sterile Gloves

Task: To apply your own sterile gloves before performing sterile procedures.

Equipment and Supplies:
• Pair of packaged sterile gloves in your size

Standards: Complete the procedure and all critical steps in _____ minutes with a minimum score of _____% within three attempts.

Scoring: Divide points earned by total possible points. Failure to perform a critical step that is indicated with an asterisk (*) will result in an unsatisfactory overall score.

Time began _____ **Time ended** _____

Steps	Possible Points	First Attempt	Second Attempt	Third Attempt
1. Perform the surgical hand scrub as explained in Procedure 56-4 before applying sterile gloves.	10			
2. Open the glove pack, being careful not to cross over the open area in the middle of the pack. Remember, a 1-inch area around the perimeter of the glove wrapper is considered not sterile.	10			
3. Glove your dominant hand first.*	10			
4. With your nondominant hand, pick up the glove for your dominant hand with your thumb and forefinger, grabbing the top of the folded cuff, which is the inside of the glove, being careful not to cross over the other sterile glove.	10			
5. Lift the glove up and away from the sterile package.	10			
6. Hold your hands up and away from your body, and slide the dominant hand into the glove.	10			
7. Leave the cuff folded.	5			
8. With your gloved dominant hand, pick up the second glove by slipping your gloved fingers under the cuff, extending the thumb up and away from the glove, so that your gloved fingers touch only the outside of the second glove.	10			

Steps	Possible Points	First Attempt	Second Attempt	Third Attempt
9. Slide your nondominant hand into the glove, without touching the exterior of the glove or any part of the gloved hand.	__10__	_____	_____	_____
10. Still holding your hands away from you, unroll the cuff by slipping the fingers into the cuff and gently pulling up and out. Do not touch your bare arm with any part of the sterile glove.	__10__	_____	_____	_____
11. Now, slip your gloved fingers up under the first cuff and unroll it, using the same technique.	__10__	_____	_____	_____

Comments:

Total Points Earned _____ Divided by _____ Total Possible Points = _____ % Score

Instructor's Signature _____

Student Name _____ Date _____ Score _____

Procedure 56-9 Prepare Patients for and Assist with Procedures, Treatments, and Minor Office Surgeries: Don a Sterile Gown

Task: To don a sterile gown before assisting with a surgical procedure.

Equipment and Supplies:
- Sterile gown and gloves (opened on a waist-high counter or Mayo stand, in an opened area to dress)

Note: A mask, goggles, and hair cover are worn.

Standards: Complete the procedure and all critical steps in _____ minutes with a minimum score of _____% within three attempts.

Scoring: Divide points earned by total possible points. Failure to perform a critical step that is indicated with an asterisk (*) will result in an unsatisfactory overall score.

Time began _____ **Time ended** _____

Steps	Possible Points	First Attempt	Second Attempt	Third Attempt
1. Scrub, using aseptic technique (Procedure 56-4). Remember to keep your hands up and above waist level.	10	_____	_____	_____
2. Grasp the sterile gown (which is packaged with the outside of the gown on the surface) by the collar and gently lift it from the sterile gown wrapper.	20	_____	_____	_____
3. Hold the gown away from your body. Allow it to gently unfold, grasping only the inside of the gown.	20	_____	_____	_____
4. Slip your hands into the sleeve openings. Remember to touch only the inside of the gown.	20	_____	_____	_____
5. The hand and forearms are advanced only to the edge of the gown cuff.	10	_____	_____	_____
6. The circulating assistant touches only the inside of the gown, pulling the gown over the scrub assistant's shoulders.	10	_____	_____	_____
7. The waistline and neck ties are tied.	10	_____	_____	_____

Comments:

Total Points Earned _____ Divided by _____ Total Possible Points = _____ % Score

Instructor's Signature _____

Student Name _____ Date _____ Score _____

Procedure 56-10 Prepare Patients for and Assist with Procedures, Treatments, and Minor Office Surgeries: Glove While Wearing a Sterile Gown

Task: To apply sterile gloves while dressed in a sterile gown before assisting with a surgical procedure.

Equipment and Supplies:
• Sterile gloves, opened on a sterile field

Note: A mask, goggles, hair cover, and a sterile gown are worn. The gloves are applied with the hands covered by the sterile gown to avoid contamination.

Standards: Complete the procedure and all critical steps in _____ minutes with a minimum score of _____% within three attempts.

Scoring: Divide points earned by total possible points. Failure to perform a critical step that is indicated with an asterisk (*) will result in an unsatisfactory overall score.

Time began _____ Time ended _____

Steps	Possible Points	First Attempt	Second Attempt	Third Attempt
1. Glove your nondominant hand first.	5	_____	_____	_____
2. Lift the glove with your major hand, and use your thumb and forefinger to grasp the top of the folded cuff. Remember, your hands are covered with the sterile gown sleeves.	10	_____	_____	_____
3. Place the glove in the palm of your non-dominant hand, with glove fingers pointing to elbows.	10	_____	_____	_____
4. Grasp the inside of the cuff with your fingers, and gently stretch the glove cuff.	10	_____	_____	_____
5. Pull the glove over your hand as you push through the gown cuff.	10	_____	_____	_____
6. Gently slide your fingers in the glove.	10	_____	_____	_____
7. With your minor gloved hand, slip your fingers under the cuff of the second glove.	10	_____	_____	_____
8. Pull the glove over your hand as you push through the gown cuff.	10	_____	_____	_____
9. The cuffs may now be adjusted.	10	_____	_____	_____

Steps	Possible Points	First Attempt	Second Attempt	Third Attempt
10. The outside sterile gown ties may now be tied with the circulator's assistance.	10			
11. The circulator grasps the red part of the tag by the corner.	5			

Comments:

Total Points Earned _____ Divided by _____ Total Possible Points = _____ % Score

Instructor's Signature _____

Procedure 56-11 Prepare Patients for and Assist with Procedures, Treatments, and Minor Office Surgeries: Assist with Minor Surgery

Task: To maintain the sterile field and to pass instruments in a prescribed sequence during a surgical procedure that involves the making of a surgical incision and the removal of a growth.

Equipment and Supplies:
- Open patient drape pack on the side counter
- Mayo stand covered with a sterile drape
- Packaged sterile gloves (two pairs)
- Needle and syringe for anesthesia medication
- Vial of local anesthetic medication
- Sterile drape
- Disposable scalpel with No. 15 blade
- Allis tissue forceps
- One skin retractor
- Three hemostats
- Supply of gauze sponges
- Biohazard waste receptacle
- Needle with suture material
- Specimen cup
- Laboratory requisitions
- Patient record

Standards: Complete the procedure and all critical steps in _____ minutes with a minimum score of _____% within three attempts.

Scoring: Divide points earned by total possible points. Failure to perform a critical step that is indicated with an asterisk (*) will result in an unsatisfactory overall score.

Time began _____ **Time ended** _____

Steps	Possible Points	First Attempt	Second Attempt	Third Attempt
1. Prep the patient's skin with surgical soap and antiseptic solution as explained in Procedure 56-3. Instruct the patient of prep procedure.	10			
2. Perform the surgical hand scrub as explained in Procedure 56-4.*	10			
3. Set up the sterile field with instruments and supplies, in the sequence to be used. If it is necessary to touch sterile supplies, apply sterile gloves as explained in Procedure 56-8 or use sterile transfer forceps as shown in Procedure 56-6. After the sterile field is set up, cover it with a sterile drape.	10			

Steps	Possible Points	First Attempt	Second Attempt	Third Attempt
4. Position the Mayo stand near the patient and the operative site, making sure the patient understands not to touch the sterile field.	**10**			
5. Apply sterile gloves, using aseptic technique.	**10**			
6. Grasp the patient drape by holding one edge or corner in each hand.	**10**			
7. Drape the surgical site without touching any part of the patient or the operating area with your gloved hands.	**10**			
8. If the physician requests medication such as a local anesthetic, a second circulating assistant holds the vial of local anesthetic so the physician can read the label. The physician withdraws the desired amount using sterile technique.	**10**			
9. The surgeon injects the local anesthetic and waits a few minutes for it to take effect.	**5**			
10. Position yourself across from the surgeon. Arrange the sterile field. Check placement location on Mayo stand.	**10**			
11. Place two sponges on the patient, next to the wound site.	**10**			
12. Grasp the scalpel blade with a hemostat, and mount the scalpel blade onto the scalpel handle if using nondisposable items. Keep all sharp equipment conspicuously placed on the sterile field.	**10**			
13. Pass the scalpel, blade down and handle first, to the surgeon or the surgeon will reach for it himself or herself. The surgeon will take the scalpel with the thumb and forefinger in the position ready for use.	**10**			
14. Grasp an Allis tissue forceps by the tips, and pass it to the surgeon to grasp a piece of the tissue to be excised.	**10**			
15. Pass the handles into the surgeon's open palm with a firm and purposeful motion. A gentle "snap" is heard as it comes in contact with the surgeon's gloved hand.	**10**			

Steps	Possible Points	First Attempt	Second Attempt	Third Attempt
16. Dispose of soiled sponges, using the biohazard waste receptacle, being careful to keep hands above your waist and not touching any nonsterile items.	10			
17. Hold clean sponges in your hand, to pat or sponge the wound, as needed.	10			
18. Safely position the specimen (if any) where it will not be disturbed on the sterile field.	10			
19. If there is a bleeding vessel, or if a hemostat is requested, pass the hemostat in the manner described in steps 14 and 15.	5			
20. Continue to sponge blood from the wound site.	10			
21. Retract the wound edge, as needed, with a skin retractor.	5			
22. Continue to monitor the sterile field and assist the surgeon as needed.	5			
23. Pass the needle and suture material to close the wound, and apply a sterile dressing as requested.	10			
24. Monitor the patient, and provide assistance as needed.	5			
25. After the physician is finished, clean the area using aseptic technique.	10			
26. Collect the specimen, place it into a labeled specimen cup, and send it to the laboratory with the proper requisitions.	10			
27. Document the procedure, wound condition, and patient education on wound care.	10			

Documentation in the Medical Record

_____

_____

_____

Comments:

Total Points Earned _____ Divided by _____ Total Possible Points = _____ % Score

Instructor's Signature _____

Student Name _____ Date _____ Score _____

Procedure 56-12 Prepare Patients for and Assist with Procedures, Treatments, and Minor Office Surgeries: Assist with Suturing

Task: To assist the surgeon in wound closure, using sterile technique.

Equipment and Supplies:
- Sterile field on Mayo stand
- Surgical scissors
- Suture material
- Sterile gloves
- Needle holder
- Gauze sponges
- Patient record

Standards: Complete the procedure and all critical steps in _____ minutes with a minimum score of _____% within three attempts.

Scoring: Divide points earned by total possible points. Failure to perform a critical step that is indicated with an asterisk (*) will result in an unsatisfactory overall score.

Time began _____ **Time ended** _____

Steps	Possible Points	First Attempt	Second Attempt	Third Attempt
Note: This procedure may be a continuation of Procedure 56-11. If done independently, you must perform the surgical scrub and glove before beginning step 1.				
1. Hold the curved needle point in your minor hand, 4 to 5 inches over the sterile field.	10	_____	_____	_____
2. With the needle holder, clamp the suture needle at the upper third of its total length.	10	_____	_____	_____
3. With your dominant hand, hold the needle holder halfway down its shaft, at the box-lock, with the suture needle point up.	10	_____	_____	_____
4. With your nondominant hand, hold the suture strand, and pass the needle holder into the surgeon's hand.	10	_____	_____	_____
5. Pick up the surgical scissors with your dominant hand and a gauze sponge with your nondominant hand.	20	_____	_____	_____
6. After the surgeon places a closure suture, knots it, and holds the two strands taut, cut both suture strands in one motion. Cut between the knot and the surgeon, at the length requested, approximately ⅛ inch.	20	_____	_____	_____

Steps	Possible Points	First Attempt	Second Attempt	Third Attempt
7. Gently blot the closure once with the gauze sponge in your nondominant hand.	10			
8. If additional strands of suture are needed, repeat the process.	10			

Comments:

Total Points Earned _____ Divided by _____ Total Possible Points = _____ % Score

Instructor's Signature _____

Procedure 56-13 Prepare Patients for and Assist with Procedures, Treatments, and Minor Office Surgeries: Apply or Change a Sterile Dressing

Task: To properly apply a sterile dressing at the completion of a surgical procedure.

Equipment and Supplies:
• Sterile dressing material or Telfa

Standards: Complete the procedure and all critical steps in _____ minutes with a minimum score of _____% within three attempts.

Scoring: Divide points earned by total possible points. Failure to perform a critical step that is indicated with an asterisk (*) will result in an unsatisfactory overall score.

Time began _____ **Time ended** _____

Steps	Possible Points	First Attempt	Second Attempt	Third Attempt
1. After surgery is completed, before the sterile drape is removed, and with sterile gloves in place, the dressing is picked up from the sterile field, placed on the wound, and held.	25	_____	_____	_____
2. The drape is then removed while switching hands to hold the dressing in place.	25	_____	_____	_____
3. The dressing is secured with paper tape and/or an appropriate bandage.	25	_____	_____	_____
4. Document the procedure in the patient's medical record.	25	_____	_____	_____

Documentation in the Medical Record

_____

_____

_____

Comments:

Total Points Earned _____ Divided by _____ Total Possible Points = _____ % Score

Instructor's Signature _____

Student Name _____ Date _____ Score _____

Procedure 56-14 Prepare Patients for and Assist with Procedures, Treatments, and Minor Office Surgeries: Remove Sutures

Task: To remove sutures from a healed incision, using sterile technique and without injuring the closed wound.

Equipment and Supplies:
- Suture removal pack containing the following:
  - Suture removal scissors
  - Gauze sponges
  - Thumb dressing forceps
  - Steri-Strips or Band-Aids
  - Skin antiseptic
- Biohazard waste container
- Sterile gloves
- Patient record

Standards: Complete the procedure and all critical steps in _____ minutes with a minimum score of _____% within three attempts.

Scoring: Divide points earned by total possible points. Failure to perform a critical step that is indicated with an asterisk (*) will result in an unsatisfactory overall score.

Time began _____ **Time ended** _____

Steps	Possible Points	First Attempt	Second Attempt	Third Attempt
1. Assemble necessary supplies.	10	_____	_____	_____
2. Wash and dry your hands. Follow standard precautions.	10	_____	_____	_____
3. Instruct patient of procedure and to lie or sit still during procedure.*	10	_____	_____	_____
4. Position patient comfortably and support the sutured area.	10	_____	_____	_____
5. Place dry towels under the site.	5	_____	_____	_____
6. Open the suture removal pack, and apply sterile gloves.	10	_____	_____	_____
7. Place a gauze sponge next to the wound site.	10	_____	_____	_____
8. Grasp the knot of the suture with the dressing forceps, without pulling.	10	_____	_____	_____
9. Cut the suture at skin level.	10	_____	_____	_____

Steps	Possible Points	First Attempt	Second Attempt	Third Attempt
10. Lift, do not pull, the suture toward the incision and out with the dressing forceps.	__10__	_____	_____	_____
11. Place the suture on the gauze sponge, and check that the entire suture strand has been removed.	__10__	_____	_____	_____
12. If any bleeding occurs, blot the area with a sterile gauze sponge before continuing.	__10__	_____	_____	_____
13. Continue in the same manner until all sutures have been removed.	__10__	_____	_____	_____
14. Remove the gauze sponge with the sutures on it, and dispose of contaminated materials in the biohazard waste container.	__10__	_____	_____	_____
15. The surgeon may apply Steri-Strips or a Band-Aid for added support, strength, and protection.	__10__	_____	_____	_____
16. The patient is instructed to keep the wound edges clean and dry and not place excessive strain on the area.	__10__	_____	_____	_____
17. Document the procedure, wound condition, and patient education on wound care.	__10__	_____	_____	_____

Documentation in the Medical Record

_____

_____

_____

Comments:

Total Points Earned _____ Divided by _____ Total Possible Points = _____ % Score

Instructor's Signature _____

Procedure 56-15 Prepare Patients for and Assist with Procedures, Treatments, and Minor Office Surgeries: Apply an Elastic Support Bandage Using a Spiral Turn

Equipment and Supplies:
• One 3- or 4-inch elastic bandage

Standards: Complete the procedure and all critical steps in _____ minutes with a minimum score of _____% within three attempts.

Scoring: Divide points earned by total possible points. Failure to perform a critical step that is indicated with an asterisk (*) will result in an unsatisfactory overall score.

Time began _____ **Time ended** _____

Steps	Possible Points	First Attempt	Second Attempt	Third Attempt
1. Choose the proper size bandage for the size of the arm you are bandaging.	10			
2. Perform a circular turn at the starting point, securing a corner of the bandage as you circle the site.	10			
3. Hold the roll so the bandage can be rolled away from you.	10			
4. Keep the roll close to the patient, and keep it facing upward. With each successive turn, overlap the previous bandage turn by one half.	10			
5. Maintain even tension and spacing as you continue to apply the bandage up the forearm.	10			
6. When crossing a joint, slightly flex the joint.	10			
7. Fasten the end of the bandage with clips or tape.	10			
8. Check the nail beds for cyanosis; ask the patient if the bandage is comfortable or feels too tight.	10			
9. Check the radial pulse.*	10			

Steps	Possible Points	First Attempt	Second Attempt	Third Attempt
10. Have the patient move his or her fingers.	10			
11. Document the procedure in the patient's medical record as well as patient instructions regarding bandage care and replacement.	10			

Documentation in the Medical Record

_____

_____

_____

Comments:

Total Points Earned _____ Divided by _____ Total Possible Points = _____ % Score

Instructor's Signature _____

Procedure 57-1 Organize a Job Search

Task: To devote adequate time to the job search and organize it in an efficient way so that proper follow-up can be conducted.

Equipment and Supplies:
- Record of a job lead form
- Record of an interview form
- Copies of resume
- List of interview questions
- Contact information for former employers and references
- Map of geographic area (e.g., printed from Internet mapping program)
- Internet access
- Computer
- Job search web links
- Local newspapers
- Contact information for friends and family

Standards: Complete the procedure and all critical steps in _____ minutes with a minimum score of _____% within three attempts.

Scoring: Divide points earned by total possible points. Failure to perform a critical step that is indicated with an asterisk (*) will result in an unsatisfactory overall score.

Time began _____ **Time ended** _____

Steps	Possible Points	First Attempt	Second Attempt	Third Attempt
1. Format the resume as an accurate, up-to-date document.	5			
2. Make copies of the record of job lead form and the record of interview form.	5			
3. Research job search websites and newspapers for job leads.	10			
4. Network and contact employers directly to obtain job leads.*	10			
5. Gather information on job leads, and complete a record of job lead form for each one.	10			
6. Prepare a targeted copy of the resume for each job lead.*	10			
7. Take the resume to the facility, and request to complete an application, *or* . . .	5			
8. Email the resume to the facility according to directions listed in the job advertisement.	5			

1103

Steps	Possible Points	First Attempt	Second Attempt	Third Attempt
9. Document all activity pertaining to each job lead.*	10			
10. Schedule interviews for as many facilities as possible.	10			
11. Keep a record of job details on the record of interview form for later reference.	5			
12. Send thank-you notes to all professionals who grant an interview when the appointment is over.*	10			
13. Compare opportunities when making a choice between offered positions.	5			

Comments:

Total Points Earned _____ Divided by _____ Total Possible Points = _____ % Score

Instructor's Signature _____

Procedure 57-2 Prepare a Resume

Task: To write an effective resume for use as a tool in gaining employment

Equipment and Supplies:
Scratch paper
- Pen or pencil
- Former job descriptions, if available
- List of addresses of former employers, schools, and names of supervisors
- Computer or word processor
- Quality stationery and envelopes

Standards: Complete the procedure and all critical steps in _____ minutes with a minimum score of _____% within three attempts.

Scoring: Divide points earned by total possible points. Failure to perform a critical step that is indicated with an asterisk (*) will result in an unsatisfactory overall score.

Time began _____ **Time ended** _____

Steps	Possible Points	First Attempt	Second Attempt	Third Attempt
1. Perform a self-evaluation by making notes about your strengths as a medical assistant. Consider job skills, self-management skills, and transferable skills.	10	_____	_____	_____
2. Explore formatting and decide on a professional resume appearance that best highlights your skills and experience. Use the templates available in word processing software or design your own.	10	_____	_____	_____
3. Place your name, address, and two telephone numbers where you can be contacted at the top of the resume.	10	_____	_____	_____
4. Write a job objective that specifies your employment goals.	10	_____	_____	_____
5. Provide details about your educational experience. List degrees and/or certifications obtained.	10	_____	_____	_____

Steps	Possible Points	First Attempt	Second Attempt	Third Attempt
6. Provide details about your work experience. Include all contact information and names of supervisors. Do not include salary expectations or reasons for leaving former jobs.	10			
7. Prepare a cover letter and a list of references. Send the references with the resume only when requested	10			

Comments:

Total Points Earned _____ Divided by _____ Total Possible Points = _____ % Score

Instructor's Signature _____

Procedure 57-3 Complete a Job Application

Task: To legibly complete an accurate, detailed job application that will help the applicant secure a job offer.

Equipment and Supplies:
- Record of job lead form
- Record of interview form
- Copies of resume
- Contact information for former employers and references
- Contact information for friends and family

Standards: Complete the procedure and all critical steps in _____ minutes with a minimum score of _____% within three attempts.

Scoring: Divide points earned by total possible points. Failure to perform a critical step that is indicated with an asterisk (*) will result in an unsatisfactory overall score.

Time began _____ **Time ended** _____

Steps	Possible Points	First Attempt	Second Attempt	Third Attempt
1. Read the entire job application before completing any portion of the document.*	10			
2. Gather any information that may be necessary to answer all questions on the application.	10			
3. Begin to complete the application legibly.*	10			
4. Answer each question on the document or write "not applicable."	10			
5. Do not leave any space blank.	10			
6. Do not write "see resume" anywhere on the document.	10			
7. Be completely honest about every fact written on the document.*	10			
8. Sign the document and date it.	10			
9. Proofread the document and make certain that no information conflicts with the resume.*	10			
10. Submit the application.	10			

Comments:

Total Points Earned _____ Divided by _____ Total Possible Points = _____ % Score

Instructor's Signature _____

Procedure 57-4 Recognize and Respond to Verbal Communications: Interview for a Job

Task: To project a professional appearance during a job interview and be able to express the reasons that the medical assistant is the best candidate for the position.

Equipment and Supplies:
- Record of job lead form
- Record of interview form
- Job application
- Copies of resume
- Contact information for former employers and references
- Contact information for friends and family
- Sample interview questions

Standards: Complete the procedure and all critical steps in _____ minutes with a minimum score of _____% within three attempts.

Scoring: Divide points earned by total possible points. Failure to perform a critical step that is indicated with an asterisk (*) will result in an unsatisfactory overall score.

Time began _____ **Time ended** _____

Steps	Possible Points	First Attempt	Second Attempt	Third Attempt
1. Prepare for the interview by studying sample interview questions, and know basic information about the facility.*	10	_____	_____	_____
2. Know all of the information that is contained on the resume so that it can be discussed confidently during the interview.*	10	_____	_____	_____
3. Prepare clothing that reflects a professional image for the facility where the medical assistant is hoping to gain employment.*	10	_____	_____	_____
4. Gather all materials that might be needed during the interview, such as copies of resumes, contact information, and copies of earned certificates.	5	_____	_____	_____
5. Arrive for the interview at least 15 minutes early.*	10	_____	_____	_____
6. Stand and shake hands with the interviewer when he or she appears.	5	_____	_____	_____
7. Listen intently to the interviewer as the position is described, and be ready to explain how you fit the requirements for the position.	5	_____	_____	_____

Steps	Possible Points	First Attempt	Second Attempt	Third Attempt
8. Answer all interview questions confidently, smiling when appropriate and displaying a positive attitude.*	10			
9. Ask intelligent questions after the interviewer finishes.*	10			
10. Determine a day and time when the next contact will be made.	5			
11. Express interest in the position.	5			
12. Send a thank-you note or letter to the interviewer within 24 hours of the interview.*	10			
13. Follow up on the interview as appropriate.*	5			

Comments:

Total Points Earned _____ Divided by _____ Total Possible Points = _____ % Score

Instructor's Signature _____

Procedure 57-5 Recognize and Respond to Verbal Communications: Negotiate a Salary

Task: To develop negotiation skills that will help the medical assistant obtain the salary and benefits that will sustain his or her family.

Equipment and Supplies:
- Record of job lead form
- Record of interview form
- Information about job offers received
- Contact name at medical facility

Standards: Complete the procedure and all critical steps in _____ minutes with a minimum score of _____% within three attempts.

Scoring: Divide points earned by total possible points. Failure to perform a critical step that is indicated with an asterisk (*) will result in an unsatisfactory overall score.

Time began _____ **Time ended** _____

Steps	Possible Points	First Attempt	Second Attempt	Third Attempt
1. Study the job offer at hand.	5	_____	_____	_____
2. Determine if the offer is sufficient as it stands.	5	_____	_____	_____
3. Make a list of what additional salary and/or benefits are needed at a minimum.*	10	_____	_____	_____
4. Arrive at the second or subsequent interview appointment to discuss the job with the hiring supervisor.	5	_____	_____	_____
5. Thank the supervisor for the offer that has been presented, and express interest in the position.*	5	_____	_____	_____
6. Express the additional salary and/or benefits desired.	10	_____	_____	_____
7. Discuss the possibilities as to whether the facility would be willing to increase the offer to match your desires.	10	_____	_____	_____
8. Express valid reasons why the additional benefits should be offered, based on past performance, experience, or other valid factors.*	10	_____	_____	_____
9. Discuss reasonable compromises regarding the additional salary and/or benefits.	10	_____	_____	_____

Steps	Possible Points	First Attempt	Second Attempt	Third Attempt
10. Ask what level or performance is expected for salary and/or benefits to be increased.	5	_____	_____	_____
11. Express interest and serious consideration of the position.	10	_____	_____	_____
12. Determine the next contact time with the supervisor.	5	_____	_____	_____
13. Weigh the offer and compromises to make a good decision about the job offer.	10	_____	_____	_____

Comments:

Total Points Earned _____ Divided by _____ Total Possible Points = _____ % Score

Instructor's Signature _____

English-Spanish Terms for the Medical Assistant

abscess   Localized collection of pus that causes tissue destruction and may be either under the skin or deep within the body.
absceso   Cantidad de pus localizada en un lugar que puede estar bajo la piel o a más profundidad en el interior del cuerpo y causa la destrucción de los tejidos.

academic degree   A title conferred by a college, university, or professional school after completion of a program of study.
grado académico   Título concedido por una, universidad o escuela profesional, tras completar un programa de estudios.

accommodation   Adjustment of the eye for seeing various sizes of objects at different distances.
acomodación   Ajuste del ojo para ver distintos tamaños de objetos a distancias diferentes.

account   A statement of transactions during a fiscal period and the resulting balance.
cuenta   Estado de transacciones durante un periodo fiscal y el saldo resultante.

account balance   The amount owed or on hand in an account.
saldo de la cuenta   Suma que se debe o que está en una cuenta.

accounts receivable ledger   A record of the income and payments due from creditors on an account.
libro mayor de cuentas por cobrar   Registro de cargos y pagos asentados en una cuenta.

accreditation   The process by which an organization is recognized for adhering to a group of standards that meet or exceed expectations of the accrediting agency.
acreditación   Proceso por el cual se reconoce a una organización por su cumplimiento de ciertos estándares en un grado que cumple o sobrepasa las expectativas de la agencia que la acredita.

act   The formal product of a legislative body; a decision or determination by a sovereign, a legislative council, or a court of justice.
ley   Producto formal de un cuerpo legislativo; decisión o determinación por un soberano, un consejo legislativo o un tribunal de justicia.

acute   Having a rapid onset and severe symptoms.
agudo   Que tiene un comienzo rápido y síntomas serios.

adage   A saying, often in metaphoric form, that embodies a common observation.
refrán   Dicho, con frecuencia metafórico, que refleja una observación común.

adhesions   Bands of scar tissue that bind together two anatomic surfaces that are normally separate.
adhesiones   Bandas de tejido de una cicatriz que unen dos superficies anatómicas que están normalmente separadas.

adrenocorticotropic hormone (ACTH)   A hormone, released by the anterior pituitary gland, that stimulates the production and secretion of glucocorticoids.
hormona adrenocorticotropina (ACTH)   Hormona, liberada por la glándula pituitaria anterior, que estimula la producción y secreción de glucocorticoides.

advent   A coming into being or use.
advenimiento   Próximo a ser o a usarse.

advocate   One who pleads the cause of another; one who defends or maintains a cause or proposal.
abogado   Persona que defiende la causa de otro; aqel que defiende o apoya una causa o propuesta.

affable   Being pleasant and at ease in talking to others; characterized by ease and friendliness.
afable   Que es agradable y tiene un trato fácil con los demás; caracterizado por su trato fácil y amistoso.

agenda   A list or outline of things to be considered or done.
agenda   Lista o resumen de cosas a considerar o a hacer.

aggression   A forceful action or procedure intended to dominate; hostile, injurious, or destructive behavior, especially when caused by frustration.
agresión   Acción o procedimiento forzado, con la intención de dominar; comportamiento hostil, injurioso o destructivo, en especial cuando es causado por frustración.

albuminuria   Abnormal presence of albumin in the urine.
albuminuria   Presencia anómala de albúmina en la orina.

aliquot   A portion of a well-mixed sample removed for testing.
alícuota   Porción de una muestra bien mezclada, separada para ser analizada.

allegation   A statement of what a party to a legal action undertakes to prove.
alegación   Declaración por una de las partes implicadas en un proceso legal para apoyar lo que dicha parte intenta probar.

allied health fields   Areas of healthcare delivery or related services in which professionals assist physicians with the diagnosis, treatment, and care of patients in many different specialty areas.
campos relacionados con la salud   Áreas del cuidado de la salud y servicios relacionados en los cuales profesionales ayudan a los médicos en el diagnóstico, tratamiento y atención de los pacientes en muchas áreas diferentes.

allocating   Apportioning for a specific purpose or to particular persons or things.
distribuir   Asignar a un fin específico o a personas o cosas en particular.

allopathy   A method of treating a disease by introducing a condition that is intended to cause a pathologic reaction that will be antagonistic to the condition being treated.
alopatía   Método de tratar una enfermedad provocando una afección con el fin de causar una reacción patológica, la cual será opuestaa la enfermedad que se está tratando.

allowed charge   The maximum amount of money that many third-party payors will pay for a specific procedure or service. Often based on the UCR fee.
cargo permitido   Cantidad máxima de dinero que muchos pagadores intermediarios pagan por una práctica o servicio especifico; con frecuencia se basa en el cargo UCR.

alopecia   Partial or complete lack of hair.
alopecia   Pérdida de cabello, parcial o total.

alphabetic filing   Any system that arranges names or topics according to the sequence of the letters in the alphabet.
archivo alfabético   Cualquier sistema que ordena los nombres o temas siguiendo la secuencia de las letras del alfabeto.

alphanumeric   Systems made up of combinations of letters and numbers.
alfanumérico   Sistema constituido por combinaciones de letras y números.

ambiguous   Capable of being understood in two or more possible senses or ways; unclear.
ambiguo   Que puede entenderse de dos o más maneras; que no es claro.

amblyopia   Reduction or dimness of vision with no apparent organic cause; often referred to as *lazy eye syndrome*.
ambliopía   Reducción o disminución de la visión sin causa orgánica aparente; con frecuencia se conoce como síndrome del ojo vago.

ambulatory   Able to walk about and not be bedridden.
ambulatorio   Capaz de caminar y no tiene que estar postrado en la cama.

amenity Something conducive to comfort, convenience, or enjoyment.
amenidad Algo que proporciona confort, comodidad o placer.

amino acids Organic compounds that form the chief constituents of protein and are used by the body to build and repair tissues.
aminoácidos Compuestos orgánicos que son los constituyentes principales de la proteína y son usados por el cuerpo para formar y reparar tejidos.

amorphous Lacking a defined shape.
amorfo Que carece de forma definida.

analyte The substance or chemical being analyzed or detected in a specimen.
analito La sustancia o producto químico que se analiza o que se detecta en una muestra.

anaphylaxis Exaggerated hypersensitivity reaction that in severe cases leads to vascular collapse, bronchospasm, and shock.
anafilaxia Reacción de hipersensibilidad exagerada, la cual, en casos graves, conduce a colapso vascular, broncospasmo y choque.

anastomosis The surgical joining together of two normally distinct organs.
anastomosis Unión quirúrgica de dos órganos normalmente diferentes.

ancillary Subordinate; auxiliary.
auxiliar Subordinado, complementario.

ancillary diagnostic services Services that support patient diagnoses (e.g., laboratory or x-ray).
servicios de diagnóstico auxiliares Servicios que apoyan el diagnóstico del paciente (como laboratorio o rayos x).

"and" In the context of ICD-9-CM, the word "and" should be interpreted as "and/or."
"y" En el contexto de ICD-9-CM, la palabra "y" debe interpretarse como "y/o."

anemia A condition marked by deficiency of red blood cells.
anemia Enfermedad caracterizada por una deficiencia de glóbulos rojos en la sangre.

angiocardiography Radiography of the heart and great vessels using an iodine contrast medium.
angiocardiografía Radiografía del corazón y los vasos sanguíneos mayores usando un medio de contraste yodado.

angiography Radiography of blood vessels using an iodine contrast medium.
angiografía Radiografía de los vasos sanguíneos usando un medio de contraste yodado.

angioplasty Interventional technique using a catheter to open or widen a blood vessel to improve circulation.
angioplastia Técnica quirúrgica que usa un catéter para abrir o hacer más ancho un vaso sanguíneo a fin de mejorar la circulación.

animate Full of life; to give spirit and support to expressions.
animar Dar vida; dar ánimo y apoyo a las manifestaciones.

annotating To furnish with notes, which are usually critical or explanatory.
anotar Añadir notas, por lo general, críticas o explicatorias.

annotation A note added by way of comment or explanation.
anotación Nota añadida a modo de comentario o explicación.

anomalies Faulty development of the fetus resulting in deformities or deviations from normal.
anomalías Desarrollo defectuoso del feto que tiene como resultado deformidades o desviaciones de lo normal.

anorexia Lack or loss of appetite for food.
anorexia Falta o pérdida del apetito.

anoxia Absence of oxygen in the tissues.
anoxia Ausencia de oxígeno en los tejidos.

anteroposterior (AP) Frontal projection in which the patient is supine or facing the x-ray tube.
anteroposterior (AP) Proyección frontal en la cual el paciente está en posición supina o frente al tubo de rayos x.

antibody   Immunoglobulin produced by the immune system in response to bacteria, viruses, or other antigenic substances.
anticuerpo   Inmunoglobulina producida por el sistema inmunológico en respuesta a bacterias, virus u otras substancias antigénicas.

anticoagulant   A chemical added to the blood after collection to prevent clotting.
anticoagulante   Producto químico que se añade a la sangre después de extraerla para que no forme coágulos.

antidiuretic hormone (ADH)   A hormone secreted at the posterior pituitary gland; causes water retention in the kidneys and an elevation of blood pressure; also known as *vasopressin*.
hormona antidiurética (ADH)   Hormona secretada por la glándula pituitaria posterior y que provoca retención de agua en los riñones y aumento de la presión sanguínea. Es conocida también como vasopresina.

antigen   Foreign substance that causes the production of a specific antibody.
antígeno   Substancia extraña que provoca la producción de un anticuerpo específico.

antimicrobial agent   A drug that is used to treat infection.
agente antimicrobiano   Substancia que se usa para tratar infecciones.

antiseptic   Pertaining to substances that inhibit the growth of microorganisms such as alcohol and betadine.
antiséptico   Perteneciente o relativo a las substancias que inhiben el crecimiento de microorganismos como el alcohol y la betadina.

antiseptic   Substance that kills microorganisms.
antiséptico   Substancia que mata microorganismos.

antiseptic   An agent that inhibits bacterial growth and that can be used on human tissue.
antiséptico   Agente que inhibe el crecimiento bacteriano y que puede usarse en los tejidos humanos.

aortagram   Radiography of the aorta using an iodine contrast medium.
aortograma   Radiografía de la aorta usando un medio de contraste yodado.

apnea   Absence or cessation of breathing.
apnea   Ausencia o cese de la respiración.

appeal   A legal proceeding by which a case is brought before a higher court for review of the decision of a lower court.
apelación   Procedimiento legal por el cual un caso se lleva ante un tribunal superior para obtener una revisión de la decisión de un tribunal inferior.

appellate   Having the power to review the judgment of another tribunal or body of jurisdiction, such as an appellate court.
de apelación   Que tiene el poder de revisar el veredicto de otro tribunal o cuerpo jurídico, como una corte de apelación.

applications   Software programs designed to perform specific tasks.
aplicaciones   Programas informáticos diseñados para realizar tareas específicas.

appraisal   To give an expert judgment of the value or merit of; judging as to quality.
evaluación   Acción de emitir un juicio experto sobre el valor o mérito de algo; juzgar la calidad de algo; evaluar el rendimiento en el trabajo.

arbitration   The hearing and determination of a cause in controversy by a person or persons either chosen by the parties involved or appointed under statutory authority.
arbitraje   Vista y resolución de una causa en conflicto por una persona o personas elegida/s por las partes implicadas o designadas por la autoridad establecida por ley.

arbitrator   A neutral person chosen to settle differences between two parties in a controversy.
árbitro   Persona neutral seleccionada para poner fin a las diferencias entre dos partes involucradas en un conflicto.

archaic   Of, relating to, or characteristic of an earlier or more primitive time.
arcaico   Perteneciente o relativo a una época anterior o más primitiva; que tiene las características de dicha época.

archive   To file or collect records or documents in or as if in an archive.
archivar   Guardar o recoger informes o documentos en un archivo o de manera similar.

arrhythmia   Abnormality or irregularity in the heart rhythm.
arritmia   Anomalía o irregularidad en el ritmo cardiaco.

arteriography   Radiography of arteries using an iodine contrast medium.
arteriografía   Radiografía de las arterias usando un medio de contraste yodado.

arthritis   Inflammation of a joint.
artritis   Inflamación de una articulación.

arthrogram   Fluoroscopic examination of the soft-tissue components of joints with direct injection of a contrast medium into the joint capsule.
artrografía   Examen fluoroscópico de los componentes de los tejidos blandos de las articulaciones con una inyección directa de un medio de contraste en la cápsula de la articulación.

articular   Pertaining to a joint.
articulatorio   Perteneciente o relativo a una articulación.

artificial intelligence   The aspect of computer science that deals with computers taking on the attributes of humans. One such example is an expert system, which is capable of making decisions, such as software that is designed to help a physician diagnose a patient, given a set of symptoms. Game-playing programming and programs designed to recognize human language are other examples of artificial intelligence.
inteligencia artificial   Parte de la informática que se ocupa de la incorporación de atributos humanos a las computadoras. Un ejemplo de esto es un sistema práctico capaz de tomar decisiones, como los programas informáticos diseñados para ayudar a los médicos a diagnosticar a un paciente dado un conjunto de síntomas. Los programas de juegos y otros programas diseñados para reconocer el lenguaje humano son otros ejemplos.

ASCII   American Standard Code for Information Interchange, a code representing English characters as numbers where each is given a number from 0 to 127.
ASCII   Estándar Americano de Codificación para el Intercambio de Información; un código que representa carácteres ingleses como números, en el cual a cada uno se le asigna un número de 0 a 127.

asepsis   Being free from infection or infectious materials.
asepsia   Que está libre del infecciones.

assault   An intentional, unlawful attempt to do bodily injury to another by force.
asalto   Intento ilícito de causar daño físico a otro usando la fuerza.

assent   To agree to something, especially after thoughtful consideration.
asentir   Aceptar algo, especialmente cuando se hace tras una detenida reflexión.

asystole   The absence of a heartbeat.
asistolia   Ausencia de latidos del corazón.

ataxia   Failure or irregularity of muscle actions and coordination.
ataxia   Fallo o irregularidad del movimiento y coordinación musculare.

atherosclerosis   A form of arteriosclerosis distinguished by fatty deposits within the inner layers of larger arterial walls.
aterosclerosis   Forma de arteriosclerosis que se distingue por la presencia de depósitos de grasa en las capas internas de las paredes de las arterias mayores.

atria   The two upper chambers of the heart.
aurículas   Las dos cavidades superiores del corazón.

atrioventricular (AV) node   Part of the cardiac conduction system located between the atria and the ventricles.
nódulo aurioventricular (AV)   Parte del sistema cardiaco que se encuentra entre las aurículas y los ventrílculos.

atrophy   Decrease in the size of a normally developed organ.
atrofia   Disminución del tamaño de un órgano desarrollado de forma normal.

atrophy   Wasting away, decreasing size.
atrofia   Desgastado, disminuido en tamaño.

attenuated   Weakened, or change in virulence of, a pathogenic microorganism.
atenuado   Cambio o debilitación en la virulencia de un microorganismo.

audiologist An allied health care professional specializing in evaluation of hearing function, detection of hearing impairment, and determination of the anatomic site of impairment.
audiólogo Profesional del cuidado de la salud que se especializa en evaluar la función auditiva, detectar las dificultades auditivas y determinar el lugar físico en el que se produce el problema auditivo.

audit A formal examination of an organization's or individual's accounts or financial situation; a methodic examination and review.
auditoría Análisis formal de las cuentas o estado financiero de una organización o un individuo; examen y revisión sistemáticos.

augment To make greater, more numerous, larger, or more intense.
aumentar Hacer mayor, más numeroso, más grande o más intenso.

aura Peculiar sensation preceding the appearance of more definite disturbance.
aura Sensación peculiar que precede a la aparición de un trastorno definido.

authorization A term used by managed care for an approved referral.
autorización Término usado en el cuido administrado para referirse a la aprobación de la referencia de un paciente de un médico a otro profesional del cuidod o de la salud.

autoimmune Development of an immune response to one's own tissues; refers to action against one's own cells to cause localized and systemic reactions.
autoinmune Desarrollo de una respuesta inmunológica a los propios tejidos; actuar contra sus propias células para originar reacciones sistémicas localizadas.

autoimmune disorder Disturbance in the immune system in which the body reacts against its own tissue. Examples of autoimmune disorders include multiple sclerosis, rheumatoid arthritis, and systemic lupus erythematosus.
trastorno autoinmune Trastorno del sistema inmunológico en el cual el cuerpo reacciona contra sus propios tejidos. Algunos ejemplos de trastornos autoinmunes incluyen la esclerosis múltiple, la artritis reumatoide y el lupus eritematoso sistémico.

axial projection Radiograph taken with a longitudinal angulation of the x-ray beam; sometimes referred to as a *semi-axial projection*.
proyección axial Radiografía que se toma con un ángulo longitudinal del haz de rayos x; a veces se llama proyección semi-axial.

azotemia Retention in the blood of excessive amounts of nitrogenous wastes.
azotemia Retención en la sangre de cantidades de desperdicios nitrogenados.

backup Any type of storage of files to prevent their loss in the event of hard disk failure.
copia de seguridad Cualquier tipo de almacenamiento de archivos para evitar que se pierdan en caso de que ocurrra un fallo en el disco duro.

bailiff An officer of some U.S. courts, usually serving as a messenger or usher, who keeps order at the request of the judge.
alguacil Funcionario de algunos tribunales estadounidenses que suele servir como mensajero o ujier y que se ocupa de mantener el orden a petición del juez.

bank reconciliation The process of proving that a bank statement and checkbook balance are in agreement.
reconciliación bancaria Proceso por el cual se prueba que un estado bancario y un saldo de una libreta de cheques concuerdan.

banners Also called *banner ads;* advertisements often found on a webpage that can be animated and attract the user's attention in hopes that he or she will click on the ad and be redirected to the advertiser's home page and will purchase from the site or gain information from the site.
viñetas Viñetas o anuncios de viñetas; anuncios, a veces animados, que se hallan, con frecuencia en las páginas web; su fin es atraer la atención del usuario con la esperanza de que éste haga clic en el anuncio, y así sea llevado a la página principal del anunciante para que compre algo en ese sitio o para que obtenga información sobre el mismo.

battery A willful and unlawful use of force or violence on the person of another. An offensive touching or use of force on a person without that person's consent.
golpiza Uso de la fuerza o violencia en contra de la persona de otro, de manera intencional e ilegítima. Tocar de manera ofensiva a una persona o usar la fuerza en contra de ella sin su consentimiento.

beneficence The act of doing or producing good, especially performing acts of charity or kindness.
beneficencia Acción de hacer o producir el bien, en especial llevando a cabo obras caritativas o bondadosas.

beneficiary The person receiving the benefits of an insurance policy. The "insured" person on a Medicare claim.
beneficiario Persona que recibe los beneficios de una póliza de seguro. La persona "asegurada" en una reclamación de Medicare.

benefits Services or payments provided under a health plan, employee plan, or some other agreement, including programs such as health insurance, pensions, retirement planning, and many other options that may be offered to employees of a company or organization.
beneficios Servicio o pago proporcionado bajo un plan de salud, un plan de empleados o algún otro acuerdo, incluyendo programas como seguros de salud, pensiones, planes de retiro y muchas otras opciones que pueden ser ofrecidas a los empleados de una compañía u organización.

benefits The amount payable by the insurance company for a monetary loss to an individual insured by that company, under each coverage.
beneficios Suma que ha de pagar la compañía aseguradora por una pérdida monetaria a un individuo asegurado por dicha compañía, bajo cada cobertura.

benign Not cancerous and not recurring.
benigno No canceroso y no recurrente.

bevel Angled tip of a needle.
bisel Punta de aguja en ángulo.

bifurcate Divide from one into two branches.
bifurcar Dividir una unidad en dos ramas.

bifurcation The point of forking or separating into two branches.
bifurcación Lugar en el que se separan dos ramas.

bilirubin Orange-colored pigment in bile, which, when it accumulates, leads to jaundice.
bilirrubina Pigmento de color naranja que se encuentra en la bilis; cuando se acumula produce ictericia.

bilirubinuria Presence of bilirubin in the urine.
bilirrubinuria Presencia de bilirrubina en la orina.

biophysical Pertaining to the science dealing with the application of physical methods and theories to biologic problems.
biofísico Perteneciente o relativo a la ciencia que trata de la aplicación de métodos y teorías físicas a los problemas biológicos.

birthday rule When an individual is covered under two insurance policies, the insurance plan of the policyholder whose birthday comes first in the calendar year (month and day—not year) becomes primary.
regla del cumpleaños Cuando un individuo está cubierto bajo dos pólizas de seguro, el plan de seguro del titular de la póliza cuya fecha de cumpleaños esté antes en el año civil (mes y día, no año) se convierte en el plan primario.

blatant Completely obvious, conspicuous, or obtrusive, especially in a crass or offensive manner; brazen.
flagrante Completamente obvio, notorio o inoportuno, en especial de una manera torpe u ofensiva; desvergonzado.

bond A durable, formal paper used for documents.
obligación Papel duradero y formal usado para documentos.

bounding pulse Pulse that feels full because of increased power of cardiac contractions or increased blood volume.
pulso saltón Pulso que se siente lleno debido a un aumento de potencia en las contracciones cardiacas o debido a un aumento del volumen de la sangre.

bradycardia A slow heartbeat; a pulse below 60 beats per minute.
bradicardia Latido lento; pulso por debajo de 60 pulsaciones por minuto.

bradypnea Respirations that are regular in rhythm but slower than normal in rate.
bradipnea Respiración que tiene un ritmo regular pero es más lenta de lo normal.

broad-spectrum antimicrobial agent A drug used to treat a broad range of infections.
agente antimicrobiano de amplio espectro Sustancia que se usa para tratar una amplia gama de infecciones.

bronchiectásis   Dilation of the bronchi and bronchioles associated with secondary infection or ciliary disfunction.
broncoectasia   Dilatación de los bronquios y bronquiolos asociada con una infección secundaria o disfunción ciliar.

bronchoconstriction   Narrowing of the bronchiole tubes.
broncoconstricción   Estrechamiento de los bronquiolos.

bruit   Abnormal sound or murmur heard on auscultation of an organ, vessel, or gland.
ruido   Sonido o murmullo anómalo que se oye al auscultar un órgano, vaso sanguíneo o glándula.

bucky   Moving grid device that prevents scatter radiation from fogging the film.
bucky   Dispositivo de rejilla móvil que evita que la difusión de la radiación empañe la película.

bundle of His   Fibers that conduct electrical impulses from AV node to ventricular myocardium.
haz de His   Fibras que conducen impulsos eléctricos del nódulo aurioventricular al miocardio ventricular.

burnout   Exhaustion of physical or emotional strength or motivation, usually as a result of prolonged stress or frustration.
agotamiento   Llegar al fin de la fortaleza o motivación física o emocional, por lo general como resultado un prolongado estado de estrés o frustración.

bursa   A fluid-filled saclike membrane that provides for cushioning and frictionless motion between two tissues.
bursa   Membrana con forma de saco llena de fluido que proporciona amortiguación y movimiento sin fricción entre dos tejidos.

byte   A unit of data that contains eight binary digits.
byte   Unidad de información que contiene ocho dígitos binarios.

C&S (culture and sensitivity)   A procedure performed in the microbiology laboratory in which a specimen is cultured on artifical media to detect bacterial or fungal growth, followed by appropriate screening for antibiotic sensitivity.
C&S (cultivo y sensibilidad)   Procedimiento llevado a cabo en el laboratorio de microbiología en el cual se cultiva un espécimen en un medio artificial para detectar el crecimiento de bacterias u hongos y después investigar su sensibilidad los antibióticos.

cache   A special high-speed storage area that can be either part of the computer's main memory or a separate storage device. One function of the cache is to store websites visited in the computer memory for faster recall the next time the website is requested.
caché   Almacenamiento especial de alta velocidad que puede formar parte de la memoria principal de la computadora o puede ser un dispositivo de almacenamiento separado. Una función del caché es almacenar las páginas Web visitadas en la memoria de la computadora para llegar a ellas con mayor rapidez la próxima vez que desee ver la página.

candidiasis   Infection caused by a yeastlike fungus that typically affects the vaginal mucosa and skin.
candidiasis   Infección causada por una levadura (una especie de hongo) que típicamente afecta la mucosa y la piel vaginal.

cannula   Rigid tube that surrounds a blunt trocar or a sharp, pointed trocar inserted into the body; when it is withdrawn, fluid may escape from the body through the cannula, depending on where it is inserted.
cánula   Tubo rígido que envuelve un trocar romo o un trocar de punta afilada que se inserta en el cuerpo; cuando se saca, puede salir fluido corporal a través de la cánula, según en donde haya sido insertada.

caption   A heading, title, or subtitle under which records are filed.
leyenda   Encabezamiento, título o subtítulo bajo el cual se archivan los informes.

carbohydrates Chemical substances, including sugars, glycogen, starches, dextrins, and celluloses, that contain only carbon, oxygen, and hydrogen.
carbohidratos Sustancias químicas, en las que se incluyen azúcares, glucógenos, almidones, dextrinas y celulosas, y están formadas sólo por carbono, oxígeno e hidrógeno.

carcinogenic A substance that is known to cause cancer.
cancerígeno Sustancia que se sabe que produce cáncer.

carcinogens Substances or agents that cause the development or increase the incidence of cancer.
carcinógeno Sustancia o agente que origina el desarrollo de cáncer o aumenta su incidencia.

cardiac arrest Condition in which cardiac contractions completely stop.
paro cardiaco Detención completa de las contracciones cardiacas.

cardiac arrhythmia Irregular heartbeat resulting from a malfunction of the electrical system of the heart.
arritmias cardiacas Pulso irregular que es resultado de un mal funcionamiento del sistema eléctrico del corazón.

cardioversion Use of an electroshock to convert an abnormal cardiac rhythm to a normal one.
cardioversión Utilización de un electrochoque para normalizar un ritmo cardiaco anómalo.

cartilage Rubbery, smooth, somewhat elastic connective tissue covering the ends of bones.
cartílago Tejido de unión similar a la goma, suave y un tanto elástico, que cubre los extremos de los huesos.

case management Process of assessing and planning patient care, including referral and follow-up to ensure continuity of care and quality management.
administración de casos Proceso de evaluación y planificación de la atención al paciente, incluyendo envío de pacientes a especialistas y seguimiento del caso para asegurar la continuidad del tratamiento y la calidad de la administración.

cash on delivery (COD) Method of payment used when an article or item is delivered; payment is expected before the item is released.
contra reembolso (COD) Método de pago usado cuando se entrega un artículo u objeto y el destinatario ha de pagar antes de recibirlo.

casts Fibrous or protein material molded to the shape of the part in which it has accumulated and thrown off into the urine in kidney disease.
cálculos Materiales fibrosos o proteínicos que han tomado la forma de la parte del cuerpo en la que han sido acumulados y que se expulsan a través de la orina en los casos de enfermedades renales.

categorically Placed in a specific division of a system of classification.
categorizado Colocado en un lugar específico dentro de una división de un sistema de clasificación.

caustic A sarcastic remark or phrase.
cáustico Comentario o frase dicha con sarcasmo.

caustic A substance that burns or destroys tissue by chemical action.
cáustico Substancia que quema o destruye tejidos por acción química.

CD burner A CD writer that is capable of writing data onto a blank CD or copying data from a CD to a blank CD.
grabador de CD Dispositivo que puede escribir datos en un CD en blanco o copiar datos de un CD a otro CD en blanco.

centrifuge An apparatus consisting essentially of a compartment spun about a central axis to separate contained materials of different specific gravities or to separate colloidal particles suspended in a liquid.
centrifugadora Aparato que consiste básicamente de un compartimiento que gira alrededor de un eje central para separar materiales con diferentes pesos específicos, o para separar partículas coloidales suspendidas en un líquido.

cerebrospinal fluid Fluid within the subarachnoid space, the central canal of the spinal cord, and the four ventricles of the brain.
fluido cerebroespinal Fluido del interior del espacio subaracnoideo, el canal central de la médula espinal y los cuatro ventrículos del cerebro.

certification   Attested as being true, as represented, or as meeting a standard; to have been tested, usually by a third party, and awarded a certificate based on proven knowledge.

certificación   Atestiguar que algo es verdadero en cuanto a lo que representa, o al cumplimiento de un estándar; que ha sido examinado, por lo general por una tercera parte, y que se le ha concedido un certificado basándose en el conocimiento del que ha dado prueba.

cerumen   A waxy secretion in the ear canal, commonly called *ear wax*.

cerumen   Secreción cerosa del canal del oído, comúnmente se conoce como cera de los oídos.

cervical   Neck region containing seven cervical vertebrae.

cervical   Región del cuello en la que hay siete vértebras cervicales.

chain of command   A series of executive positions in order of authority.

cadena de mando   Serie de puestos ejecutivos en orden de autoridad.

channels   A means of communication or expression; a way, course, or direction of thought.

canales   Medios de comunicación o de expresión; vía, curso o dirección del pensamiento.

characteristic   A distinguishing trait, quality, or property.

característica   Rasgo, cualidad o propiedad distintiva.

chief complaint   Reason for seeking medical care.

problema principal   Razón por la cual un paciente solicita atención médica.

chiropractic   A medical discipline in which a chiropractic physician focuses on the nervous system and manually and painlessly adjusts the vertebral column in order to affect the nervous system, resulting in healthier patients.

quiropráctica   Disciplina médica en la que los médicos quiroprácticos se centran en el sistema nervioso y ajustan la columna vertebral manualmente y sin dolor, para lograr un efecto sobre el sistema nervioso, dando como resultado pacientes más sanos.

cholesterol   Substance produced by the liver, found in plant and animal fats, that can produce fatty deposits or atherosclerotic plaques in the blood vessels.

colesterol   ustancia que produce el hígado y que se halla en las grasas animales y vegetales, y que puede producir depósitos grasos o placas ateroscleróticas en los vasos sanguíneos.

chronic   Persisting for a prolonged period of time.

crónico   Que persiste por largo tiempo.

chronic bronchitis   Recurrent inflammation of the membranes lining the bronchial tubes.

bronquitis crónica   Inflamación recurrente de las membranas que recubren los tubos bronquiales.

chronologic order   Of, relating to, or arranged in or according to the order of time.

orden cronológico   Perteneciente o relativo al orden en el tiempo; organizado según el orden en el tiempo.

circumvent   To manage to avoid something, especially by ingenuity or stratagem.

circunvenir   Lograr evitar algo usando ingeniosidad o estratagemas.

cite   To quote by way of example, authority, or proof, or to mention formally in commendation or praise.

cita   Que se nombra para servir de ejemplo, autoridad o prueba o para hacer una mención formal como recomendación o alabanza.

claims clearinghouse   A centralized facility (sometimes called a *third-party administrator* or TPA) to which insurance claims are transmitted and that checks and redistributes claims electronically to various insurance carriers.

centro de reclamaciones   Establecimiento centralizado (algunas veces conocido como administrador mediador o TPA) al cual se transmiten las reclamaciones de seguros y que se encarga de verificar y redistribuir las reclamaciones electrónicamente a varias compañías de seguros.

clarity   The quality or state of being clear.

claridad   Calidad o estado de claro.

clause   A group of words containing a subject and predicate and functioning as part of a complex or compound sentence.
cláusulas   Conjunto de palabras que incluye un sujeto y un predicado y que funciona como miembro de una oración compuesta.

clean claim   An insurance claim form that has been completed correctly (with no errors or omissions) and can be processed and paid promptly.
reclamación limpia   Formulario de reclamación de seguro que ha sido llenado correctamente (sin errores ni omisiones) y que puede procesarse y pagarse prontamente.

clearing houses   Networks of banks that exchange checks with one another.
sistema de compensación   Redes bancarias que intercambian cheques entres sí.

clinical trials   A research study that tests how well new medical treatments or other interventions work in the subjects, usually human beings.
ensayos clínicos   Estudio de investigación que prueba cómo actúan los nuevos tratamientos médicos u otras intervenciones en los sujetos, normalmente en los seres humanos.

clitoris   Small, elongated erectile body situated above the urinary meatus at the superior point of the labia minora.
clítoris   Órgano eréctil pequeño y alargado situado sobre el meato urinario a la altura de los labios menores.

clubbing   Abnormal enlargement of the distal phalanges (fingers and toes), associated with cyanotic heart disease or advanced chronic pulmonary disease.
hipocratismo digital (dedos en palillo de tambor)   Engrosamiento anómalo de las falanges distales (en los dedos de las manos y de los pies), relacionado con una enfermedad cardiaca cianótica o una enfermedad pulmonar crónica avanzada.

coagulate   Capable of being formed into clots.
coagular   Formar coágulos.

"code also"   When more than one code is necessary to fully identify a given condition, "code also" or "use additional code" is used.
"código adicional"   Cuando se necesita más de un código para identificar por completo una afección (enfermedad) determinada, se usa "código adicional" o "usar código adicional."

Code of Federal Regulations (CFR)   The Code of Federal Regulations (CFR) is a coded delineation of the rules and regulations published in the *Federal Register* by the various departments and agencies of the federal government. The CFR is divided into 50 Titles, which represent broad subject areas, and further into chapters, which provide specific detail.
Código de Regulaciones Federales (CFR)   El Código de Regulaciones Federales (CFR) es un resumen codificado de las normas y regulaciones publicadas en el Registro Federal por los diferentes departamentos y agencias del gobierno federal. El CFR se divide en 50 Títulos que representan amplias áreas temáticas, los cuales, a su vez, se subdividen en capítulos que proporcionan detalles específicos.

cognitive   Pertaining to the operation of the mind process by which we become aware of perceiving, thinking, and remembering.
cognitivo   Perteneciente o relativo a la operación del proceso mental por el cual nos damos cuenta de cómo, percibimos, pensamos y recordamos.

cohesive   Sticking together tightly; exhibiting or producing cohesion.
cohesivo   El estado de estar estrechamente unidos; mostrar o producir cohesión.

coitus   Sexual union between male and female; also known as *intercourse*.
coito   Unión sexual entre un macho y una hembra.

collagen   Protein that forms the inelastic fibers of tendons, ligaments, and fascia.
colágeno   Proteína que forma las fibras no elásticas de los tendones, los ligamentos y la fascia.

collodion   Preparation of cellulose nitrate that, when applied to the skin, dries to a strong, thin, protective, transparent film.
colodión   Preparación de nitrato de celulosa que, cuando se aplica a la piel, se seca formando una película fina resistente, protectora y transparente.

colloidal   Pertaining to a gluelike substance.
coloidal   Perteneciente o relativo a una substancia parecida a la cola.

colostrum   Thin, yellow, milky fluid secreted by the mammary glands a few days before and after delivery.
calostro   Fluido lácteo poco espeso y amarillo que segregan las glándulas mamarias unos días antes y después del parto.

coma   An unconscious state from which the patient cannot be aroused.
coma   Estado inconsciente del cual el paciente no puede ser despertado.

comfort zone   A mental state in which an individual feels safe and confident.
zona de bienestar   Un lugar en la mente en el que un individuo se siente seguro y confiado.

commensurate   Corresponding in size, amount, extent, or degree; equal in measure.
equiparable   Que es equivalente en tamaño, cantidad o grado; de igual medida.

commercial insurance   Plans (sometimes called *private insurance)* that reimburse the insured (or his or her dependents) for monetary losses resulting from illness or injury according to a specific schedule as outlined in the insurance policy and on a fee-for-service basis. Individuals insured under these plans are normally not limited to any one physician and can usually see the healthcare provider of their choice.
seguro comercial   Planes (a veces llamados seguros privados) que reembolsan al asegurado (o a sus dependendientes) por pérdidas monetarias debidas a enfermedad o lesión siguiendo una escala específica que se explica en la póliza de seguro y cobrando un cargo por cada servicio. Los individuos asegurados bajo estos planes, por lo general, no están limitados a un solo médico y suelen poder acudir al proveedor del cuidado de la salud que elijan.

comorbidities   Preexisting conditions that will, because of their presence with a specific principal diagnosis, cause an increase in length of stay by at least 1 day in approximately 75% of cases.
patologías coexistentes   Enfermedades preexistentes que, debido a su presencia junto al diagnóstico principal, causan un aumento en la duración de la estadía de al menos un día en aproximadamente 75% de los casos.

competence   The quality or state of being competent; having adequate or requisite capabilities.
competencia   Capacidad o aptitud de quien es competente en algo; tener las capacidades necesarias o cumplir con los requisitos necesarios para hacer algo.

competent   Having adequate abilities or qualities; having the capacity to function or perform in a certain way.
competente   Que tiene ciertas capacidades o cualidades; que tiene la capacidad de funcionar o actuar de un modo determinado.

complications   Conditions that arise during the hospital stay that prolong the length of stay by at least 1 day in approximately 75% of the cases.
complicaciones   Condiciones que surgen durante la permanencia en el hospital que prolongan el tiempo de la estadía en al menos un día en aproximadamente 75% de los casos.

compression   The state of being pressed together.
compresión   Condición de estar apretado.

computed tomography (CT)   Computerized x-ray imaging modality providing axial and three-dimensional scans.
tomografía asistida por computadora (TAC)   Modalidad de formación computarizada de imágenes de rayos x que proporciona imágenes de escáner axiales y tridimensionales.

computer   A machine that is designed to accept, store, process, and give out information.
computadora (u ordenador)   Máquina diseñada para aceptar, almacenar, procesar y emitir información.

concise   Expressing much in brief form.
conciso   Que expresa mucho en forma breve.

concurrently   Occurring at the same time.
concurrente   Que ocurre al mismo tiempo.

cones   Structures found in the retina that make the perception of color possible.
conos   Estructuras que se encuentran en la retina y que hacen posible la percepción del color.

congruence   Consistency between the verbal expression of the message and the sender's nonverbal body language.
congruencia   Expresión verbal del mensaje que corresponde al lenguaje corporal no verbal del emisor.

congruent   Being in agreement, harmony, or correspondence; conforming to the circumstances or requirements of a situation.
congruente   Que está en acuerdo, armonía o correspondencia; conforme a las circunstancias o requisitos de una situación.

connotation   An implication; something suggested by a word or thing.
connotación   Implicación; lo que sugiere una palabra o una cosa.

contaminated   Soiled with pathogens or infectious material; nonsterile.
contaminado   Manchado con materiales patógenos o infecciosos; no estéril.

contamination   Becoming unsterile by contact with any nonsterile material.
contaminación   Pasar al estado de no estéril por contacto con cualquier material no estéril.

contamination   To make impure or unclean; to make unfit for use by the introduction of unwholesome or undesirable elements.
contaminación   Volver impuro o sucio; hacer que algo sea inadecuado para el uso por la introducción de elementos insalubres o indeseables.

continuation pages   The second and following pages of a letter.
paginas de continuación   En una carta, la segunda página y las siguientes.

continuing education credits (CEUs)   Credits for courses, classes, or seminars related to an individual's profession, designed to promote education and to keep the professional up to date on current procedures and trends in his or her field; often required for licensing.
créditos de educación continua (CEU)   Créditos por cursos, clases o seminarios relacionados con la profesión de un individuo y que tienen la finalidad de promocionar la educación y mantener al profesional al corriente de los procedimientos y tendencias actuales en su campo; con frecuencia son obligatorios para obtener una licencia.

continuity of care   Care that continues smoothly from one provider to another so that the patient receives the most benefit and no interruption in care.
continuidad de la atención   Atención que continúa sin interrupciones de un proveedor a otro, de manera que el paciente recibe los máximos beneficios sin que haya una interrupción de la atención sanitaria.

contralateral   Pertaining to the opposite side of the body.
colateral   Perteneciente o relativo a la parte opuesta del cuerpo.

contrast media   Substances used to enhance visualization of soft tissues in imaging studies.
medios de contraste   Substancias usadas para mejorar la visualización de los tejidos blandos en estudios de formación de imágenes.

contributory negligence   Statutes in some states that may prevent a party from recovering damages if he or she contributed in any way to the injury or condition.
negligencia concurrente   Estatutos existentes en algunos estados que impiden que una parte sea recompensada por daños si esta parte ha contribuido en algún modo a provocar la lesión o enfermedad.

cookies   Messages sent to the hard drive from the Web server that identify users and allow preparation of custom Web pages for them, possibly displaying their name on return to the site.
cookies   Mensaje que se envía al navegador de la red desde el servidor, el cual identifica a los usuarios y puede preparar páginas web especiales para ellos, posiblemente, mostrando su nombre la próxima vez que visiten el sitio.

coordination of benefits   The mechanism used in group health insurance to designate the order in which multiple carriers are to pay benefits to prevent duplicate payments.
coordinación de beneficios   Mecanismo usado en seguros de enfermedad de grupo para designar el orden en el que varias compañías de seguros tienen que pagar los beneficios para evitar pagos dobles.

copayment   Also called *coinsurance;* a policy provision frequently found in medical insurance whereby the policyholder and the insurance company share the cost of covered losses in a specified ratio (e.g., 80/20—80% by the insurer and 20% by the insured).
co-pago   Un co-pago (o co-seguro) es una provisión frecuente de la póliza en los seguros médicos, por la que el titular de la póliza y la compañía aseguradora comparten el costo de las pérdidas cubiertas en una proporción determinada (ej.: 80/20—80% por parte del asegurador y 20% por parte del asegurado).

COPD (chronic obstructive pulmonary disease) A progressive and irreversible lung condition that results in diminished lung capacity.
COPD (enfermedad pulmonar obstructiva crónica)   Enfermedad pulmonar progresiva e irreversible que conlleva una reducción de la capacidad pulmonar.

copulation   Sexual intercourse.
copulación   Cópula sexual.

coronal plane   Plane that divides the body into anterior and posterior parts.
plano coronal   Plano que divide el cuerpo en una anterior y una posterior.

corticosteroids   Antiinflammatory hormones, natural or synthetic.
corticosteroides   Hormonas antiinflamatorias, naturales o sintéticas.

costal   Pertaining to the ribs.
costal   Perteneciente o relativo a las costillas.

coulombs per kilogram (C/kg)   International unit of radiation exposure.
culombios por kilogramo (C/kg)   Unidad internacional de exposición a la radiación.

counteroffer   A return offer made by one who has rejected an offer or job.
contraoferta   Oferta-respuesta hecha por quien ha rechazado una oferta o trabajo.

creatinine   Nitrogenous waste from muscle metabolism excreted in urine.
creatinina   Residuo nitrogenado del metabolismo muscular que se excreta en la orina.

credentialing   The act of extending professional or medical privileges to an individual; the process of verifying and evaluating that person's credentials.
concesión de credenciales   Acción de conceder privilegios profesionales o médicos a un individuo; proceso de verificar y evaluar los credenciales de esa persona.

credibility   The quality or power of inspiring belief.
credibilidad   Calidad de creíble; facilidad para ser creído.

credit   An entry on an account constituting an addition to a revenue, net worth, or liability account; the balance in a person's favor in an account.
crédito   Dato que se entra en una cuenta y que constituye una adición a los ingresos, ganancia neta o cuenta de pasivo; saldo a favor de una persona en una cuenta.

crenate   Forming notches or leaflike scalloped edges on an object.
crenar   Formar muescas o bordes en forma de concha o de hoja en un objeto.

crepitation   Dry, crackling sound or sensation.
crepitación   Sonido o sensación seca y crujiente.

critical thinking   The constant practice of considering all aspects of a situation when deciding what to believe or what to do.
razonamiento crítico   Práctica constante de considerar todos los aspectos de una situación al decidir qué creer o qué hacer.

cross-training   Training in more than one area so that a multitude of duties may be performed by one person, or so that substitutions of personnel may be made when necessary or in emergencies.
entrenamiento cruzado   Entrenamiento en más de un área, de modo que una persona pueda desempeñar varias labores o que se puedan realizar sustituciones de personal cuando sea necesario o en caso de emergencia.

cryosurgery   Technique of exposing tissue to extreme cold to produce a well-defined area of cell destruction.
criocirugía   Técnica que consiste en exponer los tejidos a un frío extremo para producir una destrucción de células en un área bien definida.

cryptogenic   Hidden origin.
criptogénico   De origen oculto.

cultivate   To foster the growth of; to improve by labor, care, or study.
cultivar   Promover el desarrollo; mejorar algo por medio de trabajo, cuidado o estudio.

curettage   Act of scraping a body cavity with a surgical instrument such as a curette.
curetaje   Acción de raspar una cavidad corporal con un instrumento quirúrgico, como una cureta o cucharilla cortante.

cursor   A symbol appearing on the monitor that shows where the next character to be typed will appear.
cursor   Símbolo que aparece en el monitor y que muestra el lugar donde aparecerá el próximo carácter que se escriba.

curt   Marked by rude or peremptory shortness.
cortante   Caracterizado por una interrupción ruda o perentoria.

cyanosis   Blue color of the mucous membranes and body extremities caused by lack of oxygen.
cianosis   Color azul de las membranas mucosas y las extremidades provocado por una falta de oxígeno.

cyberspace   The nonphysical space of the online world of computer networks.
ciberespacio   Palabra que se usa para describir el espacio no-físico del mundo en linea de las redes informáticas.

cyst   A small capsule-like sac that encloses certain organisms in their dormant or larval stage.
quiste   Pequeño saco en forma de cápsula que encierra ciertos organismos en estado letárgico o larval.

damages   Loss or harm resulting from injury to person, property, or reputation; monetary compensation imposed by law for losses or injuries.
daños   Pérdidas o perjuicios que resultan de injuriar a una persona, atentar contra una propiedad o una reputación; compensación monetaria impuesta por ley en casos de pérdidas o injurias.

database   A collection of related files that serves as a foundation for retrieving information.
base de datos   Conjunto de archivos relacionados que sirven de base para la recuperación de información.

debit   An entry on an account constituting an addition to an expense or asset balance, or a deduction from a revenue, net worth, or liability balance.
débito   Dato que se entra en una cuenta y que constituye una adición a los gastos o a una cuenta de activo o una deducción de un ingreso, ganancia neta o cuenta de pasivo.

debit card   A card similar to a credit card with which money may be withdrawn or the cost of purchases paid directly from the holder's bank account without the payment of interest.
tarjeta de débito   Tarjeta similar a la de crédito pero con la cual se puede retirar dinero o pagar compras directamente de la cuenta bancaria del titular sin tener que pagar intereses.

debridement   Removal of foreign material and dead, damaged tissue from a wound.
desbridamiento   Eliminación de materiales extraños y tejidos muertos y deteriorados de una herida.

decedent   A legal term used to represent a deceased person.
difunto   Término legal usado para referirse a una persona muerta.

decode   To convert, as in a message, into intelligible form; to recognize and interpret.
decodificar   Convertir la información, como en un mensaje, de modo que sea inteligible; reconocer e interpretar.

decubitus ulcer   A sore or ulcer over a bony prominence that is caused by ischemia from prolonged pressure; a bed sore.
úlcera por decúbito   Llaga o úlcera sobre una prominencia ósea debida a una isquemia por presión prolongada; escara.

deductible   A specific amount of money a patient must pay out of pocket, up front, before the insurance carrier begins paying. Often this amount is in the range of $100 to $1000. This deductible amount must be met on a yearly or per incident basis.
deducible   Cantidad de dinero específica que un paciente debe pagar de su bolsillo antes de que la compañía de seguros comience a pagar. Con frecuencia esta suma está entre 100 y 1000 dólares. Esta cantidad deducible ha de satisfacerse—anualmente o por caso.

default   A failure to pay financial debts, especially a student loan.
incumplimiento   Dejar de pagar deudas financieras, especialmente en un préstamo de estudiante.

defense mechanisms   Psychologic methods of dealing with stressful situations that are encountered in day-to-day living.
mecanismos de defensa   Métodos psicológicos de hacer frente a situaciones tensas que surgen en la vida diaria.

deferment   A postponement, especially of payment of a student loan.
aplazamiento   Postergación de un pago, especialmente en un préstamo de estudiante.

defibrillator   Machine used to deliver electroshock to the heart through electrodes placed on the chest wall.
desfibrilador   Máquina usada para dar un electrochoque al corazón por medio de electrodos colocados en la pared torácica.

deficiencies   Conditions caused by a below-normal intake of a particular substance.
deficiencias   Estados causados por un consumo menor del normal de una sustancia específica.

demeanor   Behavior toward others; outward manner.
conducta   Comportamiento hacia los demás; comportamiento que se exterioriza.

demographic   The statistical characteristics of human populations (as in age or income), used especially to identify markets.
dato demográfico   Característica estadística de la población humana (como edad o ingresos), que se usa sobre todo para identificar mercados.

detrimental   Harmful or damaging.
perjudicial   Que es obvio que causa daño o perjuicio.

device driver   A computer program or set of commands that enables a device connected to the computer to function. For instance, a printer may come equipped with software that must be loaded onto the computer first, so that the printer will work.
controlador de dispositivo   Programa que controla un dispositivo conectado a una computadora y que hace que dicho dispositivo pueda funcionar. Por ejemplo, una impresora puede estar equipada con un programa que primero ha de cargarse en la computadora para que ésta funcione.

diabetes mellitus type 2   Condition in which the body is unable to use glucose for energy because of either a lack of insulin production in the pancreas or resistance to insulin on the cellular level.
diabetes mellitus tipo 2   Incapacidad de utilizar la glucosa para producir energía, debido a una falta de producción de insulina en el páncreas o a una resistencia a la insulina en el nivel celular.

diagnosis   Concise technical description of the cause, nature, or manifestations of a condition or problem. *Initial diagnosis:* Physician's temporary impression, sometimes called a *working diagnosis.* *Differentiated diagnosis:* comparison of two or more diseases with similar signs and symptoms. *Final diagnosis:* Conclusion physician reaches after evaluating all findings, including laboratory and other test results.
diagnóstico   Descripción técnica y concisa de la causa, naturaleza o manifestaciones de una enfermedad o problema. *Inicial:* Impresión momentánea del médico, a veces se llama diagnóstico de trabajo. *Diagnóstico diferenciado:* comparación de dos o más enfermedades con signos y síntomas similares. *Final:* Conclusión médica a la que se llega tras evaluar todos los datos, incluyendo los resultados de análisis de laboratorio y otras pruebas.

"diagnosis"   The determination of the nature of a disease, injury, or congenital defect.
"diagnóstico"   Determinación del origen de una enfermedad, lesión o defecto congénito.

diaphoresis   The profuse excretion of sweat.
diaforesis   Excreción profusa de sudor.

diaphysis   Middle portion of a long bone containing the medullary cavity.
diafisis   Parte intermedia de un hueso largo en la que está la cavidad medular.

dictation   The act or manner of uttering words to be transcribed.
dictado   Acción de pronunciar palabras para que sean transcritas.

diction   The choice of words, especially with regard to clearness, correctness, and effectiveness.
dicción   Acción de elegir las palabras, especialmente para lograr claridad, corrección y eficacia en el discurso.

digestion   Process of converting food into chemical substances that can be used by the body.
digestión   Proceso de transformar alimentos en sustancias químicas que pueden ser usadas por el cuerpo.

Digital Subscriber Lines (DSL)   High-speed, sophisticated modulation schemes that operate over existing copper telephone wiring systems; often referred to as "last-mile technologies" because DSL is used for connections from a telephone switching station to a home or office and not between switching stations.

Línea de Abonado Digital (DSL)   Sofisticado sistema de modulación de alta velocidad que opera en sistemas de cableado telefónicos de cobre ya existentes; con frecuencia se habla del DSL como "tecnología de las últimas millas" porque se utiliza para conexiones entre un centro de conmutación telefónica y un hogar u oficina, y no entre centros de conmutación.

Digital Versatile Disk (DVD)   The DVD is an optical disk that holds approximately 28 times more information than a CD and is most commonly used to hold full-length movies. Compared with a CD, which holds approximately 600 megabytes, a DVD has the capacity to hold approximately 4.7 gigabytes.

Disco Digital Versátil (DVD)   El DVD es un disco óptico con capacidad para almacenar unas 28 veces más información que un CD; su uso más común es para guardar películas de larga duración. Mientras que un CD puede almacenar unos 600 megabytes, un DVD tiene una capacidad aproximada de almacenamiento de 4.7 gigabytes.

dilatation   Opening or widening the circumference of a body orifice with a dilating instrument.
dilatación   Proceso de abrir o ensanchar un orificio corporal con un instrumento dilatador.

dilation   The opening of the cervix through the process of labor, measured as 0 to 10 centimeters dilated.
dilatación   Ensanchamiento del cuello del útero durante el proceso del parto, se mide en centímetros, de 0 a 10.

dilation and curettage   The widening of the cervix and scraping of the endometrial wall of the uterus.
dilatación y curetaje   Proceso de hacer más ancho el cuello del útero y raspar su pared endometrial.

diluent   A liquid used to dilute a specimen or reagent.
diluyente   Líquido usado para diluir un espécimen o un reactivo.

dingy claim   A claim that is put on hold because it lacks certain adjunction that allows it to be processed, often because of system changes.
reclamación oscura   Reclamación en espera de ser procesada debido a que se necesita alguna información o elemento adicional, con frecuencia, debido a cambios en el sistema.

diplopia   Double vision.
diplopía   Visión doble.

direct filing system   A filing system in which materials can be located without consulting an intermediary source of reference.
sistema directo de archivo   Sistema de archivo en el cual los materiales pueden ser localizados sin consultar una fuente de referencia intermedia.

dirty claim   Claims that contain errors or omissions that cannot be processed or that must be processed by hand because of OCR scanner rejection.
reclamación sucia   Reclamación con errores u omisiones que no puede procesarse o que debe procesarse manualmente debido a que el escáner OCR la rechaza.

disbursements   Funds paid out.
desembolsos   Dinero o fondos que se pagan.

discretion   The quality of being discrete; having or showing good judgment or conduct, especially in speech.
discreción   Calidad de discreto; tener sensatez o tacto al obrar, especialmente al hablar.

disease   Pathologic process having a descriptive set of signs and symptoms.
enfermedad   Proceso patológico que tiene una serie descriptiva de signos y síntomas.

disinfection   Destruction of pathogens by physical or chemical means.
desinfección   Destrucción de agentes patógenos con medios físicos o químicos.

disk   A magnetic surface that is capable of storing computer programs.
disco   Superficie magnética capaz de almacenar programas de computadora.

disk drives   Devices that load a program or data stored on a disk into the computer.
unidades de discos   Dispositivos que cargan en la computadora un programa o datos almacenados en un disco.

disorder   A disruption of normal system functions.
trastorno   Interrupción de las funciones normales de un sistema.

disparaging   Speaking slightingly about something or someone, with a negative or degrading tone.
menospreciar   Hablar con desdén de algo o alguien, con un tono negativo o degradante.

disposition   The tendency of something or someone to act in a certain manner under given circumstances.
disposición   Tendencia de algo o alguien a actuar de un modo específico en determinadas circunstancias.

disruption   A breaking down, or throwing into disorder.
disrupción   Interrupción o creación de un estado de trastorno.

dissect   To cut or separate tissue with a cutting instrument or scissors.
diseccionar   Cortar o separar tejidos con tijeras u otro instrumento cortante.

dissection   To separate into pieces and expose parts for scientific examination.
disección   Separar en piezas y dejar las partes a la vista para realizar un estudio científico.

disseminate   To disperse throughout.
diseminar   Dispersar, esparcir.

disseminate   To disburse; to spread around.
diseminado   Suelto, esparcido.

diurnal rhythm   Patterns of activity or behavior that follow day-night cycles.
ritmo diurno   Patrones de actividad o comportamiento que siguen a los ciclos nocturnos.

docket   A formal record of judicial proceedings; a list of legal causes to be tried.
orden del día   Registro formal de procesos judiciales; lista de causas legales a juzgar.

domestic mail   Mail that is sent within the boundaries of the United States and its territories.
correo nacional   Correo que se envía dentro de los límites de Estados Unidos y sus territorios.

dosimeter   Badge for monitoring exposure of personnel to radiation.
dosímetro   Placa para controlar la exposición a la radiación del personal.

drawee   Bank or facility on which a check is drawn or written.
librado   Banco o entidad contra la que se gira o emite un cheque.

due process   A fundamental, constitutional guarantee that all legal proceedings will be fair and that one will be given notice of the proceedings and an opportunity to be heard before the government acts to take away life, liberty, or property; a constitutional guarantee that a law will not be unreasonable or arbitrary.
proceso debido   Garantía fundamental constitucional de que todos los procesos legales serán justos, que las partes implicadas serán notificadas de los procedimientos y que se les dará la oportunidad de ser escuchados rantes que el gobierno les quite su vida, libertad o propiedad; garantía constitucional de que la ley no irá en contra de la razón ni será arbitraria.

duty   Obligatory tasks, conduct, service, or functions that arise from one's position, as in life or in a group.
deber   Tareas, conducta, servicio o funciones de carácter obligatorio que conlleva el ocupar un puesto, en la vida o como miembro de un grupo.

dyspnea   Difficult or painful breathing.
disnea   Respiración difícil o dolorosa.

ebanking   Electronic banking via computer modem or over the Internet.
banca electrónica   Operaciones bancarias a través del módem de una computadora o en Internet.

ecchymosis   A hemorrhagic skin discoloration, commonly called *bruising*.
equimosis   Descoloramient o hemorrágico de la piel comúnmente conocido como magulladura.

ecommerce   A term used to describe the sale and purchase of goods and services over the Internet; doing business over the Internet; an abbreviation for *electronic commerce*.
comercio electrónico   Expresión que se usa para describir la compra y venta de bienes y servicios a través de Internet; hacer negocios a través de Internet. Se conoce también con la abreviatura de comercio-e.

edema Abnormal accumulation of fluid in the interstitial spaces of tissue; swelling between layers of tissue.

edema Acumulación anómala de fluido en los espacios intersticiales de los tejidos; inflamación entre capas de tejidos.

effacement The thinning of the cervix during labor, measured in percentages from 0% to 100% effaced.

borramiento Adelgazamiento del cuello del útero durante el parto. Se mide en porcentaje, borrado de 0 a 100 por ciento.

elastic pulse Pulse with regular alterations of weak and strong beats, without changes in cycle.

pulso elástico Pulso con alteraciones regulares de latidos fuertes y débiles sin cambios en el ciclo.

elastin Essential part of elastic connective tissue that, when moist, is flexible and elastic.

elastina Parte esencial del tejido conectivo elástico que cuando está húmedo es flexible y elástico.

electrodesiccation Destructive drying of cells and tissue by means of short, high-frequency electrical sparks.

electrodesecación Secado destructivo de células y tejidos por medio de cortas descargas eléctricas de alta frecuencia.

electrolytes Small molecules that conduct an electrical charge. Electrolytes are necessary for proper functioning of muscle and nerve cells.

electrolitos Pequeñas moléculas que conducen una carga eléctrica. Los electrolitos son necesarios para un funcionamiento correcto de los músculos y las células nerviosas.

electronic claims Claims that are submitted to insurance processing facilities using a computerized medium such as direct data entry, direct wire, dial-in telephone digital fax, or personal computer download and upload.

reclamación electrónica Reclamaciones enviadas al lugar de procesamiento de la compañía aseguradora usando un sistema computarizado, tales como entrada de datos directa, cable directo, fax digital con marcado telefónico, o a través de una computadora personal.

email Communications transmitted via computer using a modem.

correo electrónico Comunicaciones transmitidas a través de una computadora usando un módem.

emancipated minor A person under legal age who is self-supporting and living apart from parents or guardian.

menor emancipado Persona que no ha alcanzado la mayoría de edad legal y que se mantiene a sí misma y vive sin la custodia de padres o tutores.

embezzlement Stealing from an employer; appropriation without permission of goods, services, or funds for personal use.

desfalco Robo a un empleador; apropiación sin permiso de bienes, servicios o fondos para uso personal.

embolization Interventional technique using a catheter to block off a blood vessel to prevent hemorrhage.

embolización Técnica de intervención usando un catéter para bloquear un vaso sanguíneo y evitar una hemorragia.

embolus Foreign material blocking a blood vessel, frequently a blood clot that has broken away from some other part of the body.

émbolo Material extraño que bloquea un vaso sanguíneo, con frecuencia un coágulo de sangre procedente de otra parte del cuerpo.

emetic A substance that causes vomiting.

emético Sustancia que causa vómito.

emisor Person who writes a check.

emisor Persona que emite un cheque.

empathy Sensitivity to the individual needs and reactions of patients.

empatía Sensibilidad ante las necesidades y reacciones individuales de los pacientes.

emphysema Pathologic accumulation of air in the tissues or organs; in the lungs, the bronchioles become plugged with mucus and lose elasticity.

enfisema Acumulación patológica de aire en los tejidos u órganos; en los pulmones, los bronquiolos se obstruyen con mucosidade y pierden elasticidad.

emulsification Dispersement of ingested fats into small globules by bile.

emulsionamiento Dispersión (llevada a cabo por la bilis) en pequeños glóbulos de las grasas ingeridas.

encode   To convert from one system of communication to another; to convert a message into code.
codificar   Convertir de un sistema de comunicación a otro; convertir un mensaje en un código.

encounter   Any contact between a healthcare provider and a patient that results in treatment or evaluation of the patient's condition; not limited to in-person contact.
encuentro   Cualquier contacto entre un proveedor de atención sanitaria y un paciente que resulta en un tratamiento o evaluación del estado del paciente; no se limita a un contacto personal.

encroachment   To advance beyond the usual or proper limits.
intrusiones   Ir más allá de los límites habituales o apropiados.

endemic   Disease or microorganism that is specific to a particular geographic area.
endémico   Enfermedad o microorganismo que es específico de una zona geográfica en particular.

endocervical curettage   The scraping of cells from the wall of the uterus.
curetaje   endocervical Raspado de células de la pared uterina.

endorser   Person who signs his or her name on the back of a check for the purpose of transferring title to another person.
endosante   Persona que firma en la parte posterior de un cheque a fin de transferir la propiedad del mismo a otra persona.

enteric-coated   An oral medication with a coating that resists the effects of stomach juices; designed so medicine is absorbed in the small intestine; drug formulation in which tablets are coated with a special compound that does not dissolve until the tablet is exposed to the fluids of the small intestine.
cubierta entérica   Capa exterior que se añade a un medicamento que se toma por vía oral, la cual es resistente a los efectos de los jugos gástricos; recubrimiento diseñado para que la medicina sea absorbida en el intestino delgado; formulación usada en medicinas en la cual las tabletas se recubren con un componente especial que no se disuelve hasta que la tableta es expuesta a los fluidos del intestino delgado.

enunciate   To utter articulate sounds; the act of being very distinct in speech.
articular   Pronunciar los sonidos de manera cuidada; hablar de una forma muy clara.

enunciation   The utterance of articulate, clear sounds; the act of being very distinct in speech.
articulación   Pronunciación cuidada, con sonidos claros.

enzymatic reaction   Chemical reaction controlled by an enzyme.
reacción enzimática   Reacción química controlada por una enzima.

enzyme   Any of several complex proteins produced by cells that act as catalysts in specific biochemical reactions.
enzima   Cualquiera de las varias proteínas complejas que producen las células y que actúan como catalíticos en reacciones bioquímicas específicas.

epiphysis   End of a long bone.
epífisis   Extremo de un hueso largo.

erythropoietin   Substance released from the kidney and liver that promotes red blood cell formation.
eritropoyetina   Sustancia liberada por los riñones y el hígado y que promueve la formación de glóbulos rojos.

essential hypertension   Elevated blood pressure of unknown cause that develops for no apparent reason; sometimes called *primary hypertension*.
hipertensión esencial   Presión sanguínea alta de causa desconocida que surge sin razón aparente; a veces se llama hipertensión primaria.

established patients   Patients who are returning to the office and who have previously seen the physician.
pacientes establecidos   Pacientes que regresan al consultorio médico que ya han sido atendidos por el médico con anterioridad.

etiology   Cause of a disorder as determined for the purpose of classifying a claim.
etiología   Clasificación de una reclamación según la causa del trastorno.

eukaryote   A single-celled or multicellular organism whose cells contain a distinct membrane-bound nucleus.
eucariote   Organismo unicelular o multicelular cuyas células tienen un núcleo diferenciado rodeado por una membrana.

euthanasia   The act or practice of killing or permitting the death of hopelessly sick or injured individuals in a relatively painless way for reasons of mercy.
eutanasia   Acción o práctica de matar o permitir la muerte de enfermos o heridos en estado terminal, de una forma relativamente sin dolor, por razones de piedad.

exacerbation   An increase in the seriousness of a disease marked by greater intensity in the signs and symptoms; worsening of disease symptoms.
exacerbación   Aumento en la gravedad de una enfermedad, caracterizado por una mayor intensidad de los signos y síntomas. Empeoramiento de los síntomas de una enfermedad.

"excludes"   Term used in insurance claims. Exclusion terms are always written in italics, and the word "Excludes" is enclosed in a box to draw particular attention to these instructions. Exclusion terms may apply to a chapter, a section, a category, or a subcategory. The applicable code number usually follows the exclusion term.
"excluye"   Las expresiones de exclusión siempre se escriben en cursiva y la palabra "Excluye" se encierra en una casilla para llamar la atención acerca de estas instrucciones. Los términos de exclusión pueden ser aplicables a un capítulo, una sección, una categoría o una subcategoría. El número de código correspondiente por lo general sigue al término de exclusión.

expediency   Haste or caution; a means of achieving a particular end.
prontitud   Situación que requiere actuar con prisa o precaución; un medio de alcanzar un fin específico.

expert witness   A person who provides testimony to a court as an expert in a certain field or subject to verify facts presented by one or both sides in a lawsuit, often compensated and used to refute or disprove the claims of one party.
testigo perito   Persona que da testimonio ante un tribunal como perito o experto en cierto campo o tema para verificar los hechos presentados por una o ambas partes en litigio, a menudo, cobrando una retribución económica, y cu yo testimonio suele usarse para refutar o impugnar las demandas de una de las partes.

external noise   Noise outside the brain that interferes with the communication process.
ruido externo   Ruido producido fuera del cerebro y que interfiere con el proceso de comunicación.

externalization   Attribution of an event or occurrence to causes outside the self.
exteriorización   Acción de atribuir a un suceso o acontecimiento causas externas al mismo.

externship/internship   A training program that is part of a course of study of an educational institution and is taken in the actual business setting in that field of study; these terms are often interchanged in reference to medical assisting.
prácticas internas/externas   Programa de entrenamiento que es parte de un curso de estudio de una institución educativa y se sigue en un lugar real de trabajo en el campo de estudio; estos términos se intercambian cuando se refieren a los asistentes médicos.

exudates   Fluids with high concentration of protein and cellular debris that has escaped from the blood vessels and has been deposited in tissues or on tissue surfaces.
exudados   Fluidos con una alta concentración de proteínas y restos celulares extravasados de los vasos sanguíneos y depositados en los tejidos o en sus superficies.

familial   Occurring in or affecting members of a family more than would be expected to occur by chance.
familiar   Que sucede o afecta a miembros de una familia más de lo que podría esperarse por azar.

fascia   Sheet or band of fibrous tissue located deep in the skin that covers muscles and body organs.
fascia   Lámina o banda de tejido fibroso localizada bajo la piel y que cubre los músculos y los órganos.

fastidious   Requiring specialized media or growth factors to grow.
exigente   Que requiere un medio o factores especiales para crecer.

fat   Substance stored as adipose tissue in the body and serving as a concentrated energy reserve.
grasa   Sustancia que se almacena como tejido adiposo en el cuerpo y sirve como reserva de energía concentrada.

fax   Abbreviation for *facsimile;* a document sent using a fax machine.
fax   Abreviatura de facsímile; documento que se envía usando una máquina de fax.

febrile   Pertaining to an elevated body temperature.
febril   Perteneciente o relativo a una temperatura corporal elevada.

fecalith   A hard, impacted mass of feces in the colon.
fecaloma   Masa de heces endurecidas e impactadas en el colon.

fee profile   A compilation or average of physician fees over a given period of time.
perfil de cargos   Recopilación o porcentaje de cargos médicos en un periodo de tiempo dado.

fee schedule   A compilation of preestablished fee allowances for given services or procedures.
escala de cargos   Recopilación de asignaciones de cargos preestablecidos para servicios o procedimientos dados.

feedback   The transmission of evaluative or corrective information about an action, event, or process to the original or controlling source.
reacciones y comentarios   Envío de información de evaluación o corrección a la fuente original o a la que ejerce el control sobre una acción, suceso o proceso.

felony   A major crime, such as murder, rape, or burglary; punishable by a more stringent sentence than that given for a misdemeanor.
crimen   Delito mayor, como asesinato, violación o robo; se penaliza con una sentencia más severa que un delito menor o falta.

fermentation   An enzymatically controlled transformation of an organic compound.
fermentación   Transformación de un compuesto orgánico controlada por enzimas.

fervent   Exhibiting or marked by great intensity of feeling.
ferviente   Que posee sentimientos de gran intensidad o que da muestra de ellos.

fibrillation   Rapid, random, ineffective contractions of the heart.
fibrilación   Contracciones cardiacas rápidas, aleatorias e inefectivas.

fidelity   Faithfulness to something to which one is bound by pledge or duty.
fidelidad   Fe en algo a lo que se está unido por juramento o deber.

filtrate   Fluid that remains after a liquid is passed through a membranous filter.
filtrado   Fluido que queda después de pasar un líquido a través de un filtro membranoso.

fine   A sum imposed as punishment for an offense; a forfeiture or penalty paid to an injured party or the government in a civil or criminal action.
multa   Suma impuesta como penalización por un delito menor; suma que se paga a una parte a la que se ha perjudicado o dañado, o al gobierno, en un proceso civil o penal.

fiscal agent   An organization or private plan under contract to the government to act as a financial representative in handling insurance claims from providers of health care; also referred to as *fiscal intermediary*.
agente fiscal   Organización o plan privado bajo contrato con el gobierno para actuar como representantes financieros en la administración de reclamaciones de seguros por parte de proveedores de atención sanitaria; también se conoce como intermediario fiscal.

fiscal intermediary   An organization that contracts with the government and other insuring entities to handle and mediate insurance claims from medical facilities.
intermediario fiscal   Organización que establece un contrato con el gobierno y otras entidades aseguradoras para administrar reclamaciones de seguro provenientes de centros médicos y para mediar en ellas.

fissures   Narrow slits or clefts in the abdominal wall.
fisuras   Grietas o hendiduras estrechas en la pared abdominal.

fistulas   Abnormal, tubelike passages within the body tissue, usually between two internal organs, or from an internal organ to the body surface.
fístulas   Pasajes anómalos en forma de tubos entre los tejidos corporales, por lo general entre dos órganos internos, o de un órgano interno a la superficie del cuerpo.

flagged Marked in some way so as to remind or remember that specific action needs to be taken.
señalado Marcado de alguna forma para recordar que se necesita que se tomen medidas al respeto.

Flash Animation technology often used on the opening page of a Web site used to draw the attention of, excite, and impress the user.
Flash Tecnología de imágenes animadas que se usa con frecuencia en la página inicial de un sitio web para llamar la atención del usuario, entusiasmarlo e impresionarlo.

flatus Gas expelled through the anus.
flato Gas expulsado a través del ano.

fluoroscopy Direct observation of the x-ray image in motion.
fluoroscopía Observación directa de una imagen de rayos x en movimiento.

flush Directly abutting or immediately adjacent, as set even with an edge of a type page or column; having no indention.
alineado Directamente contiguo o inmediatamente adyacente, ordenado de forma regular en relación con un borde de una página o columna; sin sangría o espacios en blanco.

follicle-stimulating hormone (FSH) A hormone secreted by the anterior pituitary; stimulates oogenesis and spermatogenesis.
hormona foliculoestimulante (FSH) Hormona que segrega la pituitaria anterior y que estimula los procesos de formación y desarrollo de óvulos y de espermatozoides.

font A design, as in typesetting, for a set of characters.
fuente tipográfica Diseño similar al de la composición para un conjunto de caracteres.

format To magnetically create tracks on a disk where information will be stored, usually done by the manufacturer of the disk.
formatear Crear pistas magnéticas en un disco destinado a almacenar información; por lo general, el fabricante del disco es quien se encarga de hacerlo.

fovea centralis A small pit in the center of the retina that is considered the center of clearest vision.
fóvea central Pequeña concavidad en el centro de la retina que se cree que es el centro de visión más claro.

frontal projection Radiographic view in which the coronal plane of the body or body part is parallel to the film plane; AP or PA.
proyección frontal Vista radiográfica en la cual el plano coronal del cuerpo o de la parte del cuerpo está paralelo al plano de la película; AP o PA.

gait Manner or style of walking.
andares Forma o estilo de caminar.

gamete A mature male or female germ cell, usually possessing a haploid chromosome set and capable of initiating formation of a new diploid individual.
gameto Célula germinal madura, tanto masculina como femenina, que por lo general tiene un conjunto cromosómico haploide y es capaz de iniciar la formación de un nuevo individuo diploide.

gangrene Death of body tissue resulting from loss of nutritive supply and followed by bacterial invasion and putrefaction.
gangrena Muerte de tejido corporal debido a la pérdida de suministro de nutrientes por invasión bacteriana y putrefacción.

gantry Doughnut-shaped portion of a scanner than surrounds the patient and that functions, at least in part, to gather imaging data.
gantry Parte de un escáner con forma de rosquilla que rodea al paciente y funciona, al menos en parte, reuniendo datos de formación de imágenes.

generic Not protected by trademark.
genéricas Medicinas que no están protegidas por una marca registrada.

genome The genetic material of an organism.
genoma El material genético de un organismo.

genuineness Expressing sincerity and honest feeling.
autenticidad Expresión de sentimientos sincera y honrada.

germicides Agents that destroy pathogenic organisms.
germicidas Agentes químicos que destruyen o matan organismos patógenos.

gigabyte Approximately one billion bytes.
gigabyte Aproximadamente, mil millones de bytes.

girth A measure around a body or item.
contorno Medida alrededor de un cuerpo o artículo.

glean   To gather information or material bit by bit; to pick over in search of relevant material.
recopilar   Reunir información o material pedazo a pedazo; examinar en busca de material pertinente.

glucagon   A hormone produced by the alpha cells of the pancreatic islets; stimulates the liver to convert glycogen into glucose.
glucagón   Hormona producida por las células alfa de los islotes pancreáticos; estimula al hígado para que convierta el glucógeno en glucosa.

glucosuria   The abnormal presence of glucose in the urine.
glucosuria   Presencia anómala de glucosa en la orina.

glycogen   The sugar (starch) formed from glucose and stored mainly in the liver.
glucógeno   Azúcar (almidón) formado a partir de la glucosa y almacenado principalmente en el hígado.

glycohemoglobin or hemoglobin A_{1c}   A type of hemoglobin that is made slowly during the 120-day life span of the red blood cell (RBC). Glycohemoglobin makes up 3% to 6% of hemoglobin in a normal RBC; in diabetes mellitus it makes up to 12%.
glucohemoglobina o hemoglobina A_{1c}   Tipo de hemoglobina que se produce lentamente durante el periodo de los 120 días de vida de los glóbulos rojos (RBC). La glucohemoglobina constituye de un 3% a un 6% de la hemoglobina en un RBC normal; en los casos de diabetes mellitus constituye hasta un 12%.

glycosuria   Presence of glucose in the urine.
glucosuria   Presencia de glucosa en la orina.

goniometer   Instrument for measuring the degrees of motion in a joint.
goniómetro   Instrumento para medir los grados de movimiento de una articulación.

government plan   An insurance or health care plan that is sponsored and/or subsidized by the state or federal government, such as Medicaid and Medicare.
plan del gobierno   Seguro o plan de atención sanitaria patrocinado y subvencionado por el gobierno estatal o federal, como Medicaid y Medicare.

grammar   The study of the classes of words, their inflections, and their functions and relations in the sentence; a study of what is to be preferred and what avoided in inflection and syntax.
gramática   Estudio de las clases de palabras, sus desinencias y sus funciones y relaciones en la oración; estudio del uso que se prefiere y de lo que hay que evitar en cuanto a desinencias y sintaxis.

gray (Gy)   International unit of radiation dose.
gray (Gy)   Unidad internacional de dosis de radiación.

grief   An unfortunate outcome; a deep distress caused by bereavement.
pesar   Resultado desafortunado; profunda aflicción causada por la pérdida de un ser querido.

group policy   Insurance written under a policy that covers a number of people under a single master contract issued to their employer or to an association with which they are affiliated.
póliza de grupo   Seguro contratado bajo una póliza que cubre a varias personas bajo un único contrato maestro establecido con su empleador o con una asociación a la que estén afiliados.

growth hormone (GH)   Also called *somatotropic hormone,* stimulates tissue growth and restricts tissue glucose dependence when nutrients are not available.
hormona del crecimiento (GH)   También llamada hormona somatotrópica, estimula el crecimiento de los tejidos y restringe la dependencia de la glucosa de los tejidos cuando no hay nutrientes disponibles.

guarantor   A person who makes or gives a guarantee of payment for a bill.
garante   Persona que paga una factura o que garantiza su pago.

guardian ad litem   Legal representative of a minor.
tutor ad litem   Representante legal de un menor.

hard copy   The readable paper copy or printout of information.
copia impresa   Copia impresa en papel o impresión de la información.

harmonious   Marked by accord in sentiment or action; having the parts agreeably related.
armonioso   Caracterizado por una armonía en los sentimientos o acciones; partes de un todo relacionadas de forma agradable.

health insurance   Protection, in return for periodic premiums, that provides reimbursement of monetary losses resulting from illness or injury. Included under this heading are various types of insurance such as accident insurance, disability income insurance, medical expense insurance, and accidental death and dismemberment insurance. Also known as *accident and health insurance* or *disability income insurance*.
seguro de enfermedad   Cobertura a cambio del pago de primas periódicas, la cual proporciona el reembolso de las pérdidas monetarias debidas a enfermedad o lesión. Bajo este nombre se incluyen varios tipos de seguros como seguro de accidente, seguro de incapacidad, seguro de gastos médicos y seguro en caso de muerte y pérdida de extremidades. También se conoce como seguro de accidente y enfermedad o seguro de incapacidad.

hematemesis   Vomiting of bright red blood, indicating rapid upper gastrointestinal bleeding, associated with esophageal varices or peptic ulcer.
hematemesis   Vómito de sangre roja brillante que indica hemorragia rápida del sistema gastrointestinal superior, relacionado con varices esofágicas o úlcera péptica.

hematocrit   The percentage by volume of packed red blood cells in a given sample of blood after centrifugation. Volume percentage of erythrocytes in whole blood.
hematocrito   Porcentaje por volumen de glóbulos rojos en una muestra de sangre dada después de ser centrifugada. Porcentaje del volumen de eritrocitos en la sangre completa.

hematoma   A sac filled with blood that may be the result of trauma.
hematoma   Sacó lleno de sangre que puede ser el resultado de una lesión.

hematuria   Blood in the urine.
hematuria   Sangre en la orina.

hemoconcentration   A situation in which the concentration of blood cells is increased in proportion to the plasma.
hemoconcentración   Situación en la cual la concentración de glóbulos rojos ha aumentado en proporción al plasma.

hemoglobin   Protein found in erythrocytes that transports molecular oxygen in the blood.
hemoglobina   Proteína que se encuentra en los eritrocitos que transportan el oxígeno en la sangre.

hemolysis   The destruction or dissolution of red blood cells, with subsequent release of hemoglobin.
hemolisis   Destrucción o disolución de los glóbulos rojos, con la subsiguiente liberación de hemoglobina.

hemolyzed   A term used to describe a blood sample in which the red blood cells have ruptured.
hemolizado   Término usado para describir una muestra de sangre en la cual los glóbulos rojos se han roto.

hepatomegaly   Abnormal enlargement of the liver.
hepatomegalia   Agrandamiento anómalo del hígado.

hereditary   Pertaining to a characteristic, condition, or disease transmitted from parent to offspring on the DNA chain.
hereditario   Perteneciente o relativo a una característica, estado o enfermedad transmitida de padres a hijos en la cadena de ADN.

hermetically sealed   Sealed so no air is allowed to enter or escape.
herméticamente sellado   Sellado de forma que el aire no pueda entrar o escapar.

HMO   An organization that provides a wide range of comprehensive health care services for a specified group at a fixed periodic payment. HMOs can be sponsored by the government, medical schools, hospitals, employers, labor unions, consumer groups, insurance companies, and hospital-medical plans.
HMO   Organización que proporciona una amplia gama de servicios completos de atención sanitaria para un grupo específico por un pago periódico fijado. Las HMO puedes estar patrocinadas por el gobierno, facultades de medicina, hospitales, patronos, sindicatos laborales, grupos de consumidores, compañías aseguradoras y planes médico-hospitalarios.

holder   Person presenting a check for payment.
portador   Persona que presenta un cheque para cobrarlo.

holistic   Related to or concerned with all of the systems of the body, rather than breaking it down into parts.
holístico   Relacionado con todos los sistemas corporales y no dividido en partes.

homeostasis   Maintenance of constant internal ambient conditions compatible with life.
homeostasis   Mantenimiento de unas condiciones ambientales internas constantes compatibles con la vida.

homeostatic   Maintaining a constant internal environment.
homeostático   Que mantiene un ambiente interno constante.

hormone   A substance, usually a peptide or steroid, produced by one tissue and conveyed by the bloodstream to another to effect physiologic activity such as growth or metabolism; a chemical transmitter produced by the body and transported to target tissue or organs by the bloodstream.
hormona   Sustancia química transmisora, por lo general un péptido o un esteroide, que es producida por un tejido y transportada por la corriente sanguínea hasta el tejido u órgano—objetivo para provocar un efecto en la actividad fisiológica, como el crecimiento o el metabolismo.

HTML   Abbreviation for *hypertext markup language,* which is the language used to create documents for use on the Internet.
HTML   Abreviatura de lenguaje de marcas de hipertexto, que es el lenguaje que se emplea para crear documentos destinados a usarse en Internet.

HTTP   Abbreviation for *hypertext transfer protocol,* which defines how messages are defined and transmitted over the Internet; when a URL is entered into the computer, an HTTP command tells the Web server to retrieve the requested Web page.
HTTP   Abreviatura de protocolo de transporte de hipertexto, que define cómo se interpretan y transmiten los mensajes en Internet; cuando un URL entra en la computadora, una orden de HTTP manda la señal al servidor web para que busque la página web que se solicita.

hub   A common connection point for devices in a network containing multiple ports, often used to connect segments of a LAN.
nodo   Punto de conexión común para dispositivos en una red de conexiones de varios puertos; suele usar se para conectar segmentos de una LAN (red de área local).

hydrocephaly   Enlargement of the cranium caused by abnormal accumulation of cerebrospinal fluid within the cerebral system.
hidrocefalia   Agrandamiento del cráneo causado por una acumulación anómala de fluido cerebroespinal en el interior del sistema cerebral.

hydrogenated   Combined with, treated with, or exposed to hydrogen.
hidrogenado   Combinado con hidrógeno, tratado con él o expuesto a él.

hyperlipidemia   Excess of fats or lipids in the blood plasma.
hiperlipemia   Exceso de grasas o lípidos en el plasma sanguíneo.

hyperplasia   An increase in the number of cells.
hiperplasia   Aumento del número de células.

hyperpnea   Increase in the depth of breathing.
hiperpnea   Aumento en la profundidad de la respiración.

hypertension   High blood pressure (systolic pressure consistently above 140 mm Hg and diastolic pressure above 90 mm Hg).
hipertensión   Presión sanguínea alta (presión sistólica continuamente por encima de 140 mm Hg y presión diastólica por encima de 90 mm Hg).

hyperventilation   Abnormally prolonged and deep breathing, usually associated with acute anxiety or emotional tension.
hiperventilación   Respiración profunda anómalamente prolongada, que suele estar asociada con una ansiedad aguda o con tensión emocional.

hypotension   Blood pressure that is below normal (systolic pressure below 90 mm Hg and diastolic pressure below 50 mm Hg).
hipotensión   Presión sanguínea que está por debajo de lo normal (presión sistólica por debajo de 90 mm Hg y presión diastólica por debajo de 50 mm Hg).

icon   A picture, often on the desktop of a computer, that represents a program or an object. By clicking on the icon, the user is directed to the program.
icono   Dibujo, con frecuencia colocado en el escritorio de la computadora, que representa un programa o un objeto. Al hacer clic sobre el icono, el usuario es llevado a dicho programa.

idealism   The practice of forming ideas or living under the influence of ideas.
idealismo   Práctica de formarse ideas o vivir bajo la influencia de ideas.

idiopathic   Of unknown cause.
idiopático   Causa desconocida.

ileocecal valve   Valve guarding the opening between the ileum and cecum; also called the *ileocolic valve*.
válvula ileocecal   Válvula que controla la abertura entre el íleo y el intestino ciego; también se llama válvula ileocólica.

ileostomy   Surgical formation of an opening of the ileum onto the surface of the abdomen through which fecal material is emptied.
ileostomía   Formación quirúrgica de una abertura del íleo en la superficie del abdomen, a través de la cual se vacían los materiales fecales.

immigrant   A person who comes to a country to take up permanent residence.
inmigrante   Persona que va a un país para vivir allí de forma permanente.

immunotherapy   Administering repeated injections of diluted extracts of the substance that causes an allergy; also called *desensitization*.
inmunoterapia   Administración de repetidas inyecciones de extractos diluidos de la substancia que provoca una alergia; también se conoce como desensibilización.

impenetrable   Incapable of being penetrated or pierced; not capable of being damaged or harmed.
impenetrable   Que no puede ser penetrado o traspasado; que no puede ser dañado o perjudicado.

implied consent   Presumed consent, such as when a patient offers an arm for a phlebotomy procedure.
consentimiento tácito   Consentimiento que se supone que ha sido dado, como cuando un paciente presenta el brazo para que se le extraiga sangre.

in vitro   Refers to conditions outside of a living body.
in vitro   Expresión que se refiere a condiciones exteriores de un ser vivo.

incentive   Something that incites or spurs to action; a reward or reason for performing a task.
incentivo   Algo que incita o impulsa a actuar; recompensa o razón para llevar a cabo una tarea.

"includes"   Term used in insurance claims. The appearance of this term under a subdivision such as a category (three-digit) code or two-digit procedure code indicates that the code and title include these terms. Other terms also classified to that particular code and title are listed in the Alphabetic Indexes.
"incluye"   La presencia de esta expresión, cuando aparece bajo una subdivisión, como una categoría (código de tres dígitos) o como un código de procedimiento de dos dígitos, indica que el código y el título incluyen estos términos. En los Índices alfabéticos se enumeran otros términos también clasificados para este código específico.

incontinence   Inability to control excretory functions.
incontinencia   Incapacidad de controlar las funciones excretoras.

indemnity plan   Traditional health insurance plan that pays for all or a share of the cost of covered services, regardless of which doctor, hospital, or other licensed health care provider is used. Policyholders of indemnity plans and their dependents choose when and where to get health care services.
plan de indemnización   Plan de seguro de enfermedad tradicional que paga todo o parte del costo de los servicios que cubre, sin importar a qué médico, hospital u otro proveedor de atención sanitaria licenciado se acuda. Los titulares de pólizas de planes de indemnización y las personas que dependen de estos titulares escogen cuándo y dónde recibir atención médica.

indicators   An important point or group of statistical values that, when evaluated, indicates the quality of care provided in a healthcare institution.
indicadores   Importante punto o grupo de valores estadísticos que al ser evaluados indican la calidad del servicio que se proporciona en una institución de atención sanitaria.

indicted   To charge with a crime by the finding or presentment of a jury according to due process of law.
acusado   Que se le imputa con un cargo criminal por conclusión o acusación de un jurado con el proceso legal debido.

indigent   Totally lacking in something of need.
indigente   Que carece totalmente de algo necesario.

indirect filing system   A filing system in which an intermediary source of reference, such as a card file, must be consulted to locate specific files.
sistema indirecto de archivo   Sistema de archivo en el cual debe consultarse una fuente de referencia intermedia, como un fichero, para localizar documentos específicos.

individual policy   An insurance policy designed specifically for the use of one person (and his or her dependents) not associated with the amenities of a group policy, namely higher premiums. Often referred to as "personal insurance."
póliza individual   Póliza de seguros destinada específicamente a ser usada por una persona (y quienes dependan de ella) y que no conlleva los beneficios de una póliza de grupo y tiene primas más altas. Con frecuencia se le llama "seguro—personal."

induration   An abnormally hard, inflamed area.
induración   Área anómalamente dura, inflamada.

infarction   Area of tissue that has died because of lack of blood supply.
infarto   Área de tejido que ha muerto debido a una falta de suministro de sangre.

infection   Invasion of body tissues by microorganisms, which then proliferate and damage tissues.
infección   Invasión de los tejidos corporales por microorganismos, los cuales entonces proliferan y dañan los tejidos.

infertile   Not fertile or productive; not capable of reproducing.
estéril   Que no es fértil o productivo; que no tiene la capacidad de reproducirse.

inflammation   Tissue reaction to trauma or disease that includes redness, heat, swelling, and pain.
inflamación   Reacción de los tejidos ante una lesión o enfermedad que incluye enrojecimiento, calentamiento, hinchazón y dolor.

inflection   A change in pitch or loudness of the voice.
inflexión   Cambio en el tono o volumen de la voz.

informed consent   A consent in which there is understanding of what treatment is to be undertaken and of the risks involved, why it should be done, and alternative methods of treatment available (including no treatment) and their attendant risks.
consentimiento informado   Consentimiento que implica la comprensión del tratamiento al que se va a ser sometido y de los riesgos que conlleva, del porqué de dicho tratamiento, así como la comprensión de los tratamientos alternativos disponibles (incluyendo la ausencia de tratamiento) y los riesgos que conllevan.

infraction   Breaking the law; a minor offense of the rules.
infracción   Incumplimiento de la ley; delito menor contra las normas establecidas.

initiative   The causing or facilitating of the beginning of; the initiation of something into happening.
iniciativa   El causar o facilitar el comienzo de algo; el hacer que algo comience a ocurrir.

innate   Existing in, belonging to, or determined by factors present in an individual since birth.
innato   Que existe en un individuo, que le pertenece o que está determinado por factores existentes en ese individuo desde el momento de su nacimiento.

input   Information entered into and used by the computer.
entrada   Información introducida en una computadora y que la computadora utiliza.

instigate   To goad or urge forward; provoke.
instigar   Incitar, exhortar, provocar.

insubordination   Disobedience to authority.
insubordinación   Desobediencia a la autoridad.

insulin   Hormone secreted by the beta cells of the pancreatic islets in response to increased levels of glucose in the blood.
insulina   Hormona que segregan las células beta de los islotes pancreáticos en respuesta a la presencia de altos niveles de glucosa en la sangre.

insured A person or organization covered by an insurance policy, along with any other parties for whom protection is provided under the policy terms.
asegurado Persona u organización que está cubierta por una póliza de seguro junto con cualquier otro a quien se proporcione cobertura bajo los términos de la póliza.

intangible Incapable of being perceived, especially by touch; incapable of being precisely identified or realized by the mind.
intangible Que no se puede percibir, especialmente que no se puede tocar; que no puede ser identificado con precisión ni ser comprendido por la mente.

integral Essential; being an indispensable part of a whole.
integral Esencial; parte indispensable de un todo.

interaction A two-way communication; mutual or reciprocal action or influence.
interacción Comunicación bidireccional; acción o influencia recíproca o mutua.

intercom A two-way communication system with a microphone and loudspeaker at each station for localized use.
intercomunicador Sistema de comunicación bidireccional con un micrófono y un altavoz en cada estación para uso local.

intermittent Coming and going at intervals; not continuous.
intermitente Que va y viene a intervalos; de forma no continua.

intermittent claudications Recurring cramping in the calves caused by poor circulation of blood to the muscles of the lower leg.
cojeras intermitentes Calambres recurrentes en las pantorrillas causados por una mala circulación de la sangre de los músculos de la parte inferior de la pierna.

intermittent pulse Pulse in which beats are occasionally skipped.
pulso intermitente Pulso en el cual de vez en cuando se salta algún latido.

internal noise Noise inside the brain that interferes with the communication process.
ruido interno Ruido en el interior del cerebro que interfiere con el proceso de comunicación.

International Classification of Diseases, Ninth Revision, Clinical Modification (ICD-9-CM) System for classifying disease to facilitate collection of uniform and comparable health information for statistical purposes, and for indexing medical records for data storage and retrieval.
Clasificación Internacional de Enfermedades, Novena Revisión, Modificación clínica (ICD-9-CM) Sistema de clasificación de enfermedades para facilitar la recopilación de información médica uniforme, tanto para fines estadísticos como para indexar informes médicos a fin de almacenar y recuperar datos.

International Classification of Diseases, Tenth Revision (ICD-10) System containing the greatest number of changes in ICD's history. To allow more specific reporting of disease and newly recognized conditions, ICD-10 contains approximately 5500 more codes than ICD-9.
Clasificación Internacional de Enfermedades, Décima Revisión (ICD-10) Sistema que contiene el mayor número de cambios en la historia de la ICD. Para permitir elaborar informes más precisos de las enfermedades y de los estados patológicos que se conocen sólo recientemente, la ICD-10 incluye aproximadamente 5,500 códigos más que la ICD-9.

international mail Mail that is sent outside the boundaries of the United States and its territories.
correo internacional Correo que se envía fuera de los límites de Estados Unidos y sus territorios.

interval Space of time between events.
intervalo Espacio de tiempo entre dos sucesos.

intolerable Not tolerable or bearable.
intolerable Que no se puede tolerar o soportar.

intravenous urogram (IVU) Radiographic examination of the urinary tract using intravenous injection of an iodine contrast medium.
urograma intravenoso (IVU) Examen radiográfico del tracto urinario usando una inyección intravenosa de un medio de contraste yodado.

intrinsic Belonging to the essential nature or constitution of a thing; indwelling, inward.
intrínseco Que pertenece a la naturaleza o constitución básica de una cosa; inherente, interno.

introspection An inward, reflective examination of one's own thoughts and feelings.
introspección Examen de nuestros propios pensamientos y sentimientos.

invariably Consistently; without changing or being capable of change.
invariablemente De forma constante; que no cambia ni puede cambiar.

invasive Involving entry into the living body, as by incision or insertion of an instrument.
invasivo Que entra en un organismo vivo, como por incisión o inserción de un instrumento.

ipsilateral Pertaining to the same side of the body.
isolateral Perteneciente a la misma parte del cuerpo.

irregular pulse Pulse that varies in force and frequency.
pulso irregular Pulso que varía en fuerza y frecuencia.

ischemia Decreased blood flow to a body part or organ, caused by constriction or plugging of the supplying artery; temporary interruption in blood supply to a tissue or organ.
isquemia Disminución del flujo sanguíneo a una parte del cuerpo u órgano provocada por la constricción o atasco de la arteria suministradora; interrupción temporal del suministro de sangre a un tejido u órgano.

islets (of Langerhans) Cells of the pancreas that produce insulin (beta cells) and glucagon (alpha cells); also called *pancreatic islets*.
islotes (de Langerhans) Células del páncreas que producen insulina (células beta) y glucagón (células alfa); también llamados islotes pancreáticos.

jargon The technical terminology or characteristic idiom of a particular group or special activity.
jerga Terminología técnica o lenguaje característico de un grupo específico o una actividad especial.

jaundice Yellowness of the skin and mucous membranes caused by deposition of bile pigment. It is not a disease, but a sign of a number of diseases, especially liver disorders.
ictericia Coloración amarilla en la piel y las membranas mucosas causada por deposición del pigmento biliar. No es una enfermedad pero es un síntoma de muchas enfermedades, sobre todo de trastornos hepáticos.

Java An object-oriented high-level programming language commonly used and well-suited for the Internet.
Java Lenguaje de programación de alto nivel y orientado a objetos que es usado ampliamente y es muy adecuado para Internet.

judicial Of or relating to a judgment, the function of judging, the administration of justice, or the judiciary.
judicial Perteneciente o relativo al juicio, los procesos jurídicos, la administración de justicia o a la judicatura.

jurisdiction A power constitutionally conferred on a judge or magistrate, to decide cases according to law and to carry sentence into execution. Jurisdiction is original when it is conferred on the court in the first instance (original jurisdiction); it is appellate when an appeal is given from the judgment of another court (apellate jurisdiction).
jurisdicción Poder constitucional otorgado a un juez o magistrado para resolver casos de acuerdo con la ley y hacer que se cumplan las sentencias. Es jurisdicción original cuando se otorga en un tribunal de primera instancia; es jurisdicción en apelación cuando existe una apelación al juicio de otro tribunal.

jurisprudence The science or philosophy of law; a system or body of law, or the course of court decisions.
jurisprudencia Ciencia o filosofía que trata sobre la ley; sistema o cuerpo legal; línea de decisiones de los tribunales.

keratin Very hard, tough protein found in hair, nails, and epidermal tissue.
queratina Proteína muy dura que se encuentra en el pelo, uñas y tejidos epidérmicos.

keratinocytes Any one of the skin cells that synthesize keratin.
queratinocitos Cualquiera de las células de la piel que sintetizan queratina.

ketosis Abnormal production of ketone bodies in the blood and tissues resulting from fat catabolism in cells. Ketones accumulate in large quantities when fat, instead of sugar, is used as fuel for energy in cells.

quetosis Producción anormal de cuerpos de quetosis en la sangre y tejidos como resultado de un catabolismo graso en las células. Los quetones se acumulan en grandes cantidades cuando se usa grasa, en lugar de azúcar, como combustible para las células.

kyphosis Abnormal convex curvature of the thoracic spine region.

cifosis Curvatura convexa anómala de la región espinal torácica.

lacrimation The secretion or discharge of tears.

lagrimeo Secreción o descarga de lágrimas.

language barrier Any type of interference that inhibits the communication process and is related to the difference in languages spoken by the people attempting to communicate.

barrera del idioma Cualquier tipo de interferencia que inhibe el proceso de comunicación y que está relacionado con la diferencia en los idiomas que hablan las personas que intentan comunicarse.

laryngoscopy Visual examination of the voice box area through an endoscope equipped with a light and mirrors for illumination.

laringoscopia Examen visual de la laringe por medio de un endoscopio equipado con una luz y espejos.

latent image Invisible changes in exposed film that will become a visible image when the film is processed.

imagen latente Cambios invisibles en la película que se convertirán en una imagen visible cuando se procese la película.

law A binding custom or practice of a community; a rule of conduct or action prescribed or formally recognized as binding or enforceable by a controlling authority.

ley Costumbre o práctica obligatoria de una comunidad; norma de comportamiento o proceder prescrita o reconocida formalmente como norma obligatoria o que se puede hacer cumplir por una autoridad encargada.

learning style The way that an individual perceives and processes information in order to learn new material.

estilo de aprendizaje Forma en la que un individuo percibe y procesa la información para aprender cosas nuevas.

leukoderma White patches on the skin.

leucodermia Manchas blancas en la piel.

liable Obligated according to law or equity; responsible for an act or circumstance.

responsable Que tiene alguna obligación según la ley o el derecho lato; responsable de un acto o circunstancia.

libel A written defamatory statement or representation that conveys an unjustly unfavorable impression.

libelo Escrito difamatorio que produce una impresión desfavorable injusta.

ligament A tough connective tissue band that holds joints together by attaching to the bones on either side of the joint.

ligamento Banda de tejido conectivo resistente que sostiene las articulaciones uniendo los huesos de cada lado de la articulación.

ligation The process of tying off something to close it—for example, a blood vessel during surgery—with a tie called a *ligature*.

ligado Proceso de atar algo, por ejemplo, un vaso sanguíneo durante una cirugía, con una atadura llamada ligadura.

limited radiography A limited-scope radiography practice, usually in an outpatient setting, that does not require the same credentials needed for professional radiologic technology; also called *practical radiography*.

radiografía limitada Práctica radiográfica de alcance limitado que se suele usar con pacientes externos y que no requiere las mismas credenciales que se necesitan para la tecnología radiográfica profesional. También se llama radiografía práctica.

lithotripsy A procedure for eliminating a stone (as in the bladder) by crushing or dissolving it in situ through the use of high-intensity sound waves.

litotripsia Procedimiento para eliminar una piedra rompiéndola o disolviéndola in situ por medio del uso de ondas sonoras de alta intensidad.

litigious   Prone to engage in lawsuits.
litigioso   Propenso a iniciar pleitos y litigios.

loading dose   A double dose of medication administered as the first dose. It is usually done with antibiotic therapy to reach therapeutic blood levels quickly.
dosis de ataque   Dosis doble de una medicación ladministrada como primera dosis. Suele hacerse con terapia antibiótica para alcanzar rápidamente los niveles terapéuticos en sangre.

lordosis   Abnormal concave curvature of the cervical and lumbar spine regions.
lordosis   Curvatura cóncava anómala de la espina cervical y lumbar.

lower GI series   Fluoroscopic examination of the colon, usually employing rectal administration of barium sulfate (also called *barium enema*) as a contrast medium.
serie GI inferior   Examen fluoroscópico del colon, por lo general usando una administración rectal de sulfato de bario (también llamado enema de bario) como medio de contraste.

lumbar   The lower back region, containing five lumbar vertebrae.
lumbar   Región posterior inferior en la que hay cinco vértebras lumbares.

lumen   An open space, such as within a blood vessel, the intestine, a needle, a tube, or an examining instrument.
lumen   Espacio abierto, como en el interior de un vaso sanguíneo, el intestino, una aguja, un tubo o un instrumento para examinar.

luteinizing hormone (LH)   A hormone produced by the pituitary gland that promotes ovulation.
hormona luteinizante (LH)   Hormona que produce la glándula pituitaria y que promueve la ovulación.

luxation   Dislocation of a bone from its normal anatomic location.
luxación   Dislocación de un hueso de su ubicación anatómica normal.

lymphadenopathy   Any disorder of the lymph nodes or lymph vessels.
linfadenopatía   Cualquier trastorno de los nódulos o de los vasos linfáticos.

macromolecules   The molecules needed for metabolism: carbohydrates, lipids, proteins, and nucleic acids.
macromoléculas   Moléculas que se necesitan para el metabolismo: carbohidratos, lípidos, proteínas y ácidos nucleicos.

magnetic resonance imaging (MRI)   An imaging modality that uses a magnetic field and radiofrequency pulses to create computer images of both bones and soft tissues, in multiple planes.
formación de imágenes por resonancia magnética (MRI)   Modalidad de formación de imágenes en la que se usa un campo magnético y pulsos de radiofrecuencia para crear imágenes computarizadas, tanto de huesos como de tejidos blandos, en planos múltiples.

major diagnostic categories (MDCs)   Broad clinical categories differentiated from all others on the basis of body system involvement and cause of disease.
categorías de diagnosis principales (MDCs)   Amplias categorías clínicas que se diferencian de todas las demás en base a la inclusión del sistema corporal y la etiología de la enfermedad.

maker (of a check)   Any individual, corporation, or legal party who signs a check or any type of negotiable instrument.
signatario (de un cheque)   Cualquier individuo, corporación o parte legal que firma un cheque o cualquier tipo de instrumento negociable.

malignant   Cancerous.
maligno   Canceroso.

managed care   An umbrella term for all healthcare plans that provide healthcare in return for preset monthly payments and offer coordinated care through a defined network of primary care physicians and hospitals.
atención administrada   Término que engloba todos los planes de atención sanitaria que proporcionan atención médica a cambio de pagos mensuales preestablecidos y atención coordinada a través de una red definida de médicos de cabecera y hospitales.

mandated   Required by an authority or law.
obligatorio   Que lo exige una autoridad o la ley.

mandatory   Containing or constituting a command.
obligatorio   Que contiene una orden o que es una orden en sí mismo.

manifestation   Something that is easily understood or recognized by the mind.
manifestación   Algo que puede ser comprendido o reconocido por la mente con facilidad.

manipulation   Moving or exercising a body part by an externally applied force.
manipulación   Mover o ejercitar una parte del cuerpo por medio de la aplicación de una fuerza externa.

mastectomy   Surgical removal of the breast that usually includes excision of lymph nodes in the axillary region.
mastectomía   Eliminación quirúrgica del seno que por lo general incluye la escisión de los nódulos linfáticos de la región axilar.

matrix   Something in which a thing originates, develops, takes shape, or is contained; a base on which to build.
matriz   Algo donde las cosas se originan, desarrollan, toman forma o están contenidas; base sobre la cual construir.

m-banking   Banking through the use of wireless devices, such as cellular phones and wireless Internet services.
banca-m   Operaciones bancarias a través de dispositivos inalámbricos, como teléfonos celulares y servicios de comunicaciones inalámbricas.

media   The term applied to agencies of mass communication, such as newspapers, magazines, and telecommunications.
medios de comunicación   Término que se aplica a las agencias de noticias o de comunicación de masas, como periódicos, revistas y telecomunicaciones.

mediastinum   The space in the center of the chest, under the sternum.
mediastino   Espacio en el centro del pecho, bajo el esternón.

medical savings account   A tax-deferred bank or savings account combined with a low-premium, high-deductible insurance policy, designed for individuals or families who choose to fund their own health care expenses and medical insurance.
cuenta de ahorros para gastos médicos   Cuenta bancaria o de ahorros de impuestos diferidos combinada con una póliza de seguro con primas bajas y deducibles altos destinada a individuos o familias que eligen financiar ellos mismos sus gastos de atención sanitaria y su seguro médico.

medically indigent   An individual who can afford to pay for his or her normal daily living expenses but cannot afford adequate health care.
médicamente indigente   Individuo que puede pagar sus gastos normales de la vida cotidiana pero que no puede abordar el pago de un servicio de atención sanitaria adecuado.

medically necessary   Criteria used by third-party payors to decide whether a patient's symptoms and diagnosis justify specific medical services or procedures; also known as *medical necessity*.
médicamente necesario   Criterio usado por pagadores intermediarios para decidir si los síntomas y el diagnóstico de un paciente justifican el uso de procedimientos o servicios médicos específicos; también se conoce como necesidad médica.

Medigap   A term sometimes applied to private insurance products that supplement Medicare insurance benefits.
Medigap   Término que se aplica algunas veces a seguros privados que complementan los beneficios del seguro Medicare.

medullary cavity   The inner portion of the diaphysis, containing bone marrow.
cavidad medular   Porción interna de la diafisis que contiene la médula ósea.

megabyte   Approximately one million bytes.
megabyte   Aproximadamente, un millón de bytes.

megahertz   A measuring unit for microprocessors, abbreviated MHz. A megahertz is a million cycles of electromagnetic current alternation per second and is used as a unit of measure for the clock speed of computer microprocessors. The hertz is a unit of measure named after Heinrich Hertz, a German physicist.
megahercio   Unidad de medida para microprocesadores, abreviada MHz. Un megahercio es un millón de ciclos de alternancia de corriente electromagnética por segundo y se usa como unidad de medida para la velocidad de los—microprocesadores de computadoras. El hercio recibe su nombre de Heinrich Hertz, un físico alemán.

melena   Black, tarry stool containing digested blood and usually the result of bleeding in the upper GI tract.
melena   Deposición negra y alquitranada que contiene sangre digerida y por lo general es le resultado de una hemorragia en el tracto gastrointestinal superior.

mentor   A trusted counselor or guide.
mentor   Consejero o guía de confianza.

metabolite   A substance produced by metabolism.
metabolito   Sustancia producida por el metabolismo.

meticulous   Marked by extreme or excessive care in the consideration or treatment of details.
meticuloso   Caracterizado por una atención exagerada o excesiva a los detalles.

microcephaly   Small size of the head in relation to the rest of the body.
microcefalia   Tamaño pequeño de la cabeza en relación con el resto del cuerpo.

microfilm   A film bearing a photographic record of printed or other graphic matter on a reduced scale.
microfilm   Película que contiene una fotografía de un documento impreso u otro elemento gráfico a escala reducida.

microorganism   An organism of microscopic or submicroscopic size.
microorganismo   Organismo de tamaño microscópico o sub-microscópico.

MIDI   The abbreviation for *musical instrument digital interface*. A MIDI interface allows computers to record and manipulate sound.
MIDI   Abreviatura para interfaz digital para instrumentos musicales. Una interfaz MIDI permite a las computadoras grabar y manipular sonido.

miotic   Any substance or medication that causes contraction of the pupil.
miótico   Cualquier sustancia o medicamento que produce una contracción de la pupila.

misdemeanor   A minor crime, as opposed to a felony, punishable by fine or imprisonment in a city or county jail rather than in a penitentiary.
falta   Delito menor, por oposición a delito mayor, se penaliza con multa o prisión en una cárcel de una ciudad o condado más bien que con prisión en una penitenciaría.

mock   To imitate or practice.
simular   Imitar o practicar.

modem   The acronym for *modulator demodulator;* a device that allows information to be transmitted over phone lines at speeds measured in bits per second (bps).
módem   Abreviatura para modulador desmodulador, un dispositivo que permite transmitir información a través de las líneas telefónicas a velocidades que se miden en bits por segundos (bps).

molecule   A group of like or different atoms held together by chemical forces.
molécula   Grupo de átomos iguales o diferentes que se mantiene unido por fuerzas químicas.

monochromatic   Having or consisting of one color or hue.
monocromático   Que tiene un solo color o tonalidad.

mononuclear white blood cell   A leukocyte having an unsegmented nucleus; monocytes and lymphocytes in particular.
glóbulo blanco mononuclear   Leucocito que tiene un núcleo sin segmentar; en particular los monocitos y linfocitos.

mons pubis   The fat pad that covers the symphysis pubis.
monte del pubis   Almohadilla de grasa que cubre la sínfisis púbica.

morale   The mental and emotional condition (such as enthusiasm, confidence, or loyalty) of an individual or group with regard to the function or tasks at hand.
moral   Estado mental y emocional (como entusiasmo, lealtad o confianza) de un individuo o grupo en cuanto al puesto que desempeña o el trabajo que realiza.

motivation   The process of inciting a person to some action or behavior.
motivación   Proceso de incitar a una persona a hacer algo o a comportarse de una forma determinada.

multimedia   The presentation of graphics, animation, video, sound, and text on a computer in an integrated way, or all at once. CD-ROMs are the most effective multimedia devices.
multimedia   Presentación de gráficos, imágenes animadas, video, sonido y texto en una computadora de forma integrada o simultánea. Los CD ROM son los dispositivos de multimedia más eficaces.

multiparous   Pertaining to women who have had two or more pregnancies.
multípara   Perteneciente o relativo a la mujer que ha tenido dos o más embarazos.

multitasking   Performing multiple tasks at one time.
multitarea   Realización de varias tareas diferentes al mismo tiempo.

municipal court   A court that sits in some cities and larger towns and that usually has civil and criminal jurisdiction over cases arising within the municipality.
Municipal corte   Se aplica al juzgado con sede en algunas ciudades y pueblos grandes y que suele tener jurisdicción civil y penal sobre casos que surgen dentro de la municipalidad.

murmur   An abnormal sound heard when auscultating the heart. It may or may not be pathologic.
murmullo   Sonido anómalo que se escucha al auscultar el corazón y que puede ser patológico o no.

myelography   Fluoroscopic examination of the spinal canal with spinal injection of an iodine contrast medium.
mielografía   Examen fluoroscópico del canal espinal con una inyección espinal de un medio de contraste yodado.

myelomeningocele   A herniation of a portion of the spinal cord and its meninges that protrudes through a congenital opening in the vertebral column.
mielomeningocele   Hernia de una parte de la médula espinal y sus meninges que sale hacia fuera a través de una abertura congénita en la columna vertebral.

myocardial   Pertaining to the heart muscle.
miocárdico   Perteneciente o relativo al músculo cardiaco.

myocardium   The heart muscle.
miocardio   Músculo cardiaco.

myoglobinuria   Abnormal presence in the urine of a hemoglobin-like chemical of muscle tissue, which is the result of muscle deterioration.
mioglobinuria   Presencia anómala en la orina de una susbtancia química del tejido muscular parecida a la hemoglobina; es el resultado de una deterioración muscular.

mysticism   The experience of seeming to have direct communication with God or the ultimate reality.
misticismo   Experiencia de parecer tener comunicación directa con Dios o una realidad superior.

nanometer   One billionth ~ (10^{-9}) of a meter.
nanómetro   Una mil millonésima parte (10^{-9}) de metro.

naturopathy   An alternative to conventional medicine in which holistic methods are used, as well as herbs and natural supplements, with the belief that the body will heal itself. Naturopathic physicians can currently be licensed in twelve states.
naturopatía   Alternativa a la medicina convencional en la que se usan métodos holísticos, así como hierbas y suplementos naturales, con la creencia de que el cuerpo sanará por sí mismo. En la actualidad, los médicos naturópatas pueden obtener la licencia en doce estados.

necrosis   Pertaining to the death of cells or tissue.
necrosis   Perteneciente o relativo a la muerte de células o tejidos.

negative feedback mechanism   A homeostatic mechanism that responds as a regulator to counteract a change.
mecanismo de respuesta negativa   Mecanismo homeostático que responde como regulador para contrarrestar un cambio.

negligence   Failure to exercise the care that a prudent person usually exercises; implied inattention to one's duty or business; implied want of due or necessary diligence or care.
negligencia   Falta de cuidado en algo que se hace; falta implícita de atención en el deber o trabajo; deseo implícito de una diligencia o cuidado necesario o merecido.

negotiable   Legally transferable to another party.
negociable   Que se puede transferir legalmente a otra parte.

networking   The exchange of information or services among individuals, groups, or institutions; meeting and getting to know individuals in the same or similar career fields, and sharing information about available opportunities.
interconexión   Intercambio de información o servicios entre individuos, grupos o instituciones; conocer a individuos del mismo campo profesional o de campos similares y compartir información acerca de oportunidades de empleo.

neural tube defect   Any of a group of congenital anomalies involving the brain and spinal column that are caused by the failure of the neural tube to close during embryonic development.
defecto del tubo neural   Cualquiera de las anomalías congénitas que afectan al cerebro y a la médula espinal y que tienen su origen en que el tubo neural no logró cerrarse durante el desarrollo embrionario.

nodule   A small lump, lesion, or swelling felt when palpating the skin.
nódulo   Pequeña protuberancia, herida o hinchazón que se siente al tocar la piel.

nomogram   A graph on which variables are plotted so that a particular value can be read on the appropriate line.
nomograma   Gráfica en la que las variables están presentadas de tal manera que se puede leer un valor específico en la línea adecuada.

nonmaleficence   Refraining from the act of harming or committing evil.
ausencia de maleficencia   No hacer el mal.

no-show   A person who fails to keep an appointment without giving advance notice.
no-acudió   Persona que no acude a una cita médica sin dar previo aviso.

nosocomial infection   Infection acquired during hospitalization or in a healthcare setting. It is often caused by *Escherichia coli,* hepatitis viruses, pseudomonas, and staphylocci microorganisms.
infección nosocomial   Infección adquirida en un establecimiento de atención sanitaria o durante una hospitalización. Con frecuencia se debe a *E. coli,* virus de hepatitis, pseudomonas y estafilococos.

nosocomial   Pertaining to or originating in the hospital; said of an infection not present or incubating before admission to the hospital.
nosocomial   Perteneciente o relativo al hospital, incubado en el hospital, dícese de la infección que no estaba presente ni en estado de incubación antes de ser ingresado al hospital.

"note"   Notes are found in both the Alphabetic Index and the Tabular List as instructions or guides in classification assignments, defining category content or the use of subdivision codes.
"nota"   Las notas se encuentran tanto en los Índices alfabéticos como en las instrucciones o guías en las Asignaciones de clasificación, para definir el contenido de la categoría o el uso de los códigos de subdivisión.

NSAIDs   Nonsteroidal antiinflammatory drugs.
NSAIDs   Medicamentos antiinflamatorios no esterioides.

nuclear medicine   An imaging modality that uses radioactive materials injected or ingested into the body to provide information about the function of organs and tissues.
medicina nuclear   Modalidad de la formación de imágenes que usa materiales radioactivos inyectados en el cuerpo o ingeridos para obtener información acerca del funcionamiento de órganos y tejidos.

obesity   An excessive accumulation of body fat (usually defined as more than 20% above the recommended body weight).
obesidad   Acumulación excesiva de grasa en el cuerpo (se suele definir como más del 20% del peso recomendado).

objective information   Information that is gathered by watching or observating a patient.
información objetiva   Información que se recoge vigilando u observando a un paciente.

oblique projection   Radiographic view in which the body or part is rotated so that the projection is neither frontal nor lateral.
proyección oblicua   Vista radiográfica en la cual que cuerpo o parte del cuerpo se gira de forma que la proyección no es frontal ni lateral.

obliteration   Making something indecipherable or imperceptible by obscuring or wearing away.
obliterar   Hacer algo indescifrable o imperceptible oscureciéndolo o desgastándolo.

obturator   A disk or plate that closes an opening.
obturador   Disco o placa que cierra una abertura.

obturator   A metal rod with a smooth rounded tip that is placed into hollow instruments to decrease destruction of the body tissues during insertion.
obturador   Varilla de metal con un extremo redondeado que se coloca en el interior de instrumentos huecos para disminuir la destrucción de los tejidos corporales durante su inserción.

occlusion   The complete blocking off of an opening.
oclusión   Cierre completo de una abertura.

"omit code"   Term used in insurance claims. This term is used primarily in Volume 3 when the procedure is the method of approach for an operation.
"omitir código"   Esta expresión se usa sobre todo en el tomo 3 cuando el procedimiento es el método de acercamiento a una operación.

opaque   Not translucent or transparent.
opaco   Que no es translúcido ni transparente.

OPIM (other potentially infectious material)   Substances or material other than blood (e.g., body fluids such as urine and semen) that have the potential to carry infectious pathogens.
OPIM (otras materias potencialmente peligrosas)   Sustancias o materias además de la sangre (como, por ejemplo, los fluidos corporales, la orina, el semen, etc.).

opinion   A formal expression of judgment or advice by an expert; the formal expression of the legal reasons and principles on which a legal decision is based.
opinión   Expresión formal de un juicio o consejo dado por un experto; expresión formal de las razones y principios legales sobre los que se basa una decisión legal.

opportunistic infection   Infection caused by a normally nonpathogenic organism in a host whose resistance has been decreased.
infección oportunista   Infección en una persona con una resistencia a las enfermedades más baja de lo normal, provocada por un organismo que en condiciones normales no resulta patógeno.

optic disc   Region at the back of the eye where the optic nerve meets the retina. It is considered the blind spot of the eye because it contains only nerve fibers and no rods or cones and therefore is insensitive to light.
papila óptica   Región en la parte posterior del ojo donde el nervio óptico se une con la retina. Se considera el punto ciego del ojo, ya que allí sólo hay fibras nerviosas y no bastoncillos ni conos, y por tanto es insensible a la luz.

optic nerve   The second cranial nerve, which carries impulses for the sense of sight.
nervio óptico   Segundo nervio del cráneo que transporta impulsos para el sentido de la vista.

optical character recognition (OCR)   The electronic scanning of printed items as images, followed by use of special software to recognize these images (or characters) as ASCII text.
reconocimiento óptico de caracteres (OCR)   Proceso de escanear electrónicamente documentos impresos como si fueran imágenes y después, usando un programa de computadora especial, reconocer esas imágenes (o caracteres) como texto ASCII.

ordinance   An authoritative decree or direction; a law set forth by a governmental authority, specifically a municipal regulation.
ordenanza   Decreto u orden de la autoridad; ley definida por una autoridad gubernamental, específicamente, una regulación municipal.

organelle   A differentiated structure within a cell, such as a mitochondrion, vacuole, or chloroplast, that performs a specific function.
organelo   Estructura diferenciada dentro de una célula, como un mitocondrio, vacuola o cloroplasto que realiza una función específica.

orthopnea   Difficulty breathing when in a supine position. The individual must sit or stand to breathe comfortably.
ortopnea   Dificultad para respirar estando en posición supina. El individuo debe estar sentado o de pie para respirar con comodidad.

orthostatic (postural) hypotension   A temporary fall in blood pressure when a person rapidly changes from a recumbent position to a standing position.
hipotensión ortostática (relacionada con la postura)   Baja temporal de la presión sanguínea cuando una persona cambia con rapidez de una posición recostada a una posición en pie.

osteopathy   A medical discipline based primarily on the manual diagnosis and holistic treatment of impaired function resulting from loss of movement in all kinds of tissues.
osteopatía   Disciplina médica que se basa primordialmente en el diagnóstico manual y el tratamiento holístico de funciones deterioradas como resultado de la pérdida de movilidad en todo tipo de tejidos.

osteoporosis   The loss of bone density. Lack of calcium intake is a major factor in its development.
osteoporosis   Disminución de la densidad de los huesos. La falta de consumo de calcio es uno de los factores principales de su desarrollo.

otitis externa   Inflammation or infection of the external auditory canal.
otitis externa   Inflamación o infección del canal auditivo externo.

otosclerosis   The formation of spongy bone in the labyrinth of the ear, often causing the auditory ossicles to become fixed and unable to vibrate when sound enters the ears.
otosclerosis   Formación de huesos parecidos a esponjas en el laberinto del oído, a menudo causando que los huesecillos auditivos queden fijos y que no puedan vibrar cuando el sonido entra en los oídos.

ototoxic   Pertaining to a substance or medication that damages the eighth cranial nerve or the organs of hearing and balance.
ototóxico   Perteneciente o relativo a una sustancia o medicamento que daña el octavo nervio craneal o los órganos auditivos y del equilibrio.

OUTfolder   A folder used to provide space for the temporary filing of materials.
Carpeta OUT   Carpeta que se usa para proporcionar espacio para archivar materiales de forma temporal.

OUTguide   A heavy guide that is used to replace a folder that has been temporarily moved from the filing space.
Guía OUT   Guía grande que se usa para reemplazar una carpeta que ha sido retirada temporalmente del archivo.

output   Information that is processed by the computer and transmitted to a monitor, printer, or other device.
salida   Información procesada por la computadora y enviada a un monitor, impresora u otro dispositivo.

over-the-counter drugs   Medications legally sold without a prescription.
medicinas de venta libre   Medicinas que se venden sin receta legalmente.

oxytocin   A hormone secreted by the posterior pituitary gland that stimulates smooth muscle contractions of the uterus or mammary glands.
oxitocina   Hormona que segrega la glándula pituitaria posterior y que estimula las contracciones del útero o de las glándulas mamarias.

palliative   An agent that relieves or alleviates symptoms without curing the disease; something that alleviates or eases a painful situation without curing it.
paliativo   Agente que calma o alivia los síntomas sin curar la enfermedad; algo que alivia o hace más soportable una situación dolorosa sin curarla.

pandemic   Affecting the majority of the people in a country or a number of countries.
pandémico   Que afecta a la mayoría de la población de un país o de varios países.

paper claims   Hard copies of insurance claims that have been completed and sent by surface mail.
reclamaciones de papel   Copias impresas de reclamaciones de seguros que han sido completadas y enviadas por correo ordinario.

papilledema   Bulging of the optic disk and dilated retinal veins seen by ophthalmoscopic examination of the retina. Papilledema is a sign of increased intracranial pressure.
edema papilar   Abultamiento de la papila óptica y de las venas retinianas dilatadas que se ven en un examen oftalmoscópico de la retina. La emeda papilar es una señal de un aumento en la presión intracraneal.

paraphrased   Pertaining to a text, passage, or work that has been restated to give the meaning in another form.
parafraseado   Perteneciente o relativo a un texto, selección u obra que ha sido expresado nuevamente para dar su significado de otra forma.

paraphrasing Expressing an idea in different wording in an effort to enhance communication and clarify meaning.
parafrasear Expresar una idea con palabras diferentes para mejorar la comunicación y hacer más claro su significado.

parenteral Referring to injection or introduction of substances into the body through any route other than the digestive tract, such as subcutaneous, intravenous, or intramuscular administration.
parenteral Inyección o introducción de sustancias en el cuerpo a través de cualquier otra vía que no sea el tracto digestivo, como administración subcutánea, intravenosa o intramuscular.

paresthesia An abnormal sensation of burning, prickling, or stinging.
parestesia Sensación anómala de ardor, escozor o aguijoneo.

paroxysmal Pertaining to a sudden, recurrent spasm of symptoms.
paroxístico Perteneciente o relativo a espasmos repentinos recurrentes o a sus síntomas.

participating provider A physician or other health care provider who enters into a contract with a specific insurance company or program and by doing so agrees to abide by certain rules and regulations set forth by that particular third-party payor.
proveedor participante Médico u otro proveedor de atención sanitaria que establece un contrato con una compañía o programa de seguro específico, y al hacerlo acepta respetar ciertas normas y regulaciones establecidas por ese pagador intermediario.

parturition The act or process of giving birth to a child.
parto Acción o proceso de dar a luz un niño.

patency The condition of a body cavity or canal that is open or unobstructed.
abertura Estado abierto de un cuerpo, cavidad o canal.

pathogen An agent that causes disease, especially a living microorganism such as a bacterium or fungus; a disease-causing microorganism.
patógeno Agente que causa enfermedades, especialmente microorganismos vivos como bacterias u hongos; microorganismos causantes de enfermedades.

pathogenic Pertaining to disease-causing microorganisms.
patogénico Perteneciente o relativo a los microorganismos causantes de enfermedades.

pathophysiology The study of biologic and physical manifestations of disease as they are related to system abnormalities and physiologic disturbances.
patofisiología Estudio de las manifestaciones biológicas y físicas de las enfermedades y cómo se relacionan con las anomalías del sistema y las alteraciones fisiológicas.

payables The balance due to a creditor on an account.
pendiente de pago Saldo que se le debe al acreedor en una cuenta.

payee The person named on a draft or check as the recipient of the amount shown.
beneficiario Persona que se nombra en una letra de cambio o en un cheque como receptor de la cantidad indicada.

payor The person who writes a check to be cashed by the payee.
pagador Persona que emite el cheque a ser cambiado por el beneficiario.

peer review organization A group of medical reviewers who are contracted by HCFA to ensure quality control and the medical necessity of services provided by a facility.
organizacione de revisión colegial Grupo de revisores médicos contrata dos por HCFA para garantizar el control de calidad y la necesidad médica de los servicios ofrecidos por un establecimiento.

pegboard system A method of tracking patient accounts that allows the figures to be proven accurate by using mathematic formulas; also called the "write-it-once" system.
sistema de tablero perforado Método de controlar las cuentas de los pacientes que permite la demostración de la exactitud de las cifras por medio de fórmulas matemáticas; también conocido como sistema "escríbelo una vez."

perceiving The process by which an individual looks at information and sees it as real.
percibir Proceso en el cual un individuo mira la información y la ve como real.

perception   A quick, acute, and intuitive cognition; capacity for comprehension; an awareness of the elements of the environment.
percepción   Conocimiento rápido, agudo e intuitivo; capacidad de comprensión; conocimiento de los elementos del medio ambiente.

pericardium   The membranous sac that encloses the heart.
pericardio   Saco membranoso que envuelve el corazón.

periosteum   The thin, highly innervated, membranous covering of a bone.
periostio   Membrana fina y sin nervios que recubre un hueso.

peristalsis   The wavelike movement by which the gastrointestinal tract moves food downward.
peristalsis   Movimiento ondulatorio por el cual el tracto gastrointestinal mueve la comida hacia abajo.

perjured testimony   Testimony involving the voluntary violation of an oath or vow, either by swearing to what is untrue or by failing to do what has been promised under oath; false testimony.
perjuro   Testimonio que comprende la violación voluntaria de un juramento o promesa, ya sea jurando algo que es falso o no cumpliendo lo que se ha prometido bajo juramento; falso testimonio.

"perks"   Perquisites; extra advantages or benefits from working in a specific job that may or may not be commonplace in that particular profession.
beneficios adicionales   Ventajas o beneficios adicionales del trabajar en un puesto de trabajo específico que pueden ser o no comunes a esa profesión en particular.

permeable   Allowing a substance to pass or soak through.
permeable   Permite el paso o penetración de una sustancia.

persona   An individual's social facade or front that reflects the role the individual is playing in life; the personality that a person projects in public.
persona   Lo que vemos de un individuo, la imagen social que refleja el papel que dicho individuo tiene en la sociedad; la personalidad que una persona proyecta en público.

pertinent   Having a clear, decisive relevance to the matter at hand.
pertinente   Que tiene una importancia clara y decisiva en el asunto que se está tratando.

petechiae   Small, purplish hemorrhagic spots on the skin.
petequia   Pequeñas manchas en la piel, hemorrágicas y de color violeta.

phenylalanine   An essential amino acid found in milk, eggs, and other foods.
fenilalanina   Aminoácido esencial que se encuentra en la leche, los huevos y otros alimentos.

philanthropist   An individual who makes an active effort to promote human welfare.
filántropo   Individuo que se ocupa activamente de promover el bienestar humano.

philosopher   A person who seeks wisdom or enlightenment; an expounder of a theory in a certain area of experience.
filósofo   Persona que busca la sabiduría o el esclarecimiento; persona que expone una teoría en cierta área de experiencia.

phlebotomy   The invasive procedure used to obtain a blood specimen for testing, experimentation, or diagnosis of disease.
flebotomía   Procedimiento invasivo que se usa para obtener un espécimen de sangre para analizar, experimentar o diagnosticar una enfermedad.

phonetic   Describing an alteration of ordinary spelling that better represents the spoken language, that employs only characters of the regular alphabet, and that is used in a context of conventional spelling.
escritura fonética   Alteración de la escritura normal que representa mejor el lenguaje hablado, emplea sólo caracteres del alfabeto normal y se usa en un contexto de escritura convencional.

phosphors   Fluorescent crystals that give off light when exposed to x-rays.
fósforos   Cristales fluorescentes que alumbran cuando se exponen a los rayos x.

photometer   An instrument for measuring the intensity of light, specifically to compare the relative intensities of different lights or their relative illuminating power.
fotómetro   Instrumento para medir la intensidad de la luz, específicamente para comparar las intensidades relativas de luces diferentes o su poder de iluminación relativo.

photophobia   Abnormal visual sensitivity to light.
fotofobia   Sensibilidad visual anómala a la luz.

physiologic noise   Physiologic interference with the communication process.
ruido fisiológico   Interferencia fisiológica con el proceso de comunicación.

pipette   A cylindric glass or plastic tube used to deliver fluids.
pipeta   Tubo cilíndrico de vidrio o plástico que se usa para distribuir fluidos.

pitch The property of a sound, especially a musical tone, that is determined by the frequency of the waves producing it; the highness or lowness of sound; the relative level, intensity, or extent of some quality or state.
tono   Propiedad de un sonido, especialmente de un tono musical, que está determinada por la frecuencia de las ondas que lo producen; cualidad alta o baja de un sonido; nivel, intensidad o extensión relativos de alguna cualidad o estado.

plaque   An abnormal accumulation of a fatty substance.
placa   Acumulación anómala de una sustancia grasa.

plasma   The liquid portion of whole blood that contains active clotting agents.
plasma   Parte líquida de la sangre completa que contiene agentes coagulantes activos.

policyholder   The person who pays a premium to an insurance company (and in whose name the policy is written) in exchange for the insurance protection provided by a policy of insurance.
titular de la póliza   Persona que paga una prima a una compañía aseguradora (y a cuyo nombre se contrata la póliza) a cambio de la cobertura que proporciona una póliza de seguro.

polycythemia vera   A condition marked by an abnormally large number of red blood cells in the circulatory system.
policitemia vera   Afección que se caracteriza por una cantidad anómalamente elevada de glóbulos rojos en el sistema circulatorio.

polydipsia   Excessive thirst.
polidipsia   Sed excesiva.

polymorphonuclear white blood cells   Leukocytes having a segmented nucleus; also known as *polymorphonuclear neutrophils* (PMNs) or *segmented neutrophils*.
glóbulos blancos polimorfonucleares   Leucocitos que tienen un núcleo segmentado; también se conocen como neutrófilos polimorfonucleares (PMN) o neutrófilos segmentados.

polyphagia   Excessive appetite.
polifagia   Aumento del apetito.

polyps   Tumors on stems frequently found in or on mucous membranes and in the mucosal lining of the colon.
pólipos   Tumores en racimos que se encuentran con frecuencia en las membranas mucosas y en el recubrimiento mucoso del colon.

polyuria   Excessive urine production; excretion of an unusually large amount of urine.
poliuria   Producción y excreción de orina excesivas.

portal hypertension   Increased venous pressure in the portal circulation caused by cirrhosis or compression of the hepatic vascular system.
hipertensión portal   Aumento de la presión venosa en la circulación portal causado por cirrosis o compresión del sistema vascular hepático.

portfolio   A set of pictures, drawings, documents, or photographs either bound in book form or loose in a folder.
portafolio   Conjunto de ilustraciones, dibujos, documentos o fotografías, organizadas ya sea archivadas en forma de libro, o sueltas en una carpeta.

posteroanterior (PA)   Frontal projection in which the patient is prone or facing the x-ray film or image receptor.
posterioanterior (PA)   Proyección frontal en la que el paciente está boca abajo o de frente a la película de rayos x o al receptor de imagen.

posting To transfer or carry from a book of original entry to a ledger; to enter figures in an accounting system.
asentar Transferir o traer desde un libro de entradas originales a un libro mayor; entrar cifras en un sistema de contabilidad.

postmortem Done, collected, or occurring after death.
postmortem Hecho, recogido o sucedido después de la muerte.

power of attorney A legal instrument authorizing a person to act as the attorney or agent of the grantor. The authority may be limited to the handling of specific procedures. The person authorized to act as the agent is known as the *attorney in fact*.
potestad legal Instrumento legal que autoriza a una persona a actuar como abogado o agente de la persona que le concede el poder. La autorización puede estar limitada al manejo de procedimientos específicos. La persona autorizada a actuar como agente se conoce como abogado de hecho.

precedence Superiority in rank, dignity, or importance; the condition of being, going, or coming ahead or in front of.
precedencia Superioridad en rango, dignidad o importancia; condición de estar, ir o venir primero o antes.

precedent A person or thing that serves as a model; something done or said that may serve as an example or rule to authorize or justify a subsequent act of the same kind.
precedente Persona o cosa que sirve como modelo; algo hecho o dicho anteriormente y que puede servir como ejemplo o norma para autorizar o justificar un acto subsiguiente del mismo tipo.

preexisting condition A physical condition of an insured person that existed before the issuance of the insurance policy.
afección preexistente Afección física de una persona asegurada que ya existía antes de la emisión de la póliza de seguro.

premium The consideration paid for a contract of insurance; the periodic (monthly, quarterly, or annual) payment of a specific sum of money to an insurance company that, in return, agrees to provide certain benefits.
prima Pago por un contrato de seguro; pago periódico (mensual, trimestral o anual) de una suma específica de dinero a una compañía aseguradora, la cual, a cambio, acepta proporcionar ciertos beneficios.

preponderance A superiority or excess in number or quantity; majority.
preponderancia Superioridad o mayor número o cantidad; mayoría.

preponderance of the evidence Evidence that is of greater weight or more convincing than the evidence offered in opposition to it; evidence that, as a whole, shows that the fact sought to be proven is more probable than not.
preponderancia de evidencia Evidencia que tiene mayor peso o que es más convincente que la evidencia con la que se confronta; evidencia que, en conjunto, muestra que el hecho que se pretende probar es más posible que imposible.

prerequisite Something that is necessary to achieve a result or to carry out a function.
requisito previo Algo que es necesario para obtener un resultado o para desempeñar una función.

present illness The chief complaint, written in chronologic sequence with dates of onset.
enfermedad actual Problema principal, descrito en secuencia cronológica con las fechas de cada acceso.

preservatives Substances added to a specimen to prevent deterioration of cells or chemicals.
preservativos Sustancias añadidas a un espécimen para prevenir el deterioro de células o sustancias químicas.

pressboard A strong, highly glazed composition board resembling vulcanized fiber; heavy card stock.
cartón prensado Cartón de composición resistente y muy satinado que se parece a la fibra vulcanizada; cartulina de gran resistencia.

primary diagnosis The condition or chief complaint for which a patient is treated in outpatient (physician's office or clinic) medical care.
diagnóstico primario Afección o problema principal por el cual se trata a un paciente con atención médica externa (en un consultorio médico o una clínica).

principal A capital sum of money due as a debt or used as a fund, for which interest is either charged or paid.
principal Capital o suma de dinero que se debe como deuda o que se usa como fondo, por el cual se cargan o se cobran intereses.

principal diagnosis A condition, established after study, that is chiefly responsible for the admission of a patient to the hospital. It is used in coding inpatient hospital insurance claims.
diagnóstico principal Enfermedad o lesión que, tras su estudio, se determina que es la causa principal por la que un paciente ingresa en el hospital. Es usado en la codificación de reclamaciones de seguros de pacientes hospitalizados.

privately owned laboratories (POLs) Laboratories owned by a private individual or corporation, such as a freestanding laboratory or the laboratory inside a physician's office.
laboratorios privados (POLs) Laboratorios cuyo propietario es un individuo o una corporación privada, como el laboratorio dentro de un consultorio médico o un laboratorio independiente.

processing How an individual internalizes new information and makes it his or her own.
procesar Forma en la que un individuo interioriza y asimila la información nueva.

procrastination Intentionally putting off the doing of something that should be done.
procrastinación Dejar a un lado o retrasar, de manera intencional, algo que debe hacerse.

professional behaviors Those actions that identify the medical assistant as a member of a healthcare profession, including dependability, respectful patient care, initiative, positive attitude, and teamwork.
comportamientos profesionales Características que identifican al asistente médico como profesional de la atención sanitaria, incluyendo confiabilidad, trato respetuoso a los pacientes, iniciativa, actitud positiva y disposición para trabajar en equipo.

professional courtesy Reduction or absence of a fee for professional associates.
cortesía profesional Reducción o supresión de un cargo para los asociados profesionales.

professionalism Characterizing or conforming to the technical or ethical standards of a profession; exhibiting a courteous, conscientious, and generally businesslike manner in the workplace.
profesionalismo Actitud que se caracteriza por cumplir o actuar de acuerdo con los estándares técnicos y éticos de una profesión; dar muestras de cortesía, meticulosidad y, en general, mostrar un comportamiento adecuado en el lugar de trabajo.

proficiency Competency as a result of training or practice.
pericia Estado de competencia en algo, que se alcanza por medio de entrenamiento o práctica.

profit sharing Offer of part of the company's profits to employees or other designated individuals or groups.
participación en los beneficios Oferta de parte de los beneficios de la compañía a los empleados u otros individuos o grupos designados.

progress notes Notes entered in the patient chart to track the progress and condition of the patient.
notas del progreso Notas escritas en historial médico del paciente para seguir el progreso y estado del mismo.

prokaryote A unicellular organism that lacks a membrane-bound nucleus.
procaryota Organismo unicelular cuyo núcleo no está unido por una membrana.

prolactin (PRL) A hormone secreted by the anterior pituitary gland that stimulates the development of the mammary gland.
prolactina (PRL) Hormona que segrega la glándula pituitaria anterior y que estimula el desarrollo de la glándula mamaria.

proofread To read text and mark corrections.
corregir pruebas Leer un texto y marcar correcciones.

prosthesis The artificial replacement for a body part.
prótesis Pieza artificial para reemplazar una parte del cuerpo.

proteins Organic compounds, occurring in plants and animals, that contain the major elements carbon, hydrogen, oxygen, and nitrogen and the amino acids essential for life maintenance.
proteínas Compuestos orgánicos que existen en plantas y animales y que contienen los elementos principales: carbón, hidrógeno, oxígeno y nitrógeno y los aminoácidos esenciales para el mantenimiento de la vida.

provider An individual or company that provides medical care and services to patients or the public.
proveedor Individuo o compañía que proporciona atenciones y servicios médicos pacientes o al público.

provisional diagnosis A temporary diagnosis made before all test results are received.
diagnóstico provisional Diagnóstico temporal llevado a cabo antes de recibir todos los resultados de las pruebas.

proxemics The study of the nature, degree, and effect of the spatial separation individuals naturally maintain.
proxemia Estudio de la naturaleza, grado y efecto de la separación espacial que los individuos mantienen de forma natural.

prudent Marked by wisdom or judiciousness; shrewd in the management of practical affairs.
prudente Caracterizado por poseer sabiduría o sensatez; hábil en el manejo de los asuntos prácticos.

psoriasis A usually chronic, recurrent skin disease marked by bright red patches covered with silvery scales.
psoriasis Enfermedad recurrente de la piel, por lo general crónica, caracterizada por manchas de color rojo brillante cubiertas por escamas plateadas.

psychosocial Pertaining to a combination of psychologic and social factors.
psicosocial Perteneciente o relativo a una combinación de factores psicológicos y sociales.

public domain The realm embracing property rights that belong to the community at large, are unprotected by copyright or patent, and are subject to appropriation by anyone.
dominio público Campo que abarca los derechos de propiedad que pertenecen a la comunidad en general, que no están protegidos por leyes de derechos de autor ni por patentes y están sujetos a apropiación por parte de cualquiera.

pulmonary consolidation In pneumonia, the process by which the lungs become solidified as they fill with exudates.
solidificación pulmonar Proceso por el cual los pulmones se vuelven rígidos a medida que se llenan con exudados en los casos de pulmonía.

pulse deficit Condition in which the radial pulse is less than the apical pulse. It may indicate peripheral vascular abnormality.
déficit del pulso Cuando el pulso radial es menor que el apical. Puede indicar una anomalía vascular periférica.

pulse pressure The difference between the systolic and the diastolic blood pressures (less than 30 points or more than 50 points is considered normal).
presión del pulso Diferencia entre las presiones sanguíneas sistólica y diastólica (menos de 30 puntos o más de 50 puede considerarse normal).

pure culture A bacterial or fungal culture that contains a single organism.
cultivo puro Cultivo de bacterias u hongos que contiene un solo organismo.

putrefaction The decomposition of organic matter that results in a foul smell.
putrefacción Descomposición de materia orgánica que da como resultado un olor fétido.

pyemia The presence of pus-forming organisms in the blood.
piemia Presencia en la sangre de organismos formadores de pus.

quackery The pretense of curing disease.
curanderismo Práctica del que finge curar enfermedades.

quality control An aggregate of activities designed to ensure adequate quality, especially in manufactured products or in the service industries.
control de calidad Conjunto de actividades destinadas a garantizar la calidad adecuada, en especial en productos manufacturados o en las industrias de servicios.

queries Requests for information from a database.
consultas Peticions de información de una base de datos.

rad The conventional unit of absorbed radiation dose.
rad Unidad convencional de dosis de radiación absorbido.

radiograph An x-ray image.
radiografía Imagen obtenida con el uso de rayos x.

radiographer A person qualified to perform radiographic examinations.
técnico de radiología Persona cualificada para realizar exámenes radiológicos.

radiography Making diagnostic images using x-rays.
radiografía Proceso de diagnosticar imágenes usando rayos x.

radiologist A physician specialist in medical imaging and/or therapeutic applications of radiation.
médico radiólogo Médico especialista en formación de imágenes o en aplicaciones terapéuticas de la radiación.

radiolucent Describing a substance that is easily penetrated by x-rays; these substances appear dark on radiographs.
transparente a la radiación Término que se aplica a una substancia que puede ser penetrada con facilidad por los rayos x; estas substancias aparecen oscuras en las radiografías.

radiopaque Describing a substance that can be easily seen on an x-ray image; describing a substance that is not easily penetrated by x-rays; these substances appear light on radiographs.
opaco a la radiación Sustancia que puede visualizarse con facilidad en la imagen de rayos x. Término que se aplica a una substancia que no puede ser penetrada con facilidad por los rayos x; estas substancias aparecen claras en las radiografías.

rales Abnormal or crackling breath sounds during inspiration.
estertores Sonidos respiratorios o crujidos anómalos durante la inspiración.

ramifications Consequences produced by a cause or following from a set of conditions.
ramificaciones Consecuencias producidas por una causa o que siguen a una serie de estados.

rapport A relationship of harmony and accord between the patient and the health care professional.
concordia Relación de armonía y acuerdo entre el paciente y el profesional de la atención sanitaria.

Raynaud's phenomenon Intermittent attacks of ischemia in the extremities resulting in cyanosis, numbness, tingling, and pain.
fenómeno de Raynaud Ataques intermitentes de isquemia en las extremidades, resultando en cianosis, entumecimiento, picazón y dolor.

RBRVS (resource-based relative value system) A fee schedule designed to provide national uniform payment of Medicare benefits after being adjusted to reflect the differences in practice costs across geographic areas.
RBRVS (sistema de valor relativo basado en recursos) Escala de cargos diseñada para proporcionar un pago de beneficios de Medicare uniforme a nivel nacional después de haber sido ajustado para reflejar las diferencias en los costos prácticos a través de áreas geográficas.

ream A quantity of paper consisting of 20 quires or variously 480, 500, or 516 sheets.
resma Una cantidad de papel que consiste de 20 manos o que varía entre 480, 500 o 516 hojas.

reasonable doubt Doubt based on reason and arising from evidence or lack of evidence; not doubt that is imagined or conjured up, but doubt that would cause reasonable persons to hesitate before acting in a manner important to themselves.
duda razonable Duda basada en la razón o que surge de evidencia o falta de evidencia; no es una duda imaginaria ni inventada, sino una duda que puede hacer que una persona razonable vacile antes de dar un paso importante.

receipts Amounts paid on patient accounts.
recibos Sumas pagadas en las cuentas de los pacientes.

recipient The receiver of some thing or item.
receptor El que recibe un artículo u objeto.

rectify To correct by removing errors.
rectificar Corregir eliminando errores.

reduction   The return to correct anatomic position, as in the reduction of a fracture.
reducción   Regreso a la posición anatómica correcta, como en el caso de reducción de una fractura.

referral (reference) laboratory   A private or hospital-based laboratory that performs a wide variety of tests, many of them specialized. Physicians often send specimens collected in the office to referral laboratories for testing.
laboratorio de referencia   Laboratorio privado o de un hospital que realiza una amplia gama de análisis, muchos de ellos especializados. Con frecuencia los médicos envían especímenes recogidos en la consulta a estos laboratorios para ser analizados.

reflection   The process of considering new information and internalizing it to create new ways of examining information.
reflexión   Proceso de estudiar información nueva e interiorizarla para crear formas nuevas de examinar información.

refractile   Capable of causing light rays to bend, thus altering or distorting an image.
refractante   Capaz de provocar la refracción de la luz, desviación alterando o distorcionando una imagen.

registered dietitian (RD)   A professionally certified person with a bachelor's degree in food and nutrition who is concerned with the maintenance and promotion of health and the treatment of diseases through proper diet.
dietista registrado (RD)   Profesional certificado persona con titulación universitaria en alimentos y nutrición y que se preocupa del mantenimiento y la promoción de la salud y el tratamiento de las enfermedades a través de la dieta adecuado.

relapse   The recurrence of disease symptoms after apparent recovery.
recaída   Recurrencia de los síntomas de una enfermedad tras una aparente recuperación.

relevant   Having significant and demonstrable bearing on the matter at hand.
pertinente   Que tiene una relación importante y demostrable con el asunto que se está tratando.

rem   The dose of ionizing radiation equivalent to one roentgen of x-ray exposure.
rem   La dosis de radiación ionizante equivalente a un roentgen de exposición a rayos x.

remission   A decrease in the severity of a disease or symptoms; the partial or complete disappearance of the clinical and subjective characteristics of a chronic or malignant disease.
remisión   Disminución de la gravedad de una enfermedad o sus síntomas; desaparición parcial o total de las características clínicas y subjetivas de una enfermedad crónica o maligna.

remittent fever   Fever in which temperature fluctuates greatly but never falls to the normal level.
fiebre remitente   Fiebre en la cual la temperatura fluctúa mucho pero nunca baja al nivel normal.

renal threshold   The level above which a substance cannot be reabsorbed by the renal tubules and is therefore excreted in the urine.
umbral renal   Nivel por encima del cual una sustancia no puede ser reabsorbida por los túbulos renales y por lo tanto es excretada en la orina.

reparations   The act of making amends, offering atonement, or giving satisfaction for a wrong or injury.
reparaciones   Acción de enmendar u ofrecer compensaciones por un error o un daño.

reprimands   Criticisms for a fault; a severe or formal reproof.
reprimendas   Críticas por una falta; reprobación severa o formal.

reproach   An expression of rebuke or disapproval; a cause or occasion for blame, discredit, or disgrace.
reproche   Expresión de crítica o desaprobación; causa o motivo de culpa, descrédito u oprobio.

requisites   Things considered essential or necessary.
requisitos   Cosas que se consideran esenciales o necesarias.

resolution   The ability of the eye to distinguish two objects that are very close together; the sharpness of an image.
resolución   Capacidad del ojo para distinguir dos objetos que están muy cerca uno del otro; nitidez de una imagen.

retention   Keeping something in possession or use; to keep someone's pay or service.
retención   El hecho de mantener en posesión o en uso; mantener a alguien a su servicio o como empleado.

retention schedule   A method or plan for retaining or keeping track of medical records and their movement from active to inactive to closed filing.
plan de retención   Método o plan para retener o guardar expedientes médicos, y el paso de los mismos del estado de expediente activo a pasivo y a cerrado.

retribution   The giving or receiving of reward or punishment; something given or exacted in recompense.
retribución   Acto de dar o recibir una recompensa o castigo; algo que se da o se cobra como recompensa.

rhinitis   Inflammation of the mucous membranes of the nose.
rinitis   Inflamación de las membranas mucosas de la nariz.

rhonchi   Abnormal rumbling sounds during expiration that indicate airway obstruction caused by thick secretions or spasms; continuous dry rattling in the throat or bronchial tube resulting from partial obstruction.
ronquido   Ruido sordo y anómalo durante la expiración que indica obstrucción de las vías respiratorias debido a secreciones espesas o a espasmos; ruido seco y continuo en la garganta o en el tubo bronquial debido a una obstrucción parcial.

rider   A special provision or group of provisions added to an insurance policy to expand or limit the benefits otherwise payable. It may increase or decrease benefits, waive a condition or coverage, or in any other way amend the original contract.
cláusula adicional   Provisión o conjunto de provisiones especiales añadidas a una póliza de seguro para ampliar o limitar los beneficios que de otro modo se pueden pagar. Puede aumentar o disminuir beneficios, anular una condición o cobertura o puede enmendar el contrato original de otra manera.

robotics   Technology dealing with the design, construction, and operation of robots in automation.
robótica   Tecnología de la automatización que se ocupa del diseño, construcción y operación de robots.

rods   Structures located in the retina of the eye that form the light-sensitive elements.
bastoncillos   Estructuras que están en la retina del ojo y constituyen los elementos sensibles a la luz.

Roentgen (R)   The conventional unit of radiation exposure.
Roentgen (R)   Unidad convencional de exposición a radiación.

router   A device used to connect any number of LANs that communicate with other routers and determine the best route between any two hosts.
direccionador   Dispositivo usado para conectar cualquier cantidad de LAN que se comunican con otros direccionadores para determinar la mejor ruta entre dos computadoras conectadas a una red.

sagittal plane   The plane that divides the body into right and left halves.
plano sagital   Plano que divide el cuerpo en la mitad derecha y la mitad izquierda.

salutation   Word or gestures expressing greeting, good will, or courtesy.
saludo   Expresión de saludo, buenos deseos o cortesía por medio de palabras o gestos.

sanitization   Reducing the number of potentially harmful microorganisms to a relatively safe level.
saneamiento   Reducción del número de microorganismos a un nivel relativamente seguro.

sarcasm   A sharp and often satiric response or ironic utterance designed to cut or give pain.
sarcasmo   Respuesta aguda y frecuentemente satírica o declaración irónica destinada a burlarse o a lastimar.

scanner   A device that reads text or illustrations on a printed page and translates the information into a form that the computer can understand.
escáner   Dispositivo que lee texto o ilustraciones de una página impresa y traduce esa información a un formato comprensible para la computadora.

sclera   The white part of the eye that encloses the eyeball.
esclerótica   Parte blanca del ojo que encierra el globo ocular.

scleroderma   An autoimmune disorder that affects the blood vessels and connective tissue, causing fibrous degeneration of the major organs.
escleroderma   Trastorno autoinmune que afecta a los vasos sanguíneos y los tejidos conectivos provocando degeneración en las fibras de los órganos principales.

sclerotherapy   The injection of sclerosing (hardening) solutions to treat hemorrhoids, varicose veins, or esophageal varices.
escleroterapia   Inyección de soluciones de esclerosis (endorecedores) para tratar hemorroides, venas varicosas o varices esofágicas.

scoliosis   Abnormal lateral curvature of the spine.
escoliosis   Curvatura lateral anómala de la columna.

scored tablet   A drug tablet manufactured with an indentation that allows it to be broken or cut into equal parts.
tableta con hendidura   Tableta que se fabrica con una hendidura que permite dividirla o romperla en partes iguales.

screen   Something that shields, protects, or hides; to select or eliminate products or applicants by comparing them with a set of desired criteria.
pantalla   Algo que actúa como escudo, que protege u oculta para permitir un proceso de selección.

search engines   Computer programs that search documents for keywords and return a list of documents containing those words.
buscadores   Programas de computadoras que buscan documentos a partir de palabras clave y proporcionan una lista de los documentos que contienen esas palabras.

seborrhea   Excessive discharge of sebum from the sebaceous glands, forming greasy scales on the skin or cheesy plugs in skin pores.
seborrea   Descarga excesiva de sebo de las glándulas sebáceas, formando escamas de grasa en la piel o tapones con aspecto de queso en los poros de la piel.

secondary hypertension   Elevated blood pressure caused by another medical condition.
hipertensión secundaria   Presión sanguínea elevada causada por otra enfermedad o afección médica.

"see"   An instruction to the coder to look in another place. This instruction must always be followed and is found in the Alphabetic Index, volumes 2 and 3.
"ver"   Instrucción que se le da a la persona encargada de la codificación para que consulte en otro lugar. Siempre debe seguirse esta instrucción; la expresión se encuentra en el Índice alfabético, tomos 2 y 3.

"see also"   An instruction to the coder to look elsewhere if the main term or subterm(s) for an entry are not sufficient for coding the information. If a code number follows, "see also" is enclosed in parentheses; if there is no code number, "see also" is preceded by a dash.
"ver también"   Instrucción que se le da a la persona encargada de la codificación para que consulte en algún otro lugar si el término o subtérminos principales para una entrada no son suficientes para codificar la información. Si "ver también" va seguido por un número de código, dicho código va entre paréntesis; si no hay número de código, "ver también" va precedido por un guión.

"see category"   An instruction to the coder to refer to a specific category (three-digit code); it must always be followed.
"ver categoría"   Instrucción que se le da a la persona encargada de la codificación para que consulte una categoría específica (código de tres dígitos); Siempre debe seguirse.

self-insured plans   Insurance plans funded by organizations having a big enough employee base that they can afford to fund their own insurance program.
planes de autoaseguración   Planes de seguros implementados por organizaciones con un número de empleados lo suficientemente grande como para permitirles financiar su propio programa de seguros.

sequentially   Happening in relation to or by arrangement in a sequence.
secuencial   Aquello que ocurre relativo a una secuencia o que es ordenado en secuencia.

serous   Pertaining to thin, watery, serum-like drainage.
seroso   Perteneciente o relativo a una materia poco espesa, acuosa, parecida al suero.

serum   The portion of whole blood that remains liquid after the blood has clotted.
suero   La porción de la sangre que queda líquida después de la coagulación.

service benefit plan A plan that provides benefits in the form of certain surgical and medical services rendered, rather than in cash. A service benefit plan is not restricted to a fee schedule.
plan de beneficios de servicio Plan que proporciona beneficios en forma de ciertos servicios médico-quirúrgicos en vez de con dinero en metálico. Un plan de servicio de beneficio no está restringido por una escala de cargos.

sheath The covering surrounding the axon of the nerve cell that acts as an electrical insulator to speed the conduction of nerve impulses.
película Recubrimiento que rodea los axones de la célula nerviosa y que se comporta como aislante eléctrico para aumentar la velocidad de conducción del impulso nervioso.

shingling A method of filing whereby each new report is laid on top of the next older report, resembling the shingles of a roof.
laminado Método de archivo en el cual cada informe nuevo se coloca encima del informe anterior, del mismo modo que se colocan las tejas en un techo.

Sievert (Sv) International unit of radiation dose equivalent.
Sievert (Sv) Unidad internacional de dosis equivalentes de radiación.

sinoatrial (SA) node The pacemaker of the heart, located in the right atrium.
nódulo sinoauricular (SA) Marcapasos del corazón que se halla en la aurícula derecha.

sinus arrhythmia Irregular heartbeat originating in the sinoatrial (pacemaker) node.
arritmia de seno Ritmo cardiaco irregular que tiene su origen en el nódulo sinoauricular (marcapasos).

socioeconomic Relating to a combination of social and economic factors.
socioeconómico Perteneciente o relativo a una combinación de factores sociales y económicos.

sociologic Oriented or directed toward social needs and problems.
sociologico Que se orienta o dirige hacia las necesidades y problemas sociales.

sonography An imaging modality that uses sound waves to produce images of soft tissues; also called *diagnostic ultrasound*.
sonografía Modalidad de formación de imágenes que usa ondas sonoras para producir imágenes de los tejidos blandos; también se conoce como ultrasonido de diagnóstico.

sound card A device that allows a computer to output sound through speakers that are connected to the main circuitry board (motherboard).
tarjeta de sonido Dispositivo que le permite a una computadora emitir sonido a través de altavoces conectados a la tarjeta principal del circuito.

specimen A sample of body fluid, waste product, or tissue that is collected for analysis and diagnosis.
espécimen Muestra de un fluido corporal, residuo o tejido que se usa para análisis y diagnósticos.

spirometer An instrument that measures the volume of inhaled and exhaled air.
espirómetro Instrumento que sirve para medir el volumen del aire inhalado y exhalado.

spores Thick-walled reproductive cells formed within bacteria and capable of withstanding unfavorable environmental conditions; thick-walled dormant forms of bacteria that are very resistant to disinfection measures.
esporas Células reproductoras de paredes gruesas que se forman dentro de las bacterias y son capaces de resistir condiciones ambientales adversas; tipos de bacterias letárgicas de paredes gruesas que son muy resistentes a las medidas de desinfección.

staff privileges Authorization for a healthcare professional to practice within a specific facility.
privilegios del personal Autorización para un profesional de atención sanitaria, para ejercer la práctica dentro de unas instalaciones específicas.

standards Items or indicators used to measure quality or compliance with a statutory or accrediting body's policies and regulations.
estándares Artículos o indicadores usados para medir la calidad o cumplimiento de las pólizas y regulaciones de un cuerpo normativo o acreditativo.

stat   Medical term meaning "immediately" or "at this moment"; an order found on a laboratory requisition indicating that the test must be done immediately (from the Latin word *statin,* meaning "at once").

stat   Abreviatura usada en medicina que significa inmediatamente o ahora mismo. Orden encontrada en un pedido de laboratorio que indica que el análisis debe llevarse a cabo inmediatamente (de la palabra latina statin, que significa "ahora"); inmediatamente.

stationers   Sellers of writing paper.

dependientes de papelería   Vendedores de artículos de papelería.

statute   A law enacted by the legislative branch of a government.

estatuto   Ley sancionada por la rama legislativa de un gobierno.

stereotactic   An x-ray procedure to guide the insertion of a needle into a specific area of the breast.

estereotáctico   Procedimiento de rayos x para guiar la inserción de una aguja en zonas específicas del pecho.

stereotype   Something conforming to a fixed or general pattern; a standardized mental picture that is held in common by many and represents an oversimplified opinion, prejudiced attitude, or uncritical judgment.

estereotipo   Algo que se ajusta a un patrón fijado o general; imagen mental estandarizada que tienen en común muchas personas y que representa opiniones simplificadas, actitudes con prejuicios o razonamientos carentes de sentido crítico.

sterilization   Complete destruction of all forms of microbial life.

esterilización   Destrucción total de toda forma de vida microbiana.

stertorous   Describing strenuous respiratory effort that has a snoring sound.

estertóreo   Esfuerzo respiratorio penoso que tiene el sonido de un ronquido.

stipulate   To specify as a condition or requirement of an agreement or offer; to make an agreement or covenant to do or forbear from doing something.

estipular   Especificar como condición o requisito de un acuerdo u oferta; establecer un acuerdo o prometer hacer, o dejar de hacer, algo.

stock option   Offer of stocks for purchase to a certain individual or to certain groups, such as employees of a for-profit hospital.

opción sobre acciones   Oferta de venta de acciones que se le hace a un ciertos individuos o grupos, como a los empleados de un hospital.

stressors   Stimuli that cause stress.

estresantes   Dícese de los estímulos que causan estrés.

stridor   A shrill, harsh respiratory sound heard during inhalation during laryngeal obstruction.

estridor   Sonido respiratorio estridente que se oye durante la inhalación en los casos de obstrucción laríngea.

stroke   Sudden paralysis and/or loss of consciousness caused by extreme trauma or injury to an artery in the brain.

apoplejía   Súbita pérdida de conocimiento y parálisis causada por una lesión o daño grave de una arteria del cerebro.

stylus   A metal probe inserted into or passed through a catheter, needle, or tube that is used for clearing purposes or to facilitate passage into a body orifice.

punzón   Sonda metálica que se inserta o pasa por medio de un catéter, aguja o tubo y que se usa para limpiar o para facilitar el paso a un orificio del cuerpo.

subjective information   Information gained by questioning the patient or taking it from a form.

información subjetiva   Información obtenida haciendo preguntas al paciente o tomándola de un formulario.

subluxation   Incomplete dislocation of a bone from its normal anatomic location.

subluxación   Dislocación incompleta de un hueso desde su posición anatómica normal.

subluxations   Slight misalignments of the vertebrae or partial dislocations.

subluxaciones   Alineamientos ligeramente defectuosos o dislocaciones parciales de las vértebras.

subordinate   Submissive to or controlled by authority; placed in or occupying a lower class, rank, or position.
subordinado   Que está sometido a una autoridad o controlado por ella; que ostenta un cargo u ocupa una clase, rango o puesto inferior.

subpoena   A writ or document commanding a person to appear in court, under penalty for failure to appear.
subpoena   Documento escrito ordenando a una persona comparecer en el juzgado bajo penalidad en caso de no comparecencia.

substance number   A number based on the weight of a ream of paper containing 500 sheets.
número de sustancia   Número basado en el peso de una resma de papel de 500 hojas.

subtle   Difficult to understand or perceive; having or marked by keen insight and the ability to penetrate deeply and thoroughly.
sutil   Difícil de comprender o percibir; que tiene perspicacia y la capacidad de penetrar a fondo y en toda su extensión en un asunto.

succinct   Marked by compact, precise expression without wasted words.
sucinto   Caracterizado por una expresión precisa y concisa sin palabras inútiles.

superfluous   Exceeding what is sufficient or necessary.
superfluos   Que exceden aquello que es suficiente o necesario.

suppurative   Forming and/or discharging of pus.
supuración   Formación o emisión de pus.

surrogate   A substitute; put in place of another.
subrogado   Sustituto; puesto en lugar de otro.

switch   In networks, a device that filters information between LAN segments, decreases overall network traffic, and increases speed and bandwidth usage efficiency.
conmutador   En las redes de comunicación, dispositivo que filtra información entre segmentos de LAN y disminuye el tráfico global de la red, aumentando la velocidad y la eficacia en el uso del ancho de banda.

syncope   Fainting; a brief lapse in consciousness.
síncope   Desmayo; lapso breve en estado de consciencia.

syndrome   A group of signs and symptoms related to a common cause or presenting a clinical picture of a disease or an inherited abnormality.
síndrome   Conjunto de signos y síntomas relacionados con una causa común o que presentan el cuadro clínico de una enfermedad o una anomalía heredada.

synopsis   A condensed statement or outline.
sinopsis   Declaración resumida; resumen.

synovial fluid   Clear fluid found in joint cavities that facilitates smooth movements and nourishes joint structures.
fluido sinovial   Fluido claro que se halla en las cavidades de las articulaciones y que facilita los movimientos suaves y nutre las estructuras articulatorias.

tachycardia   Rapid but regular heart rate exceeding 100 beats per minute.
taquicardia   Ritmo cardiaco rápido pero regular que sobrepasa los 100 latidos por minuto.

tachypnea   Respiration that is rapid and shallow; hyperventilation.
taquipnea   Respiración rápida y profunda; hiperventilación.

tactful   Having a keen sense of what to do or say in order to maintain good relations with others or avoid offense.
tacto   Tener un sentido de lo que se debe hacer o decir para mantener buenas relaciones con los demás y evitar ofenderlos.

target organ   The organ that is affected by a particular hormone.
órgano objetivo   Órgano afectado por una hormona específica.

target tissue   A group of cells that are affected by a particular hormone.
tejido objetivo   Grupo de células afectadas por una hormona específica.

targeted to   Directed or used toward a target; directed toward a specific desire or position.
dirigido a   Dirigido a un fin o meta específico, usado hacia un fin; dirigido hacia un deseo o un puesto específico.

TCP/IP Abbreviation for Transmission Control Protocol/Internet Protocol; a suite of communications protocols used to connect users or hosts to the Internet.
TCP/IP Abreviatura de protocolo de control de transmisión/protocolo Internet; conjunto de protocolos de comunicación que se usa para conectar usuarios o computadoras a Internet.

tedious Tiresome because of length or dullness.
tedioso Que cansa porque es demasiado largo o aburrido.

telecommunications The science and technology of communication by transmission of information from one location to another via telephone, television, telegraph, or satellite.
telecomunicaciones Ciencia y tecnología de la comunicación basada en la transmisión de información de un lugar a otro por teléfono, televisión, telégrafo o satélite.

telemedicine The use of telecommunications in the practice of medicine, allowing great distances between healthcare professionals, colleagues, patients, and students.
telemedicina Uso de las telecomunicaciones en la práctica médica, permitiendo la comunicación entre profesionales de atención sanitaria, colegas, pacientes y estudiantes que se hallan a grandes distancias.

teleradiology The use of telecommunications devices to enhance and improve the results of radiologic procedures.
telerradiología Uso de dispositivos de telecomunicación para mejorar y perfeccionar los resultados de procedimientos radiológicos.

tendon A tough band of connective tissue connecting muscle to bone.
tendón Banda resistente de tejido conectivo que conecta los músculos con los huesos.

teratogen Any substance that interferes with normal prenatal development.
teratógeno Cualquier sustancia que interfiere con el desarrollo prenatal normal.

teratogenic A substance that is known to cause birth defects.
teratogénico Sustancia que se sabe que provoca defectos de nacimiento.

testimony A solemn declaration usually made orally by a witness under oath in response to interrogation by a lawyer or authorized public official.
testimonio Declaración solemne, por lo general oral, hecha por un testigo bajo juramento como respuesta a una pregunta (o preguntas) de un abogado o un funcionario público autorizado.

thanatology The description or study of the phenomena of death and of psychologic methods of coping with death.
tanatología Descripción o estudio del fenómeno de la muerte y de los métodos psicológicos para hacerle frente.

third-party payor An entity (usually an insurance company) that makes a payment on an obligation or debt but is not a party to the contract that created the debt.
pagador mediador Entidad (por lo general una compañía aseguradora) que hace un pago de una obligación o deuda pero que no es parte del contrato que ha creado dicha deuda.

third-party payor Someone other than the patient, spouse, or parent who is responsible for paying all or part of the patient's medical costs.
pagador mediador Alguien ajeno al paciente, cónyuge, padre o madre que es responsable del pago de todo o parte de los gastos médicos del paciente o de parte de ellos.

thixotropic gel A material that appears to be a solid until subjected to a disturbance such as centrifugation, when it becomes a liquid.
gel tisotrópico Material que parece ser sólido hasta el momento en que se somete a una alteración como la centrifugación, cuando se convierte en líquido.

thoracic Pertaining to the region of the back containing 12 thoracic vertebrae, between the neck and low back.
torácica Perteneciente o relativo a región de la espalda entre el cuello y la región lumbar inferior en la que hay 12 vértebras torácicas.

thready pulse Pulse that is scarcely perceptible.
pulso débil Pulso que es apenas perceptible.

thrombus Blood clot.
trombo Cóagulo de sangre.

thyroid-stimulating hormone (TSH)   A hormone secreted by the anterior lobe of the pituitary gland that stimulates the secretion of hormones produced by the thyroid gland.
hormona estimulante de la tiroides (TSH)   Hormona que segrega el lóbulo anterior de la glándula pituitaria y que estimula la secreción de hormonas producidas por la glándula tiroides.

tickler file   A chronologil file used as a reminder that something must be taken care of on a certain date.
archivo cronológico   Archivo que se usa para recordar que algo que debe llevarse a cabo en una fecha determinada.

tinea   Fungal skin disease that results in scaling, itching, and inflammation.
tinea   Enfermedad de la piel causada por hongos y que produce descamación, picazón e inflamación.

tissue culture   The technique or process of keeping tissue alive and growing in a culture medium.
cultivo de tejidos   Técnica o proceso de mantener un tejido vivo y en fase de crecimiento en un medio de cultivo.

toxemia   An abnormal condition of pregnancy characterized by hypertension, edema, and protein in the urine.
toxemia   Característica anómala del embarazo, con presencia de hipertensión, edema y proteínas en la orina.

tracer   A radioactive substance administered to a patient undergoing a nuclear medicine imaging procedure.
trazador   Sustancia radioactiva que se administra al paciente para someterlo a procedimientos de formación de imágenes en medicina nuclear.

tracheostomy   A surgical opening through the neck into the trachea, to facilitate breathing.
traqueotomía   Abertura realizada quirúrgicamente en el cuello a la altura de la tráquea para facilitar la respiración.

transaction   An exchange or transfer of goods, services, or funds.
transacción   Intercambio o transferencia de bienes, servicios o fondos.

transcription   A written copy made either in longhand or by machine.
transcripción   Copia escrita de algo, hecha a mano, o con la ayuda de una máquina.

transducer   The part of the sonography machine in contact with the patient that sends high-frequency sound waves and receives the sound echoes that return from the patient's body.
transductor   Parte de una máquina de sonografía que está en contacto con el paciente envía ondas sonoras de alta frecuencia y recibe los ecos de los sonidos que regresan del cuerpo del paciente.

transection   A cross-section; division by cutting across.
sección transversal   División cortando a través.

transient ischemic attack   Temporary neurologic symptoms caused by gradual or partial occlusion of a cerebral blood vessel.
ataque isquémico transitorio   Síntomas neurológicos temporales causados por una oclusión gradual o parcial de un vaso sanguíneo del cerebro.

transillumination   Inspection of a cavity or organ by passing light through its walls.
diafanoscopia   Inspección de una cavidad u órgano haciendo pasar luz a través de sus paredes.

transport medium   A medium used to keep an organism alive during transport to the laboratory.
medio para transporte   Medio usado para mantener un organismo vivo durante el transporte al laboratorio.

transverse plane   Plane that divides the body into superior and inferior parts.
plano transversal   Plano que divide el cuerpo en parte superior e inferior.

trauma   Physical injury or wound caused by an external force or violence.
trauma   Lesión física o herida causada por una fuerza externa o violencia.

treatises   Systematic expositions or arguments in writing, including methodic discussion of the facts and principles involved and the conclusions reached.
tratados   Exposiciones sistemáticas o argumentos escritos que incluyen una descripción metódica de los hechos y principios involucrados y las conclusiones a las que se ha llegado.

triage   Responding to requests for immediate care and treatment after evaluating the urgency of the need and prioritizing the treatment; the sorting and allocation of treatment to patients according to a system of priorities designed to maximize the number of survivors and treat the sickest patients first.

criterio de selección   Responder a peticiones de atención y tratamiento inmediato tras evaluar la urgencia de la necesidad y establecer prioridades de tratamiento. Clasificación y asignación de tratamiento a pacientes según un sistema de prioridades destinado a maximizar el número de sobrevivientes y tratar primero a los pacientes más enfermos.

triglycerides   Fatty acids and glycerols that are bound to proteins and form high- and low-density lipoproteins.

triglicéridos   Ácidos grasos y gliceroles que se unen a las proteínas y forman lipoproteínas de alta y baja densidad.

truss   An elastic, canvas, or metallic device for retaining a reduced hernia within the abdominal cavity.

braguero   Malla elástica o dispositivo metálico para retener una hernia reducida dentro de la cavidad abdominal.

turgor   Resistance of the skin to being grasped between the fingers and released; normal skin tension that is decreased in dehydration and increased with edema.

turgor   Resistencia de la piel a ser pellizcada; tensión normal de la piel que disminuye con la deshidratación y aumenta con el edema.

type and cross-match   Tests performed to assess the compatibility of blood to be transfused.

prueba de tipo y RH   Análisis que se realizan para evaluar la compatibilidad de la sangre que va a ser usada en una transfusión.

unequal pulses   Pulses in which the beats vary in intensity.

pulso desigual   Pulso en el cual los latidos varían en intensidad.

Uniform Commercial Code   A unified set of rules covering many business transactions; often referred to simply as the UCC, it has been adopted in all 50 states, the District of Columbia, and most U.S. territories.

Código de Comercio Uniforme (UCC)   Conjunto de normas unificadas que cubren muchas transacciones comerciales; se conoce simplemente como UCC y ha sido adoptado en los 50 estados, el Distrito de Columbia y la mayoría de los territorios estadounidenses.

unique identifiers   Codes used as part of a method of anonymous HIV testing in which the code is used, instead of a name, to protect the confidentiality of the patient.

identificadores únicos   Método de prueba de VIH (HIV) anónimo en el cual se usa un código en lugar de nombres, para proteger la confidencialidad del paciente.

unit dose   A method used by the pharmacy to prepare individual doses of medications.

dosis unitaria   Método usado por la farmacia para preparar dosis individuales de medicamentos.

universal claim form   The form developed by the Health Care Financing Administration (HCFA, now known as the Centers for Medicare and Medicaid Services, or CMS) and approved by the AMA for use in submitting all government-sponsored claims.

formulario de reclamación universal   Formulario desarrollado por la Administración financiera de la atención sanitaria (HCFA, ahora conocida como Centros de servicios de Medicare y Medicaid, o CMS) y aprobado por AMA para usarse al someter todas las reclamaciones subvencionadas por el gobierno.

upper GI series   Fluoroscopic examination of the esophagus, stomach, and duodenum using oral administration of barium sulfate as a contrast medium.

serie GI superior   Examen fluoroscópico del esófago, estómago y duodeno usando una administración oral de sulfato de bario como medio de contraste.

urea The major nitrogenous end product of protein metabolism and the chief nitrogenous component of the urine.
urea Principal producto final nitrogenado del metabolismo de las proteínas y el principal componente nitrogenado de la orina.

urease An enzyme that catalyzes the hydrolysis of urea to form ammonium carbonate.
ureasa Enzima que cataliza la hidrólisis de la urea para formar carbonato de amonio.

uremia A toxic renal condition characterized by an excess of urea, creatinine, and other nitrogenous end products in the blood.
uremia Enfermedad renal tóxica que se caracteriza por un exceso de urea, creatinina y otros productos finales en la sangre.

urgency A sudden, compelling desire to urinate and the inability to control the release of urine.
urgencia Deseo repentino y apremiante de orinar y la incapacidad de controlarlo.

URL Abbreviation for *Uniform Resource Locator;* the global address of documents or information on the Internet. The URL provides the IP address and the domain name for the web page, such as "microsoft.com."
URL Abreviatura de localizador universal de recursos; la dirección a nivel mundial, de documentos o de información en Internet. El URL proporciona la dirección IP y el nombre del dominio de una página web, como por ejemplo: "microsoft.com."

urticaria A skin eruption creating inflamed wheals; hives.
urticaria Erupción cutánea que produce ampollas imflamadas.

"use additional code" This term appears only in volume 1 in those subdivisions where the user should add further information by means of an additional code to give a more complete picture of the diagnosis. In some cases you will find "if desired" following the term. For the purpose of coding in military medical treatment facilities, the "if desired" phrase will not be used. Therefore when the term "use additional code... if desired" appears, you will disregard "if desired" and assign the appropriate additional code.
"usar código adicional" Esta expresión aparece sólo en el tomo 1, en aquellas subdivisiones en las que el usuario debe añadir más información por medio de un código adicional para proporcionar un cuadro más completo del diagnóstico. En algunos casos, se verá "si se desea" tras el término. En la codificación en establecimientos militares de tratamiento médico, no se usará la expresión "si se desea." Por lo tanto, cuando aparezca el término "usar código adicional...si se desea," no se tendrá en cuenta "si se desea" y se asignará el código adicional correspondiente.

utilization review The review of individual cases by a committee to make sure that services are medically necessary and to study how providers use medical care resources.
revisión de utilización Revisión de casos individuales por un comité, para asegurarse de que los servicios son médicamente necesarios y estudiar cómo los proveedores usan los recursos de cuidados de salud.

Valsalva's maneuver Occurs when one strains to defecate and urinate, uses the arms and upper trunk muscles to move up in bed, or strains during laughing, coughing, or vomiting. It causes a trapping of blood in the great veins, preventing it from entering the chest and right atrium, which may cause heart attack and death.
maniobra de Valsalva Ocurre cuando uno hace fuerza para defecar y orinar, usa los brazos y los músculos de la parte superior del tronco para levantarse de la cama, o hace fuerza al reír, toser o vomitar. Causa una retención de sangre en las venas mayores, impidiendole que entre en el pecho y la aurícula derecha y puede provocar un ataque al corazón y la muerte.

vasodilation   Increase in the diameter of a blood vessel.
vasodilatación   Aumento en el diámetro de un vaso sanguíneo.

vector   An organism, such as an insect or tick, that transmits the causative organisms of disease.
vector   Organismos, tales como un insecto o garrapata, que transmite los organismos que provocan enfermedades.

ventricles   The two lower chambers of the heart.
ventrículos   Las dos cavidades inferiores del corazón.

veracity   Devotion to or conformity with the truth.
veracidad   Compromiso o conformidad con la verdad.

verdict   The finding or decision of a jury on a matter submitted to it in trial.
veredicto   Conclusión o decisión de un jurado en un asunto sometido a juicio.

versatile   Embracing a variety of subjects, fields or skills; having a wide range of abilities.
versátil   Que abarca diferentes sujetos, campos o destrezas; que tiene una amplia gama de destrezas.

vertigo   Dizziness; a sensation of faintness or an inability to maintain normal balance.
vertigo   Mareo; sensación de desmayo o de incapacidad de mantener el equilibrio normal.

vested   Granted or endowed with a particular authority, right, or property; having a special interest in something.
conferirido   Concedido o dotado con una autoridad, derecho o propiedad particular; que tiene un interés especial en algo.

viable   Capable of living, developing, or germinating under favorable conditions.
viable   Capaz de vivir, desarrollarse o germinar bajo condiciones favorables.

virtual reality   An artificial environment experienced by a computer user, often by using special gloves, earphones, and goggles to enhance the experience, that feels as if it were a real environment.
realidad virtual   Entorno artificial que experimenta el usuario de una computadora, muchas veces usando guantes especiales, audífonos y lentes para mejorar la experiencia, y que parece ser un ambiente real.

virulent   Exceedingly pathogenic, noxious, or deadly.
virulento   Excesivamente patógeno, nocivo o mortal.

viscosity   The quality of being thick and lacking the capability of easy movement.
viscosidad   Cualidad de espeso e incapaz de moverse con facilidad.

vocation   The work in which a person is regularly employed.
profesión   Trabajo en el que una persona está empleada regularmente.

volatile   Referring to a flammable substance's capacity to vaporize at a low temperature. Easily aroused; tending to erupt in violence.
volátil   Referente a la capacidad de una sustancia flamable para evaporarse a baja temperatura. Que reacciona con facilidad y tiene tendencia a entrar en erupción de forma violenta.

vulva   The external female genitalia, which begins at the mons pubis and terminates at the anus.
vulva   Zona genital exterior femenina que comienza en el monte púbico y termina en el ano.

watermark   A mark in paper resulting from differences in thickness usually produced by pressure of a projecting design in the mold or on a processing roll, and visible when the paper is held up to the light.
filigrana   Marca en un papel que resulta de diferencias de espesor, por lo general se produce presionando un diseño en relieve en el molde o en un rodillo de procesamiento, y es visible por transparencia.

wet mount A slide preparation in which a drop of liquid specimen is protected by a coverslip and observed with a microscope.
montaje húmedo Preparación de una lámina en la que una gota de espécimen líquido por ejemplo, se protege con una cubierta de vidrio y se observa con un microscopio.

wheal Localized area of edema, or a raised lesion.
roncha Área localizada de un edema o una lesión protuberante.

"with" In the context of ICD-9-CM, the term "with," "with mention of," or "associated with" in a title dictates that both parts of the title must be present in the statement of the diagnosis in order to assign the particular code.
"con" En el contexto de la ICD-9-CM, las expresiones "con", "con mención de" y "asociado con" en un título exigen que ambas partes del título estén presentes en la descripción del orden de diagnóstico para asignar el código específico.

workers' compensation Insurance against liability imposed on certain employers to pay benefits and furnish care to employees injured, and to pay benefits to dependents of employees killed in the course of or in a situation arising out of their employment.
compensación laboral Seguro contra la responsabilidad impuesta a ciertos patronos para pagar beneficios y proporcionar atenciones a los trabajadores lesionados, y pagar beneficios a las personas que dependan de trabajadores que mueran en el trabajo o a causa de él.

Zip drive A small and portable disk drive that is primarily used for backing up information and archiving computer files; a 100-megabyte Zip disk will hold the equivalent of about 70 floppy disks.
unidad Zip Unidad de un disco pequeño y portátil que se usa principalmente para hacer copias de seguridad de información y para guardar archivos electrónicos. Un disco Zip de 100 megabytes tiene una capacidad equivalente a la de unos 70 disquetes.